Handbook of
PSYCHOLOGICAL SERVICES
for CHILDREN
and ADOLESCENTS

Handbook of
PSYCHOLOGICAL SERVICES
for CHILDREN
and ADOLESCENTS

Edited by

JAN N. HUGHES
ANNETTE M. LA GRECA
JANE CLOSE CONOLEY

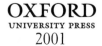

OXFORD
UNIVERSITY PRESS
2001

OXFORD
UNIVERSITY PRESS

Oxford   New York

Athens   Auckland   Bangkok   Bogotá   Buenos Aires   Calcutta
Cape Town   Chennai   Dar es Salaam   Delhi   Florence   Hong Kong   Istanbul
Karachi   Kuala Lumpur   Madrid   Melbourne   Mexico City   Mumbai
Nairobi   Paris   São Paulo   Shanghai   Singapore   Taipei   Tokyo   Toronto   Warsaw

and associated companies in
Berlin   Ibadan

Copyright © 2001 by Oxford University Press, Inc.

Published by Oxford University Press, Inc.,
198 Madison Avenue, New York, New York 10016

Oxford is a registered trademark of Oxford University Press.

Library of Congress Cataloging-in-Publication Data
Handbook of psychological services for children and adolescents / edited by
Jan N. Hughes, Annette M. La Greca, Jane Close Conoley.
p. cm.
Includes bibliographical references and index.
ISBN 0-19-512523-1
1. Child mental health services—Handbooks, manuals, etc.   2. Teenagers—Mental health
services—Handbooks, manuals, etc.   I. Hughes, Jan N., 1949-   II. La Greca, Annette, M.
(Annette Marie)   III. Conoley, Jane Close.
RJ499.3 .H3665   2000
362.2'083—dc21   00-020682

1 3 5 7 9 8 6 4 2

Printed in the United States of America
on acid-free paper

CONTRIBUTORS

Adrienne Akers, M.S.
Early Intervention Research Institute, Utah State University, Logan, UT 84322-6580

Arthur D. Ánastopoulos, Ph.D.
Department of Psychology, University of North Carolina at Greensboro, Greensboro, NC 27412

Pamela J. Bachanas, Ph.D.
Emory University School of Medicine, 341 Ponce DeLeon Ave., Atlanta, GA 30308-2012

Christopher S. Baglio, M.S.
Director of Behavioral Health, Shapiro Developmental Center, 100 E. Jeffery St., Kankakee, IL 60901

Victor Bernstein, Ph.D.
Department of Psychiatry, University of Chicago, MC 3077, 5841 S. Maryland Ave., Chicago, Illinois 60618

Ron Brown, Ph.D.
Emory University, Medical University of South Carolina, Department of Pediatrics, 171 Ashley Ave., Charleston, SC 29425

Sally Campbell, LCSW
Healthy Families Alexandria, 5249 Duke St., Suite 308, Alexandria, VA 22304

Timothy A. Cavell, Ph.D.
Department of Psychology, Texas A&M University, College Station, TX 77843-4225

Patricia Chamberlain, Ph.D.
Oregon Social Learning Center, 107 East 5th Ave., Suite 202, Eugene, OR 97401

Sandra L. Christenson, Ph.D.
University of Minnesota, 350 Elliott Hall, 75 East River Rd., Minneapolis, MN 55455

Angelika Hartl Claussen, Ph.D.
Department of Psychology, University of Miami, Linda Ray Intervention Center, 750 NW 15 Street, Miami, FL 33136

Colleen A. Conoley
Department of Educational Psychology, Texas A&M University, College Station, TX 77843-4225

Jane Close Conoley, Ph.D.
College of Education, Texas A&M University, College Station, TX 77843-4222

Patricia M. Crittenden, Ph.D.
Family Relations Institute, 9481 SW 147 St., Miami, FL 33176

Julie J. Desai, M.A.
River Centre Clinic, 5465 Main St., Sylvania, OH 43560

Dennis Drotar, Ph.D.
Department of Psychology, Case Western Reserve University, Cleveland, OH 44106-7123

Susan T. Ennett, Ph.D.
Department of Health Behavior and Health Education, School of Public Health, University of North Carolina, 311 Rosenau Hall, CB #7400, Chapel Hill, NC 27599-7400

Robert Friedman, Ph.D.
Louis de la Parte Florida Mental Health Institute, University of South Florida, 13301 N. 30th St., Tampa, FL 33612

David M. Garner, Ph.D.
7261 W. Central Ave., Toledo, OH 43617-1100

Maribeth Gettinger, Ph.D.
Department of Educational Psychology, University of Wisconsin, 1025 W. Johnson St., Madison, WI 53706

Yvonne Godber, Ed.S.
School Psychology Program, University of Minnesota, 350 Elliott Hall, 75 East River Road, Minneapolis, MN 55455

Arnold P. Goldstein, Ph.D.
Counseling and Human Services, Center for Research on Aggression, Syracuse University, 805 S. Crouse Ave., Syracuse, NY 13210-1714

Scott W. Henggeler, Ph.D.
Family Services Research Center, Medical University of South Carolina, Department of Psychiatry and Behavioral Sciences, 171 Ashley Ave., Charleston, SC 29425

Stephen R. Hooper, Ph.D.
Center for Development and Learning, University of North Carolina, CB #7255 BSRC, Chapel Hill, NC 27599

Stanley J. Huey, Jr.
Family Services Research Center, Department of Psychiatry and Behavioral Sciences, Medical University of South Carolina, 67 President St., Suite CPP, PO Box #250861, Charleston, SC 29425

Jan N. Hughes, Ph.D.
Dean's Office, College of Education, Texas A&M University, College Station, TX 77843-4222

Nadine J. Kaslow, Ph.D.
3110 Pine Heights Dr. NE, Atlanta, GA 30324-2843

Erika E. Klinger, M.A.
Department of Psychology, University of North Carolina at Greensboro, Greensboro, NC 27412

Rebecca Koscik
Department of Educational Psychology, University of Wisconsin, 1025 W. Johnson St., Madison, WI 53706

William M. Kurtines, Ph.D.
Department of Psychology, Florida
International University, Miami,
FL 33199

Annette M. LaGreca
P.O. Box 249229,
5665 Ponce De Leon Blvd.,
2nd floor, University of Miami,
Coral Gables, FL 33124
(or 33146 for st. address)

Andrea Landini, M.D.
Via Terrachini, 14, 42100 Reggio
Emilia, Italy

Michelle Macias, M.D.
Department of Pediatrics, Medical
University of South Carolina,
135 Rutledge Ave.,
PO Box 250 522,
Charleston, SC 29425

Barbara T. Meehan, M.S.
Department of Psychology, Texas
A&M University, College Station,
TX 77843-4235

LaAdelle Phelps, Ph.D.
Department of Counseling
and Educational Psychology,
State University of New York
at Buffalo, 409 Baldy Hall,
Buffalo, NY 14260

Robert C. Pianta, Ph.D.
Curry School of Education, University of Virginia, 405 Emmet Street,
147 Ruffner Hall, Charlottesville,
VA 22093

Cynthia A. Riccio, Ph.D.
Department of Educational Psychology, Texas A&M University, College Station, TX 77843-4225

Stephen R. Shirk, Ph.D.
Child Study Center, University of
Denver, University Park, Denver,
CO 80208

Wendy Silverman, Ph.D.
Department of Psychology, Florida
International University, Miami,
FL 33199

Peter G. Sprengelmeyer
Oregon Social Learning Center,
107 East 5th Ave., Suite 202,
Eugene, OR 97401

E. Paige Temple, M.A.
Department of Psychology, University of North Carolina at Greensboro, Greensboro, NY 27412

Lynn Zagorski
Department of Psychology,
Case Western Reserve University,
Cleveland, OH 44106-7123

CONTENTS

PART I

*Framing
the
Issues*

ROBERT M. FRIEDMAN

The Practice of Psychology with Children, Adolescents, and Their Families

A Look to the Future

The practice of psychology with children, adolescents, and their families in the future promises to be both increasingly important and a great challenge. This chapter presents some of the demographic and epidemiologic issues likely to affect that practice, then discusses some of the rapidly changing clinical, financial, and system issues and the implications that they are likely to have.

Demographics of Children

The first issue is the overall growth in the population of children (defined as individuals under the age of 18). According to the 1998 *Kids Count Data Book* (Annie E. Casey Foundation, 1998), the population of children under age 18 in the United States was slightly over 69 million in 1996, and it is expected to increase by about 4% to almost 72 million by year 2005. Even more significant is the fact that the population of children between the ages of 13 and 17 is expected to increase by 12% during this same time period (from 18,973,200 to 21,223,800). Because it is the adolescent population that is most likely to be the recipient of mental health and other related services, this by itself speaks to an increasing need.

The *Kids Count Data Book* (Annie E. Casey Foundation, 1998) also indicates that in 23 states and the District of Columbia an increase of 10% or more is projected in the population of children between 13 and 17 years of age from 1996 to 2005. Of the five states that have the largest populations of children (California, Texas, New York, Florida, and Illinois), the growth rate during this time period for 13- to 17-year-olds will be 16% or greater in four states (the exception is Illinois, where the growth is projected to be 4%). The growth in these five states alone will account for over one third of the growth in the nation in this population group. Because these are all states with large urban areas and because the projected increase in less urban states is not as great, the data address what is likely to be an increased need for services, based on population growth alone, that will be particularly marked in urban areas.

Although the fastest growing age group in the country is adolescents, overall children of color are the fastest growing population group. Specifically, children of color — African American, Latino, Asian American and Pacific Islanders, Native American and Alaska Natives — constituted 19% of the population of children under the age of 19 in 1990, and that number was expected to grow to 33% by 2000 and to 40% by 2020 (Children's Defense Fund, 1991). It has been estimated that the Latino community will become the largest ethnic group in the United States (Household and Family Characteristics, 1990). The 1997 *Kids Count* (Annie E. Casey Foundation, 1997) report projects a growth between 1996 and 2005 of 8% in the number of African American children, of 30% in the number of Latino children, of 39% in the number of Asian and Pacific Island children, and of 6% in the number of Native American children (Annie E. Casey Foundation, 1997). For the same time period, a decrease of 3% is projected in the number of Caucasian children. This combination of rapid growth of children of color and slight decrease of Caucasian children will not only produce a much more diverse society but also create special opportunities and challenges for psychologists and other mental health professionals.

One reason that this presents a special challenge is that historically children of color and their families have been underserved or inappropriately served not only within mental health systems but also in other health and social service systems (Hernandez, Isaacs, Nesman, & Burns, 1998; Isaacs-Shockley, Cross, Bazron, Dennis, & Benjamin, 1996). Several reviewers of research on the appropriateness of mental health service delivery for minorities indicate that such services often do not adequately address culturally based perceptions and behaviors, such as value orientation, ethnic identity, natural supports, issues of biculturalism, language difficulties, socioecological conditions, acculturation issues, religious beliefs, and family structure (Gibbs & Huang, 1989; Hernandez et al., 1998; Rosado & Elias, 1993).

There has been a movement within the children's mental health field over the past ten years to develop "culturally competent" systems of care and services (Cross, Bazron, Dennis, & Isaacs, 1989; Hernandez & Isaacs, 1998; Isaacs & Benjamin, 1991; Isaacs-Shockley et al., 1996). Within this concept, culture is defined as "the integrated pattern of human behavior that includes thoughts, communication styles, actions, customs, beliefs, values, and institutions of a racial, ethnic, religious or social group" (Cross et al., 1989, p. 13). This movement was initiated out of a belief that the importance of culture in shaping attitudes, feelings, and behavior has been under-emphasized in the children's mental health field.

This is a view that has been reinforced by the recent report of the Task Force on Professional Child and Adolescent Psychology (1998) of the American Psychological Association's Board of Professional Affairs. This task force emphasized the need to understand behavior in a broad socioecological context and the need to develop both outreach approaches and interventions that reflect the values and culture of diverse groups of children and families. Similarly, as a report of an earlier task force of the Center for Mental Health Services on training of psychologists to provide child and adolescent services indicates:

> Psychologists need to appreciate the broad sociocultural perspectives with regard to diversity of beliefs, values, expectations, and social status of the child and family as they relate to the following: cultural norms in the determination of psychopathology, interactions between the provider and the patient and his or her family, the match between the child's and the family's view of the problem and the provider's treatment theory and methods, service delivery systems and agencies, acculturation for the patient and psychologist, and the development of ethnic identity. (Roberts et al., 1998, p. 297)

Hernandez and colleagues (1998) also point out that service providers need to recognize that many children of color are especially adversely affected by poverty, poor nutrition, lack of health care, geographic isolation, and institutionalized discrimination.

This brief analysis of demographic trends suggests that although the population of children overall will be growing in the United States, this growth will be particularly marked for adolescents and for children of color. This fact creates a special challenge for psychologists and other mental health professionals in the future to examine their own knowledge of culture and its impact on values, feelings, and behavior; to further examine their own attitudes about cultural differences; and to strengthen their skills in working in cross-cultural and multicultural situations. It also creates a challenge for the entire field of psychology to ensure that models for understanding behavior and intervening include an appropriate emphasis on the sociocultural, ecological context in which behavior develops and occurs (Cross et al., 1989; Koss-Chioino & Vargas, 1999; Roberts et al., 1998; Task Force on Professional Child and Adolescent Psychology, 1998).

Epidemiological Findings

Recent reviews of the prevalence of emotional and mental disorders in children and adolescents that meet the criteria for a diagnosis, according to either the *DSM-III-R* (American Psychiatric Association, 1987) or *DSM-IV* (American Psychiatric Association, 1994) system, suggest that approximately 20% of children have or have had such a disorder within the past six months (Brandenburg, Friedman, & Silver, 1990; Costello, 1989; Friedman, Katz-Leavy, Manderscheid, & Sondheimer, 1996; Roberts, Attkisson, & Rosenblatt, 1998). Among the most common disorders are affective disorders such as anxiety and depression, disruptive disorders such as oppositional defiant disorder and conduct disorder, and attention-deficit/hyperactivity disorder.

Since the beginning of the Child and Adolescent Service System Program, initiated by the National Institute of Mental Health (NIMH) in 1984 and continued by the Center for Mental Health Services (CMHS; Stroul & Friedman, 1986), a major focus has been on children with "serious emotional disturbance." These are children who "have had a diagnosable mental, behavioral, or emotional disorder of sufficient duration to meet diagnostic criteria specified within the *DSM-III-R*, that resulted in functional impairment that substantially interferes with or limits the child's role or functioning in family, school, or community activities" (Substance Abuse and Mental Health Services Administration, 1993, p. 29425). This definition of "serious emotional disturbance" was developed by a work group of CMHS, following a 1992 Congressional mandate that such a definition be developed and used as a basis for allocating federal mental health block grant monies to states (Pub. L. No. 102-321). The emphasis on this group of children at the federal level and in states across the country has been a reflection of the public policy position that the primary responsibility of the public system should be to serve those with the most serious disorders (Friedman, Kutash, & Duchnowski, 1996).

Although "serious emotional disturbance" is not a specific diagnosis, it does place a strong emphasis on functional impairment, a concept that until recently has not received extensive attention (Hodges & Gust, 1995). A work group convened by CMHS in response to PL 102-321 reviewed existing epidemiological studies to estimate the prevalence of serious emotional disturbance. This group operationalized the concept of "substantial functional impairment" as a score of 60 or lower on the Child Global Assessment Scale (C-GAS) and, based on this definition, concluded that from 9% to 13% of children between the ages of 9 and 17 had a serious emotional disturbance (Friedman, Katz-Leavy, Manderscheid, & Sondheimer, 1996, 1998). This group further determined that data were not adequate to make a projection of the prevalence rate for children under the age of 9. It also indicated that data were inadequate to make separate prevalence estimates by racial or ethnic groups but that it was clear that prevalence estimates were higher, in fact often twice as high, for children living in poverty than for children from middle- and upper-class backgrounds. The development of effective outreach and service delivery approaches to meet the needs of children in poverty and their families represents another part of the challenge facing psychologists interested in working with children, particularly because there has been a sizeable growth in the number of poor children. Between 1976 and 1996, the number of poor children in the United States increased by approximately 3.6 million (Annie E. Casey Foundation, 1996).

Although there are not many studies on prevalence of diagnosable disorders in preschool children, a large-scale community epidemiological study recently completed in the Chicago area determined that 21.4% of 2- to 5-year-olds had an Axis I disorder (Lavigne et al., 1996). Moreover, whereas 13.6% of 2-year-olds had a diagnosable disorder, the comparable figures were 26.5% of 3-year-olds, 25% of 4-year-olds, and 21.9% of 5-year-olds. The most common disorder was oppositional defiant disorder, already present in 16.8% of children aged 2 through 5 years. Using a C-GAS of 60 or below as an indicator of severe functional impairment, this group found that 9.1% of the children in their study group qualified as having a serious emotional disturbance. These figures suggest that there is both a need and an opportunity for psychologists interesting in working with very young children and their families.

Another important epidemiological development in recent years has been the increasing recognition of the frequency of comorbidity of disorders (Angold, Costello, & Erkanli, 1999; Caron & Rutter, 1991; Greenbaum, Prange, Friedman, & Silver, 1991; Kessler, 1994). This is particularly the case with the most common groups of disorders affecting children and adolescents: anxiety and depressive disorders, attention-deficit/hyperactivity disorders, oppositional defiant and conduct disorders, and substance abuse. Although the field is still a long way from a full understanding of the developmental, diagnostic, assessment, and treatment implications of this phenomenon, it is clear that comorbidity between disorders occurs much more frequently than could be accounted for by the rate of occurrence of the individual disorders in the general population.

The high rate of comorbidity is compounded by the consistent finding that children with serious emotional disturbances often show deficits as well in other important domains of functioning such as intellectual and educational functioning and social and adaptive skills (Friedman, Kutash, & Duchnowski, 1996; Quinn & Epstein, 1998). Also, they have frequently experienced major losses in their lives through death, divorce, and separation and exposure to violence in their communities, in their families, and certainly in the media (Friedman, 1992). In speaking of the relationship between emotional and behavioral functioning and academic performance, for example, Quinn and Epstein (1998) indicate that, "the solution to the reciprocal interaction of learning and behavior problems in the classroom and school remains a critical but apparently elusive aspect of the total treatment effort" (p. 104).

The finding of a high rate of comorbidity within the emotional/behavioral domain, along with a high level of co-occurrence of difficulties in other important life domains and exposure to significant losses and to violence, adds to the complexities for the psychological practitioner. It calls for a need to be able to look comprehensively at children and families, as well as a need once again to buttress a traditional psychological perspective with a resilience focus and more of a contextual, ecological perspective.

Service Utilization

Another challenge to practitioners is to effectively engage children in need of assistance and their families in receiving services and to retain them in services. Research, for example, indicates that there is typically a lag of several years between the time that parents identify that a problem is present and the time at which they seek assistance (Lardieri, Greenbaum, & Pugh, 1996).

Two recent studies have produced findings that are consistent in reflecting the relative lack of specialty mental health services provided to children with special needs. Leaf and colleagues (1996) examined the use of services in the Methodological Epidemiological Catchment Area (MECA) study. Their sample was 1,285 youngsters between the ages of 9 and 17 from four different communities. They report that although the prevalence rate of a diagnosable disorder in the sample was 32.2%, within the 12 months prior to the study only 14.9% of the youngsters received mental health services. Further, of the total sample, 8.1% received services in the specialty mental health sector, 8.1% received services in the schools, 2.9% received services in the medical sector, 1.6% received services from a social services agency, 1.2% received services from clergy, and 0.7% received services from other sources.

Burns and colleagues (1995) report on data from the Great Smoky Mountain study, a community epidemiological study done in western North Carolina. Their sample consisted of 1,015 youngsters, approximately equally divided between 9-, 11-, and 13-year-olds. In this study, 20.3% of the sample received a diagnosis based on a structured diagnostic interview, and, in the three months preceding participation in the study, 16% received mental health services. However, of those who received mental health services, 75% received them through the schools, whereas only 4% received services from the specialty mental health sector.

Taken together, the findings from these two community studies indicate that only a small percentage of children with diagnosable disorders are receiving services from the specialty mental health sector. More are receiving services from the school, a finding that led the Great Smoky Mountain group to conclude that "the major player in the de facto system of care was the education sector" (Burns et al., 1995, p. 155). Similarly, after reviewing these findings, as well as the findings from other studies, Hoagwood and Erwin (1997) also conclude that schools are the primary provider of mental health services for children.

Because the studies by Leaf et al. (1996) and Burns et al. (1995) were both based on community samples, they cover service utilization in both the public and private mental health sectors. A recent report focused specifically on the private sector, examining use of mental health services by children and adults in mental health plans under the auspices of United Behavioral Health, a private managed care company (Gresenz, Liu, & Sturm, 1998). This study reports on 600,000 enrollees (including 172,000 children) in 108 different plans. Overall, less than 1% of children aged 5 and under, 3.19% of children between 6 and 12 years of age, and 5.03% of children between 13 and 17 years of age used outpatient services in a 12-month period.

The phenomenon of relatively low intensity use of outpatient services by children has been found in other studies as well. Armbruster and Fallon (1994) indicate that the majority of children who enter outpatient treatment attend for only one or two sessions. In the Great Smoky Mountain study, the mean number of outpatient visits over a two-year period after the initial interview ranged from a low of 0.6 for youngsters with no diagnosis who had private or no insurance to a high of 11.7 for children with serious emotional disturbances who had public insurance (Burns et al., 1997). Children in the Great Smoky Mountain study who had private insurance averaged 4.4 visits, and children with no insurance averaged 7.8 visits. Interestingly, in this study the greatest use of both outpatient and inpatient services was by children with public insurance, followed by the uninsured group; the lowest use was by the privately insured group.

The problem of premature termination from treatment, also referred to as dropping out or attrition, has long held the attention of the mental health field. One estimate is that among families who begin treatment, 40% to 60% terminate prematurely (Kazdin, Holland, & Crowley, 1997). One of the explanations for the high rate of dropping out and for failure to keep the first appointment is that referrals for children and adolescents are often made not by themselves but by their parents, the schools, the courts, or other agencies and that the youngsters themselves are less interested in services. Kazdin, Holland, and Crowley (1997) have developed a "Barriers to Treatment Participation Scale" and have identified three main factors involved in premature termination: stressors and obstacles associated with treatment (e.g., cost, transportation), perceptions that treatment is not very relevant, and a poor relationship with the therapist. Earlier research in which parents were directly surveyed about reasons for termination found that the most common reason, cited in 19.2% of the cases, was "Child did not want to come back" (Gould, Shaffer, & Kaplan, 1985).

Although the findings on failure to complete treatment raise a significant concern, several recent studies offer encouragement that this tendency can be changed. In two separate studies using random assignment procedures, Szapocznik and his colleagues were able to demonstrate decreased rates of premature termination using "strategic structural-systems engagement" (SSSE; Santisteban et al., 1996; Szapocznik et al., 1988). In the comparison condition, engagement as usual, the therapist would have a phone contact with the family, during which the therapist would be empathetic and supportive of the caller and schedule the first appointment. In the SSSE procedure, the therapist would go beyond this to try to determine concerns about therapy not only on the part of the caller but also on the part of other family members. The therapist might then make extra phone calls or appointments to try to respond to the concerns or help the caller to frame the use of therapy in a way that would make it acceptable to all family members.

Koroloff, Elliott, Koren, and Friesen (1996) also successfully improved engagement in treatment with low-income families who had a child with a serious emotional disturbance. The successful intervention used in this study was having a trained and experienced parent, called a "family associate," work with the referral family to answer questions, offer support, and help them negotiate the system and make the arrangements to receive help. Similarly, children with serious emotional disturbances whose families were assigned a specialized case manager were more likely to be still in treatment at the end of one year than children whose families, through a random assignment procedure, were assigned to a condition in which the therapist was also expected to provide case management (Burns, Farmer, Angold, Costello, & Behar, 1996).

The work of Catron and Weiss (1994) on the impact of school-based mental health services also offers encouragement for retention in treatment. Youngsters who were identified in school as being in need of treatment were randomly assigned either to school-based treatment or to treatment in the community. Of those to whom services were offered in the school, 98% entered services, and almost all completed treatment. Of those whose families were encouraged, and even assisted, to seek services outside of the school, only 17% received services.

These findings suggest collectively that although engagement and retention in treatment remain an issue, it is possible to increase engagement and retention through approaches that provide extra support and assistance to families or increase accessibility of services. Implementing such procedures is part of the challenge of increasing appropriate utilization of services by children in need of such services and their families.

Systems of Care

As indicated earlier, in the 1980s there was clearly a shift in public mental health systems at both the federal and state levels toward identifying children with serious emotional disturbances and their families as the priority population. This shift was built partly on the research of Knitzer (1982), who reported, after a survey of states around the country, that most states had very few services to offer children with emotional disorders other than outpatient or out-of-home care; that only seven states had the beginnings of a continuum of care; that children with serious emotional disturbances were not only in the mental health sector but also in other service sectors such as child welfare, juvenile justice, and special education; and that these sectors, rather than working collaboratively on behalf of children, were more often working independently or even competitively, trying to pass on to each other the responsibility for and cost of care.

Based on these findings and on the recognition that children with serious emotional disturbances had multiple needs that required assistance from various service sectors, NIMH, through its Child and Adolescent Service System Program (CASSP), promoted the concept of a "community-based system of care" as a strategy for improving care and outcomes for these children (Stroul & Friedman, 1986, 1996). A system of care was defined as "a comprehensive spectrum of mental health and other necessary services which are organized into a coordinated network to meet the multiple and changing needs of severely emotionally disturbed children and adolescents" (Stroul & Friedman, 1986, p. 3). The system of care did not represent a specific model but rather a philosophy based on a set of core values and guiding principles. The core values, for example, emphasized that the system of care should be child centered and family focused, with the needs of the child and family rather than the needs of a provider or a funding agency determining the services to be provided; that the services should be community based; and that services should be culturally competent. It was also emphasized that children should have access to a comprehensive array of services that address their physical, emotional, social, and educational needs and that they should receive individualized services in accordance with their unique needs and potentials.

In addition to office-based outpatient treatment and inpatient care, the system-of-care model emphasized the importance of home-based services, day treatment, case management, crisis services, and a variety of types of out-of-home care, including care provided in specialized therapeutic foster homes, therapeutic group homes, and residential treatment centers. It also emphasized the importance of services and supports provided by the health sector, the schools, social services, recreation, and the vocational area. The original monograph on systems of care (Stroul & Friedman, 1986) described a number of innovative services that in fact had been developed partly or fully by psychologists (Friedman & Duchnowski, 1990).

In a parallel and important effort, systems of care have emphasized developing partnerships between parents and professionals (DeChillo, Koren, & Mezera, 1996; Friesen & Huff, 1996; Koroloff, Friesen, Reilly, & Rinkin, 1996), and a national parent advocacy organization has been developed. This organization, called the Federation of Families for Children's Mental Health, has chapters throughout the country and is becoming increasingly influential in advocating not only for increased funding for services but also for the development of systems of care in which the voices of parents are represented and listened to at the policy and at the practice levels. Together with the National Alliance for the Mentally Ill, another family organization that is primarily focused on adults with mental illness, the influence of family organizations over mental health policy and practice has grown enormously.

As the concept of a system of care evolved and states began to implement it, the concept of individualized care came into sharper focus. Although the concept was not new to the mental health field and was a part of the core philosophy for systems of care, researchers have pointed out that the actual power and potential of the approach has developed "beyond anything imagined in 1986" (Lourie, Katz-Leavy, & Stroul, 1996). In the public mental health field, this approach, which was first called "wraparound" by Lenore Behar (1985), a psychologist who has been a leader in this field for many years, has become widespread. In fact, following in the footsteps of a major children's mental health initiative developed and supported by the Robert Wood Johnson Foundation (Cole & Poe, 1993) and a second one supported by the Annie E. Casey Foundation (King & Meyers, 1996), the U.S. Congress in 1992 authorized a national children's mental health initiative, to be operated by CMHS (Publ. L. 102-321), specifically to establish community-based systems of care in which children with serious emotional disturbances would receive individualized care through a wraparound process. This initiative has now grown to the point that it has provided funding in 65 sites across the country and has an annual budget of more than $80 million.

A special issue of the *Journal of Child and Family Studies* has been devoted to research on wraparound (Clark & Clarke, 1996) and a monograph describing the concepts, values, and use of wraparound throughout the country and research results has been published (Burns & Goldman, 1999). Within a wraparound process, a team of individuals, including the child (if at an appropriate developmental stage), parents, members of the family's natural support systems, usually a case manager, and other professionals who have contact with the family, come together to develop a comprehensive plan. The group examines the needs and the strengths of the family across many life domains (e.g., emotional/behavioral, educational, physical health, economic, recreational, spiritual, safety) and develops an individualized plan of support and assistance for the family. If needed supports and services are not available, the team typically has flexible financial resources so that they may be created. If, for example, a youngster is about to be discharged from a residential program and his family needs support and assistance during a transition time, then the team can purchase services from one or more individuals who will spend time on a daily basis in the home assisting the family. If a child's strongest interest is in a particular area, such as music, theater, computers, or sports, and the team believes that it would help the child to be able to build on this, then the flexible money can be used to enable this to happen. If a family has no transportation because they have no money to fix their car and therefore cannot get to needed services, then the flexible money can be used to repair the car. These examples illustrate the different life domains that can be addressed by the plan, the intensity of services that can be provided, and the way in which flexible dollars can be used. In addition to these services, the child may be receiving medication, special education, social skills training, or a combination of all of these to address other needs.

The process of developing the plan is participatory, and a major emphasis is on listening to the needs of the family and ensuring that they, along with all of the other participants, are committed to the plan that is developed. This is very much a collaborative model between parents and professionals, between representatives of different systems, and between individuals in the natural support system and the formal service system.

Although the specifics of an "individualized" model such as wraparound are not easy to determine, the following "essential" elements were identified at a recent consensus conference: wraparound efforts must be based in the community; services and supports must be individualized, build on strengths, and meet the needs of children and families across multiple life domains; the process must be culturally competent; families must be full and active partners in every level of the process; it must be a team-driven process; teams must have flexible approaches with adequate flexible funding; plans must include a balance of formal services and informal supports; community agencies and team must make an unconditional commitment to serve the child and the family; the plan must be developed based on an inter-agency, community-neighborhood collaborative process; and outcomes must be determined and measured for each goal that is established (Goldman, 1999).

This model obviously differs enormously from traditional mental health practice, which is office based: it is based on a model of the clinician as the expert and the family as the client that needs to be fixed, is based almost exclusively on deficits, not on strengths, and is focused largely on the emotional/behavioral domain. Although it may not be possible or necessary to incorporate all elements of the wraparound approach with all children and families, particularly with those whose problems are less complex, the approach has tremendous implications for the practice and the funding of mental health services for children and families. It calls for a very different training approach, a collaborative, community-oriented model, and a heightened level of creative response to potential service options. It calls for a continual emphasis on cultural competence and natural supports, for a partnership with families, and for identifying and building on strengths and not just focusing on problems.

Research on wraparound is still in early stages, although the results of the early studies are encouraging (Burns & Goldman, 1999). It has strong support from parent organizations, such as the Federation of Families for Children's Mental Health, and has expanded to service systems other than mental health. It is a movement whose influence continues to grow and to affect the practice of psychology with children and families. This is likely to be a very positive development despite the fact that many of its concepts are inconsistent with the traditional practice of psychology. Its focus on individualization is very consistent with the values of psychologists and offers an important addition to the manner in which psychology is practiced. This is recognized in the recent report of the Task Force on Professional Child and Adolescent Psychology (1998) and is reflected more and more in day-to-day practice.

Although this trend is a growing one, another trend leads the field in a very different direction, but one that also has much to offer. This trend is discussed in the next section, after which an attempt is made to integrate the approaches.

Empirically Supported Treatments

The 1990s has seen a major movement within psychology and the mental health field in general to identify empirically supported treatments (American Psychological Association, 1995; Chambless & Hollon, 1998; Lonigan, Elbert, & Johnson, 1998). As Kazdin and Weisz (1998) point out, the vast majority of treatments for children and adolescents have not been investigated, and "there is a need to identify and to develop validated treatments and to foster their application in clinical settings" (p. 31). Special issues of the *Journal of Clinical Child Psychology*, the *Journal of Consulting and Clinical Psychology*, and the *Journal of Pediatric Psychology* have all been devoted to this topic.

The focus of this effort is to look at standardized, manualized treatments for children and adolescents with identifiable disorders that have been found to produce significant improvements relative to other accepted treatments in well-controlled studies and/or in a series of carefully controlled single case experiments (Chambless & Hollon, 1998). It is not intended "to deny the importance of other factors such as the therapeutic alliance, as well as client and patient variables that affect the process and outcome of psychological therapies" (Chambless & Hollon, 1998, p. 7), but it is an effort to study standardized treatments.

In this regard, it represents a very different direction from the system-of-care movement just described, with its emphasis on highly individualized interventions. This dilemma is referred to in an article on a multisite clinical trial on attention-deficit/hyperactivity disorder, a study called "the largest, most intensive, and longest treatment study of a childhood disorder that has ever been conducted" (Pelham, Wheeler, & Chronis, 1998, p. 201). This study, supported by NIMH, compares the effects of pharmacological treatment, an intensive psychosocial treatment package, a combination of pharmacological treatment with psychosocial treatment, and a community comparison group on 566 clinic-referred children between the ages of 7 and 9. In describing this study, the investigators indicate that it introduces a "tension between competent clinical care and scientific rigor. Good clinical treatment is individualized, compatible with the clinician's style, intuitive as well as logical, and attentive to the affective relationship. Good science requires that the treatment be uniform, manualized, explicit, and logical, with the patient-clinician relationship a variable to be examined" (Arnold et al., 1997, p. 868). In an effort to combine the requirements of good science with the requirements of good clinical practice, the investigators allow for some level of individualization in this study in both the pharmacological and psychosocial interventions. Although the level of individualization allowed does not meet, or even approach, the requirements for the wraparound approach, it would appear to exceed the level included in almost all of the studies reviewed as part of the effort to identify empirically supported treatments.

In identifying weaknesses of the empirically supported treatment approach, with its emphasis on manualized treatment, Kaslow and Thompson (1998), who authored the article on empirically supported treatments for child and adolescent depression, indicate that "rigid application of a manualized treatment protocol may result in difficulty establishing rapport with a depressed youth and ineffective dissemination of psychological services due to the therapist's inability to attend to the distinctive mood or context of each session or the child's current concerns" (p. 153). They also indicate that the manualized approach makes it difficult to address individual differences, to deal with comorbid psychological conditions and environmental influences, and to attend to important aspects of the child's background. They also identify several strengths of the empirically supported treatment approach: it is systematic and focused, it enables more mental health professionals to be trained in effective methods, it increases the likelihood of detecting differences between treatment conditions, and it has a greater likelihood of replication.

It is perhaps helpful to appreciate that the system-of-care movement with its focus on highly individualized care originated in the field, whereas the empirically supported treatment movement has its roots in the laboratory and specialized clinic. As Weisz and Hawley (1998) indicate, although the APA Task Force was created largely to identify treatments that might warrant use in naturalistic clinical settings, "most of the child treatments identified thus far (and possibly most of the adult treatments, as well) have been tested neither in conventional clinics nor under conditions that very much resemble clinical practice. As a consequence, we actually know little about whether these treatments will be effective in clinical use, despite the fact that they have empirical support" (p. 212). Some of the differences identified by Weisz and Hawley between conditions of clinical practice and the conditions under which the clinical research has been done have to do with the level of severity and motivation of the clients, the extent of comorbidity, and the unpredictability of real life in clinics, where children typically do not stay in treatment long enough to complete a manualized program. They point out, for example, that their own research in child outpatient community clinics has found that the average number of diagnoses per child, as determined through a standardized diagnostic interview, is 3.5, clearly a much higher level than for children seen in most clinical research studies. The concern of Weisz and Hawley is echoed by others as well (Kaslow & Thompson, 1998; Kazdin & Kendall, 1998; Kazdin & Weisz, 1998). Brestan and Eyberg (1998), who reviewed the findings on treatments for conduct disorder, raise a concern that the characteristics of the children studied in the clinical research are not representative of the population of conduct-disordered children on age, gender, race, and ethnicity.

As the practice of psychology with children and adolescents progresses through the next decade, clearly one of the challenges is to bring the strengths and experiences of the system-of-care movement, with its extensive experience in dealing with children with very complex problems in naturalistic community settings and its focus on wraparound approaches, together with the strengths and experience of the clinical research movement, with its extensive experience in testing interventions under well-controlled conditions. The Multimodal Treatment Study of Children with Attention Deficit/Hyperactivity Disorder (Arnold et al., 1997; Greenhill et al., 1996; Richters et al., 1995) represents one well-controlled research effort to do this on a large scale. Until more research is done on effectiveness of interventions in natural settings with regularly referred children and their families, however, the challenge for practicing psychologists and other mental health professionals is how to combine the features of competent clinical care, including developing effective relationships with children and families and working in partnership with them and others of importance in the child's life, with adequate knowledge of the most promising interventions. Mental health professionals will frequently find that they work with youngsters who do not fit neatly into a single diagnostic category and that the youngsters and their families have many strengths as well; despite this, it will still be important to understand the state-of-the-art interventions for specific disorders, even though the state-of-the-art may not yet be based on well-conducted effectiveness studies. A challenge for the system-of-care movement is to be better able to describe the overall intervention process, including the decision-making approach that is used, so that others can be trained in it and so that it can be replicated and eventually tested.

This challenge of bringing together the system-of-care movement with the clinical research–empirically supported treatment approach will need to take place in the context of major changes in the financing of mental health services. Significant changes have already taken place and are likely to continue. The next section briefly addresses these changes.

Financing of Services

The 1990s have clearly been a time of rapid change from "fee for service" arrangements for health care in both the public and private sectors to "managed care" arrangements. The managed care arrangements have taken a variety of forms. One of the most common is "health maintenance organizations" (HMOs), which are essentially organizations that provide health care services in exchange for a prepaid, fixed fee. Whereas there were 166 HMOs nationally in 1975 that enrolled 5.8 million persons, by 1995 there were about 600 HMOs that enrolled more than 51 million members nationally (Dial, Bergsten, Kantor, Buck, & Chalk, 1996; Group Health Association of America, 1995), and the number of enrollees has grown considerably since then.

In the public sector, state Medicaid agencies, the largest funding source for children's mental health services, have moved dramatically to managed care, either through HMOs or through mental health (or behavioral health) "carve outs." A carve out is an arrangement in which the financing and administration of mental health services is separate from the financing and administration of physical health services. As of late 1997 and early 1998, nearly all states were engaged in some health care reform activity involving Medicaid. Of the 43 managed care reforms either underway or being planned at that time, 28 (65%) involved carve outs, whereas the remaining 15 (35%) were "integrated," which is defined as a reform in which the financing and administration of physical and behavioral health are integrated (Pires, Armstrong, & Stroul, 1999).

Although managed care has taken different forms in different states, some aspects have been consistent and should continue to have a major impact on the practice of psychology with children:

- A major focus is on cost containment.
- There is a dramatic reduction in the autonomy of the individual practitioner, with many requirements for review and approval before particular services can be offered or continued.
- There is a greater emphasis on short-term treatment.
- There is also a greater focus on diagnosis-based practice or treatment standards or guidelines, which, although conceptually consistent with the movement toward empirically supported treatment, are more frequently based on expert judgment than on empirical findings.
- The pathway to referrals is through participating in one or more practice networks, and the networks are most likely to make referrals to those practitioners who adhere to their guidelines.

As a federally initiated work group points out, "practice guidelines (or provider guidelines) are gaining in importance because of improved knowledge in health care delivery, economic and political pressure for accountability, and related attempts to delimit the type and amount of care to be provided, and concerns about access to care, quality assurance, and service outcomes" (Zubritsky & Hadley, 1998, p. 71). The term *practice or provider guidelines* and the related term *clinical competencies* have been defined as a set of patient care strategies developed to assist clinicians in clinical decision making and patient management (Zarin, McIntyre, & Pincus, 1996).

Although there is much discussion about practice standards and guidelines and about clinical competencies, a recent report of a group that examined these issues specifically related to children concluded that there is not yet a consensus about the framework of practice standards, that different stakeholder groups have different priorities, and that the fact that such guidelines and protocols are typically organized around specific diagnoses has "limited usefulness to the broad population of children with mental health needs or to children with multiple, complex needs, thereby reinforcing the fragmented, categorical nature of current system functions" (Goldman, Irvine, & Davis, 1999, p. v). This group, the Child, Adolescent, and Family Panel for the Mental Health Managed Care and Workforce Training Project, identified a set of principles that it believes should guide the development of protocols. These principles, similar to those for systems of care (Stroul & Friedman, 1986), emphasize family involvement, individualized and strengths-based care, cultural competence, a developmental perspective, and care coordination.

As the health care field has moved to managed care, an increased emphasis has been placed on quality assurance and assessment of outcomes (Boothroyd, Skinner, Shern, & Steinwachs, 1998; Campbell, 1998; Hernandez, Hodges, & Cascardi, 1998). Although much work has yet to be done in this area, it is clear that one direction involves the inclusion of consumers and families in the process of developing outcome-based accountability systems. As Campbell points out, consumers have typically been omitted from the process of developing outcome systems, but "the transformation of the health care delivery system to a managed care environment may provide mental health consumers with the opportunity to take responsibility for their own lives in the medical marketplace, and to be truly seen as customers"

(Campbell, 1998, p. 15). This increased emphasis on both quality assurance and accountability for outcomes may prove to be one of the most positive aspects of the changes in financing that have taken place and that are likely to continue to take place for a while.

Summary

It is clear from the demographic and epidemiological data that a major need exists for psychological and other mental health services for children and that this need is only likely to grow in the future. With the increasing racial and ethnic diversity of our population and the higher prevalence of emotional disorders in children who live in poverty, a special need is going to exist for professionals who are trained and skilled in working with and understanding the impact of cultural and contextual issues. It is also clear that the existing utilization of mental health services is very low in relation to need and that the mental health field has to devise ways to more effectively reach out to those in need. This may very well involve working even more closely with other systems, such as the schools, health care, child welfare, child care, and juvenile justice; the system-of-care framework that has dominated the public mental health field for the past 15 years provides an important approach to doing that.

At the practice level, there is a growing need to build on the strengths of the individualized-care, wraparound approach that has emerged from the system-of-care framework while incorporating some of the positive features of the movement to identify empirically supported treatments. The individualized-care approach has its roots in the field and focuses on children with complex problems and needs that cut across many life domains in addition to mental health; the empirically supported treatment movement has its roots in clinical research, is diagnosis based, and needs to test its wings in more naturalistic community settings. At the same time as efforts are taking place to build on the strengths of these two often conflicting approaches, the reality of practice is that with the growth of managed care and cost containment strategies, practitioners are being asked to do more in less time and are given less autonomy in how they go about doing it.

It may be that the new accountability approaches that are developed with strong input and involvement from consumers and families will facilitate a proper balance between the cost containment efforts and the requirements of effective care. It may also be that eventually effectiveness research efforts will help clarify the proper relationship between individualized care on the one hand and more manualized, standardized care on the other. Given the complexities of research in naturalistic settings with the types of children and families who are typically seen in these settings, it may in fact be that the process of identifying effective interventions for children in community settings with multiple and complex needs will continue to be elusive. Given this, practitioners will face the challenge of being knowledgeable about and competent in individualized care approaches, being competent as well with empirically supported treatments, being able to develop an approach to combining the two, and gathering systematic outcome data that is an appropriate match for the children and families they are serving.

REFERENCES

American Psychiatric Association (1987). *Diagnostic and Statistical Manual of Mental Disorders, 3rd edition-revised (DSM-III-R)*. Washington, DC: American Psychiatric Association.

American Psychiatric Association (1994). *Diagnostic and Statistical Manual of Mental Disorders, 4th edition (DSM-IV)*. Washington, DC: American Psychiatric Association.

American Psychological Association, Task Force on Promotion and Dissemination of Psychological Procedures, Division of Clinical Psychology (1995). Training in and dissemination of empirically validated psychological treatments: Report and recommendations. *Clinical Psychologist, 48*, 3–23.

American Psychological Association, Task Force on Professional Child and Adolescent Psychology (1998). *Task force report*. Washington, DC: Board of Professional Affairs.

Angold, A., Costello, E. J., & Erkanli, A. (1999). Comorbidity. *Journal of Child Psychology and Psychiatry, 40*, 57–87.

Annie E. Casey Foundation (1996, 1997, 1998). *Kids count data book*. Baltimore: Author.

Armbruster, P., & Fallon, T. (1994). Clinical, sociodemographic, and systems risk factors for attrition in a children's mental health clinic. *American Journal of Orthopsychiatry, 64*, 577–585.

Arnold, L. E., Abikoff, H. B., Cantwell, D. P., Conners, C. K., Elliott, G., Greenhill, L. L., Hechtman, L., Hinshaw, S. P., Hoza, B., Jensen, P. S., Kraemer, H. C., March, J. S., Newcorn, J. H., Pelham, W. E., Richters, J. E., Schiller, E., Severe, J. B., Swanson, J. M., Vereen, D., & Wells, K. C. (1997). National Institute of Mental Health collaborative multimodal treatment study of children with ADHD (the MTA). *Archives of General Psychiatry, 54*, 865–870.

Behar, L. (1985). Changing patterns of state responsibility: A case study of North Carolina. *Journal of Clinical Child Psychology, 14*, 188–195.

Boothroyd, R. A., Skinner, E. A., Shern, D. L., & Steinwachs, D. M. (1998). Feasibility of consumer-based outcome monitoring: A report from the National Outcomes Roundtable. In R. W. Manderscheid & M. J. Henderson (Eds.), *Mental health, United States, 1998* (pp. 29–43). Rockville, MD: Substance Abuse and Mental Health Services Administration.

Brandenburg, N. A., Friedman, R. M., & Silver, S. E. (1990). The epidemiology of childhood psychiatric disorders: Prevalence findings from recent studies. *Journal of the American Academy of Child and Adolescent Psychiatry, 29*, 76–83.

Brestan, E. V., & Eyberg, S. M. (1998). Effective psychosocial treatments of conduct-disordered children and adolescents: 29 years, 82 studies, and 5,272 kids. *Journal of Clinical Child Psychology, 27*, 180–189.

Burns, B. J., Costello, E. J., Angold, A., Tweed, D., Stangl, D., Farmer, E. M. Z., & Erkanli, A. (1995). Children's mental health service use across service sectors. *Health Affairs, 14*, 148–159.

Burns, B. J., Costello, E. J., Erkanli, A., Tweed, D. L., Farmer, E. M. Z., & Angold, A. (1997) Insurance coverage and mental health service use by adolescents with serious emotional disturbance. *Journal of Child and Family Studies, 6*, 89–111.

Burns, B. J., Farmer, E. M. Z., Angold, A., Costello, E. J., & Behar, L. (1996). A randomized trial of case management for youth with serious emotional disturbances. *Journal of Clinical Child Psychology, 25*, 476–486.

Burns, B. J., & Goldman, S. K. (1999). *Systems of care: Promising practices in wraparound for children with serious emotional disturbance and their families.*

Rockville, MD: Substance Abuse and Mental Health Services Administration.

Campbell, J. (1998). Consumerism, outcomes, and satisfaction: A review of the literature. In R. W. Manderscheid & M. J. Henderson (Eds.), *Mental health, United States, 1998* (pp. 11–28). Rockville, MD: Substance Abuse and Mental Health Services Administration.

Caron, C., & Rutter, M. (1991). Comorbidity in child psychopathology: Concepts, issues and research strategies. *Journal of Child Psychology and Psychiatry, 32,* 1063–1080.

Catron, T., & Weiss, B. (1994). The Vanderbilt School-Based Counseling Program. *Journal of Emotional and Behavioral Disorders, 2,* 247–253.

Chambless, D. L., & Hollon, S. D. (1998). Defining empirically supported therapies. *Journal of Consulting and Clinical Psychology, 66,* 7–18.

Children's Defense Fund. (1991). *The state of America's children.* Washington, DC: Author.

Clark, H. B., & Clarke, R. T. (1996). Research on the wraparound process and individualized services for children with multi-system needs. *Journal of Child and Family Studies, 5,* 1–5.

Cole, R. F., & Poe, S. (1993). *Partnerships for care: Systems of care for children with serious emotional disturbances and their families.* Washington, DC: Washington Business Group on Health.

Costello, E. J. (1989). Developments in child psychiatric epidemiology: An epidemiologic study of behavior characteristics in children. *Journal of the American Academy of Child and Adolescent Psychiatry, 28,* 836–841.

Cross, T. L., Bazron, B. J., Dennis, K. W., & Isaacs, M. R. (1989). *Towards a culturally competent system of care: Vol. I. A monograph on effective services for minority children who are severely emotionally disturbed.* Washington, DC: Georgetown University Child Development Center.

DeChillo, N. D., Koren, P. E., & Mezera, M. (1996). Families and professionals in partnership. In B. A. Stroul (Ed.), *Children's mental health: Creating systems of care in a changing society* (pp. 389–407). Baltimore: Brookes.

Dial, T. H., Bergsten, C., Kantor, A., Buck, J. A., & Chalk, M. E. (1996). Behavioral health care in HMOs. In R. W. Manderscheid & M. A. Sonnenschein (Eds.), *Mental health, United States, 1996* (pp. 45–58). Rockville, MD: Substance Abuse and Mental Health Services Administration.

Friedman, R. M. (1992). Mental health and substance abuse services for adolescents: Clinical and service system issues. *Administration and Policy in Mental Health, 19,* 191–206.

Friedman, R. M., & Duchnowski, A. J. (1990). Service trends in the children's mental health system: Implications for the training of psychologists. In P. R. Magrab (Ed.), *National conference on clinical training in psychology: Improving psychological services for children and adolescents with severe mental disorders* (pp. 35–41). Washington, DC: Georgetown Child Development Center.

Friedman, R. M., Katz-Leavy, J. W., Manderscheid, R. W., & Sondheimer, D. L. (1996). Prevalence of serious emotional disturbance in children and adolescents. In R. W. Manderscheid & M. A. Sonnenschein (Eds.), *Mental health, United States, 1996* (pp. 71–89). Rockville, MD: Substance Abuse and Mental Health Services Administration.

Friedman, R. M., Katz-Leavy, J. W., Manderscheid, R. W., & Sondheimer, D. L. (1998). Prevalence of serious emotional disturbance: An update. In R. W. Manderscheid & M. J. Henderson (Eds.), *Mental health, United States, 1998* (pp. 110–112). Rockville, MD: Substance Abuse and Mental Health Services Administration.

Friedman, R. M., Kutash, K., & Duchnowski, A. J. (1996) The population of concern: Defining the issues. In B. A. Stroul (Ed.), *Children's mental health:*

Creating systems of care in a changing society (pp. 69–96). Baltimore: Brookes.

Friesen, B. J., & Huff, B. (1996). Family perspectives on systems of care. In B. A. Stroul (Ed.), *Children's mental health: Creating systems of care in a changing society* (pp. 41–67). Baltimore: Brookes.

Gibbs, J. T., & Huang, L. N. (1989). *Children of color: Psychological interventions with minority youth*. San Francisco: Jossey-Bass.

Goldman, S. K. (1999). The conceptual framework for wraparound. In B. J. Burns & S. K. Goldman (Eds.), *Systems of care: Promising practices in wraparound for children with serious emotional disturbance and their families* (pp. 9–16). Rockville, MD: Substance Abuse and Mental Health Services Administration.

Goldman, S. K., Irvine, M. D., & Davis, C. (1999). *Report of the child, adolescent, and family panel for the mental health managed care and workforce training project*. Washington, DC: Georgetown University Child Development Center.

Gould, M. S., Shaffer, E., & Kaplan, D. (1985). The characteristics of dropouts from a child psychiatry clinic. *Journal of the American Academy of Child and Adolescent Psychiatry, 24*, 316–328.

Greenbaum, P. E., Prange, M. E., Friedman, R. M., & Silver, S. E. (1991). Substance abuse prevalence and comorbidity with other psychiatric disorders among adolescents with severe emotional disturbances. *Journal of the American Academy of Child and Adolescent Psychiatry, 30*, 575–583.

Greenhill, L. L., Abikoff, H. B., Arnold, L. E., Cantwell, D. P., Conners, C. K., Elliott, G., Hechtman, L., Hinshaw, S. P., Hoza, B., Jensen, P. S., March, J. S., Newcorn, J., Pelham, W. E., Severe, J. B., Swanson, J. M., Vitiello, B., & Wells, K. (1996). Medication treatment strategies in the MTA study: Relevance to clinicians and researchers. *Journal of the American Academy of*

Child and Adolescent Psychiatry, 34, 1304–1313.

Gresenz, C. R., Liu, X., & Sturm, R. (1998). Managed behavioral health services for children under carve-out contracts. *Psychiatric Services, 49*, 1054–1058.

Group Health Association of America (1995). *Patterns in HMO enrollment (5th ed,)*. Washington, DC: Author.

Hernandez, M., Hodges, S., & Cascardi, M. (1998). The ecology of outcomes: System accountability in children's mental health. *Journal of Behavioral Health Services and Research, 25*, 136–150.

Hernandez, M., & Isaacs, M. R. (1998). (Eds.). *Promoting cultural competence in children's mental health services*. Baltimore: Brookes.

Hernandez, M., Isaacs, M. R., Nesman, T., & Burns, D. (1998). Perspectives on culturally competent systems of care. In M. Hernandez & M. R. Isaacs (Eds.), *Promoting cultural competence in children's mental health services* (pp. 1–25). Baltimore: Brookes.

Hoagwood, K., & Erwin, H. D. (1997). Effectiveness of school-based mental health services for children: A 10-year research review. *Journal of Child and Family Studies, 6*, 435–454.

Hodges, K., & Gust, J. (1995). Measures of impairment for children and adolescents. *Journal of Mental Health Administration, 22*, 403–413.

Household and Family Characteristics. (1990). Series P-20. Washington, DC: U.S. Government Printing Office.

Isaacs, M., & Benjamin, M. P. (1991). *Towards a culturally competent system of care: Vol. II. Programs which utilize culturally competent principles*. Washington, DC: Georgetown University Child Development Center.

Isaacs-Shockley, M., Cross, T., Bazron, B. J., Dennis, K., & Benjamin, M. P. (1996). Framework for a culturally competent system of care. In B. A. Stroul (Ed.), *Children's mental health: Creating systems of care in a changing society* (pp. 23–39). Baltimore: Brookes.

Kaslow, N. J., & Thompson, M. P. (1998). Applying the criteria for empirically supported treatments to studies of psychosocial interventions for child and adolescent depression. *Journal of Clinical Child Psychology, 27*, 146–155.

Kazdin, A. E., Holland, L., & Crowley, M. (1997). Family experiences of barriers to treatment and premature termination from child therapy. *Journal of Consulting and Clinical Psychology, 65*, 453–463.

Kazdin, A. E., & Kendall, P. C. (1998). Current progress and future plans for developing effective treatments: Comments and perspectives. *Journal of Clinical Child Psychology, 27*, 217–226.

Kazdin, A. E., & Weisz, J. R. (1998). Identifying and developing empirically supported child and adolescent treatments. *Journal of Consulting and Clinical Psychology, 66*, 19–36.

Kessler, R. C. (1994). The National Comorbidity Survey of the United States. *International Review of Psychiatry, 6*, 365–376.

King, B., & Meyers, J. (1996). The Annie E. Casey Foundation's mental health initiative for children. In B. A. Stroul (Ed.), *Children's mental health: Creating systems of care in a changing society* (pp. 249–261). Baltimore: Brookes.

Knitzer, J. (1982). *Unclaimed children: The failure of public responsibility to child and adolescents in need of mental health services.* Washington, DC: Children's Defense Fund.

Koroloff, N. M., Elliott, D. J., Koren, P. E., & Friesen, B. J. (1996). Linking low-income families to children's mental health services: An outcome study. *Journal of Emotional and Behavioral Disorders, 4*, 2–11.

Koroloff, N. M., Friesen, B. J., Reilly, L., & Rinkin, J. (1996). The role of family members in systems of care. In B. A. Stroul (Ed.), *Children's mental health: Creating systems of care in a changing society* (pp. 409–426). Baltimore: Brookes.

Koss-Chioino, J. D., & Vargas, L. A. (1999). *Working with Latino youth: Culture, development and context.* San Francisco: Jossey-Bass.

Lardieri, S., Greenbaum, P. E., & Pugh, A. M. (1996, February). Parent reports of problem behavior onset among children and adolescents with serious emotional disturbances. Paper presented at the Annual System of Care Research Conference, Tampa, FL.

Lavigne, J. V., Gibbons, R. D., Christoffel, K. K., Arend, R., Rosenbaum, D., Binns, H., Dawson, N., Sobel, H., & Isaacs, C. (1996). Prevalence rates and correlates of psychiatric disorders among preschool children. *Journal of the American Academy of Child and Adolescent Psychiatry, 35*, 204–214.

Leaf, P. J., Alegria, M., Cohen, P., Goodman, S. H., Horwitz, S. M., Hoven, C. W., Narrow, W. E., Vaden-Kiernan, M., & Regier, D. A. (1996). Mental health service use in the community and schools: Results from the four-community MECA study. *Journal of the American Academy of Child and Adolescent Psychiatry, 35*, 889–897.

Lonigan, C. J., Elbert, J. C., & Johnson, S. B. (1998). Empirically supported psychosocial interventions for children: An overview. *Journal of Clinical Child Psychology, 27*, 138–145.

Lourie, I. S., Katz-Leavy, J. K., & Stroul, B. A. (1996). Individualized services in a system of care. In B. A. Stroul (Ed.), *Children's mental health: Creating systems of care in a changing society* (pp. 429–452). Baltimore: Brookes.

Pelham, W. E., Wheeler, T., & Chronis, A. (1998). Empirically supported psychosocial treatments for attention deficit hyperactivity disorder. *Journal of Clinical Child Psychology, 27*, 190–205.

Pires, S. A., Armstrong, M. I., & Stroul, B. A. (1999). *Health care reform tracking project: Tracking state managed care reforms as they affect children and adolescents with behavioral health disorders and their families.* Tampa, FL: University of South Florida.

Public Law 102-321, 1992.

Quinn, K. P., & Epstein, M. H. (1998). Characteristics of children, youth, and families served by local interagency systems of care. In M. H. Epstein, K. Kutash, & A. Duchnowski (Eds.), *Outcomes for children and youth with behavioral and emotional disorders and their families* (pp. 81–114). Austin, TX: Pro-Ed.

Richters, J. E., Arnold, L. E., Jensen, P. S., Abikoff, H., Conners, C. K., Greenhill, L. L., Hechtman, L., Hinshaw, S. P., Pelham, W. W., & Swanson, J. M. (1995). NIMH collaborative multisite multimodal treatment study of children with ADHD: Background and rationale. *Journal of the American Academy of Child and Adolescent Psychiatry, 34,* 987–1000.

Roberts, M. C., Carlson, C. I., Erickson, M. T., Friedman, R. M., La Greca, A. M., Lemanek, K. L., Russ, S. W., Schroeder, C. S., Vargas, L. A., & Wohlford, P. F. (1998). A model for training psychologists to provide services to children and adolescents. *Professional Psychology: Research and Practice, 29,* 293–299.

Roberts, R. E., Attkisson, C. C., & Rosenblatt, A. (1998). Prevalence of psychopathology among children and adolescents. *American Journal of Psychiatry, 155,* 715–725.

Rosado, J. W., & Elias, N. J. (1993). Ecological and psychocultural mediators in the delivery of services for urban, culturally diverse Hispanic clients. *Professional Psychology: Research and Practice, 24,* 450–459.

Santisteban, D. A., Szapocznik, J., Perez-Vidal, A., Kuartines, W. M., Murray, E. J., & LaPerriere, A. (1996). Efficacy of intervention for engaging youth and families into treatment and some variables that may contribute to differential effectiveness. *Journal of Family Psychology, 10,* 35–44.

Stroul, B. A., & Friedman, R. M. (1986). *A system of care for seriously emotionally disturbed children and youth.* Washington, DC: Georgetown University Child Development Center.

Stroul, B. A., & Friedman, R. M. (1996). The system of care concept and philosophy. In B. A Stroul (Ed.), *Children's mental health: Creating systems of care in a changing society* (pp. 3–21). Baltimore: Brookes.

Substance Abuse and Mental Health Services Administration. (1993). Final notice establishing definitions for (1) Children with a serious emotional disturbance, and (2) adults with a serious mental illness. *Federal Register, 58,* 29422–29425.

Szapocznik, J., Perez-Vidal, A., Brickman, A. L., Foote, F. H., Santisteban, D., & Hervis, O. (1988). Engaging adolescent drug abusers and their families in treatment: A strategic structural systems approach. *Journal of Consulting and Clinical Psychology, 56,* 552–557.

Weisz, J. R., & Hawley, K. M. (1998). Finding, evaluating, refining, and applying empirically supported treatments for children and adolescents. *Journal of Clinical Child Psychology, 27,* 206–216.

Zarin, D. A., McIntyre, J. S., & Pincus, H. A. (1996). The role of psychotherapy in the treatment of depression: Review of two practice guidelines. *Archives of Behavioral Psychiatry, 53,* 291–293.

Zubritsky, C., & Hadley, T. R. (1998). The managed behavioral health care workforce initiative: Standards, guidelines, and competencies for behavioral health care. In R. W. Manderscheid & M. J. Henderson (Eds.), *Mental Health, United States, 1998* (pp. 70–81). Rockville, MD: Substance Abuse and Mental Health Services Administration.

2

ROBERT C. PIANTA

Implications of a Developmental Systems Model for Preventing and Treating Behavioral Disturbances in Children and Adolescents

Early detection of risk and the design and delivery of risk-reducing and health-promoting interventions are essential functions for child and adolescent psychologists (Adelman & Taylor, 1998; Carlson, Tharinger, Bricklin, DeMers, & Paavola, 1996), in addition to traditional functions such as diagnosis and treatment of mental disorders. A theory of behavior change and of the ways in which schools, families, therapists, and other contexts figure in behavior change is essential to achieving a comprehensive system of mental-health promotion for children and adolescents. One source of ideas on behavior change that has until recently received fairly limited attention from applied child and adolescent psychologists is developmental theory (Tharinger & Lambert, 1998) — in particular, developmental systems theory, in which the role of contexts with respect to developmental processes is explicitly illuminated.

Developmental systems theory (e.g., Ford & Lerner, 1992; Sameroff, 1995) has certain advantages for understanding the ways in which developmental resources present in a variety of contexts (home, school, neighborhood, therapy) can be located and harnessed both before (prevention) and after (remediation) the emergence of serious behavioral disturbance. Developmental systems theory offers a way to think about the multiple inputs that shape development across domains of mental health, achievement, and socialization outcomes and, in particular, describes overarching principles by which contexts influence these outcomes. In turn, these principles provide child and adolescent psychologists with a set of ideas to guide practice, recognizing that the essential features of practice with children and adolescents involve observation and manipulation of the interdependencies of context and child behavior (see Nastasi, 1998, for more details).

Context, Time, and Local Politics

In developing a theoretical framework to understand behavioral change as it may be influenced by preventive and remedial psychological interventions, three realities of behavioral change must be acknowledged. These are the role of context in the development and amelioration of risk and pathology; the role of time in the process of change; and the constraints on intervention replication due to local factors. Developmental systems perspectives address all three of these realities.

Context

The influences of context on behavior is the core of psychological practice, regardless of whether the behavioral concern is driven by biological processes (as might be the case with autism) or whether it is wholly contextually driven (as is the case in coercive family processes and aggression). From this point of view, intervention in child and adolescent psychology involves rearranging contextual inputs to the child in order to achieve a desired outcome (Nastasi, 1998). It is increasingly recognized that interventions applied in the context or contexts in which a problem occurs can be more effective agents of change than efforts at change that take place in an office or in a context remote from the problem at hand (e.g., Henggeler, 1994; Henggeler, Schoenwald, Bordun, Rowland, & Cunningham, 1998; Nastasi, 1998). Rarely is it the case that children in need of mental health services display problems only at home or only in contexts other than school, and a key aspect of efforts to change a behavioral pattern is the extent to which intervention plans engage processes that regulate the development of the behavioral pattern in those contexts in which the pattern is of concern.

Thus the design of treatment plans for child and adolescent problem behavior ideally recognizes these multiple contexts and produces change as a function of manipulating contextual inputs to the child (Adelman, 1996; Henggeler et al., 1998; Roberts, 1996). In some ways, applied child and adolescent psychologists adopt the role of "context manager" by designing interventions to be carried out by others in natural contexts (parents, teachers, peers), by training the intervenors, and by monitoring progress (Adelman, 1996; Henggeler et al., 1998; Johnson, Malone, & Hightower, 1997; Nastasi, 1998). In short, if a theory of behavioral change is to be relevant for prevention and intervention efforts of psychologists, it must facilitate an appreciation of the role of various contexts and identify processes by which psychologists can influence contexts and, in turn, help shape child development (Tharinger & Lambert, 1998).

Developmental Time: Pathways

One lesson learned from developmental research is that there is no single, linear, one-to-one mapping of early risk (or nonrisk) status onto problem (or competent) outcomes. Instead, it may be helpful to adopt Sroufe's (1989) use of Waddington's metaphor of development and a branching tree, with many possible outcomes possible depending on the path one takes from trunk to branches. Because not all impulsive first-graders become aggressive sixth-graders, understanding the relation between risk and outcome depends on understanding the processes that shape developmental pathways. Targeting these processes for intervention could be key to interrupting the relation between risk and later problems (Loeber, 1990) by creating "branches" along developmental pathways.

How do parents, psychologists, or teachers play a role in creating and sustaining these branching pathways? A developmental systems approach to intervention (Pianta, 1999) emphasizes vulnerability and protective mechanisms (Rutter, 1987) that influence the response to risk (for better or worse) within a window of opportunity, or a period of relative plasticity, when responses to risk are being formulated. Understanding variations in individuals' responses to risk factors and how contexts shape those responses, either by supporting the individual or by acting directly on the risk factor(s) that affect the individual, is a key aspect of delivering health-promoting services.

Local Politics

Despite efforts to develop standardized treatment protocols and documentation of their effectiveness, local factors (e.g., a teacher's willingness to change, a parent's compliance with a behavior management system, a child's regular attendance at appointments) always constrain the applicability of any intervention or practice (Molnar & Lindquist, 1990). Rather than treating these local constraints as "nuisance" or "noise" factors, child and adolescent psychologists need tools to understand how to integrate these nuisance factors with validated principles of behavior change enacted in context.

At the local level — in homes, classrooms, neighborhoods, or clinics — pressure is high to find solutions (Pianta & Walsh, 1996). This pressure forces a focus on effective practices that are enacted most often on the basis of their having demonstrated an association with behavioral improvement in a clinical trial. Replicating such trials under local constraints is nearly impossible (Henggeler, 1994), and if the putative effective intervention is not strongly theory based, with convincing arguments for why it should or should not work under a given set of circumstances, then the practitioner is left with little basis for choosing the next step. Approaches to intervention with children and adolescents must somehow recognize the realities of local constraints and local pressures while embracing a validated knowledge base that can inform choices about intervention strategies and techniques.

As just one example, Diaz and Berk (1995) argued that the widespread use of office-based "cognitive-behavioral interventions" for children with impulsivity problems neglects the literature on how links between cognition, emotion, and behavior develop into self-regulation. Two specific shortcomings are evident with regard to the local politics issue. First, the vast majority of cognitive-behavioral interventions were developed by comparing already-identified impulsive (or depressed, etc.) children with unidentified or undiagnosed children. These retrospective studies showed differences in aspects of cognition that then became the basis for the range of programmatic treatments targeted at reducing these differences. However, the literature on the development of self-regulation demonstrates fairly convincingly that over time children's emotions and emotional behaviors, in the context of interactions with adults, come increasingly under the mediational control of cognition. Thus cognition is a latecomer to the mediation of emotional experience.

Second, although self-regulation can be taught as a discrete skill or set of skills, it develops naturally in contexts in which child-adult relationships provide emotion-regulating experiences. When end products of developmental processes are taught (as in cognitive-behavioral therapy) as discrete skills in an office-based context, in contrast to providing relationship experiences in which self-regulation typically develops, such interventions lack grounding in developmental and contextual underpinnings. In the view of Diaz and Berk (1995), use of a practice with scores of supporting effectiveness studies without an accompanying understanding of developmental processes that underlie the problem to which the practice is directed accounts for the fact that cognitive-behavioral interventions have limited effects on problems with self-control or emotion regulation on playgrounds or in lunchrooms. As a further example of the need to integrate theory in real-life contexts, Doll (1996) recommends that if psychologists are to intervene helpfully in the peer problems of children (e.g., rejection, aggression), they must participate in peer interactions on the playground and in the lunchroom!

Theory about the development of problem behavior — the processes that produce the problem under consideration, particularly the role of context in shaping behavioral patterns — can provide a useful guide for local-level applications of treatment protocols. Theory-based knowledge used in this way should be well validated and can serve as a means for practitioners to make the many important local decisions they face. Developmental systems theory provides child and adolescent psychologists with a set of principles by which behavior change in context can be understood, an asset to local decision-making processes (Molnar & Lindquist, 1990).

Developmental Systems Theory

Designing solutions for the behavioral and emotional problems of children is complex. General systems theory provides a set of principles that can help child and adolescent psychologists make sense of the multiple transactions of contexts, local constraints, and time involved in influencing developmental pathways.

For the purposes of this discussion, *systems* is defined as units composed of sets of interrelated parts that act in organized, interdependent ways to promote the adaptation and survival of the whole. Families, classrooms, child-parent and child-teacher relationships, self-regulatory behaviors, and peer groups are systems of one form or another. The work of child and adolescent psychologists involves these and many other systems.

General systems theory (GST) has a long history in the understanding of biological, ecological, and other complex living systems (e.g., Ford & Ford, 1987; Ford & Lerner, 1992) and has been applied to child development by Ford and Lerner (1992) and Sameroff (1995) in what is called developmental systems theory (DST). DST can be applied to the broad array of systems involved in the practice of psychology with children and adolescents (Pianta, 1999). The principles of DST help integrate analysis of the multiple factors that influence young children, such as families, communities, social processes, cognitive development, schools, teachers, and peers or conditions such as poverty.

One essential feature of DST is acknowledgment of the various contexts, or systems, that affect development. These systems have influences ranging from distal (governments) to proximal (families); they include culture, small social groups, dyads, the child, behavioral systems, and genetic and biological systems. These contexts play key roles in the regulation of developmental change — how development is orderly, organized, and planned as opposed to random, chaotic, or unpredictable (Sameroff, 1995). According to Sameroff, contexts contain regulatory mechanisms that, like thermostats, maintain organization and calibration of certain developmental functions. Knowledge of these contexts and their regulatory functions is essential for understanding and shaping developmental pathways.

As will be discussed later, child-adult relationships play a key regulatory function for children's experience in home and classroom settings. Child-parent and child-teacher relationships provide stability to children's emotional experience (Lynch & Cicchetti, 1992), provide structure and guides for interactions with peers (Howes, Hamilton, & Matheson, 1994), serve as a source of security that supports exploration and mastery, and involve interactions that help shape the child's self-regulation (Birch & Ladd, 1997; Pianta, 1997, 1999).

Sameroff (1995) identifies systems and adult-child relationships that regulate development in specific ways. These systems (or contexts) contain codes that prescribe regulatory actions of the system vis-à-vis the child. These regulatory actions shape the proximal context in which the child must adapt. For example, schools (as systems) have rules that govern the behavior of teachers and children. These rules constrain the kinds of interactions that take place in classrooms (e.g., teachers cannot hit students, students cannot hit teachers).

Cultures and Large Communities

Cultures and communities regulate the behavior of individuals and smaller social groups by creating, organizing, and maintaining roles within the larger group (Boulding, 1985). For example, cultures help define the roles of parents in terms of acceptable and unacceptable discipline practices.

The set of culture-level codes that affect development can be called a *developmental agenda* (Sameroff, 1995). One way of thinking about a culture's developmental agenda is as the shared timetable for developmental milestones or generally held beliefs and expectations for child development. The developmental agenda is a series of culturally defined points in the child's life when the child-rearing context is restructured to provide different experiences to the child. These restructurings include toilet training, entering school, and adolescent rites of passage (e.g., getting a driver's license). Many, if not all, enactments of cultural codes tend to be keyed to the chronological age of children in that culture, not to the developmental level of an individual child. These restructurings are large-scale, long-term actions called *macroregulations* in Sameroff's model.

Macroregulations may produce opportunity or trigger failure of one sort or another. Powerful challenges (learning academic subjects, dating) are enacted based on chronological age (or some proxy such as grade in school) and may challenge the child's or family's capacity to adapt. These macroregulations may require certain skills or capacities or may assume previous developmental successes that are not part of the child's life history or present status.

For example, when a child with little preparation is placed in an elementary classroom with demanding teachers and high expectations for performance, such placement policies can produce "child failure" or "school failure," which is better characterized as a failure of the system rather than of the child (Pianta & Walsh, 1996). Careful scrutiny of policies and regulations that operate as a community's or culture's developmental agenda and changing these policies to ensure more developmentally sensitive challenges with adequate supportive resources is one avenue for enacting wide-ranging preventive intervention strategies.

Families and Small Social Groups

Families and small social groups (peer groups, gangs, church groups, schools, classrooms) are concerned with the regulation of the individual child's behavior toward the goal of producing individuals who adequately fulfill roles in the larger social structure (culture). For example, families influence children's behavior in ways that produce competent self-regulation and help the child become a functional member of groups outside the family.

Small-group codes trigger behaviors of the group that operate within a shorter time span than cultural-level codes and often reflect the colliding demands of living together in small social groups and meeting the larger developmental agenda. Sameroff calls these *miniregulations*: caregiving practices such as feeding, discipline, expectations for performance, and patterns of emotional expression allowed within the group that are enacted through regulatory interactions with adults. This form of regulation allows the group to function as a cohesive social unit in order to accomplish its purpose in a social structure. Family- and classroom-code influences are apparent, for example, in family expectations for performance and discipline practices in school. Fundamental to the functioning of these small social groups is that these codes are enacted through behavioral interactions with children.

Interpersonal Relationships

Child-parent, child-peer, and teacher-child relationships are dyadic systems that play key roles in regulation of child behavior within small social groups (Hinde, 1987). Regulation at the relationship level is enacted through individual codes, according to Sameroff (1995). With respect to relationships between adults and children, these codes involve the adult's (parent, teacher) accumulated feelings and beliefs about their behaviors with children — what works and does not work — their motivation styles, and their goals for interaction (Pianta, 1999). These individual codes can be described in terms of the adult's (or child's) "internal working model" or "representational model" of himself or herself and the relationship (Zeanah et al., 1993).

Representations, feelings, and beliefs are enacted in very brief, often subtle aspects of moment-to-moment interaction with children (microregulations). The qualities of this interaction are described both by what is being done by the adult or child (i.e., feeding, punishing, attending) and also by how it is being done. Aspects of dyadic behavioral interactions such as reciprocity, sensitivity, coordination, and synchrony are frequently used to describe relationships between parents and children (e.g., Egeland, Pianta & O'Brien, 1993; Rogoff, 1990) and even teachers and children (Howes & Hamilton, 1992; Pianta, Nimetz, & Bennett, 1998). A parent and child sharing a laugh (mutuality or synchrony) or a teacher who reads a child's subtle frustration cues and slides a puzzle piece closer to the child's hand (sensitivity) are examples of the qualitative aspects of interaction in which the regulatory influence of individual-level codes are enacted. Individual codes can enhance or erode the ways in which that relationship context is a developmental resource. For example, a teacher's aloof, businesslike style of relating to children may trigger a negative emotional and behavioral response from a child who seeks emotional contact with such a teacher and is rebuffed (Lynch & Cicchetti, 1992).

Because adult-child relationships are asymmetric (the adult is more mature and has greater weight in determining the quality of the relationship), they play key roles in determining how a child will adapt in a specific situation — home or classroom (e.g., Birch & Ladd, 1996; Howes & Hamilton, 1992). As a consequence, child competence is embedded in and a property of relationships with adults. In the early years, relationships with adults, primarily parents (usually mothers) but often child-care providers or other family members, form the infrastructure of development that supports nearly all of what a child is asked to do in and outside of the family — relate to other people, be persistent and focused, be motivated to perform, be compliant or assertive, communicate, and explore the world.

In the school years, this infrastructure is carried forward, with evidence suggesting that relationships with adults are a valuable resource to healthy development through adolescence (Resnick et al., 1997; Werner & Smith, 1980).

The Child as a System

The developing child is also a system. From this point of view, motor, cognitive, social, and emotional development are not independent entities on parallel paths but are integrated within organized, dynamic processes.

Psychological practices (assessment or intervention) that focus solely on one of these domains (e.g., cognition, personality, attention span, aggression, or reading achievement) can reinforce the notion that developmental domains can be isolated from one another and from the context in which they are embedded. Taking a developmental systems perspective, many argue that child assessment should focus on broad indices that reflect integrated functions across a number of behavioral domains as they are observed in context (e.g., Greenspan & Greenspan, 1991; Sroufe, 1989). Terms such as *adaptation* have been used to capture these broad qualities of behavioral organization, and, although fairly abstract, they call attention to a focus on how children use the range of resources available to them (including their own skills and the resources of peers, adults, and materials) to respond to internal and external demands.

Biological Systems

Increasing attention is being paid to biological systems (e.g., genetics, neuroanatomy, neurophysiology) as explanations for risk and psychiatric disorder. Biological "causes" have been offered for such functional problems as reading failure, overactivity and attention problems, and conduct problems (Pennington & Ozonoff, 1991; Riccio, Hynd, Cohen, & Gonzalez, 1993). Yet research pointing to biological or genetic reasons for many forms of problem outcomes is too often misinterpreted to suggest a "causal" role for biology and ignores the reality that biological systems are embedded in and interact with other systems (Gottlieb, 1991; Greenough & Black, 1991). At best, these studies must be viewed in light of evidence that biochemical and genetic activity are affected by experiential and environmental parameters (Gottlieb, 1991; Greenough & Black, 1991) and that biological influences on behavior operate within the larger systems influences described previously. Recent evidence has, in fact, made it very clear that neurophysiology and neuroanatomy can be affected by qualities of interaction between young children and parents, predictability of routines, and the emotional climate of the home (see Young, 1994).

Finally, it must be recognized that the systems (or contexts) previously described interact with one another in ways that also provide regulation and structure to developmental activity. In the context of these interactions, relationships with adults are midlevel systems—strongly affected by forces from all directions while influencing the child's development. These relationships are like the keystone or linchpin of development—they are in large part responsible for developmental success under conditions of risk, and more often than not they transmit those risk conditions to the child (National Institute of Child Health and Human Development [NICHD] Early Child Care Research Network, 1999).

Principles That Influence the Behavior and Analysis of Developmental Systems

The previous section described for the most part the topography or landscape of development—the systems or contexts involved in developmental change. Yet it is the behavior of these systems—how they regulate development, for example—that is of greatest interest and that holds promise for understanding behavior change. The behavior of developmental systems is best understood in the context of a number of principles by which systems can be analyzed.

Units of Analysis

From a developmental systems perspective, the behavior of "smaller" systems (such as children's self-regulation) is understood in terms of its function in the context of "larger" systems (such as child-adult relationships). The unit of analysis is at a macrolevel. In terms of parts and wholes, interest is in the whole. In this way, the focus of attention is often at a level higher than the one in which the initial question is framed. Thus to understand the discipline-related behavior of a teacher in her classroom, one must know something about the school, school system, and community in which they are embedded and about the teacher's history of experience in relation to behavioral expectations in the classroom. Similarly, it is not possible to understand why a parent has difficulty maintaining behavioral expectations (the part) without knowing how that activity relates to the purpose of these other concerns (the whole). One cannot understand or explain a student's task orientation without understanding the meaning of the task, preparedness for the task, interactions with the teacher that support performance, and so forth. Behaviors (e.g., attention, motivation) of a child in a context are often best understood in relation to the interactions of the child and the elements of that context and how those interactions function or do not function to support the child. The whole gives meaning to the activity of the parts.

Functional Relations between Parts and Wholes

Systems are embedded within other systems. What is a unit in one system — for example, the child in the family or peer group — is also a system itself. Relations between systems and their component units can be analyzed in terms of differentiation and integration.

Differentiation refers to the fact that over time, in response to internal and external pressures, one of the ways in which systems adapt is by the emergence of subunits. These subunits take on different roles in order for the system as a whole to function. Conversely, integration refers to the fact that in order for the system as a whole to maintain its integrity and identity, differentiated subunits must also be integrated, or connected, with one another to accomplish the primary function of the system. In a developing system there is always a tension between differentiation and integration. This tension is a consequence of relations between units that are active and in contact with one another.

Differentiation and integration allow systems to behave efficiently. In a system in which units are both differentiated (serving different functions) and integrated (the right hand knows what the left is doing), the system can adapt to pressure in a much wider variety of ways than if units were redundant and not connected. Thus parents instruct, discipline, and comfort. It is not necessary for a different adult to take on each of these functions.

Psychology and education are often involved in approaches (assessment, intervention) that promote differentiated functions. For example, the typical ways in which psychological services are offered to children reflect a highly differentiated approach through which children are seen for services outside of contexts in which they live, enrolled in programs, or placed in residential treatment. Although directed toward enhancing some segment of child competence or experience, the end product of separating intervention resources from the contexts or processes in which problems occur may be little functional improvement for the child (Henggeler et al., 1998; Wang & Kovach, 1995). Similarly, assessment practices very frequently seek answers through which to describe or predict functioning by assessing processes and subprocesses, using tests of increasingly isolated skills or functions.

Motivation

Systems theory offers alternative views of the locus of motivation and change. Within behavioral perspectives, change and motivation to change are often viewed as derived extrinsically from being acted on by positive or negative reinforcement or reinforcement history. Maturationist or biological views of change posit that the locus of change is the unfolding of genetic programs, or chronological age. From both perspectives the child is a somewhat passive participant in change — change is something that happens to the child, whether from within or without.

In developmental systems theory the motivation to change is an intrinsic property of a system, inherent within that system's activity. Developmental change follows naturally as a consequence of the activity of interacting systems. That children are active can be seen in the ways they continually construct meaning, seek novelty and challenges, or practice emergent capacities. Furthermore, the child acts within contexts that are dynamic and fluid. Motivation, or the "desire" to change, is derived from the coaction of systems, of child and context.

Maturationist or biological views of the motivation for developmental change can result in "transitional" grades that delay entry into formal schooling for a year of maturation or in the use of medication as a means to address a lack of fit between child and classroom (e.g., Riccio et al., 1993; Shepard & Smith, 1986). Strongly behavioral views of motivation focus solely on contingencies while failing to acknowledge the meaning of target behaviors and contextual responses to the child's goals, leading to a disjunction between how the child perceives his or her fit in the world and how "helpers" may be attempting to facilitate change. Views of motivation informed by systems theory acknowledge that behavioral adaptation is a process embedded in contexts; for example, within relationships between child and adult or child and peers.

Change

Developmental change occurs when systems reorganize and transform under pressure to adapt. In this view, change is not simply a function of acquiring skills but a reorganization of skills and competencies in response to internal and external challenges and demands.

Self-stabilization and *adaptive self-reorganization* are terms that help us understand both stability and adaptive change of a complex system. Self-stabilization refers to the gyroscopic property of systems that can respond to perturbations or demands while not undergoing reorganization. The self-stabilizing system adapts to pressure without altering its basic structure or identity. Self-stabilization is a very important property of systems. It preserves their identity in the face of contextual pressures or demands and ensures that major change, or reorganization, occurs at a slow, regulated pace. If it were not for self-stabilization, the behavior of systems and individuals would be unpredictable and unstable. In some intervention situations, self-stabilizing properties of systems are viewed as resistance to change, or the tendency toward homeostasis and equilibrium. However, these self-preserving tendencies of systems are critical to incorporate in treatment plans; they constrain the intervenor's efforts for good reason and force treatment to take into account the systems' (child, family, teacher) perspective on the change being targeted.

Adaptive self-reorganization refers to the response of a system to more constant or intense environmental (or internal) pressures or demands. Under these circumstances, the self-stabilizing properties of the system are inadequate to meet demands, and the system must reorganize in order to achieve fit.

Prediction in Assessment and Intervention

Psychologists devote considerable effort to prediction, usually in the context of assessing children's skills or progress in treatment. From a systems perspective, prediction is fraught with uncertainty, a lot like forecasting the weather. This is also true for the problem of replicability, as when a clinician attempts to replicate a standard treatment protocol under highly variable local conditions. In these situations, general systems theory reminds professionals that the rules that govern the relations between predictors and outcomes rely on probabilities generated by observing many individual cases but that they rarely explain any single case.

Two equally important principles of systems theory are helpful in relation to considering the problem of prediction. As was described earlier, the developmental progress of individuals can be thought of as a branching tree (Sroufe, 1989) in which paths overlap at the start (looking like a trunk) but that over time will branch and deviate from one another. Thus individuals with the same starting point may end up with a range of outcomes. This is known as the principle of multifinality (Ford & Lerner, 1992), which embodies the uncertainty of making specific predictions about individuals. For example, among children who demonstrate extreme levels of externalizing behavior in the early grades, some develop a range of psychiatric diagnoses in adolescence, whereas others among the group are functioning quite well (Egeland, Pianta, & O'Gawa, 1996).

Alternatively, a specific outcome, such as a diagnosis of depression or conduct disorder, can be traced backward to a range of risk or potentiating conditions that varies widely across the set of individuals with the diagnosis (Egeland et al., 1996). This phenomenon is known as the principle of equifinality and emphasizes that different starting points may lead to similar outcomes; again an example of the uncertainties of prediction.

The discussion now turns to ways in which these principles of developmental systems can be observed in the context of relationships between adults and children. More specifically, I identify ways in which developmental systems theory provides implications for how relationships can function as resources for development that in turn can be harnessed in preventive and remedial intervention.

Social Processes, Relationships, and Prevention

A central focus of developmental systems perspectives, particularly within the field of developmental psychopathology, has been on the role of social processes in the development of problem outcomes in children. Social relationships regulate much of what develops in children — cognition, language, self-regulation, knowledge of emotions, self-esteem, and work habits (see Sroufe, 1989). Children as active systems interact with contexts, exchanging information, material, energy, and activity (Ford & Ford, 1987). As was noted earlier, the embeddedness of children's competence in contexts is such that properties that appear to "reside" in the child (such as cognition, attention, social competence, problem behaviors) are actually distributed across the child and these contexts (e.g., Campbell, 1994; Hofer, 1994; Resnick, 1994).

The concept of affordance embodies the idea that contexts contain resources for the child that can be activated to sustain the child's adaptation to the demands of that setting. A context can be evaluated on the basis of high or low affordance by examining it in relation to how it helps children adapt to these developmental challenges. Importantly, the affordance of a context has to be accessed by interactions with the child.

Thus any discussion of the child's competencies is qualified by knowledge of the contextual supports for those competencies. Inferences about diagnostic status or etiology are inaccurate or premature without a full understanding of the contribution of context, both concurrently and over time, to a child's competencies.

As noted earlier, a central facet of children's experiences in context are their relationships with socialization agents and caregivers — parents, teachers, and others. In fact, the very nature of risk, for many so-called at-risk children, is bound up in the inability of social contexts (mostly relationships with parents and in the family) to appropriately regulate the child's emotional and social development vis-à-vis the key themes described previously. It is in these social processes, mostly involving relationships between child and adults, that risk can be recognized and can be transmitted so easily to the child (and further exacerbated by school and peer contexts). In this view, adult-child relationships are a cornerstone of development, and intervention involves the intentional structuring or harnessing of developmental resources (such as adult-child relationships) or the skilled use of this context to developmental advantage (Lieberman, 1992).

This is inherently a prevention-oriented view (Consortium on School-Based Promotion of Social Competence [CSBPSC], 1994; Henggeler, 1994; Roberts, 1996) that depends on professionals' understanding the mechanisms responsible for altering developmental pathways and emulating (or enhancing) these influences in preventive interventions (e.g., Hughes, 1992; Lieberman, 1992). The developmental salience of relationships between children and adults and their near-universal presence in children's lives make them ideal targets for preventive intervention (Pianta, 1999), and these relationships, as well as the child's relationships with professionals such as psychologists, figure prominently in remedial interventions for diagnosed children.

Relationships between children and adults play a prominent role in the development of competencies in the preschool, elementary, and middle-school years (Birch & Ladd, 1996; Pianta & Walsh, 1996; Wentzel, 1996). They form the "developmental infrastructure" on which later experiences build. Child-adult relationships play an important role in adaptation of the child within the context in which that relationship resides — home or classroom (e.g., Howes, Hamilton, & Matheson, 1994; Howes, Matheson, & Hamilton, 1994). The key qualities of these relationships appear to be related to the ability or skill of the adult to read the child's emotional and social signals accurately, to respond contingently based on these signals (e.g., to "follow the child's lead"), to convey acceptance and emotional warmth, to offer assistance as necessary, to model regulated behavior, and to enact appropriate structures and limits for the child's behavior. These qualities determine that relationship's affordance value.

Relationships with adults also figure prominently in developmental pathways toward behavior problems and psychopathology (Campbell, 1994; Greenberg, Speltz, & DeKleyn, 1993; Toth & Cicchetti, 1996). A disturbed parent-child relationship places a child at risk for developing conduct problems in the early school years, with a well-established link between controlling, hostile behavior by parents and disruptive behavior problems in early childhood (Campbell, 1994; Greenberg et al., 1993). Few contexts or systems have been as widely linked to child psychopathology, especially in childhood, as the child-parent relationship, largely because this relationship figures so prominently in the development of self-regulation, difficulties with which are hallmarks of problem behavior.

Qualities of the mother-child relationship also affect the quality of a child's relationship with a teacher (Cohn, 1990; Motti, 1986), and, in turn, child-teacher relationships can be key influences for school-aged children. Maltreated and non-maltreated children's perceptions of their relationships with mothers were related to their needs for closeness with their teachers (Lynch & Cicchetti, 1992) and to the teachers' ratings of child adjustment (Toth & Cicchetti, 1996).

This link between the quality of child-parent relationships and the relationships a child forms with a teacher confirms Bowlby's (1969) contention that the mother-child relationship establishes for the child a set of internal guides for interacting with adults that are carried forward into subsequent relationships and affect behavior in those relationships (Sroufe, 1983). These representations can affect the child's perceptions of the teacher (Lynch & Cicchetti, 1992), the child's behavior toward the teacher and the teacher's behavior toward the child (Motti, 1986), and the teacher's perceptions of the child (Pianta, 1999; Toth & Cicchetti, 1996). Presumably, these processes are also evident in the context of a therapeutic relationship with a professional.

As was noted above, relationships with teachers are a source of influence on many outcomes related to the school context (Birch & Ladd, 1996; Howes, Matheson, & Hamilton, 1994; Pianta, 1999; Wentzel, 1996), confirming this view that child-adult relationship systems are central to understanding and influencing development in context. Teacher-child relationships influence children's competencies with peers in the classroom (e.g., Howes, Hamilton, & Matheson, 1994) and trajectories toward academic success or failure in the early grades and beyond (Birch & Ladd, 1996; Lynch & Cicchetti, 1992; Pianta, Steinberg, & Rollins, 1995).

The dimensions of child-teacher conflict, closeness, and overdependency consistently appear in samples that vary by age, ethnicity, and economic status (see Pianta, 1999), are fairly stable, and correlate with concurrent and future teacher-reported measures of adjustment, grade retention, and special education referrals (Birch & Ladd, 1997; Pianta et al.,1995). Furthermore, Wentzel (1996) reported that middle-school students benefited from relationships with teachers that were characterized by open communication and a sense of closeness, suggesting that this is a relational context with salience for children beyond the early grades and preschool years.

Finally, a recent national survey of adolescents revealed that the single most common factor associated with healthy outcomes across all domains assessed was that youth reported having a relationship that they experienced as supportive with an adult (Resnick et al., 1997). In particular, these relationships were described as being emotionally supportive — the youth could count on the adult to understand and offer advice. Note the similarities in these child-reported features of positive relationships to those features of sensitive caregiving described earlier with respect to child-parent relationships. Parents, teachers, mentors, and coaches were among those adults mentioned most frequently as the source of this support. Importantly, relationships with adults functioned in this way for all adolescents sampled in this large survey of a normative population, not just those at high risk for problems.

Relationships, as dyadic systems, involve multiple components and processes, each of which can be a focus of intervention designed to enhance relationship quality. Pianta (1999) has outlined in detail the ways in which these can be altered using specific intervention techniques for child-teacher relationships in the context of school-based consultations. Interestingly, Barkley's (1987) behaviorally focused intervention for use with parents and children relies heavily on relationship-building components.

Clearly, relationships embody features of the individuals involved. These features include biologically predisposed characteristics (e.g., temperament), personality factors, and the individual's developmental history. But a key feature is how an adult's history of being cared for affects the way she interprets and attends to a child's emotional behavior and cues (Zeanah et al., 1993). An individual's "internal working model" or "representational model" of a relationship (Bowlby, 1969) is the set of stored feelings and beliefs about a relationship that in turn guides feelings, perceptions, and behavior in that, or in a different, relationship. These models are open systems; the information stored in them, although fairly stable, is open to being changed based on new experience. The open nature of representational models is illustrated in home-based interventions with young mothers that aim to alter their perceptions of self and others (Zeanah et al., 1993) and in teacher-focused consultations that address views of the child and the self in relation to the child (Pianta, 1999).

Relationship systems often must meet multiple demands. For example, a parent must be a teacher, confidante, provider, caregiver, and role model in a number of different situations. A flexible relationship system is able to respond to a wide range of contextual conditions and internal pressures. Flexible relationships between adults and children accommodate a range of children's needs; they function across many contexts (home, classroom, playground); and they support the child in a number of ways (emotionally, with respect to instruction and learning, in relation to peers). Thus one measure of a relationship's functional value for a child, in addition to how well it supports competence in a particular setting, is its flexibility to provide support in multiple contexts and across multiple demands.

Relationships can also be understood in terms of the feedback processes that involve exchanges between the two individuals (adult and child). These processes are most easily observed in interactive behaviors but also include other means by which information is conveyed from one person to another. What people do with, say or gesture to, and perceive about one another are also major components of feedback mechanisms. For example, how a child communicates about needs and desires (whiny and petulant or direct and calm), how an adult selectively attends to different cues, or how these two individuals interpret their behavior toward each other are each involved in feedback processes that can be legitimate targets of psychological interventions. Rich, varied, contingent, multimodal feedback loops that are reciprocal and mutual make for the kind of relationship system that can function as a regulator of development.

Summary

It has been argued that the future of applied child and adolescent psychology depends in part on the degree to which psychologists become involved in the design and delivery of prevention services that promote health among children and families (CSBPSC, 1994; Henggeler, 1994; Roberts, 1996). Services considered "psychological," such as counseling, behavioral consultation, and assessment, will become usurped by personnel who are often less well trained, using techniques that are less well grounded in psychological and developmental principles (Adelman, 1996; Tharinger & Lambert, 1998). The changing landscape of third-party payment, increasing use of paraprofessionals in direct service to children and families, and emerging knowledge on best practices in intervention come together to create opportunities to reexamine and redesign how services are delivered to children (Henggeler, 1994; Roberts, 1996).

As experts in development and behavior, psychologists can formulate theory-driven responses to the challenges posed by children struggling to succeed, and to do so they must take seriously theories of developmental change, not just rely on technical expertise in assessment or application of intervention protocols. Developmental systems theory is a particularly useful theoretical framework for the purposes of informing and designing preventive interventions for children and adolescents, particularly because developmental systems theory addresses key issues in psychological practice, such as the role of context, how competence changes as a function of time, and how local constraints must be embodied and embraced rather than controlled out of efforts to intervene.

The importance of adopting a systems theory perspective on development cannot be overemphasized. To the extent that children's problem behaviors are located solely in "child," "home," or "school" causes, a preventive intervention orientation will be impossible. Current models of training for helping professionals (including most child and adolescent psychologists) too frequently oversimplify models of development and overemphasize categorical diagnoses of child psychopathology rather than a developmental pathways–based perspective (e.g., Tharinger & Lambert, 1998). Such perspectives are narrow and likely to truncate alternatives available to children. Systems theory counters these oversimplified views of development and, although complex and uncertain to some degree, offers a view of development that opens up possibilities for preventive intervention.

Within a systems-oriented intervention framework, child-adult relationships are an ideal resource for preventive intervention. They are available to all children, a range of options exist for strengthening and intensifying their benefits to children, and in many contexts systems are already in place that can influence these relationships (e.g., early intervention home visitor programs, Head Start, family-based services, teacher-training requirements). These "natural" resources for children have been underutilized in many formal models of intervention for children and families that have focused on inducing change as a function of office-based work with professionals. From this perspective, preventive service delivery that utilizes child-adult relationships as a resource capitalizes on the distributed nature of development during childhood and harnesses resources for shaping developmental pathways toward positive outcomes.

ACKNOWLEDGMENTS   The work reported herein was supported under the Educational Research and Development Centers Program, PR/Award No. R307A60004, as administered by the Office of Educational Research and Improvement, U.S. Department of Education. However, the contents do not necessarily represent the positions or policies of the National Institute on Early Childhood Development and Education, the Office of Educational Research and Improvement, or the U.S. Department of Education, and endorsement by the Federal government should not be assumed. Address correspondence to the author at University of Virginia, P.O. Box 9051, Charlottesville, VA 22906-9051.

REFERENCES

Adelman, H. S. (1996). Restructuring education support services and integrating community resources: Beyond the full service school model. School Psychology Review, 25, 431–445.

Adelman, H. S., & Taylor, L. (1998). Mental health in schools: Moving forward. School Psychology Review, 27, 175–190.

Barkley, R. (1987). Defiant children: A clinician's manual for parent training. New York: Guilford Press.

Birch, S., & Ladd, G. (1996). Interpersonal relationships in the school environment and children's early school adjustment. In K. Wentzel & J. Juvonen (Eds.), Social motivation: Understanding children's school adjustment (pp. 199–225). Cambridge: Cambridge University Press.

Birch, S., & Ladd, G. (1997). The teacher-child relationship and children's early school adjustment. Journal of School Psychology, 35, 61–79.

Boulding, K. E. (1985). The world as total system. Beverly Hills, CA: Sage.

Bowlby, J. (1969). Attachment and loss: Vol. 1. Attachment. New York: Basic Books.

Campbell, S. B. (1994). Hard-to-manage preschool boys: Externalizing behavior, social competence, and family context at two-year follow-up. *Journal of Abnormal Child Psychology, 22,* 147–166.

Carlson, C. I., Tharinger, D. J., Bricklin, P. M., DeMers, S. T., & Paavola, J. C. (1996). Health care reform and psychological practice in schools. *Professional psychology: Research and practice, 27,* 14–23.

Cohn, D. A. (1990). Child-mother attachment of six-year-olds and social competence at school. *Child Development, 61,* 152–162.

Consortium on the School-Based Promotion of Social Competence. (1994). The school-based promotion of social competence: Theory, research, practice, and policy. In R. J. Haggerty, L. Sherrod, N, Garmezy, & M. Rutter (Eds.), *Stress, risk, and resilience in children and adolescents: Processes, mechanisms, and interventions* (pp. 268–316). New York: Cambridge University Press.

Diaz, R. M., & Berk, L. E. (1995). A Vygotskian critique of self-instructional training. *Development and Psychopathology, 7,* 369–392.

Doll, B. (1996). Children without friends: Implications for practice and policy. *School Psychology Review, 25,* 165–183.

Egeland, B., Pianta, R. C., & O'Brien, M. (1993). Maternal intrusiveness in infancy and child maladaptation in early school years. *Development and Psychopathology, 5,* 359–370.

Egeland, B., Pianta, R. C., & O'Gawa, J. (1996). Pathways from early behavior problems to psychiatric diagnoses in adolescence. *Development and Psychopathology, 8,* 735–750.

Ford, D. H., & Ford, M. E. (1987). *Humans as self-constructing living systems.* Hillsdale, NJ: Erlbaum.

Ford, D. H., & Lerner, R. M. (1992). *Developmental systems theory: An integrative approach.* Newbury Park, CA: Sage.

Gottlieb, G. (1991). Experimental canalization of behavioral development: Theory. *Developmental Psychology, 27,* 4–13.

Greenberg, M. T., Speltz, M. L., & DeKleyn, M. (1993). The role of attachment in the early development of disruptive behavior disorders. *Development and Psychopathology, 5,* 191–213.

Greenough, W. T., & Black, J. E. (1991). Induction of brain structure by experience: Substrates for cognitive development. In M. Gunnar & C. A. Nelson (Eds.), *Minnesota symposia on child psychology: Vol. 24. Behavioral developmental neuroscience.* Hillsdale, NJ: Erlbaum.

Greenspan, S. I., & Greenspan, N. (1991). *Clinical interview of the child* (2nd ed.). Madison, CT: International Universities Press.

Henggeler, S. W. (1994). A consensus: Conclusions of the APA task force report on innovative models of mental health services for children, adolescents and their families. *Journal of Clinical Child Psychology, 23,* 3–6.

Henggeler, S. W., Schoenwald, S. K., Bordun, C. M., Rowland, M. D., & Cunningham, P. B. (1998). *Multisystemic treatment of antisocial behavior in children and adolescents.* New York: Guilford Press.

Hinde, R. (1987). *Individuals, relationships, and culture.* New York: Cambridge University Press.

Hofer, M. A. (1994). Hidden regulators in attachment, separation, and loss. In N. A. Fox (Ed.), *The development of emotion regulation: Biological and behavioral considerations. Monographs of the Society for Research in Child Development, 59* (Serial No. 240, pp. 192–207).

Howes, C., & Hamilton, C. E. (1992). Children's relationship with child-care teachers: Stability and concordance with parental attachments. *Child Development, 63,* 867–878.

Howes, C., Hamilton, C. E., & Matheson, C. C. (1994). Children's relationships with peers: Differential associations with aspects of the teacher-child relationship. *Child Development, 65,* 253–263.

Howes, C., Matheson, C. C., & Hamilton, C. E. (1994). Maternal, teacher, and child-care history correlates of children's relationships with peers. *Child Development, 65,* 264–273.

Hughes, J. N. (1992). Social psychology foundations of consultation. In F. J. Medway & T. P. Cafferty (Eds.), *School psychology: A social psychological perspective* (pp. 269–304). Hillsdale NJ: Erlbaum.

Johnson, D. B., Malone, P. J., & Hightower, A. D. (1997). Barriers to primary prevention efforts in the schools: Are we the biggest obstacle to the transfer of knowledge? *Applied and Preventive Psychology, 6,* 81–90.

Lieberman, A. F. (1992). Infant-parent psychotherapy with toddlers. *Development and Psychopathology, 4,* 559–574.

Loeber, R. (1990). Development and risk factors of juvenile antisocial behavior and delinquency. *Clinical Psychology Review, 10,* 1–41.

Lynch, M., & Cicchetti, D. (1992). Maltreated children's reports of relatedness to their teachers. In R. C. Pianta (Ed.), *Relationships between children and nonparental adults: New directions in child development* (pp. 81–108). San Francisco: Jossey-Bass.

Molnar, A., & Lindquist, B. (1990). *Changing problem behavior in schools.* San Francisco: Jossey-Bass.

Motti, F. (1986). Relationships of preschool teachers with children of varying developmental histories. Unpublished doctoral dissertation, University of Minnesota.

Nastasi, B. K. (1998). A model for mental health programming in schools and communities: Introduction to the miniseries. *School Psychology Review, 27,* 165–174.

National Institute of Child Health and Human Development, Early Child Care Research Network (1999). Chronicity of maternal depressive symptoms, maternal sensitivity, and child functioning at 36 months: Results from the NICHD Study of Early Child Care. *Developmental Psychology, 35*(5), 1297–1310.

Pennington, B. F., & Ozonoff, S. (1991). A neurological perspective on continuity and discontinuity in developmental psychopathology. In D. Cicchetti & S. L. Toth (Eds.), *Rochester Symposium on Developmental Psychopathology: Vol 3. Models and integrations* (pp. 117–160). Rochester, NY: University of Rochester.

Pianta, R. C. (1997). Adult-child relationship processes and early schooling. *Early Education and Development, 8,* 11–26.

Pianta, R. C. (1999). *Enhancing relationships between children and teachers.* Washington, DC: American Psychological Association.

Pianta, R. C., Nimetz, S. L., & Bennett, E. (1998). Mother-child relationships, teacher-child relationships and adjustment in preschool and kindergarten. *Early Childhood Research Quarterly, 12,* 263–280.

Pianta, R. C., Steinberg, M., & Rollins, K. (1995). The first two years of school: Teacher-child relationships and deflections in children's classroom adjustment. *Development and Psychopathology, 7,* 297–312.

Pianta, R. C., & Walsh, D. (1996). *High-risk children in the schools: Creating sustaining relationships.* New York: Routledge.

Resnick, L. B. (1994). Situated rationalism: Biological and social preparation for learning. In L. Hirschfield & S. Gelman (Eds.), *Mapping the mind: Domain specificity in cognition and culture* (pp. 474–493). Cambridge, England: Cambridge University Press.

Resnick, M. D., Bearman, P. S., Blum, R. W., Bauman, K., Harris, K. M., Jones, J., Tabor, J., Beuhring, T., Sieving, R. E., Shew, M., Ireland, M., Behringer, L. H. & Udry, J. R. (1997). Protecting adolescents from harm: Findings from the National Longitudinal Study of Adolescent Health. *Journal of the American Medical Association, 278,* 823–832.

Riccio, C. A., Hynd, G. W., Cohen, M. J., & Gonzalez, J. J. (1993). Neurological basis of attention deficit hyperactivity disorder. *Exceptional Children, 60,* 118–124.

Roberts, M. C. (1996). *Model programs in child and family mental health.* Hillsdale, NJ: Erlbaum.

Rogoff, B. (1990). *Apprenticeship in thinking: Cognitive development in social context.* New York: Oxford University Press.

Rutter, M. (1987). Psychosocial resilience and protective mechanisms. *American Journal of Orthopsychiatry, 57,* 316–331.

Sameroff, A. J. (1995). General systems theory and developmental psychopathology. In D. Cicchetti & D. J. Cohen (Eds.), *Developmental psychopathology: Risk, disorder, and adaptation* (Vol. 1, pp. 659–695). New York: Wiley.

Shepard, L. A., & Smith, M. L. (1986). Synthesis of research on school readiness and kindergarten retention. *Educational Leadership, 44,* 78–86.

Sroufe, L. A. (1983). Infant-caregiver attachment and patterns of adaptation in preschool: The roots of maladaptation and competence. In M. Perlmutter (Ed.), *Minnesota Symposium on Child Psychology: Vol. 16.* Hillsdale, NJ: Erlbaum.

Sroufe, L. A. (1989). Pathways to adaptation and maladaptation: Psychopathology as developmental deviation. In D. Cicchetti (Ed.), *Emergence of a discipline: Rochester Symposium on Developmental Psychopathology* (pp. 13–40). Hillsdale, NJ: Erlbaum.

Tharinger, D. J., & Lambert, N. M.

(1998). The application of developmental psychology to school psychology practice: Informing assessment, intervention, and prevention efforts. In C. Reynolds & T. Gutkin (Eds.), *Handbook of School Psychology* (3rd ed., pp. 137–166). New York: Wiley.

Toth, S., & Cicchetti, D. (1996). The impact of relatedness with mother on school functioning. *Journal of School Psychology, 34,* 247–266.

Wang, M., & Kovach, J. (1995). Bridging the achievement gap in urban schools: Reducing educational segregation and advancing resilience-promoting strategies. *Closing the achievement gap: A vision to guide change in beliefs and practice* (pp. 9–24). Washington, DC: U.S. Department of Education Regional Educational Laboratory Network.

Wentzel, K. (1996). Effective teachers are like good parents: Understanding motivation and classroom behavior. Paper presented at the annual meeting of the American Educational Research Association, New York.

Werner, E., & Smith, R. (1980). *Vulnerable but invincible.* New York: Wiley.

Young, K. T. (1994). *Starting points: Meeting the needs of our youngest children. The report of the Carnegie Task Force on Meeting the Needs of Young Children.* New York: Carnegie Foundation.

Zeanah, C. H., Benoit, D., Barton, M., Regan, C., Hirschberg, L., & Lipsitt, L. (1993). Representations of attachment in mothers and their one-year-old infants. *Journal of the American Academy of Child and Adolescent Psychiatry, 32,* 278–286.

3

STEPHEN R. SHIRK

The Road to Effective Child Psychological Services

Treatment Process and Outcome Research

One way to characterize the history of child psychotherapy research is through the assumptions that have guided investigations of treatment. Early research was based on the uniformity assumptions of psychotherapy (Kiesler, 1966); distinctions among types of patients, variations in treatments, and differences across therapists were minimized (Shirk & Russell, 1996). A corollary of this assumption was that distressed children who received the "same" treatment would show comparable outcomes. Given this assumption, it is not surprising that early child treatment investigators, like their adult counterparts, were preoccupied with the efficacy of child psychotherapy in general.

Over the years, however, uniformity assumptions have gradually given way to assumptions of specificity. Paul's (1967) well-known reframing of the central question for psychotherapy researchers — "*What* treatment, delivered by *whom*, is most effective for *what* problem, under *which* set of circumstances?" — prompted a new emphasis on the heterogeneity of patients, therapists, and treatments. Treatment samples that once contained children with poorly defined or diverse problems have been replaced by more homogeneous samples; for example, typically only children who meet diagnostic criteria for a specific disorder are included in a clinical trial. Similarly, on the therapy side, substantial attention has been directed to the specification of treatments, often through manualization of therapy and monitoring therapist adherence to treatment techniques. This stands in sharp contrast to early studies that rarely examined therapist behaviors in sessions and frequently defined treatment in terms of the professed orientation of the therapist (Russell & Shirk, 1998).

Reflecting this shift in assumptions, recent child treatment research has required the application of a well-defined treatment delivered by well-trained therapists to a set of children with well-demarcated problems. The fruits of embracing the specificity assumptions have been the identification of empirically supported treatments for children and adolescents with different disorders. In fact, the field appears to be ready to deliver these fruits to market, poised to "transport" empirically supported treatments from the lab to the clinic (Lonigan, Elbert, & Bennett Johnson, 1998). Such a prospect is not without controversy. Some have suggested that the fruit is not sufficiently ripe, whereas others have warned that the road to market may be so long that the crop will spoil before delivery. Whether or not one believes that (1) more research is needed before treatment transportation or (2) that the distance between the lab and clinic is so vast that treatment generalization is unlikely, from a service perspective, a central issue of our time revolves around the implementation of empirically supported treatments in clinical settings.

The primary aim of this chapter is to examine recent child treatment research as it bears on the issue of implementing empirically supported therapies in clinical service contexts. To this end, limitations of existing outcome research will be considered, and the potential contribution of process research will be examined. It is proposed that successful transportation of empirically supported treatments from research contexts to clinical settings will require a new line of investigation on processes that impede or facilitate engagement in treatment by clinic-referred children and families.

Child and Adolescent Treatment Outcomes

The promise of child psychotherapy has changed markedly since Levitt (1957) concluded that "until additional evidence from well-planned investigations becomes available, a cautious, tongue-in-cheek attitude toward child psychotherapy is recommended" (p. 157). Roughly four decades and three hundred outcome studies later, one finds a strikingly different assessment of the benefits of child therapy.

In contrast to early narrative or "box score" reviews of the outcome literature, recent efforts to summarize child treatment outcomes have relied on meta-analytic procedures (Casey & Berman, 1985; Kazdin, Bass, Ayers, & Rodgers, 1990; Weisz, Weiss, Alicke, & Klotz, 1987; Weisz, Weiss, Han, Granger, & Morton, 1995). By converting diverse outcomes across studies to a common metric, the effect size, a more precise quantitative measure of treatment outcome is obtained compared with relatively crude tallies of positive or negative effects. In brief, the effect size represents, under most circumstances, the posttreatment mean on a given outcome measure for the treated group minus the posttreatment mean of the control group divided by the standard deviation of the outcome measure. The effect size, then, provides an estimate in standard deviation units of the magnitude and direction of treatment effects. Effect sizes of .20, .50, and .80 reflect small, medium, and large effects, respectively (Cohen, 1988).

Four successive broadband meta-analyses of child psychotherapy have yielded uniformly positive results; average effect sizes aggregated across diverse treatments and varied disorders have ranged between .71 to .88 (Casey & Berman, 1985;

Kazdin et al., 1990; Weisz et al., 1987; Weisz, Weiss, et al., 1995). These results point to relatively large treatment effects for child psychotherapy in general, or, stated differently, the average treated child is better off than about 75% to 80% of untreated comparison children. Such recurrent findings appear to provide compelling support for the usefulness of child psychotherapy. However, it is important to note that such a conclusion sounds strangely consistent with the old uniformity assumptions of psychotherapy. By aggregating across treatments, patients, problems, and outcomes, the evaluation of the impact of specific treatments for specific patients with specific problems is lost. As Weisz, Huey, and Weersing (1998) have observed, one of the main limitations of meta-analysis involves the confounding of independent variables; for example, certain problems tend to be treated with certain methods. Compounding this problem is the fact that some treatments rarely have been evaluated, and when they have, the studies often have been poorly executed (Shirk & Russell, 1992). Consequently, even by analyzing interactions between treatment and patient characteristics, it can be difficult to reach definitive conclusions about the relative efficacy of specific treatments for specific disorders when using meta-analysis.

This conclusion, however, is not equivalent to accepting the "Dodo Bird verdict" (Luborsky, Singer, & Luborsky, 1975) that "all have won and all must have prizes" (p. 995). In fact, evidence from the most recent meta-analysis (Weisz, Weiss, et al., 1995) suggests that treatments are not equally efficacious. The specificity problem is not inherently a meta-analytic problem; instead, current meta-analyses are only as good as the studies that constitute the data. Because too few published studies have been based on well-defined treatments for well-demarcated disorders, by necessity current meta-analyses have aggregated results at a relatively broad level of analysis. Analyses of treatment by problem-by-patient interactions have focused on broad-band treatments (e.g., behavioral versus nonbehavioral), broadband problems (e.g., internalizing versus externalizing disorders), and broad age groups (e.g., children versus adolescents). Such criticisms are not intended to minimize the importance of recent meta-analyses of child treatment. Clearly, such efforts have provided some of the best evidence for the potential usefulness of child and adolescent therapy. But the implementation of empirically supported treatments in clinical settings requires a level of specification of treatments, problems, and patients not currently available to meta-analysts.

The Search for Efficacious Treatments

In an effort to move beyond generic claims that psychological treatments benefit the majority of patients, researchers have advanced criteria for defining empirically supported therapies for specific disorders (Chambless & Hollon, 1998). In order for a treatment to be considered an efficacious psychosocial intervention, the therapy, preferably manualized, must be shown to be superior to pill placebo or alternative treatment in two well-designed clinical trials conducted by different investigative teams. Alternatively, a large series of single-case design studies that are experimentally sound and that compare the treatment to an alternative therapy also will suffice. In both cases, the clinical sample must be clearly specified.

Treatments that have been shown to be superior to no-treatment controls (e.g., wait-list controls) in two studies or that have been shown to be more effective than placebo or alternative treatment in two studies but have not been independently replicated are classified as *probably efficacious*. Although this approach to identifying efficacious treatments has stirred considerable controversy (Beutler, 1998; Garfield, 1998), it is consistent with the specificity assumptions of psychotherapy. In brief, the emphasis is on identifying specific treatments that are beneficial for patients with specified disorders or problems.

To this end, special issues of the *Journal of Clinical Child Psychology* and the *Journal of Consulting and Clinical Psychology* have provided reviews guided by the aforementioned criteria. The aim of this work is intended to be descriptive rather than prescriptive (Lonigan et al., 1998); that is, it is not the goal to produce a restrictive set of treatment guidelines but to identify treatments with the best evidentiary support. It is beyond the scope of this chapter to describe the results of each of these reviews; however, it is important to note that evidence for treatment efficacy varies by disorder and that no single form of treatment is uniformly effective across disorders. With regard to variation in evidence, there appears to be stronger support for the efficacy of specific interventions for various externalizing disorders than for internalizing disorders. For example, among the therapies for child and adolescent depression, only two treatments were classified as *probably efficacious* (Kaslow & Thompson, 1998), whereas two treatments were deemed well established and ten were labeled as *probably efficacious* for child conduct problems (Brestan & Eyberg, 1998). It is likely that this pattern reflects differences in the number of treatment studies that target internalizing versus externalizing problems (Kazdin et al., 1990) and underscores the need for additional treatment research on internalizing disorders.

With regard to variations in the types of treatments that appear promising, there is little doubt that behaviorally based approaches fared far better than nonbehavioral treatments in these reviews. For none of the reviewed disorders was a nonbehavioral treatment (e.g., psychodynamic therapy, play therapy, or client-centered therapy) identified as probably efficacious. It is possible that the failure of these approaches to meet criteria reflects the paucity of research on nonbehavioral therapies and the lack of clear parameters for defining treated samples in many nonbehavioral outcome studies (Shirk & Russell, 1992). However, these results parallel recent meta-analytic findings that indicate that nonbehavioral treatments for children tend to yield smaller treatment effects than behaviorally derived therapies (Weisz, Weiss, et al., 1995) and that such differences cannot be adequately explained as an artifact of methodological quality (Weiss & Weisz, 1995). Furthermore, a recent randomized trial of traditional child psychotherapy failed to demonstrate significant treatment effects over and above those obtained through supportive academic tutoring (Weiss, Catron, Harris, & Phung, 1999). Thus, despite their widespread use in clinical practice (Kazdin et al., 1990; Koocher & Pedulla, 1977), nonbehavioral forms of child therapy currently have very little evidentiary support. This is not to say that such treatments could not be shown to be efficacious for certain problems. For example, Fonagy and colleagues (Fonagy & Target, 1994; Moran, Fonagy, Kurtz, Bolton, & Brook, 1991) have shown that psychoanalytically oriented therapy relative to standard medical hospitalization can improve the diabetic control of hospitalized children. Similarly, several studies have indicated that nonbehavioral approaches have potential for the reduction of child anxiety and phobias (Miller, Barrett, Hampe, & Noble, 1972; Milos & Reiss, 1982). Yet the absence of systematic programs of research on nonbehavioral therapies for children, especially the lack of studies on children with specific disorders, has resulted in a patchwork of potentially efficacious treatments that lack consistent empirical support.

Simply to conclude that behaviorally based treatments fared better than nonbehavioral treatments obscures the fact that many subtypes of behavior therapy were shown to be efficacious or probably efficacious. It is not the case that generic behavior therapy is uniformly efficacious across disorders; instead, specific treatment packages and procedures derived from behavioral principles are differentially efficacious with different problems. For example, parent management training based on operant principles was shown to be efficacious for child conduct problems (Brestan & Eyberg, 1998), whereas in vivo desensitization and live modeling were found to be efficacious for childhood phobias (Ollendick & King, 1998). Thus, even within behavior therapy, treatment specificity prevails at the level of techniques and procedures tailored for specific problems.

This degree of specificity and focus is one of the most striking features that distinguishes behavioral treatments from nonbehavioral child therapies. In the latter, one finds continued reliance on generic treatment processes such as emotion expression, relational support, or insight that are often only weakly related to conceptualizations of pathogenic process (Shirk & Russell, 1996). Increasingly, treatments that produce beneficial effects for children and adolescents utilize interventions that target specific deficits or distortions that have been identified in basic developmental psychopathology research. As Kazdin (1997) has maintained, treatment development should follow from research on processes related to dysfunction, and corresponding interventions should be conceptually related to remediating such processes. In essence, models of intervention should be tightly linked to models of developmental psychopathology (Shirk & Russell, 1996). The assumption of treatment specificity, then, follows from the growing recognition among developmental psychopathologists that unique sets of pathogenic processes differentially contribute to different disorders, that there may be multiple pathways to the same disorder, and that many rather than a few, pathogenic processes typically contribute to the development of a disorder (Kazdin & Kagan, 1994).

Limitations of the Current Approach

It is worth noting some of the limitations of the current approach to identifying empirically supported treatments. For some problems, such as anxiety or depression, supportive evidence often comes from studies conducted with nonreferred children who may or may not meet diagnostic criteria for a specific disorder. For many of the identified problems, the boundary conditions for the efficacy of specific treatments is poorly defined. As Brestan and Eyberg (1998) note:

> [The] typical conduct-disordered child in treatment is a nine-year-old Caucasian boy from a lower middle income background, whose mother may or may not be participating

in his cognitive-behavioral treatment for conduct problems. In our review, we found little information from which to know whether this boy would do better, or worse, in his particular treatment if he were a girl or from a minority background, or if his family (or his therapist) belonged to a higher or lower economic group. (p. 187)

Across most disorders, relatively little attention has been directed to the developmental parameters of specific interventions. Some years ago, Kendall, Lerner, and Craighead (1984) observed that "children" is not a homogeneous category and that treatments designed for this diverse class of individuals extend the uniformity assumptions of psychotherapy. Instead, it is likely that children with different developmental capacities will not respond uniformly to a standardized treatment. Differential outcomes in child treatment are likely to result from the interplay of specific therapeutic tasks (e.g., self-monitoring) with emerging developmental capacities (e.g., perspective-taking ability; Shirk, 1988). In fact, growing evidence indicates that treatments are moderated by child age, a crude index for developmental level. For example, the effects of cognitive interventions are positively related to age (Durlak, Fuhrman, & Lampman, 1991), whereas behavior management training shows the opposite trend (Dishion & Patterson, 1992). Such findings suggest that therapeutic processes are embedded in and at times constrained by developmental processes (Shirk, 1988). It is important to remember that these developmental processes are not restricted to the individual child but also involve the child's changing relationships with parents and peers (Shirk, 1998).

In addition to these concerns, the current method for identifying empirically supported treatments could be strengthened in several ways. First, as Weisz and Hawley (1998) have pointed out, the current approach relies heavily on qualitative evaluations of outcome studies that may differ significantly across reviewers. Few specific criteria have been provided to determine what constitutes a "well conducted" study, a "specified" sample, or even a clearly defined "treatment." Of equal if not greater importance, the criteria for empirical support are ambiguous. Although the standard of two studies that demonstrate greater efficacy for treatment than for comparison conditions appears relatively simple, no provisions have been made for studies that (1) show beneficial effects on some but not all measures of outcome, (2) show immediate posttreatment effects but no benefits at follow-up, and (3) show statistically significant group effects but fail to produce clinically significant results (Weisz & Hawley, 1998). Finally, it is not clear what one should do with treatments that produce beneficial effects in two studies but fail to do so in others. Clearly, simple tallies of positive results could yield a misleading portrait of therapeutic efficacy if null or negative results are not given appropriate weight (Weisz & Hawley, 1998). Thus the current approach to identifying empirically supported treatments represents an important step toward specifying efficacious treatments for particular disorders, but continued progress will require clearer parameters for defining treatments, patients, and outcomes.

The Gap between Treatment Efficacy and Effectiveness

Based on both meta-analytic and specific narrative reviews, it seems reasonable to conclude, with certain caveats, that a variety of psychosocial treatments can produce beneficial effects for children and adolescents with a range of emotional or behavioral problems. I emphasize, however, that they *can* rather than *do* produce benefi-cial effects. In striking contrast to research on the *efficacy* of child treatment, there is precious little evidence to support the *effectiveness* of child therapy in real-life clinical contexts. As noted by Weisz et al. (1998), most of the more than three hundred studies that have been reviewed in meta-analyses have been conducted with nonreferred children under conditions that may not be representative of clinical practice. Among the characteristics that define what has been dubbed *research therapy* are: (1) recruited rather than clinic-referred samples, (2) homoge-neous samples with a specific focal problem targeted for treatment, (3) therapists who receive substantial training and ongoing supervision in a specific treatment protocol, (4) limited caseloads that are the focus of clinical practice, and (5) therapy that is highly structured and often guided by a manual and monitored for adherence (Weisz et al., 1998). In contrast, *clinic therapy*, whether in outpatient, hospital, or school settings, often departs from research therapy on most or all of the foregoing conditions. In their review of the effects of clinically representative therapy, Shadish et al. (1997) reported only one study from the 1987 meta-analysis by Weisz and colleagues that was (1) conducted in a nonuniversity setting, (2) involved patients who were referred through usual channels, and (3) involved experienced therapists with typical caseloads rather than therapists who were specifically trained to deliver a research treatment. Fewer than a handful of such studies have emerged over the past 10 years. Thus evidence for the effectiveness of child therapy is sparse indeed, and what little evidence exists suggests that child therapy delivered under clinically representative conditions is less than optimal (Hoagwood, Hibbs, Brent, & Jensen, 1995, 1996; Weisz, Donenberg, Han, & Kauneckis, 1995). In fact, one estimate (Weisz, Donenberg, et al., 1995) of the effectiveness of clinic therapy indicates that such therapy is not effective at all (with an average effect size of .01). Although this unhappy outcome might be attributed to pervasive methodological flaws that plague existing clinic-based research, a recent well-designed and controlled study of traditional outpatient child psychotherapy failed to produce positive effects rela-tive to an academic tutoring intervention (Weiss et al., 1999).

The major question, then, is what accounts for the disparity between the promis-ing results of research therapy and the pessimistic findings from clinic-based therapy? Four sets of variables could contribute to this gap: (1) patient characteristics, (2) treatment characteristics, (3) therapist characteristics, and (4) setting characteristics.

Patient Characteristics

In terms of patient characteristics, the primary focus has been on the prevalence of comorbid disorders in clinical practice relative to clinical trials. Weisz and Hawley (1998) have noted that research on clinic-based treatment indicates that the average number of disorders per referred child is 3.5. This stands in contrast to many clinical trials in which children may not meet diagnostic criteria for a single disorder but instead present with elevated symptoms or in which children with comorbid disorders are excluded from the study sample. This important difference is not consistent across disorders. For example, many clinical trials for ADHD have used children who meet diagnostic criteria and who have comorbid disruptive behavior problems (Pelham, Wheeler, & Chronis, 1998).

Of course, diagnostic comparability does not mean that research and clinic groups are equivalent in terms of severity of impairment. The degree to which a child's everyday functioning is compromised can and should be distinguished from level of symptomatology (Green, Shirk, Hanze, & Wanstrath, 1994), but the assessment of impairment in various domains of functioning has been overshadowed in most clinical trials by a narrow focus on symptoms (Kazdin, 1997). Interestingly, it is level of impairment rather than symptoms that predicts referral for treatment (Bird et al., 1990) and that may distinguish clinic-referred children from recruited children in clinical trials. In fact, there is some evidence to suggest that families who volunteer to participate in research have children with fewer social, emotional, or academic problems than those who do not participate (LaGreca & Silverman, 1993; Phares & Lum, 1996). Research has not directly addressed potential biases in participant consent in child clinical trials, nor whether such a bias might result in there being less-impaired children in recruited than in referred samples. Again, there are exceptions to this potential problem. Perhaps the best example comes from clinical trials of multisystemic therapy for juvenile offenders (Henggeler, Schoenwald, & Pickrel, 1995). Here there is little doubt that samples are composed of adolescents with serious problems and impairments that are comparable to those encountered in clinical practice.

Finally, it is important to consider other patient characteristics that may distinguish participants in clinical trials from those in clinical practice. Most of the focus has been child centered, but children in treatment are embedded in their families or other systems of care, and these caregiving contexts could distinguish referred from recruited children. In general, outcome research needs to move beyond its myopic concern with symptoms in individual children to a wide-angle consideration of parent, family, and caregiving characteristics that impede or facilitate change. It is not uncommon to hear practitioners express less concern about children's presenting problems than about contextual factors, for example, parental psychopathology, family stress, and fractured school systems, that undermine adaptive functioning and represent significant obstacles in child clinical practice.

Treatment Characteristics

In terms of treatment characteristics, it appears that one of the most striking differences between research therapy and clinic-based therapy involves the differential use of behaviorally derived interventions. The vast majority of child clinical trials have evaluated subtypes of behavior therapy, whereas surveys of child practitioners typically reveal an eclectic therapeutic orientation with a strong emphasis on nonbehavioral techniques (Kazdin, Siegel, & Bass, 1990; Koocher & Pedulla, 1977). Given the large gap between outcomes for clinic therapy versus research therapy, Weisz, Donenberg, Han, & Kauneckis (1995) have concluded that the underutilization of behavioral methods in clinical practice may be responsible for the poor showing of clinic-based therapy. It is interesting to note, however, that surveys indicate that many practitioners include behavioral methods in their treatment armamentarium (cf. Kazdin, Siegel, & Bass, 1990; Milam, Russell, & Ash, 1982). Furthermore, Weisz and Weiss (1989) failed to find differential outcomes for children treated primarily with behavioral versus nonbehavioral methods in their study of clinic-based psychotherapy.

Taken together, these results suggest that treatment method alone may not be sufficient to account for the disparity between research and clinic outcomes. It may be the case that any intervention, including behavioral interventions, is more difficult to implement in clinical practice because of severity or scope of child problems or the lack of parental cooperation. Alternatively, the strength of treatments, including behavioral treatments, may be weakened when delivered along with other types of interventions. Eclectic interventions may be especially difficult to deliver, possibly because such treatments have multiple foci or entail very different treatment principles that are potentially incompatible (Shirk, 1999).

Finally, there is growing evidence that treatment adherence is related to effectiveness of interventions (Henggeler, Melton, Brondino, Scherer, & Hanley, 1997). Substantial differences between research therapy and clinic-based therapy in training, supervision, and monitoring could result in differential adherence to treatment methods and in corresponding differences in outcomes.

Therapist Characteristics

The third potential contributor to differential outcomes between research and clinic-based therapy involves therapist characteristics. It is worth noting that therapist characteristics is one of the most neglected variables in treatment research, especially with children, despite findings indicating that different therapists who deliver the "same" treatment, even in manualized clinical trials, produce widely different mean levels of improvement in their caseloads (Lambert & Okiishi, 1997; Luborsky, McLellan, Diguer, Woody, & Seligman, 1997). Such findings suggest that characteristics associated with either research or clinic therapists may be responsible for differential outcomes.

One possibility is that research therapists, relative to clinic therapists, are more effective because they receive specialized training, often just prior to delivering interventions. Weisz, Donenberg, et al. (1995) examined this possibility in studies from their meta-analytic sample and found a nonsignificant trend in the opposite direction. That is, studies involving pretreatment training yielded smaller effect sizes than studies involving no such training, though the difference was statistically unreliable.

Results from the adult literature suggest that therapists who produce better outcomes are more skillful at engaging patients and are more likely to adhere to treatment protocols (Luborsky et al., 1997). Both processes, engagement and adherence, may be more likely to occur in research therapy than in clinic therapy as a function of both patient and therapy characteristics. In brief, clinic-referred patients may be more difficult to engage, and clinic therapy may lack the focus that allows for close adherence to a treatment protocol.

Setting Characteristics

Finally, setting characteristics may contribute to differential outcomes. Therapists in clinical settings such as schools, hospitals, and outpatient clinics are often faced with heavy caseloads, substantial variation in types of cases, and limited supervision or collateral consultation. Furthermore, settings vary in their degree of supportiveness, leadership, and organization, which could indirectly affect treatment outcomes through their impact on staff morale and investment. Although Weisz, Donenberg, and colleagues (1995) did not find a reliable difference in effect sizes derived from studies that treated children in clinic settings compared with those delivered in other contexts, it is unclear how many of the studies conducted in clinics actually involved clinically representative conditions (i.e., involved patients referred through usual channels, therapists with regular caseloads, and treatments that were not specifically designed for the study). Obviously, the location and conditions of a research study are not equivalent to those under which treatment is delivered in the real world. In order to evaluate the potential impact of setting on treatment outcomes, identification and measurement of dimensions, above and beyond physical location, that characterize variations in treatment settings must be considered.

Summary of Outcome Research

Although the focus of efficacy trials has been on *what* treatment for *which* disorder, the specificity assumptions of psychotherapy demand more. The gap between efficacy and effectiveness will be narrowed when investigators also begin to consider carefully *who* delivers treatment under *which* set of circumstances.

Clearly, the next step is to study empirically supported treatments under real-world conditions (Weisz & Hawley, 1998). It would be naïve to assume that most treatments can be successfully delivered without modifications that account for critical differences in patient, therapist, and setting characteristics. Obviously, the mere provision of a treatment manual to overloaded therapists who treat resistant, multiproblem patients with little supervisory support is unlikely to improve outcomes in clinical settings. In fact, one treatment that shows considerable promise as an effective therapy, multisystemic therapy (Henggeler & Borduin, 1990), was explicitly designed to generalize to community settings. Developed for juvenile offenders, the treatment involves a comprehensive empirically based intervention that can be tailored to the nuances of individual families in varying social circumstances. Specific training in the approach is essential, after which ongoing supervision can be delivered in an efficient manner that accommodates many setting constraints (Heneggler et al., 1995). Such features increase the likelihood that an intervention can be implemented in real-world settings. In summary, successful transportation of efficacious treatments will require close examination of factors that could interfere with the implementation and utilization of empirically supported therapies in clinical settings.

Process Research and the Development of Effective Treatments

Psychotherapy process research is concerned with the substance of therapy, that is, the techniques, exchanges, and contents of therapy sessions, and with the relationship between these therapy components and processes that are assumed to mediate change, such as improved parenting, better problem solving, or enhanced emotion regulation. The evolution of child therapy process research has been reviewed elsewhere (Russell & Shirk, 1998; Shirk & Russell, 1996). Here the focus will be on processes that are central to implementing empirically supported treatments in clinical settings.

It is evident that successful transportation of efficacious treatments from research to clinical contexts will entail numerous hurdles, including retraining or recruiting staff who can deliver the interventions, providing adequate supervision to ensure treatment integrity, and devising strategies to deal with comorbid patient problems. However, one of the most significant challenges will involve the engagement and retention of children and families in treatment. Research on attrition from child and family therapy indicates that approximately 40% to 60% of families who begin treatment terminate prematurely (Armbruster & Kazdin, 1994; Gould, Shaffer, & Kaplan, 1985). Often termination is early in treatment, but even when it is not, therapy attendance can be sporadic. From a service perspective, lack of engagement and attrition exacerbates the gap between the need for and the provision of clinical services. In terms of implementing empirically supported treatments, early dropout and marginal involvement are likely to reduce treatment strength and compromise effectiveness.

Research on early termination has identified a number of child, family, and logistic characteristics that predict dropout, although the literature contains numerous inconsistent findings (Armbruster & Kazdin, 1994). In part, these inconsistent results appear to be rooted in uniformity assumptions about attrition that fail to consider type of disorder and type of setting. Recent studies that have examined attrition by type of disorder indicate that some characteristics are predictive across disorders (e.g., single parent family and minority status), whereas others are not (e.g., parent education and severity of child symptoms; Kendall & Sugarman, 1997). One factor that has received considerable attention as a predictor of engagement, parent motivation for treatment, has been supported in numerous studies, but the strength of the relationship appears to vary as a function of assessment method (Armbruster & Kazdin, 1994).

Remarkably few studies have taken a process-oriented perspective on engagement and attrition. Instead, most studies have focused on broad characteristics that provide little insight into possible mechanisms that influence involvement (Kazdin, Holland, & Crowley, 1997).

One noteworthy exception is the barriers-to-treatment model (Kazdin et al., 1997). According to this model, "families experience multiple barriers associated with participating in treatment and that these experiences increase the risk for dropping out" (p. 454). Barriers include: (1) practical obstacles and stressors such as conflict about participating, (2) treatment demands such as cost, difficulty, and relevance, and (3) relationship characteristics such as the alliance with the therapist. In a study of treatment for antisocial youth, Kazdin et al. (1997) found that all three types of barriers distinguished treatment completers from dropouts and that perceived barriers mediated the association between child and family risk characteristics (social class, minority status) and treatment completion. A major advantage of this approach is that it points to possible mechanisms that may influence level and duration of treatment participation. In this case, perceived relevance of treatment was especially important for treatment completion.

Studies that have examined parents' reasons for early termination also shed light on possible processes that contribute to disengagement. It may be surprising to find that not all reasons are negative. In fact, one of the most frequent reasons given is that "help is no longer needed" (Gould et al., 1985; Kendall & Sugarman, 1997). Thus ideas about what constitutes satisfactory improvement and grounds for termination might differ considerably between parents and practitioners.

On the other hand, one of the most important negative reasons given by parents for terminating treatment is child resistance (Gould et al., 1985; Kendall & Sugarman, 1997). This finding suggests that child patients have an impact on parental decision making about continuing treatment and that increased conflict between parent and child resulting from treatment participation may be a significant barrier to treatment continuation.

In addition, this finding suggests that the alliance between child and therapist may influence parents' decisions to continue or drop out. Children who form a positive relationship with their therapist are likely to be less resistant and less difficult for parents to bring to treatment than those who lack a solid alliance. In fact, our own research suggests that these processes are linked. The adolescent-therapist alliance in individual therapy has been shown to be associated with parent commitment to treatment, though the direction of effect is ambiguous (Raney, Shirk, Sarlin, Kaplan, & During, 1991). This perspective suggests that processes that contribute to forming alliances with children may complement parental processes, such as the perception of treatment relevance, in predicting treatment engagement and continuation.

By taking a process-oriented perspective, these approaches begin to identify loci for interventions aimed at improving treatment involvement. Over the years, one recurrent target has been parent and child expectations about therapy (see Shirk & Russell, 1998, for a review). A variety of therapy preparation techniques have been developed and tested. Most show that prepared children and parents evince greater knowledge about therapy than their unprepared counterparts, but it is not clear that greater knowledge translates into increased engagement (Shirk & Russell, 1998). One problem with these interventions is that they have not been derived from conceptual or empirical models that identify specific types of cognitions or expectations that could undermine treatment participation.

Promoting Treatment Engagement

A limited number of studies have evaluated variations in treatment procedures in relation to treatment engagement. In one study of family-based behavior therapy for antisocial children, Prinz and Miller (1994) adapted conventional parent management training by including supportive discussions of issues not directly related to parent-child interaction. This enhanced form of behavior management therapy produced a significantly lower dropout rate than conventional behavior therapy, particularly for families faced with high levels of adversity. One interpretation of the finding is that the supportive components of therapy enabled high-adversity families to cope with stress sufficiently to continue treatment. Given that high levels of adversity are often found among clinic-referred families and that disruptive life events often prompt referrals (Jensen, Bloedau, & Davis, 1991), effective clinic-based parent management training may require integration of conventional prescriptive interventions along with adult-focused supportive interventions.

Another noteworthy approach to improving engagement has been evaluated by Szapocznik and colleagues (Szapocznik et al., 1988; Santisteban et al., 1996). Drawing on structural family therapy methods, these investigators examined pre-treatment and early treatment interventions aimed at engaging families with drug-abusing adolescents. The procedure — restructuring family interactions related to treatment involvement — was evaluated relative to usual clinic procedures in a randomized trial. Results indicated that the structural therapy intervention improved entry into treatment and reduced attrition. Although it would be unwise to generalize to other treatments, these findings suggest that it might be useful to couple specific involvement interventions with existing treatment packages in order to promote treatment participation in clinic settings.

Finally, virtually no research has addressed therapist interventions or behaviors that contribute to child or family alliance formation. Preliminary results from a study of family therapy with adolescent substance abusers showed that therapists' interventions early in treatment were related to alliance formation (Diamond, Liddle, Dakof, & Hogue, 1997). Specifically, therapists who focused on the adolescent's experience, formulated goals that were meaningful to the adolescent, and presented themselves as the adolescent's ally were more successful in building positive alliances than therapists who were lower on these behaviors. It is possible that these behaviors are critical to engagement across a wide range of therapies; however, until child therapy research begins to systematically evaluate within-session transactions, such practical insights will remain elusive.

In summary, process research can play an important role in the development of effective treatments. It is likely that one of the greatest challenges to implementing empirically supported therapies in clinical settings will involve overcoming obstacles to treatment engagement. Successful transportation of therapies from the lab to the clinic will require an understanding of the processes that mediate treatment engagement and retention.

Summary

From a service perspective, one of the major challenges of our time involves the implementation of empirically supported treatments in clinical settings. Although some have argued that the assumption of nongeneralizability of treatments from research contexts to clinical settings may be unwarranted (Lonigan et al., 1998), substantial differences in patient, therapist, and setting characteristics across these contexts suggest otherwise. In brief, the assumption of nongeneralizability follows from the specificity assumptions that have guided recent treatment research. Rather than expecting uniform outcomes across settings, one assumes that outcomes will vary as a function of the setting in which they are delivered.

Clearly, this is an empirical question that can only be answered through effectiveness trials. However, research on attrition suggests that obstacles to patient engagement must be addressed in order to successfully transport empirically supported treatments from research to clinical settings. No treatment can be effective if families and children cannot be sufficiently engaged in the process of therapy. Failure to understand the processes that mediate treatment engagement in clinic-referred children and families will undermine the road to effective child psychological services.

REFERENCES

Armbruster, P., & Kazdin, A. (1994). Attrition in child psychotherapy. In T. Ollendick & R. Prinz (Eds.), *Advances in clinical child psychology* (Vol. 16, pp. 81–108). New York: Plenum.

Beutler, L. (1998). Identifying empirically supported treatments: What if we didn't? *Journal of Consulting and Clinical Psychology, 66,* 113–120.

Bird, H., Yager, T., Staghezza, B., Gould, M., Canino, G., & Rubio-Stipec, M. (1990). Impairment in the epidemiological measurement of psychopathology in the community. *Journal of the American Academy of Child and Adolescent Psychiatry, 29,* 796–803.

Brestan, E., & Eyberg, S. (1998). Effective psychosocial treatments of conduct-disordered children and adolescents: 29 years, 82 studies, and 5,272 kids. *Journal of Clinical Child Psychology, 27,* 180–189.

Casey, R. J., & Berman, J. (1985). The outcome of psychotherapy with children. *Psychological Bulletin, 98,* 388–400.

Chambless, D., & Hollon, S. (1998). Defining empirically supported therapies. *Journal of Consulting and Clinical Psychology, 66,* 7–18.

Cohen, J. (1988). Statistical power analysis for the behavioral sciences (2nd ed.). Hillsdale, NJ: Erlbaum.

Diamond, G., Liddle, H., Dakof, G., & Hogue, A. (1997, December). Therapists' alliance building techniques with adolescents in family therapy. Poster presented at the meeting of the Society for Psychotherapy Research, Tucson, AZ.

Dishion, T., & Patterson, G. (1992). Age effects in parent training outcome. *Behavior Therapy, 23,* 719–729.

Durlak, J., Fuhrman, T., & Lampman, C. (1991). Effectiveness of cognitive-behavioral therapy for maladapting: A meta-analysis. *Psychological Bulletin, 110,* 204–214.

Fonagy, P., & Target, M. (1994). The efficacy of psychoanalysis for children with disruptive disorders. *Journal of the American Academy of Child and Adolescent Psychiatry, 33,* 45–55.

Garfield, S. (1998). Some comments on empirically supported treatments. *Journal of Consulting and Clinical Psychology, 66,* 121–125.

Gould, M., Shaffer, D., & Kaplan, D. (1985). The characteristics of dropouts from a child psychiatry clinic. *Journal of the American Academy of Child and Adolescent Psychiatry, 24,* 316–328.

Green, B., Shirk, S., Hanze, D., & Wanstrath, J. (1994). The Children's Global Assessment Scale in clinical practice: An empirical evaluation. *Journal of the American Academy of Child and Adolescent Psychiatry, 33,* 1158–1164.

Henggeler, S., & Borduin, C. (1990). *Family therapy and beyond: A multisystemic approach to treating the behavior problems of children and adolescents.* Pacific Grove, CA: Brooks/Cole.

Henggeler, S., Melton, G., Brondino, M., Scherer, D., & Hanley, J. (1997). Multisystemic therapy with violent and chronic juvenile offenders and their families: The role of treatment fidelity in successful dissemination. *Journal of Consulting and Clinical Psychology, 65,* 821–833.

Henggeler, S., Schoenwald, S., & Pickrel, S. (1995). Multisystemic therapy: Bridging the gap between university- and community-based treatment. *Journal of Consulting and Clinical Psychology, 63,* 709–717.

Hoagwood, K., Hibbs, E., Brent, D., & Jensen, P. (1995). Introduction to special section: Efficacy and effectiveness in studies of child and adolescent psychotherapy. *Journal of Consulting and Clinical Psychology, 63,* 683–687.

Jensen, P., Bloedau, L., & Davis, H. (1991). Children at risk: II. Risk factors and clinic utilization. *Journal of the American Academy of Child and Adolescent Psychiatry, 29,* 804–812.

Kaslow, N., & Thompson, M. (1998). Applying the criteria for empirically supported treatments to psychosocial interventions for child and adolescent depression. *Journal of Clinical Child Psychology, 27,* 146–155.

Kazdin, A. (1997). A model for developing effective treatments: Progression and interplay of theory, research, and practice. *Journal of Clinical Child Psychology, 26,* 114–129.

Kazdin, A. E., Bass, D., Ayers, W. A., & Rodgers, A. (1990). Empirical and clinical focus of child and adolescent psychotherapy research. *Journal of Consulting and Clinical Psychology, 58(6),* 729–740.

Kazdin, A., Holland, L., & Crowley, M. (1997). Family experience of barriers to treatment and premature termination from child therapy. *Journal of Consulting and Clinical Psychology, 65,* 453–463.

Kazdin, A., & Kagan, J. (1994). Models of dysfunction in developmental psychopathology. *Clinical Psychology: Science and Practice, 1,* 35–52.

Kazdin, A., Siegel, T., & Bass, D. (1990). Drawing upon clinical practice to inform research on child and adolescent psychotherapy. *Professional Psychology: Research and Practice, 21,* 189–198.

Kendall, P., Lerner, R., & Craighead, W. (1984). Human development and intervention in child psychopathology. *Child Development, 55,* 71–82.

Kendall, P., & Sugarman, A. (1997). Attrition in the treatment of childhood anxiety disorders. *Journal of Consulting and Clinical Psychology, 65,* 883–888.

Kiesler, D. (1966). Some myths of psychotherapy research and a search for a paradigm. *Psychological Bulletin, 65,* 110–136.

Koocher, G., & Pedulla, B. (1977). Current practices in child psychotherapy. *Professional Psychology, 8,* 275–287.

LaGreca, A., & Silverman, W. (1993). Parent reports of child behavior problems: Bias in research participation. *Journal of Abnormal Child Psychology, 29,* 89–101.

Lambert, M., & Okiishi, J. (1997). The effects of the individual psychotherapist and implications for future research. *Clinical Psychology: Science and Practice, 4,* 66–75.

Levitt, E. E. (1957). The results of psychotherapy with children: An evaluation. *Journal of Consulting Psychology, 21(3),* 189–196.

Lonigan, C., Elbert, J., & Bennett Johnson, S. (1998). Empirically supported psychosocial interventions for children: An overview. *Journal of Clinical Child Psychology, 27,* 138–145.

Luborsky, L., McLellan, A., Diguer, L., Woody, G., & Seligman, D. (1997). The psychotherapist matters: Comparison of outcomes across twenty-two therapists and seven patient samples. *Clinical Psychology: Science and Practice, 4,* 53–65.

Luborsky, L., Singer, B., & Luborsky, L. (1975). Comparative studies of psychotherapies. *Archives of General Psychiatry, 42*, 995–1008.

Milam, D., Russell, R., & Ash, M. (1982). A look at psychologists and their intervention efforts with children. *Journal of Clinical Child Psychology, 11*, 268–272.

Miller, L., Barrett, C., Hampe, E., & Noble, H. (1972). Comparison of reciprocal inhibition, psychotherapy, and waiting list control for phobic children. *Journal of Abnormal Psychology, 79*, 269–279.

Milos, M., & Reiss, S. (1982). Effects of three play conditions on separation anxiety in children. *Journal of Consulting and Clinical Psychology, 50*, 389–395.

Moran, G., Fonagy, P., Kurtz, A., Bolton, A., & Brook, C. (1991). A controlled study of the psychoanalytic treatment of brittle diabetes. *Journal of the American Academy of Child and Adolescent Psychiatry, 30*, 926–935.

Ollendick, T., & King, N. (1998). Empirically supported treatments for children with phobic and anxiety disorders. *Journal of Clinical Child Psychology, 27*, 156–167.

Paul, G. (1967). Strategy of outcome research in psychotherapy. *Journal of Consulting Psychology, 31*, 109–118.

Pelham, W., Wheeler, T., & Chronis, A. (1998). Empirically supported psychosocial treatment for attention deficit hyperactivity disorder. *Journal of Clinical Child Psychology, 27*, 190–205.

Phares, V., & Lum, J. (1996). Family demographics of clinically-referred children: What we know and what we need to know. *Journal of Abnormal Child Psychology, 24*, 787–801.

Prinz, R., & Miller, G. (1994). Family based treatment for childhood anti-social behavior: Experimental influences on dropout and engagement. *Journal of Consulting and Clinical Psychology, 62*, 645–650.

Raney, D., Shirk, S., Sarlin, N., Kaplan, D., & During, L. (1991, March). Parent collaboration as a predictor of adolescent inpatient treatment process and progress. Paper presented at the meeting of the Society for Adolescent Medicine, Denver, CO.

Russell, R., & Shirk, S. (1998). Child psychotherapy process research. In T. Ollendick & R. Prinz (Eds.), *Advances in clinical child psychology* (Vol. 20, pp. 93–124). New York: Plenum Press.

Santisteban, D., Szapocznik, J., Perez-Vidal, A., Kurtines, W., Murray, E., & LaPerriere, A. (1996). Efficacy of intervention for engaging youth and families into treatment and some variables that may contribute to differential effectiveness. *Journal of Family Psychology, 10*, 35–44.

Shadish, W., Matt, G., Navarro, A., Siegle, G., Crits-Christoph, C., Hazelrigg, M., Joem, A., Lyons, L., Nietzel, M., Prout, H., Robinson, L., Smith, M., Svartberg, M., Weiss, B. (1997). Evidence therapy works in clinically representative conditions. *Journal of Consulting and Clinical Psychology, 65*, 355–365.

Shirk, S. (1998). Developmental therapy. In T. Ollendick & W. Silverman (Eds.), *Developmental issues in the clinical treatment of children* (pp. 60–73). Needham Heights, MA: Allyn & Bacon.

Shirk, S. (1999). Integrated child psychotherapy: Treatment ingredients in search of a recipe. In S. Russ & T. Ollendick (Eds.), *Handbook of psychotherapies with children and families* (pp. 369–384). New York: Kluwer Academic/Plenum Publishers.

Shirk, S. (Ed.)(1988). *Cognitive development and child psychotherapy*. New York: Plenum Press.

Shirk, S., & Russell, R. (1992). A re-evaluation of estimates of child therapy effectiveness. *Journal of the American Academy of Child and Adolescent Psychiatry, 31*, 703–709.

Shirk, S., & Russell, R. (1996). *Change processes in child psychotherapy: Revitalizing treatment and research*. New York: Guilford Press.

Shirk, S., & Russell, R. (1998). Process is

sues in child psychotherapy. In A. Bellack & M. Hersen (Eds.), *Comprehensive clinical psychology* (pp. 57–82). London: Pergamon.

Szapocznik, J., Perez-Vidal, A., Brickman, A., Foote, F., Santisteban, D., Hervis, O., & Kurtines, W. (1988). Engaging adolescent drug abusers and their families into treatment: A strategic structural systems approach. *Journal of Consulting and Clinical Psychology, 56,* 552–557.

Weiss, B., Catron, T., Harris, V., & Phung, T. (1999). The effectiveness of traditional child psychotherapy. *Journal of Consulting and Clinical Psychology, 67,* 82–94.

Weiss, B., & Weisz, J. (1995). Relative effectiveness of behavioral versus nonbehavioral child psychotherapy. *Journal of Consulting and Clinical Psychology, 63,* 317–320.

Weisz, J., Donenberg, G., Han, S., & Kauneckis, D. (1995). Child and adolescent psychotherapy outcomes in experiments versus clinics: Why the disparity? *Journal of Abnormal Child Psychology, 23,* 83–106.

Weisz, J., & Hawley, K. (1998). Finding, evaluating, refining, and applying empirically supported treatments for children and adolescents. *Journal of Clinical Child Psychology, 27,* 206–216.

Weisz, J., Huey, S., & Weersing, V. (1998). Psychotherapy outcome research with children and adolescents: The state of the art. In T. Ollendick & R. Prinz (Eds.), *Advances in clinical child psychology* (Vol. 20, pp. 49–91). New York: Plenum Press.

Weisz, J. R., & Weiss, B. (1989). Assessing the effects of clinic based psychotherapy with children and adolescents. *Journal of Consulting and Clinical Psychology, 57,* 741–746.

Weisz, J., Weiss, B., Alicke, M., & Klotz, M. (1987). Effectiveness of psychotherapy with children and adolescents: A meta-analysis for clinicians. *Journal of Consulting and Clinical Psychology, 55,* 542–549.

Weisz, J., Weiss, B., Han, S., Granger, D., & Morton, T. (1995). Effects of psychotherapy with children and adolescents revisited. A meta-analysis of treatment outcome studies. *Journal of Consulting and Clinical Psychology, 117,* 450–468.

PART II

*Delivering
Psychological Services
in Diverse Settings*

4

CYNTHIA A. RICCIO
JAN N. HUGHES

Established and Emerging Models of Psychological Services in School Settings

This chapter provides an orientation to delivering psychological services in school settings for those psychologists who are not familiar with this context of service delivery. School-based models for psychological services can facilitate both student access to services and the interaction between the context in which problems may occur and the intervention/treatment program (Davis, 1999). A number of advantages to school-based services have been identified, including the opportunities for collaboration or consultation with school staff, opportunities for primary and secondary prevention interventions, elimination of barriers of transportation, and the decreased stigma that may be associated with accessing psychological services in schools as compared with outpatient settings (Armbruster, Gerstein, & Fallon, 1999). In particular, it has been suggested that children from minority cultures will be more likely to utilize services within the school setting (Comer, 1985). Finally, the practice and science of psychology address the need for the integration of educational and health services, as well as for more comprehensive service delivery to children and families (Talley, 1995; Talley & Short, 1996).

In describing the delivery of psychological services in schools, there are a number of issues to be considered. These include various existing models for the organization and administration of school psychological services, ethical considerations that come into play when functioning within the school system, and legal issues, as well as the differing taxonomies that are used in schools as opposed to the private sector. In addition, credentialing issues and other differences that may come to bear on the ability to provide services within the school setting, the myriad models for the provision of psychological services, and avenues for employment by a school system are discussed. In addition to these general topics and identification of those competencies that are specific to the established practice of psychology in the schools, future directions for innovative service, as well as funding possibilities for school-based psychological services, are discussed. Finally, we identify the challenges facing psychologists who provide services in schools.

Organization and Administration of School Psychological Services

The administration of psychological services in most settings tends to be done by the administrators of the setting itself. In contrast, psychological services within the schools are administrated from a variety of levels with many possible configurations. Psychological services in schools, as well as the operations of schools in general, are governed to some extent by state departments of education (SDOE). The extent of governance varies considerably from state to state but may include restrictions on the types of therapies or testing measures that can be used by psychologists working within the public schools. Administrative regulation at the state level is broad based and general, often in the form of regulations or policy statements. At the next level, in some states, there may be a regional level of educational administration in the form of regional assistance centers. These regional offices or centers generally provide support and continuing education opportunities for professionals employed in the schools, as opposed to actual governance; however, practices vary by state.

The next, more immediate, level of administration is the local education agency (LEA) as run by the school district superintendent and board of education. Identifying the administrative structure of the school district is important in that the organizational structure defines the communication and collaboration patterns of individual school and school district personnel in meeting and defining the goals of the district and the individual schools (Podemski, Marsh, Smith, & Price, 1995). In some cases this may be a county-wide system, as in Alabama or Georgia, or it may be at the town or city level, as in Connecticut. In a number of states, school districts in rural areas are made up of a number of towns or townships in a cooperative regionalized agreement. The superintendent of schools and the board of education are not only responsible for budgetary considerations but also set the most global level of policy with regard to discipline, to services deemed as essential, and so forth for the schools under their jurisdiction, within the constraints set by federal and state legislation and regulations. In larger school districts, at the upper management level, in addition to the superintendent of schools, there are often additional administrators with differing responsibilities with regard to budget, transportation, and so on. In smaller school districts, responsibilities for budget, transportation, curriculum coordination, and other business concerns are handled by the superintendent or assistant superintendent. Although there is an increasing emphasis on site-based management with more responsibility and freedom occurring at the school level (Podemski et al., 1995), final decisions regarding the hiring of personnel continue to occur at the levels of the boards of education and superintendencies.

Of particular importance is the administrative assignment for psychological services and personnel at the district level. Depending on the school district, psychological services may be housed under pupil personnel services (PPS), with a director of psychological services. In this scenario, another individual would be the director of special education; another might be the director of speech and language services, and so forth. In smaller school districts, all pupil services personnel may be grouped together under the director of special education, and psychological service personnel may be granted varying degrees of autonomy. Psychological services within a school district may be made of up personnel with varying levels of formal education. Depending on state regulations and the school district, psychological services personnel may include master's-level psychometrists or psychological examiners (also referred to as educational diagnosticians), advanced master's-level or specialist-level school psychologists, and doctoral-level psychologists. The structure of supervision within psychological services varies and is likely to change over time (Tally & Short, 1996). Similarly, the extent to which job responsibilities for service delivery differ by degree level also varies by setting and is influenced by regulations of the SDOE, as well as the state licensing laws.

It is the district-level administrator with responsibility for psychological services who determines the assignments of the personnel and the activities that they will engage in. Although there is little likelihood that the superintendent would attempt to micromanage how a psychologist spends his or her time, the immediate supervisor (director of psychological services, PPS, or special education) will have direct impact on the activities engaged in by a psychologist employed in that district. Placement of psychological services in the organizational structure of the school district may or may not determine the populations served by the full-time psychologists; this depends on how tied to the budgetary designations (special education, regular education) the position becomes. The extent to which psychologists are involved with special or regular education can have an impact on the services they provide. Within special education, the financial resources are available for services, and the population to be served is delineated, often reflecting the extremes of behavior or emotional problems within the school. Service delivery is generally constricted to identification and intervention for children who already demonstrate significant difficulty. In contrast, within regular education, there are opportunities to have a broader impact through implementation of preventive and educative programs, as well as a wider range of options for service delivery (Oakland & Cunningham, 1999). At the same time, the availability of financial resources for service delivery in regular education may not be available on a consistent basis. In some districts, centralization and management of personnel is maximized by having all psychologists and related services staff (e.g., speech/language pathologists, social workers) maintain offices within a central administration building; in other districts, psychologists are assigned to specific schools with an office in one or more of these schools.

Regardless of how centralized or decentralized the administration, provision of services in the schools requires that psychologists work in the individual schools. From a systems perspective, the psychologist must be aware not only of the system operating at the larger community level (the school board) but also of the immediate system in each school (Woody, LaVoie, & Epps, 1992). With educational reform moving toward site-based management or decentralization, more decisions are being made at the level of the individual school by the building-level administrators, teachers, and parents (Ingwerson, 1990; Lange, 1993). At each school, the principal, with assistance from the Parent-Teacher Association in some cases, sets the tone for the provision of services and expectations of students and staff. Increasingly, principals are exercising more control at the local school level in terms of curriculum, as well as discipline. Norms, beliefs, and attitudes at the school level are generally found in the school mission statement (Podemski et al., 1995). Understanding and recognizing the differing cultures of individual schools within a school district is important, as these beliefs and attitudes underlie the behaviors and expectations of the administrator and staff of each building.

How successful a psychologist is in providing services in a school setting will depend in part on her or his acceptance by the teachers and building-level administration (Davis, 1999). Psychologists functioning within the school need to understand the mission and goals of the school and find ways to tie psychological services to meeting these goals. Many schools have handbooks that are given to students and parents to acquaint them with the policies and procedures to be followed by students or parents in their specific school. These handbooks often communicate the values, goals, and "personality" of the individual schools, as well as identifying key concerns. The need for each school to develop its own handbook underscores the potential differences that one may encounter in working at differing schools with differing administrative philosophies. In addition to getting a broad sense of the school philosophy, it is helpful for psychologists to introduce themselves and to address teachers and staff by name, as well as to involve teachers and staff in developing plans for services if not in identifying the services needed (Kelly, 1995). It is important for psychologists to maintain good relationships with faculty, administrators, and staff, as well as to keep track of the emotional climate of the school. This can be facilitated by attending faculty meetings and school social functions (Kelly, 1995). In many ways, functioning in the schools requires the psychologist to implement good public relations skills at a variety of levels. Working in the schools further requires that the professional be aware of educational reforms that are having impact on teachers, children, and families. Task forces have been established by the American Psychological Association's (APA) Division of School Psychology to study those reform issues that have had potential impact on school psychology in the past (Talley, 1995), and such task forces will likely continue to be established in the future.

Within each school, there is yet another systemic layer that becomes evident in working with children who may be in need of psychological services. Regardless of employment category, within the school setting, most referrals are generated by teachers, and most decision making with regard to service delivery to students is done as a "team." As a result, functioning within the school setting requires that the psychologist be able to work as part of the various teams in order to generate referrals for services and be viewed as a "team player." Some schools have a standing committee or team that serves as the building-level assistance team or intervention assistance team. Additional terms used for these committees or teams include "teacher assistance team," "pupil assistance team," "child study team," and so on. The intent of this team is to address any concerns a teacher, multiple teachers, or a parent may have with regard to a child's behavior or academic functioning and to provide a mechanism for problem solving (Graden, 1989). In ideal situations, the purpose is to identify appropriate interventions, alternative solutions, or modifications that will foster the desired outcomes for the student. The possible intervention or solution for a given child may include any psychological services (i.e., conjoint consultation, therapy) provided within regular education or referral for services through special education.

Originally introduced as an alternative to traditional in-service training, the building-based assistance team also may serve as an alternative to traditional one-to-one consultation (Ross, 1995). The components that serve the needs of continuing education include providing structured support and assistance to teachers, as well as practice in employing group problem-solving processes. Teachers who participate in the team are presumed to be able to apply the skills gained in addressing the problems of one student to other students who may have difficulty. Thus participation is seen as an impetus for teacher growth and as a means to enable teachers to meet a broader range of pupil needs. Psychological perspectives are an important aspect of the problem-solving process, and psychologists should be involved in building-based assistance teams whenever possible (Ross, 1995).

Ethical Dilemmas Associated with
Psychological Services in Schools

Although the same ethical principles that apply to the practice of psychology in general also apply to the practice of psychology in the schools, the relationships between psychologists, teachers, parents, and children may be less easily defined or misunderstood by those receiving services. Whenever one is concerned, for example, with issues of confidentiality and work with children, there is a need to clearly define to whom the confidentiality applies. This becomes more of an issue when the principal or teacher has been the one who initiated the referral and who may feel he or she has a right to know specifics of the treatment. Similar issues can arise in consulting with teachers when the principal then solicits information regarding the teacher's response to suggestions and ability to implement them. Jacob-Timm and Hartshorne (1994, 1998) provide a number of such situations that are not likely to occur in other settings. In cases in which psychologists function as employees of the school district, providing direct and indirect services to children, families, and teachers, it is extremely important to identify the client and to clearly delineate and define the relationships of those involved, as well the limits of confidentiality, at the onset of any service delivery or relationship (Bowser, 1995).

Another issue that comes into play in school-based practice is that of self-determination and autonomy. As may occur in other settings, the child may not have the option of deciding when or if to engage in services, and respect for their rights in this area may be problematic (Jacob-Timm & Hartshorne, 1998). In school settings, in which a child is actively engaging in problem behavior, parents may not feel that they have the autonomy to decline services, either. Similarly, teachers may be required or strongly encouraged to participate in in-service activities or consultation activities by direction of administrators, resulting in some question of the extent of "voluntariness" of their consent. These factors need to be given additional consideration within the school setting. Similarly, psychologists, as employees of the school district, may be directed to take part in activities or may be limited in activities they can take part in by administration. Identifying in advance (i.e., at the time of hire) the need for autonomy within one's area of expertise can help to avert some difficulties (Bowser, 1995).

Another area of concern specific to the school setting is that of maintaining integrity in professional relationships, as well as avoiding dual relationships. It is not uncommon for teachers who work in a school district to have children of their own in that school district. This can present a conflict of interest for psychologists who have a social or professional relationship with an individual as a teacher and who are asked to provide services to the child and family of the same individual. Similarly, teachers receiving consultation may indicate an interest in pursuing a more therapeutic relationship once a positive relationship has been established in the consultation process. As with other ethical issues, identifying limits in advance can avoid problems later on.

Within the school setting, a number of professionals, including school counselors or social workers, may provide some type of services. In many instances, the school handbook or other notice has informed parents or provided notice that children may be seen by these professionals at some point during the school year. To many teachers, as well as principals, this blanket notice may be seen as including psychologists due to a shared vested interest in mental health. In keeping with ethical, as well as legal, considerations, however, this type of notice is not sufficient for a child to be seen by a psychologist (Jacob-Timm & Hartshorne, 1998). In practice, if a child is referred directly to the psychologist (by the child him- or herself or someone else), the sole activity of a first session should be to identify the presenting problem and explain the need for informed consent by parents for services.

Under the Family Educational Rights and Privacy Act (FERPA; Pub. L. No. 93-380), access to pupil records is limited to those in the school setting with legitimate need. "Legitimate need" is often subjectively defined and does not necessarily result in a formal release of information. This means that if progress notes and treatment plans are to be considered part of the child's school records, control of the information, although limited, is much more available or open than would be the case in any other setting. Arrangements may be needed whereby full and detailed psychological records are maintained separately from the child's educational records and the need for increased control of access to these records is established with school administration well in advance.

Identified here are only some of the more global ethical issues and dilemmas that are more likely to occur in a school-based setting, as compared with other settings. APA ethical principles apply to psychologists; other personnel in the school may not be aware of them and are not bound by them. As such, it is not safe to assume that they understand them or the psychologist's position in upholding them. As indicated, the best practice for avoiding ethical dilemmas and resulting problems would dictate a proactive explanation of the ethical principles at all levels of service delivery (Bowser, 1995; Jacob-Timm & Hartshorne, 1998).

Legal and Regulatory Aspects of Service Delivery

Traditionally, the roles and functions of school psychologists have included assessment, consultation, provision of teacher and staff in-service workshops, and short-term therapy (Tharinger, 1995). In conjunction with assessment and eligibility decisions related to special education, the psychologist who completes the evaluation usually participates in the team decision-making process. A number of legal actions have constricted the extent to which psychologists engage in these practices, however. Legal influences on the practice of psychology in the schools stem from a variety of sources, including constitutional law, federal education legislation and regulations, state rules for implementing legislation, and case law (Reschly & Bersoff, 1999). Of these, special education legislation beginning in the 1970s and continuing through the 1990s has had the greatest influence on the practice of psychology in the schools. What originated as the Education for All Handicapped Act (Pub. L. No. 94-142) has been amended twice as the Individuals with Disabilities Education Act Amendments (IDEA; 1990, 1997) and includes mandates for a free and appropriate public education for all children. Psychological services related to this act have traditionally focused on the requirement for the comprehensive individual assessment of children to determine eligibility for special education services. It is generally recognized, if not mandated by state law, that psychologists are the personnel with the requisite training to conduct some portion, if not all, of these assessments. Because of this requirement that assessment precede access to services, responsibilities of psychologists in schools have centered on the assessment process (Benson & Hughes, 1985; Phillips, Boysen, & Schuster, 1997; Talley & Short, 1996).

The eligibility process, although it parallels the assessment process that would enable diagnostic decision making in other practice settings, is very different, and again mandated by federal education legislation, as well as the various state regulations on the implementation of the federal legislation. Under IDEA, there are 13 disability areas or exceptionalities identified by category. Although identified by category in IDEA, categorical labels are not required by IDEA but are used by 48 of 50 states; in Massachusetts, for example, special education services are noncategorical, and eligibility is for "special education" services in general. How eligibility is determined (any quantification) is not specified in IDEA but rather is determined by state regulations and varies considerably from state to state. In many instances, even similar "labels" have differing criteria as compared with the *Diagnostic and Statistical Manual of Mental Disorders* (DSM-IV; American Psychiatric Association, 1994); not all *DSM-IV* diagnoses are necessarily covered by IDEA categories and not all categories coincide with a *DSM-IV* diagnosis (e.g., traumatic brain injury).

Following legally mandated procedure, teams of teachers and other professionals participate in the eligibility decision. These team meetings are held to determine eligibility for services, to make a placement decision, to develop an individualized education plan (IEP), or to review progress on goals set in the IEP. These teams may be referred to as IEP teams, planning and placement teams (PPT), staffing teams, multidisciplinary eligibility teams, and so forth depending on the state, but the participants and timing of these meetings are generally governed by federal and state law. Depending on the state and school district, psychologists may either participate in all aspects of the process (eligibility, program planning, IEP development) or may participate only in specific aspects of the process.

In addition to differences in the interaction level of participants, the locations of meetings vary as well. In more centralized systems, staffings or team meetings may be held in the central office, with limited representation of the staff from the school the child attends. In less centralized systems, meetings may be held at the building level, with attempts made to include as many teachers and other professionals who know the child as possible. Even at the building level, someone from central administration with budgetary power, or a designee, will participate in or orchestrate the meeting. Meetings held at the building level facilitate and encourage the participation of all teachers who may be directly or indirectly involved with the child, as well as facilitating a team approach before, during, and after the assessment and placement decision.

The "eligibility" decision and categorical label (if used), as opposed to "diagnosis," serve the purpose of accessing funds and services. Although the eligibility decision often results in assigning a categorical label to a child, as previously stated, the labels and criteria for assigning a label are not necessarily synonymous with diagnostic categories used by psychologists in other settings. For example, the criteria for diagnosis of a specific learning disability, although including documentation of a significant discrepancy between ability and achievement in virtually all contexts, varies considerably from state to state and differs considerably from the criteria for a developmental disorder based on DSM-IV. In the area of emotional disturbance as defined by federal legislation, there are no subcategories of disorders, nor is diagnosis of a psychological disorder as defined by DSM-IV needed. Instead, the child must meet one of five criteria stipulated by the education legislation, but not solely as the result of social emotional maladjustment. These are only a few examples of the types of differences in language that a psychologist not well grounded in the educational nosology will be expected to understand.

Special education law also provides for the provision of related services, including psychological services. Related services may include developmental, corrective, and supportive services that are deemed necessary to ensure that a child can benefit from his or her educational program. Related services can take the form of therapy with the child or family, of parent training, or of teacher or conjoint consultation. Another decision-making process has evolved within special education law as it relates to discipline. When the misbehavior is such that the response to a child's behavior is expulsion or suspension of more than 10 consecutive days or 10 nonconsecutive days that constitute a pattern, IDEA mandates that a team decide whether or not the misbehavior in question is related to, or a manifestation of, the child's disability. This requires a review of the child's program by the IEP team and "other qualified personnel" (e.g., a psychologist) who are familiar with the behaviors associated with various disorders. Finally, a child with a disability can be moved to an alternative educational setting for up to 45 days for engaging in specific behaviors (e.g., carrying a weapon to school, possession or sales of controlled substances). Federal mandates further stipulate that there must be some type of behavioral assessment and a therapeutic or behavioral program designed to decrease the likelihood of the target behavior while the child is at the alternative setting.

In addition to special education legislation, antidiscrimination legislation is having an increased effect on services in the schools. Section 504 of the Rehabilitation Act of 1973 prohibits discrimination against any otherwise qualified individual solely on the basis of a handicapping condition. Although the purpose of 504 was to eliminate discrimination on the basis of handicap in any program that receives federal financial assistance, Subpart D applies to preschool, elementary, and secondary education programs and requires schools to make special accommodations for students with handicaps to ensure educational opportunity equal to that of their nonhandicapped peers. Under Section 504, schools cannot deny aid, benefit, or service (direct or indirect) on the basis of handicap; schools cannot deny pupils with handicaps an opportunity to participate in or benefit from any of the services or benefits it affords to others; and schools must provide equal opportunities for students with handicaps to obtain the same outcomes as other students (Jacob-Timm & Hartshorne, 1998). For students to receive services under Section 504, the student does not have to be determined eligible for special education, nor does he or she have to meet criteria for disability based on *DSM-IV*. Under Section 504, a disabled person is defined as: "any person who (i) has a physical or mental impairment which substantially limits one or more of such person's major activities, (ii) has a record of such an impairment, or (iii) is regarded as having such an impairment" (Rehabilitation Act of 1973). The broader definition of "handicapped" under Section 504 includes a number of students who do not qualify as "disabled" under IDEA or *DSM-IV*, with learning included as a major life activity (Prasse, 1995; Jacob-Timm & Hartshorne, 1998). For example, students with communicable diseases or addictions who may not be eligible under IDEA may be eligible for services to help them achieve similar positive outcomes. Those services provided under Section 504 vary depending on the nature of the disability condition but could include therapeutic components.

Credentialing and Licensure Issues

The credentialing of psychologists for employment within the school setting has been described as complex (Fagan & Wise, 1994). For doctoral-level clinicians, the practice of psychology in the schools may in fact require dual credentials. In addition to becoming licensed as a psychologist through the respective state board of examiners for psychologists, in most states school-based practice requires approval of the state department of education, which may or may not recognize the psychology license. In most states, the state department of education issues a certificate that serves as the credential for the provision of psychological services in the schools. Increasingly, there is a trend to move this function to the state board of examiners (e.g., in Texas), but this still may result in psychologists having to obtain a second credential.

Some notable differences exist between the license for psychology and the certification for school psychologists. Whereas obtaining licensure is facilitated by program accreditation of the American Psychological Association (APA) and requires the applicant to pass the Examination for Professional Practice of Psychology

(EPPP), obtaining the school-based certification or license is generally facilitated by program accreditation of the National Council for Accreditation of Teacher Education (NCATE) and the National Association of School Psychologists (NASP). Depending on the state, the school-based credential may require that the applicant pass an exam, but in this case it would be the National School Psychology Exam (NSPE) or what is now referred to as the Praxis II Exam. In the 1980s, NASP instituted the Nationally Certified School Psychologist (NCSP) credential in an attempt to establish standards for practice in the schools. The Praxis II is one component of this credentialing process, and even in those states that may not have adopted the NCSP as the state credential, a passing score on the Praxis II may be required. As of 1990, Brown (1990) reported that 24 states had established reciprocity with the NCSP; although it is voluntary, by the early 1990s more than 16,000 school psychologists had attained the NCSP (NASP, 1991, 1994). Because NASP endorses the specialist level as entry level to the profession, the NCSP and Praxis II are geared to this level of training (Pryzwansky, 1999). At the same time, NASP has established standards of training for school psychology that are reflected in its record review, as well as in the content of the Praxis II. Also, in contrast to the EPPP, the Praxis II is specific to the specialty area of school psychology and may be construed as needed to demonstrate knowledge and competence within the specialty area. Although the American Board of Professional Psychology (ABPP) offers a specialty credential for school psychology (Przywansky, 1999), at this time the ABPP has not gained the acceptance by the state departments of education that is enjoyed by the NCSP as a "specialty" credential.

New and Expanded Opportunities for Psychologists in Schools

Schools as Sites for Integrated Services

The decade of the 1990s has been one of remarkable change in the prevalent models for providing psychological services to children and families. These changes are a result of many interactive factors. Prominent within this mix is an increase in the sheer number of children who, due to adverse child-rearing circumstances or other vulnerabilities, either experience significant mental or emotional disorders or are at significant risk for such disorders. For example, poverty is associated with a number of adverse child-rearing conditions. Although the overall percentage of children living in poverty has remained fairly stable at about 20%, in 1998 the number of families with children who lived in poverty despite being headed by someone who worked full-time year round rose to the highest it has been in the 24 years that the data have been kept (Children's Defense Fund, 1999a). A growing number of children experience the ill effects of child abuse and neglect, violence and aggression, substance abuse, homelessness, lack of appropriate and accessible health care, and lack of adequate child care. The statistics on the status of today's children presented in Table 4.1 only begin to tell the story of risk, because risk factors tend to co-occur, and the probability of significant dysfunction increases exponentially with each increase in the number of risk factors (Sameroff, Seifer, & Bartko, 1997).

TABLE 4.1   The Status of Children's Well-Being

Despite a booming economy and the lowest unemployment figures in 25 years, there has been a significant increase in the number of children living in working-poor families (in which at least one parent worked 26 or more weeks during the year yet family income was below poverty level). The number of children living in working-poor families increased from 4.3 million in 1989 to 5.6 million in 1997.[2]

Nearly 1 in 5 children (19%) lived in poverty in 1997. The child poverty level for the United States is not only the highest among developed countries but was also 50% higher than the next highest rate.[2]

In 1996, 30% of children lived with parents who did not have full-time, year-round employment.[2]

In 1998, almost one-fourth (23%) of children lived with only their mothers, 4% lived with only their fathers, and 4% lived with neither of their parents. Wide geographical differences exist in the percentage of children living in households headed by a single parent, ranging from a low of 14% in Utah to 62% in the District of Columbia.[1]

In 1994, 12.3% of children aged 5–17 had significant functional impairments (difficulty performing at least one of four everyday tasks).[1]

In 1995, 2.4 million (5%) of children aged 5–17 spoke a language other than English at home and had difficulty speaking English. This number is up from 1.3 million in 1979. This percentage is likely to increase sharply due to the rapid increase in the percentage of Hispanic children. Thirty-one percent of children of Hispanic origin had difficulty speaking English in 1995, compared with 1% of white non-Hispanic or black non-Hispanic children. By 2002, it is projected that more than one in five children in the United States will be of Hispanic origin.[1]

In 1997, 32% of all births were to unmarried women. The percentage of all births to unmarried women rose sharply from 18% in 1980 to 33% in 1994 and has remained relatively stable since 1994.[1]

In 1997, 29% of children in families living in poverty had not received the recommended series of vaccines.[1]

In 1996, 8% of all adolescents aged 12–17 lacked a usual source of medical care. Over 27% of uninsured adolescents in this age group lacked a usual source of care.[1]

The percentage of infants born at low birth weight continues to rise. In 1997, this percentage was the highest in over 20 years, at 7.5%.[1]

In 1997, 9% of eighth-grade children reported smoking tobacco daily during the previous 30 days.[1]

In 1997, 24% of 10th-grade students reported having five or more alcoholic beverages in a row in the past two weeks. In this age group, 22% reported having used illicit drugs in the previous 30 days.[1]

In 1998, 8% of teens aged 16–19 were not attending school and not working.[2]

Based on the report *Indicators of School Crime and Safety*, published jointly by the U.S. Departments of Justice and Education in 1998, in 1996 5% of all 12th-graders reported being injured with a weapon such as a knife, gun, or club during the prior 12 months while they were at school, and 12% reported that they had been injured intentionally without a weapon while at school.[3]

The 1995 Youth Risk Behavior Survey found that 10% of high school students had carried a weapon (e.g., gun, knife, or club) on school property in the month preceding the survey.

1. National Maternal and Child Health Clearinghouse (1999). *America's children: Key national indicators of child well-being 1998.* Retrieved October 1999 from the World Wide Web: http://childstats.gov/ac1999/poptxt.as. (Available from U.S. Government Printing Office, Publication No. 065-000-01162-0).

2. Annie E. Casey Foundation (1999). *Kids Count data online.* Retrieved October 5, 1999 from the World Wide Web: http://aecf.org/kidscount/kc1999/findings2.htm.

3. Children's Defense Fund (1999). *Violence in Schools.* Retrieved October 5, 1999 from the World Wide Web: http://www.childrensdefense.org/youthviolence/violenceschools.htm.

4. Office of Juvenile Justice and Delinquency (1998). *Juvenile Offenders and Victims: 1997 Update on Violence.* As cited in (Children's Defense Fund (1998). *Keeping children safe in school: A resource for states,* p. 11. Author: Washington, DC.)

The magnitude of the needs of today's youth has strained the capacity of families and systems that provide care to children and families. The crisis orientation and single-focus nature of family support systems, combined with a lack of coordination among services, has undermined their capacity to meet the multiple needs of a large segment of today's youth (Knitzer, 1997). The publication of a few startling accounts of the failure of child and family support systems to meet the needs of children and families (Knitzer, 1982; Schorr & Schorr, 1988) propelled legislative initiatives at the state and national levels aimed at establishing comprehensive and coordinated systems of care for our nation's most vulnerable youth. In 1984, Congress established the Child and Adolescent Services System Program (CASSP) of the National Institute of Mental Health to develop a child mental health facility in each state by funding a CASPP director and facilitating coordinated systems of care at the state level for youth with serious emotional disturbances (Day & Roberts, 1991). CASPP was successful in stimulating improvements in the coordination, breadth, and accessibility of child mental health services and in raising attention at the state level for the need for greater coordination across agencies that provide health and related services to children (Day & Roberts, 1991).

Concern with the educational outcomes of our nation's schools has led to similar demands for reform (National Commission on Excellence in Education, 1983). The goals of educational reform are best represented in the Goals 2000: Educate America Act (1994), which established goals within eight broad areas: school readiness; school completion; student achievement and citizenship; teacher education and professional development; mathematics and science; adult literacy and lifelong learning; safe, disciplined, and alcohol- and drug-free schools; and parental participation. Importantly, policymakers appreciate that achieving many of these educational goals requires addressing the health and mental health needs of children and families. Indeed, the need for comprehensive and coordinated education, health, and social services to address the many risks faced by today's youth is a common theme in both health care and educational reform initiatives (Talley & Short, 1996).

As previously noted, schools are viewed as a logical location for integrated education and health services, especially for health promotion and prevention programs (Dryfoos, 1994). The promotion of "life skills," including health competencies, is central to the mission of schools. Schools possess structures that support universal health promotion efforts, such as a health curriculum for kindergarten through Grade 12, and provide an existing, community infrastructure for the delivery of integrated health, education, and social services for children most in need of comprehensive and integrated services. Because schools are the most stable caregiving system in many children's lives, they can support coordination of care across time. School-based clinics are an important vehicle for increasing the health status of children and adolescents without easy access to primary health care.

New Roles for Psychologists in Integrated School Health

Psychologists are well qualified to take leadership roles within school-based and school-linked integrated-services models (Kolbe, Collins, & Cortese, 1997; La Greca & Hughes, 1999; Talley & Schrag, 1999). Their expertise in developmental psychology is relevant to the design of school health curricula and to the development of schoolwide violence and substance abuse prevention programs. As a result of their training, psychologists have the ability to view behavior as the result of the complex interplay of biological, sociological, and environmental influences and to develop treatment and prevention plans that take into account the complex nature of children's difficulties. They also possess skills in a range of intervention methods, including individual and group counseling, family and teacher consultation, social skills interventions, parent education and training, and crisis intervention. Perhaps most important is their commitment to making decisions on the basis of data.

Increasingly, funding for services and programs is linked to demonstration of reliance on empirically supported treatment and prevention interventions and to strong program evaluation efforts. Psychologists' expertise in research and evaluation design, measurement, and their knowledge of and ability to interpret studies that document intervention efficacy are highly valued in today's climate of increased demand for accountability. In today's marketplace, service delivery programs are increasingly evaluated on the basis of systemic outcome measures, such as the number of children in out-of-home placements or the number of children who pass state-mandated tests of minimal educational competencies, rather than on individual measures of child performance. Consequently, competencies in assessing such systemic outcomes are highly valued. Program evaluators are called on to provide not only data on program outcomes but also data that leads to improvements in the treatment provided. Psychologists who can use data to test the assumptions and theories that underlie a program and to identify program elements responsible for desired changes are in a position to play critical roles in enhancing program effectiveness.

Increasingly, direct mental health services are often provided by paraprofessionals and mental health practitioners prepared at the master's level. Psychologists have essential roles to play in supervision and training of these front-line providers. For example, volunteer mentoring programs to at-risk children and adolescents can significantly reduce substance use and early school withdrawal (Tierney, Grossman, & Resch, 1995). Essential to the success of such programs is the care with which paraprofessionals are recruited, trained, and supervised (Fleming, Oliver, & Bolton, 1996; Musick & Stott, 1990). For example, Henggeler, Melton, Bondino, Scherer, and Hanley (1997) demonstrated the importance of supervision to outcomes for clients receiving multisystemic therapy provided by master's-level therapists in a community setting. Specifically, when weekly feedback from an expert regarding treatment fidelity was withdrawn, adherence to treatment principles suffered, resulting in poorer client outcomes. These authors provided convincing data that the incremental costs of weekly supervision resulted in significant cost savings due to improved program outcomes. Data such as these convince policy makers of the cost efficiencies of providing front-line providers with quality training and supervision.

Legislative and Funding Supports for Integrated Services for Children

During the 1990s, a broad consensus was achieved concerning the need for integrated educational, health, and social services (National Commission on Children,

1991). As the decade and the century end, legislation that mandates — or at least encourages — integrated educational and health services is changing the landscape for providing health and education services from one of predominantly fragmented services that are categorically funded to one of integrated, flexible services that are supported by a combination of government and private-sector funds. Schools are envisioned as key partners in many of these legislative and social policy initiatives. Next, a few of the major legislative and funding supports at the federal level for integrated services are reviewed.

IDEA

Discussed previously in terms of mandated psychological services (primarily assessment and related services students need to benefit from educational services), this legislation specifies national guidelines for educational services for children with disabilities. Although coordination of services and multidisciplinary teams have always been emphasized in IDEA and its predecessors, the highly bureaucratic nature of services provided under this legislation, strict requirements for a determination of eligibility for services, and auditing provisions that required schools to demonstrate that IDEA-funded personnel did not provide incidental benefits to nondisabled students have historically worked against coordination of services. The IDEA amendments of 1997 have attempted to promote greater coordination of special education services with regular education, as well as with health and social services (Individuals with Disabilities Education Act Analysis, 1997), with greater flexibility in the use of funds granted to states. For example, local education agencies can use up to 5% of funds to develop and implement coordinated services, and states can provide services to children up to age 9 under a broad category of "developmental delay" rather than requiring a specific handicapping condition. The amendments strengthened the ability of an educational agency to seek reimbursement from Medicaid programs and other federal or state agencies for psychological and other health services it provides and that of mandated interagency councils to coordinate services integration. States also are required to develop systems for assessing outcomes for disabled students in terms of specified performance goals. Services to children from birth to age 3 years provided under Part C of IDEA must be delivered to the extent possible in children's natural environments. Funds under Part C can also be used to serve "at-risk" infants and toddlers through collaborative efforts with public and private groups.

Elementary and Secondary Education Act (ESEA)

When ESEA was passed in 1965, it heralded a new role for the federal government in public education. ESEA authorizes the expenditure of federal dollars to improve public education. When reauthorized in 1994 as the Improving America's Schools Act (IASA), it established a new Title XI, Coordinated Services, allowing a local school district or school consortia to use funds received under the law for coordinating projects to provide students and their families better access to social, health, and education services. Furthermore, it mandated parent involvement and coordination among other federal programs. Several programs funded under ESEA require or encourage partnerships between local education agencies and community-based organizations (e.g., Even Start Family Literacy Program, Catalogue of Federal Domestic Assistance, no, 84.213).

ESEA is the authorizing legislation for the Safe Schools/Healthy Students initiative, a program funded through a joint agreement among the U.S. Departments of Education, Health and Human Services, and Justice [see Federal Register, 1999 64 (241) pp. 5814–5815]. These discretionary grants are awarded to local education agencies to develop community-wide approaches to creating safe and drug-free schools and promoting healthy childhood development. Programs are intended to prevent violence and the illegal use of drugs and to promote safety and discipline through an integrated, comprehensive strategy that comprises at least six general elements: school safety; alcohol and other drug and violence prevention and early-intervention programs; school and community mental health preventive and treatment intervention services; early childhood psychosocial and emotional development programs; education reform; and safe school policies. The plan must be developed by a partnership comprising the local education agencies or consortia, local public mental health authority, local law enforcement agency, family members, students, and juvenile justice officials. In September 1999 the White House announced the first awards under the Safe School, Healthy Students initiatives. These 54 awards, each covering a three-year period, totaled more than $100 million. Abstracts of two of these funded proposals (Table 4.2) illustrate the program's emphasis on integrated services.

The 21st Century Community Learning Centers program, also authorized under ESEA, is a discretionary grant program that funds after-school programs for children who would otherwise be unsupervised in an effort to increase the safety of children, reduce their risk-taking behaviors, and improve learning. The programs must be based on such empirically supported strategies as mentoring, problem-solving skills training, and tutoring. Schools must demonstrate collaboration with other public and nonprofit agencies, organizations, local businesses, postsecondary institutions, scientific and cultural institutions, and other community partners. In its first year, 1998, a total of $40 million was awarded under this initiative. In 1999, 176 schools were awarded a total of $200 million. In his proposed fiscal year 2000 budget, President Clinton has requested $600 million for this program (U.S. Department of Education, 1999).

Block Grant Programs

Behavioral patterns established in youth are the leading cause of the most serious and costly health and social problems that affect our nation, and school-based health programs are recognized by policy experts as the most effective means of addressing such behavioral patterns as tobacco and alcohol use, risky sex, pregnancy, poor nutrition, and obesity (Kolbe et al., 1997). Thus it is not surprising that a number of federal block grant programs support comprehensive school-based or school-linked health services. Block grants are awarded to states on a formula basis and are then distributed to local communities. Table 4.3 presents a brief description

New Haven, Connecticut

Partners: New Haven Board of Education, Connecticut State Department of Children and Families, and New Haven Department of Police Services.

The New Haven initiative is an expansion of a current partnership with the Department of Police Services, Juvenile Probation Office, and the Yale Child Study Center. A District Student Support Team consisting of these partner members and numerous other allied agencies will coordinate service delivery, monitor efficiency of services, and establish cross-agency procedures for referral and points of entry. The goal of the New Haven initiative is to create an infrastructure of collaboration and to expand current efforts to improve school safety and child well-being. Early childhood needs will be addressed through the addition of a Family Resource Center, two additional Children and Parents Succeeding sites, and home-based mental health and case management services. Parent leadership training and an Early Childhood Resource Van will supplement these efforts. To improve the school climate and reduce/prevent alcohol and drug abuse and violence, a social development curriculum will be updated and on-going teacher training provided. Schools will provide outreach coordinators to link students and families to services. At least 150 students will be paired with adult mentors. These mentors and other staff will assist students making transitions from alternative placements back to regular-education settings. All schools will have either a part-time or full-time mental health clinician, and all K–5 students will be screened by trained teachers for problem behaviors requiring further intervention. A School Safety Policy Work Group will convene to review current policies and revise them as warranted. Law enforcement will play a major role in reducing truancy through enforcement and home visits. A police athletic league will be also expanded to provide youth with prosocial adult role models.

Louisville, Kentucky

Partners: Jefferson County Public Schools, Seven Counties Services, Inc., and the Louisville Police Department.

The Jefferson County Public Schools (JCPS) District is the largest district in Kentucky. Located in an urban area that includes inner-city Louisville . . . more than one-half of the students are economically disadvantaged. . . . Truancy, low academic performance, and disciplinary problems are of concern. . . . The goals of Project SHIELD are to: (1) strengthen community partnerships that support safe, disciplined, and drug-free schools; (2) help students develop skills and emotional resilience to achieve positive mental health, engage in pro-social behavior, and avoid violence and drug use; and (3) ensure that students are able to learn in a safe, disciplined, and drug-free environment. To support early childhood development, a Primary Mental Health Program will be conducted, providing individual interactive play sessions for children who are beginning to show adjustment difficulties. . . . Existing drug and violence prevention and early intervention programs will be integrated and augmented with science-based model programs, including Second Step, Skills Mastery and Resistance Training (SMART), Big Brothers/Big Sisters (a model program of case managed mentoring), and Preparing for Drug-Free Years. To enhance mental health prevention and intervention, the following science-based programs will be implemented: Functional Family Therapy (FFT), a model program for youth ages 11–18; and Multi-Systemic Therapy (MST), a model program for chronic, violent, or substance abusing juvenile offenders ages 12–18. . . . Teacher training will focus on classroom behavior management. To support school safety, teams at the district and school level will be trained on Crime Prevention Through Environmental Design (CPTED), the effective use of the physical environment to reduce crime.

From U.S. Department of Education (1999). President Clinton announces more than $100 million in community grants to prevent violence among youth (Press release). Washington, DC: Author. Retrieved October 8, 1999 from *http://www.ed.gov/pressreleases/09-1999/schools.htm*.

TABLE 4.3   Examples of Federal Block Grants That Support Integrated
School Health Programs

Maternal and Child Health Services Block Grant program

The Health Resources and Services Administration at the Department of Health and Human Services administers the Maternal and Child Health Services Block Grant. This grant enables states and territories to maintain and strengthen health care for pregnant women, mothers, infants, and children, including children with special health care needs. Beginning in fiscal year 1991, states must demonstrate that they use at least 30% of their federal allotment under this program for preventive and primary care services for children and at least 30% for services for children with special health care needs.

Community Mental Health Services Block Grant

The Substance Abuse and Mental Health Services Administration in the Department of Health and Human Services disseminates the Community Mental Health Services Block Grant. This grant provides financial assistance to states and territories to carry out the state's plan for providing comprehensive community mental health services to adults with a serious mental illness and to children with a serious emotional disturbance.

Community Prevention Grant

The Office of Juvenile Justice and Delinquency Prevention at the Department of Justice disseminates this grant. Also known as Title V: Delinquency Prevention Program Community Prevention Grant, this grant increases the capacity of state and local governments to support effective prevention programs and improve the juvenile justice system. State advisory boards channel funds to local governmental agencies who partner with youth, parents, social service providers, law enforcement, and others to implement local delinquency prevention programs. Although funds to states are based on a formula, funds to local governments are awarded on a competitive basis. In 1997 $20 million in funds were awarded, with the average grant approximately $56,000.

Community Services Block Grant

The Office of Community Services, Administration for Children and Families, U.S. Department of Health and Human Services funds the Community Services Block Grant. This grant supports states' efforts to provide services and activities having a measurable and potential major impact on causes of poverty in the community. Funds can be targeted to improve the educational attainment of low-income individuals. For example, local programs that attempt to maintain pregnant and parenting teens in schools would be eligible for funding under this program. Funds may be used to coordinate and establish linkages between governmental and other social services programs to assure the effective delivery of health and educational services to low-income individuals.

Substance Abuse Prevention and Treatment Block Grant

The Substance Abuse and Mental Health Services Administration at the Department of Health and Human Services disseminates the Substance Abuse Prevention and Treatment Block Grant. This grant provides financial assistance to states and territories to support projects for the development and implementation of prevention, treatment, and rehabilitation activities directed to the diseases of alcohol and drug abuse. A minimum of 20% of the funds must be spent for community-based prevention programs such as school-based universal programs, as well as programs that target individuals most at risk for substance abuse.

The Safe and Drug-Free Schools and Communities State Grants

This formula program is disseminated through the U.S. Office of Education and complements the discretionary Safe and Drug-Free Schools Program and the Safe Schools/Healthy Students initiative. Funds are allocated to the states on a formula basis and then distributed by states in line with state priorities. The program was created to meet the National Education Goal that, by the year 2000, every school in the United States will be free of drugs, violence, and the unauthorized presence of firearms and alcohol and offer a disciplined environment conducive to learning. Programs must involve parents and be coordinated with related federal, state, and community efforts and resources.

From National Conference of State Legislatures (1999). *Funding School Health Programs. Block Grant Survey* [on line]. Available: http://www.ncsl.org/programs/health/pp/bgsurey.htm.

79

of seven block grant programs that are used to support school-based health programs. Block grant programs encourage or require states to grant considerable discretion to local communities in developing programs that address the objectives of the block funds yet are tailored to the unique needs and resources of the community. For example, school-based health center programs in Texas that receive funding from the Texas Department of Health (which is funded through federal block grants and state funds) must be planned and organized by a local community advisory group made up of parents, school administrators, school nurses, teachers, students, local health care providers, religious leaders, business leaders, and representatives from youth and family service agencies.

In 1991, the Centers for Disease Control and Prevention (CDC) began providing fiscal and technical support for state departments of education and state departments of health to jointly help local school districts implement the eight components of school health programs: (1) health services; (2) psychological, counseling, and social services; (3) health education; (4) nutrition services; (5) physical education and other physical activities; (6) the psychosocial and biophysical environment; (7) health programs for faculty and staff; and (8) integrated efforts of schools, families, and communities to improve the health of students and staff (Allensworth & Kolbe, 1987). The CDC provides support for each state to hire senior-level policy experts to mobilize and integrate the various resources of the federal and state programs to help schools improve these eight components.

State Children's Health Insurance Program (SCHIP)

The Balanced Budget Act of 1997 established the State Children's Health Insurance Program (P.L. 105–33, 1997). By giving grants to states to provide health insurance coverage to uninsured children living at up to 200% of the federal poverty level, SCHIP goes a long way in achieving the goal of universal children's insurance coverage. States may provide this coverage by expanding Medicaid or by expanding or creating a state children's health insurance program. States can also select the benefit plan it offers within specified options that ensure fairly comprehensive health coverage.

Many states have used the opportunity SCHIP provides to further the integration of education and health services to children and families. For example, states have eased enrollment barriers by having similar eligibility criteria for free or reduced-cost lunch programs and for SCHIP and by making schools a key component in efforts to enroll students in the program and to refer students to community-based providers. The Chicago Public Schools (CPS), the Illinois Department of Human Services, and the Illinois Department of Public Aid have forged a successful partnership for enrolling children and linking children and families with appropriate providers (Children's Defense Fund, 1999c). Every fall and spring the parents of children attending Chicago public schools are required to pick up their child's report card in person. The CPS used this opportunity to assist eligible families with the enrollment process. In fall 1999 the Chief Executive Officer of CPS sent every family whose children were eligible for free or reduced-cost lunch programs a letter urging them to use the school's assistance on "Report Card Pick Up Day" to submit their applications for KidCare (the Illinois SCHIP). Included with the letter was a KidCare application and information on eligibility and outreach assistance programs. Teachers received training in the outreach strategies, one of which was having a team of individuals at each school who assisted with filling out the applications. Throughout the year, six KidCare centers located within the schools assist parents with the enrollment process. Denise Taylor, coordinator for these outreach efforts, said a primary benefit of these outreach efforts is greater access to health services that affect a child's learning, including vision and hearing screening and services, preventive and corrective dental services, screening and assessment of mental and emotional disorders, primary health care, and mental health services (personal communication, October 8, 1999). An additional benefit of these school-based efforts to increase children's access to health care is enhanced communication between school and community providers, as well as greater involvement of community providers in the schools.

Federal Discretionary Grant Programs

A number of federal agencies administer discretionary (i.e., competitive) grant programs that provide funds that can be used to support school-based, integrated health services. For example, since 1991 the Health Resources and Services Administration has funded the Rural Health Outreach Grant Program, which provides funds for rural health outreach demonstration projects. In order to qualify for the program, applicants are required to develop network arrangements among three or more health care and/or social service organizations. In fiscal year 1998, many of the 98 projects funded under this program involved collaborative agreements between schools and other community agencies in meeting the health needs of rural children and their families. Two programs highlighted in Table 4.4 illustrate the diversity of collaborators among successful grantees.

Challenges for Psychologists

New and emerging models of psychological health care for children require knowledge and skills that may not have been emphasized in a psychologist's training (La Greca & Hughes, 1999). For example, although government and private sector funds to support school-based and school-linked services are more readily available, accessing these funds requires skills in locating potential sources of funds, writing successful proposals (including budgets), administering programs, and documenting program processes and outcomes. New models adopt a collaborative approach to working with families versus an expert approach. Skills in establishing collaborative relationships with families and in building on family strengths are key to success in these models. Whereas psychologists may have been trained in interviewing skills essential to diagnosing pathology, they may be less prepared to conduct an interview that identifies family strengths and assets as a basis for collaboratively developing intervention goals and methods. Providers in systems of care are expected to collaborate with other professionals and to treat clients as "whole" beings versus simply treating clients' problems. This change means that professional boundaries

TABLE 4.4   Examples of Integrated Programs Funded Under the Rural Health Outreach Grant Program

---

Central Peninsula Counseling Services. Kenai, Alaska

The overall thrust of the Kenai Peninsula Family Support Program is to provide high-risk seriously emotionally disturbed (SED) youth with easier access to behavioral health services. The project proposes to bring the services to the youth in their homes, schools, and local community settings. The Kenai Peninsula Borough is located in a remote (3–6 hours south of Anchorage) portion of southern Alaska. It covers an area as large as West Virginia and has 32 separate rural communities and Alaska Native villages and over 40,000 residents. It is estimated that over 700 SED youth are located in this area. The services are provided through the placement of full-time family support counselors, employed by the participating mental health service providers, in 17 public schools owned by the borough and are offered in both school and home settings as group or individual counseling. The network includes the Central Peninsula Counseling Services, Kenai Peninsula Borough School District, Seward Life Action Council, South Peninsula Community Mental Health Center, Central Peninsula General Hospital, and the Center for the Study and Teaching of At-Risk Students. Fiscal Year 1998 funding amount was $197,000.

Tattnall County Board of Health. Reidsville, Georgia

The project provides direct delivery of health care services, focusing on the prevention of teen pregnancy at Tatnall County High School, located in rural southeast Georgia. These objectives are being attained through the use of comprehensive ongoing adolescent case management for at-risk high school students; through the availability of on-site mental health/substance abuse counseling services; through the provision of resource mothers for interested pregnant female high school students; and through the establishment of a male mentoring program for at-risk male adolescents. The population of the county high school for the school year 1995–96 was 841, including 63.3% white, 33.7% African American, and 3.1% Hispanic and other ethnic groups. The network members are the Tattnall County Board of Health, the county board of education, mental health outpatient services, family services, the male mentoring program, and a county hospital. Fiscal Year 1998 funding amount was $197,115.

From Federal Office of Rural Health Policy (1999). Rural Health Outreach Grantee Directory FY 1998. Washington, DC: Author. Retrieved October 8, 1999 from World Wide Web: http://www.nal.usda.gov/orhp/orgrante.htm.

are less defined and more permeable as professionals provide a broader range of services in order to treat the "whole" client. For example, nurses may provide mental health counseling services to adolescents who visit a school-based health clinic, and psychologists perform case management functions (e.g., as in multiple systemic therapy; see chapter 15, by Huey and Henggeler this volume). New service models require interprofessional collaboration, including skills in working across agencies and disciplines in providing coordinated interventions.

Psychologists most familiar with clinic-based services need to learn about the structures and mores of schools, as discussed previously. Certainly knowledge of the legal and regulatory basis for the provision of educational and related services is essential. Psychologists venturing into schools may also need to develop skills in ecologically based assessments such as classroom-based structured behavioral observations and curriculum-based assessment procedures. They may require skills in classroom-based interventions such as the Good Behavior Game (Kellam, Rebok, Ialongo, & Mayer, 1994), peer mentoring/tutoring (Jason et al., 1992), behavioral consultation (Kratochwill & Bergan, 1990), and affective education (Greenberg, Kusche, Cook, & Quamma, 1996).

Psychologists may have received little training in developing, implementing, and evaluating programs that target groups such as homeless children, pregnant teens, or aggressive children. The expansion of health care to heretofore uninsured children of the "working poor" through managed care programs that combine state, federal, and local funds has blurred the distinction between public and private sector care and altered the demographic characteristics of children served by child psychologists, as well as the setting for services (e.g., schools versus clinics). Children served in the public sector are likely to have multiple problems that require comprehensive and integrated services, and psychologists trained in single modality treatments, especially office-based treatments, will find their tools a poor match for the needs of these children and families. The ability to take the perspective of the client, to view a situation from different perspectives, to listen nonjudgmentally, and to distinguish between cultural influences and individual psychopathology are essential to providing culturally responsive and appropriate psychological services.

Summary

Psychologists have important roles to perform in providing psychological services to children in school-based and school-linked settings. This chapter has attempted to serve as a "primer" in terms of the diversity of roles psychologists perform in school-based and school-linked services. Psychological services in schools encompass both the provision of mandated psychological services to children with disabilities and the provision of discretionary psychological services. The potential for growth in school-based psychological services lies in discretionary services. Whereas child and adolescent psychologists may have many skills relevant to these new and expanded roles, most will need to develop new competencies in order to assume leadership roles in these new and emerging models for the delivery of psychological health services in schools (American Psychological Association Task Force on Professional Child and Adolescent Psychology, 1999). These roles include the development and evaluation of prevention and treatment programs for specific populations of at-risk or disabled youth, administration and coordination of health, education, and social services, provision of clinical supervision, treatment of complex cases, staff development, and grant writing. For psychologists with the prerequisite interests and skills, today is a time of unparalleled opportunities for enhancing the well-being of children and families through school-based models of psychological practice.

REFERENCES

Allensworth, D., & Kolbe, L. (1987). The comprehensive school health program: Exploring an expanded concept. *Journal of School Health, 57*, 409–473.

American Psychiatric Association (1994). *Diagnostic and statistical manual of mental disorders* (4th ed.). Washington, DC: Author.

American Psychological Association Task Force on Professional Child and Adolescent Psychology (1999). *Final report to the Board of Professional Affairs.* Washington, DC: American Psychological Association.

Annie E. Casey Foundation (1999). *Kids Count* [on-line]. Available: www (World Wide Web): http://aecf.org/kidscount/kc1999/findings2.htm (October 5, 1999).

Armbruster, P., Gerstein, S. H., & Fallon, T. (1997). Bridging the gap between service need and service utilization: A school-based mental health program. *Community Mental Health Journal,* 33(3), 199–211.

Benson, A. J., & Hughes, J. (1985). Perceptions of role definition processes in school psychology: A national survey. *School Psychology Review, 14,* 64–74.

Bowser, P. (1995). Professional conduct: Meeting NASP's ethical standards. In A. Thomas & J. Grimes (Eds.), *Best practices in school psychology III* (pp. 33–39). Washington, DC: National Association of School Psychologists.

Brown, D. T. (1990). Professional regulation and training in school psychology. In T. B. Gutkin & C. R. Reynolds (Eds.), *Handbook of school psychology* (2nd ed., pp. 991–1009). New York: Wiley.

Children's Defense Fund (1998). *Keeping children safe in school: A resource for states.* Washington, DC: Author.

Children's Defense Fund (1999a). *Despite strong economy, a record high number of working families with children are living in poverty* [on-line]. Available: www (World Wide Web): http://childrensdefense.org/release990930.htm (October 5, 1999).

Children's Defense Fund (1999b). *Violence in schools* [on-line]. Available: www (World Wide Web): http://www.childrensdefense.org/youthviolence/violenceschools.htm. (October 5, 1999).

Children's Defense Fund (1999c). *Sign them up! What is working for children's health* [on-line]. Available www (World Wide Web): http://childrensdefense.

org/whatsworking/1999-0824.htm (October 7, 1999).

Comer, J. P. (1985). The Yale-New Haven Primary Prevention project: A follow-up study. *Journal of the American Academy of Child and Adolescent Psychiatry, 24,* 154–160.

Davis, W. E. (1999, August). Meeting mental health needs of children, adolescents, and their families. Paper presented at the annual convention of the American Psychological Association, Boston, MA.

Day, C., & Roberts, M. C. (1991). Activities of the Child and Adolescent Service System Program for improving mental health services for children and families. *Journal of Clinical Child Psychology, 20,* 340–350.

Dryfoos, J. G. (1994). *Full-service schools: A revolution in health and social services for children, youth, and families.* San Francisco: Jossey-Bass.

Education for All Handicapped Children Act of 1975, Pub. L. No. 94-142 (1975).

Fagan, T. K., & Wise, P. J. (1994). *School psychology.* New York: Longman.

Family Educational Rights and Privacy Act of 1974, a part of Pub. L. No. 93-380 (1974).

Federal Office of Rural Health Policy (1999). Rural Health Outreach Grantee Directory FY 1998 [on-line]. Available: www (World Wide Web): http://www.nal.usda.gov/orhp/orgrante.htm (October 8, 1999).

Federal Register (1999). Notice of Intent To Make Funds Available for School Violence Prevention and Early Childhood Development Activities Under the Safe Schools/Healthy Students Initiative [on-line]. *Federal Register,* 64(241), pp. 5814–5815. Available: www.wais.access.gpo.gov (October 7, 1999).

Fleming, R. K., Oliver, J. R., & Bolton, D. B. (1996). Training supervisors to train staff: A case study in a human service organization. *Journal of Organizational Behavior Management, 16,* 3–25.

Goals 2000. Educate America Act, Pub. L. No. 103-227 (1994).

Graden, J. L. (1989). Redefining "prereferral" intervention as intervention assistance: Collaboration between general and special education. *Exceptional Children, 51*, 487–496.

Greenberg, M. T., Kusche, C. A., Cook, E. T., & Quamma, J. P. (1996). Promoting emotional competence in school-aged children: The effects of the PATHS curriculum. *Development and Psychopathology, 7*, 117–136.

Henggeler, S. W., Melton, G. B., Brondino, M. J., Scherer, D. G., & Hanley, J. H. (1997). Multisystemic therapy with violent and chronic juvenile offenders and their families: The role of treatment fidelity in successful dissemination. *Journal of Consulting and Clinical Psychology, 65*, 821–833.

Improving America's Schools Act of 1994, Elementary and Secondary Education Amendments of 1993, Pub. L. No. 103-382 (1994).

Individuals with Disabilities Education Act, Pub. L. No. 101-476; 20 U.S.C. Chapter 33 (1990).

Individuals with Disabilities Education Act Amendments of 1997, Pub. L. No. 105-17 (1997).

Ingwerson, D. W. (1990). A superintendent's view: Learning to listen and trust each school faculty. Personal reflections on shared decision-making. *School Administrator, 47*, 8–11.

Jacob-Timm, S., & Hartshorne, T. S. (1994). *Ethics and law for school psychologist* (2nd ed.). New York: Wiley.

Jacob-Timm, S., & Hartshorne, T. S. (1998). *Ethics and law for school psychologist* (3rd ed.). New York: Wiley.

Jason, L. A., Weine, A. M., Johnson, J. H., Warren-Sohlberg, L., Filippelli, L. A., Turner, E. Y., & Lardon, C. (1992). The School Transitions Project: A comprehensive preventive intervention. *Journal of Emotional and Behavioral Disorders, 1*(1), 65–70.

Kellam, S. G., Rebok, G. W., Ialongo, N., & Mayer, L. S. (1994). The course and malleability of aggressive behavior from early first grade into middle schools: Results of a developmental epidemiologically based prevention trial. *Journal of Child Psychology and Psychiatry, 35*, 259–281.

Kelly, C. (1995). Building-level public relations. In A. Thomas and J. Grimes (Eds.), *Best practices in school psychology III* (pp. 269–278). Washington, DC: National Association of School Psychologists.

Knitzer, J. (1982). *Unclaimed children: The failure of public responsibility to children and adolescents in need of mental health services.* Washington, DC: Children's Defense Fund.

Knitzer, J. (1997). Service integration for children and families: Lessons and questions. In R. J. Illback, C. T. Cobb, & H. M. Joseph, Jr. (Eds.), *Integrated services for children and families: Opportunities for psychological practice* (pp. 3–21). Washington, DC: American Psychological Association.

Kolbe, L. J., Collins, J., & Cortese, P. (1997). Building the capacity of schools to improve the health of the nation: A call for assistance from psychologists. *American Psychologist, 52*, 256–265.

Kratochwill, T. R., & Bergan, J. R. (1990). *Behavioral consultation in applied settings: An individual guide.* New York: Plenum Press.

La Greca, A. M., & Hughes, J. N. (1999). United we stand, divided we fall: The education and training needs of clinical child psychologists. *Journal of Clinical Child Psychology, 28*, 435–447.

Lange, J. T. (1993). Site-based, shared decision-making: A resource for restructuring. *National Association of Secondary School Principals Bulletin, 76*, 98–107.

Musick, J. S., & Stott, F. M. (1990). Paraprofessionals, parenting, and child development: Understanding the problems and seeking solutions. In S. J. Meisels & J. P. Shonkoff (Eds.), *Handbook of early childhood intervention* (pp.

651–667). Cambridge: Cambridge University Press.

National Association of School Psychologists. (1991, November). Recertification deadline draws near. *NASP Communique*, 1, 10.

National Association of School Psychologists. (1992). *Intervention assistance teams: A model for building level instructional problem solving*. Silver Spring, MD: Author.

National Association of School Psychologists. (1994). *Standards for the credentialing of school psychologists*. Silver Spring, MD: Author.

National Commission on Children (1991). *Beyond rhetoric: A new American agenda for children and families*. Washington, DC: U.S. Government Printing Office.

National Commission on Excellence in Education. (1983). *A nation at risk: The imperative for educational reform*. Washington, DC: U. S. Government Printing Office.

National Maternal and Child Health Clearinghouse (1999). *America's children: Key national indicators of child well-being 1998* [on-line]. Available: www (World Wide Web): http://child stats.gov/ac1999/poptxt.as. (Also available from U.S. Government Printing Office, Publication No. 065-000-01162-0)

Oakland, T., & Cunningham, J. (1999). The future of school psychology: Conceptual models for its development and examples of their applications. In C. R. Reynolds, & T. B. Gutkin (Eds.), *Handbook of school psychology* (3rd ed., pp. 34–51). New York: Wiley.

Phillips, V., Boysen, T. C., & Schuster, S. A. (1997). Psychology's role in statewide education reform. *American Psychologist*, 52, 250–255.

Podemski, R. S., Marsh, G. W., II, Smith, T. E. C., & Price, B. J. (1995). *Comprehensive administration of special education* (2nd ed.). Englewood Cliffs, NJ: Prentice-Hall.

Prasse, D. P. (1995). School psychology and the law. In A. Thomas & J. Grimes (Eds.), *Best practices in school psychology III* (pp. 41–50). Washington, DC: National Association of School Psychologists.

Pryzwansky, W. B. (1999). Accreditation and credentialing systems in school psychology. In C. R. Reynolds & T. Gutkin (Eds.), *Handbook of school psychology* (3rd ed., pp. 1145–1158). New York: Wiley.

Rehabilitation Act of 1973, Pub. L. No. 93-112, 34 C. F. R. Part 104 (1996).

Reschly, D. J., & Bersoff, D. N. (1999). Law and school psychology. In C. R. Reynolds & T. Gutkin (Eds.), *Handbook of school psychology* (3rd ed., pp. 1077–1110). New York: Wiley.

Ross, R. P. (1995). Best practices in implementing intervention assistance teams. In A. Thomas & J. Grimes (Eds.), *Best practices in school psychology III* (pp. 227–238). Washington, DC: National Association of School Psychologists.

Sameroff, A. J., Seifer, R., & Bartko, W. T. (1997). Environmental perspectives on adaptation during childhood and adolescence. In S. S. Luthar, J. A. Burack, D. Cicchetti, & J. R. Weisz (Eds.), *Developmental psychopathology: Perspectives on adjustment, risk, and disorder* (pp. 507–526). New York: Cambridge University Press.

Schorr, L. B., & Schorr, D. (1988). *Within our reach: Breaking the cycle of disadvantage*. New York: Anchor.

State Children's Health Insurance Program. Title XXI of the Social Security Act. Pub. L. No. 105-33 (1997).

Talley, R. (1995). APA policy and advocacy for school psychology practice. In A. Thomas & J. Grimes (Eds.), *Best practices in school psychology III* (pp. 191–202). Washington, DC: National Association of School Psychologists.

Talley, R. C., & Schrag, J. A. (1999). Legal and public policy foundations supporting service integration for students with disabilities. *Journal of Educational and Psychological Consultation, 10,* 229–249.

Talley, R. C., & Short, R. J. (1996). Social reforms and the future of school practice: Implications for American psychology. *Professional Psychology: Research and Practice, 27,* 5–13.

Tharinger, D. (1995). Roles for psychologists in emerging models of school-related health and mental health services. *School Psychology Quarterly, 10,* 203–216.

Tierney, J. P., Grossman, J. B., & Resch, N. L. (1995). *Making a difference: An impact study of Big Brothers/Big Sisters.*

(Available from Public/Private Ventures, 2005 Market Street, Suite 900, Philadelphia, PA, 19103).

U.S. Department of Education (1999). President Clinton announces more than $100 million in community grants to prevent violence among youth [online press release]. Available: www (World Wide Web): http://www.ed.gov/pressreleases/09-1999/schools.htm (October 8, 1999).

Woody, R. H., LaVoie, J. C., & Epps, S. (1992). *School psychology: A developmental and social system approach.* Boston: Allyn & Bacon.

5

DENNIS DROTAR
LYNN ZAGORSKI

Providing Psychological Services in Pediatric Settings in an Era of Managed Care

Challenges and Opportunities

Psychologists in pediatric settings provide services to a great many children, adolescents, and their families in primary care settings and in acute and chronic care hospitals (Drotar, 1995; Singer & Drotar, 1989). Relevant clinical issues in providing such services have been described in a number of publications (Drotar, 1993, 1995; Schroeder & Mann, 1991). On the other hand, there have been few, if any, comprehensive descriptions of the programmatic and professional issues that arise in providing psychological services to children and families in pediatric settings, especially in an era of managed care. The purpose of this chapter is to provide an overview of the challenges and opportunities of implementing a program of pediatric psychological services to children and their families in an academic medical setting. Based on the senior author's (Drotar) 27 years of clinical experience and the junior author's (Zagorski) time and energy-intensive experience as a clinical services coordinator, this chapter describes key issues in the development, management, and administration of psychological services in pediatric settings.

What Clinical Problems Are Typically Seen in Pediatric Settings?

The specific psychological and behavioral problems that are seen by psychologists in pediatric settings vary widely as a function of the type of setting in which such care is provided. In primary care settings, pediatric psychologists see an extraordinary range of behavioral and developmental problems (Schroeder & Mann, 1991). For example, Charlop, Parrish, Fenton, and Cataldo (1987) described the referral problems of 100 patients who received outpatient behavioral treatment during a one-year period. Parents of children in this sample ranked behavioral noncompliance (16.2%), tantrums (12.8%), and aggression (8.1%) as the three behaviors of greatest concern.

Psychologists who provide services to pediatric inpatients encounter very different clinical populations that involve a high frequency of emergency/crisis situations, as well as mental health and family problems that are associated with chronic health conditions (Drotar & Bush, 1985). For example, in Olson and colleagues' (1989) description of 740 hospitalized children who were referred to a pediatric psychology service at Oklahoma Health Sciences Center over a 4½-year period, the largest number of referral problems ($n = 145$) were related to depression and/or suicide attempts. Relatively large numbers of children were also seen for adjustment to chronic illness ($n = 92$), behavioral problems ($n = 69$), psychosomatic problems ($n = 61$), and pain management ($n = 57$). The heterogeneous nature of clinical problems seen in pediatric settings raises difficult questions related to the management of psychological services. For example, is it feasible to provide comprehensive coverage of psychological services across these diverse populations? If not, which populations should receive priority?

Challenges in Service Delivery

Psychologists who provide services to children, adolescents, and their families in pediatric settings face the challenges of responding to requests for consultation from a large number of pediatric colleagues, of providing evaluative and treatment services for patients who are referred, and of funding these services in a managed care environment.

Deployment of Services

Decisions concerning the deployment of psychological services in pediatric settings are complicated because there are many more requests from patients and providers for such services than can be met. In our setting, 5 full-time PhDs, 1 full-time MD, two master's-level psychologists, one bachelor's-level assistant, three graduate students, and two psychology fellows provide psychological/behavioral services to the patients of a full-time pediatric faculty of more than one hundred, as well as to community pediatricians. Referral problems run the gamut from intensive supportive services for children and families undergoing highly specialized medical procedures such as bone marrow transplantation to services for children with highly prevalent problems such as attention-deficit/hyperactivity disorder (ADHD) who are referred from primary care providers.

Given the extensive variation in the types of clinical problems that are encountered, one difficult question for pediatric psychology service providers is, How comprehensive as opposed to specialized should their services be? Comprehensive, broad-based deployment of services has the advantage of reaching the largest number of pediatric consumers of services and, of course, children and families. By contrast, a very broad-based deployment of pediatric psychological services is unrealistic given the limited resources of most departments. Moreover, a broad spectrum program of psychological services does not take advantage of the specialized expertise of pediatric psychologists in such areas as neuropsychology or mental health interventions for children with chronic illness. A clear advantage of specialization is that pediatric psychologists can use their training and expertise to their fullest advantage and provide services that are not offered elsewhere in the community. The disadvantage of specialized deployment of pediatric psychological services is that many children present with complex and comorbid problems that are not easily managed within specialized service patterns. Moreover, to the extent that a program of psychological services is mandated to provide services to the patients of community primary care practitioners, a highly specialized program will not be sufficiently responsive to the needs of these patients and their providers.

Challenges Imposed by Managed Care

Managed care has changed the patterns of delivery of psychological services, and pediatric psychological services are no exception. For a more extensive discussion of managed care and the implications for psychologists, readers are referred to Roberts's and Hurley's (1997) excellent description. Several of the managed care issues most salient to pediatric psychology services are discussed here. In pediatric and in other settings, managed care has reduced the number of reimbursed contacts and hence has challenged providers to provide shorter term services. Although short-term, crisis-oriented interventions have long been an integral part of pediatric psychologists' repertoires (Drotar, 1977), the challenges of providing such services are extraordinary: pediatric psychologists need to develop expertise in identifying the child's key problems and either managing them or providing quick triage to community providers. To best accomplish this difficult task, pediatric psychologists need to define their areas of expertise and interest clearly (e.g., Who are they most qualified to treat? Who are they most interested in treating?). Pressures that make the task of referring patients to other providers very difficult include the realities that chronic and comorbid problems do not always lend themselves to short-term intervention and that some pediatric colleagues prefer that their favorite psychologists personally handle the problems that they refer.

A related challenge is that reduction in the overall level of reimbursement for mental health services by insurance companies has forced pediatric psychologists, as is also true for their medical colleagues, to increase their frequency of contact hours to sustain their salaries; in other words, work harder for less money. A clear downside to this fact of professional life is the increased risk for burnout and disruption in quality of care. As a working guideline, several pediatric psychology programs in academic medical settings that we know of require their full-time providers to provide at least 25 hours of direct patient contact time per week. However, this contact time requirement does not include time spent on reports to pediatricians and schools, on the phone, or on contacts with pediatricians and other professionals, most of which is not reimbursed. Although one can always work more efficiently, there are limits to human endurance. As providers in pediatric settings are required to see more and more patients, the quality of their clinical work and their ability to contribute to teaching and research programs, as well as the quality of their lives, may suffer.

Managed care has also increased the competition among mental health providers in communities, and pediatric psychologists are part of this. Hospital and community providers each want to achieve a more optimal "payer mix," which can be defined as serving a greater proportion of patients whose families have better insurance relative to those who are either underinsured or uninsured. The fact that managed care companies do not necessarily differentiate among psychologists with specialized expertise in treating pediatric populations when selecting mental health providers for their panels reduces pediatric psychologists' competitive edge.

To help attract a broad range of consumers, especially those with more optimal insurance coverage, and for consumer convenience, psychological services in many pediatric settings are now being offered in offsite locations known as satellite clinics, which are often more convenient for families than hospital settings. Although deployment of psychologists in satellite clinics has the clear advantage of increasing consumer satisfaction, it has the disadvantage of fragmenting services and limiting pediatric psychologists' ability to manage hospital-based services that they have traditionally provided. As an example, in our setting, because so many of our psychologists are providing services at satellite clinics, it has been difficult for us to sustain adequate coverage for inpatients, some of whom require daily and intensive intervention and consultation with staff.

Challenges in Providing Collaborative Psychological Services

One of the most important issues in providing psychological services in pediatric settings is the fact that these services need to be integrated with the work of other professionals, not only pediatricians but also many others (Drotar, 1995). The overall impact of psychologists' efforts in pediatric hospitals can be enhanced by the quality of their collaborations with the many professionals who provide services to children and their families in these settings. These include: nursing staff who administer treatments to children and provide emotional support; child life staff who enhance the emotional support and coping abilities of hospitalized children and their families; social workers who provide support to families, assessment of relevant family problems, coordination of care, and follow-up with community agencies; child psychiatrists who see children with mental health disorders; and professionals from speech pathology, occupational and physical therapy, respiratory therapy, and so forth. All of these professionals contribute to the care that is provided to children and their families in hospital settings.

Although collaborative and coordinated delivery of psychological services can be most helpful to children and families, there are many challenges and obstacles to providing such care (Drotar, 1995). One of these is the overlap in the kinds of behavioral and family problems that are seen by psychologists, child psychiatrists, and social workers and in the kinds of services that are provided by these professionals. In order to avoid interprofessional conflicts and confusion on the part of pediatricians who make referrals, as well as of families who receive services, there is a continuing need to clarify professional roles (Drotar & Sturm, 1996).

In some instances, interprofessional conflicts may reflect a discrepancy in what colleagues expect from one another. Pediatricians typically want concrete practical advice from psychologists that is immediately helpful to their management of patients. When they do not receive such service, they can be frustrated. As an example, a psychologist evaluated a child with a learning problem who had been referred by a pediatrician. The test report focused on the nature of the child's information-processing deficits but provided little information concerning remediation. The referring pediatrician became quite annoyed because the psychologist did not recommend management strategies or help the parents decide about the child's placement. The potential for frustration based on not meeting collaborators' expectations, as shown in this example, heightens the need for psychologists to communicate effectively with their pediatric and other professional collaborators concerning their expectations from referrals.

Coordination of Care

One of the continuing dilemmas in providing collaborative psychological services in pediatric settings involves coordination of care with medical and other professionals. Although coordinated care is necessary to avoid duplication of effort and to limit confusion on the part of pediatricians and families, there are many obstacles. One of these is that the separate administrative structure, organization, and cultures of separate professional disciplines in pediatric settings can interfere with collaborative planning. Other obstacles relate to the realities of practice. For example, given the significant financial and time pressures associated with the practice of modern pediatric medicine and pediatric psychology, it is increasingly difficult to find the time for mutual dialogue with physicians about their patients, let alone to provide the type of comprehensive care or systems-level interventions that may be needed for optimal treatment planning and follow-up, at least for some children (Drotar, 1995; Mullins, Gillman, & Harbeck, 1992).

For example, significant clinical dilemmas are often raised by children with chronic illness and comorbid mental health problems that require comprehensive, collaborative care, as shown by the following example: Sally is a 15-year-old with diabetes of several years' duration whose endocrinologist has become very concerned because the management of her blood sugar has threatened her health, necessitating two hospitalizations. It has recently come to light that Sally has developed an eating disorder that has a profound impact on her ability to manage her diabetes. Having become highly invested in being thin, Sally deliberately runs her blood sugars high. Her endocrinologist refers her to a mental health provider who has extensive clinical experience with adolescents with diabetes and, together with the family, they work out a coordinated strategy for Sally's management.

In order to implement coordinated care for patients such as Sally, mental health services need to be covered by insurance. A significant obstacle to such coordinated care among pediatric psychologists and medical and other professionals relates to limitations in insurance coverage. Managed care insurance companies often subcontract mental health coverage with a designated mental health insurance company. In many pediatric hospital settings, those who contract with managed care insurance companies are often unaware that their pediatric psychology col-leagues may not have a contract with the mental health company associated with the medical company. This discrepancy in contracting makes it difficult for medical professionals to refer their patients to a pediatric psychologist who works in the same setting, thus jeopardizing continuum of care for some children and their families.

Challenges Related to Administering and Organizing Psychological Services in Pediatric Settings

Important ingredients in developing and sustaining psychological services in pediat-ric settings reflect the leadership, organization, and administration of these psycho-logical services. The functions of the administrator of a program of psychological services include the following: planning for delivery and deployment of psychologi-cal services (e.g., in what setting? with what populations?); hiring and supervising psychologists, professional development and mentoring of staff; helping faculty with difficult decisions concerning clinical care and consultation; and coordinating planning for services with other professionals.

Many pediatric psychology service programs are administered by a section or division chief who is a psychologist. However, the specific lines of administrative authority and responsibility for program development vary considerably across set-tings. Depending on the setting, a chief of a pediatric psychology program could report to the chair of pediatrics, of psychiatry, or of psychology or to a hospital administrator. Divisions of psychology may be based in departments of pediatrics, psychiatry, or psychology/behavioral science (Drotar, 1995). Each of these adminis-trative arrangements has advantages and disadvantages. A primary advantage of basing services in a department of pediatrics includes greater prospects for a close communication and working relationship with pediatric faculty. One potential disadvantage, which is true of all arrangements in which psychologists are adminis-tered by medical departments, is that professional autonomy may be challenged.

Basing psychological services within a department of psychiatry has been the traditional model of administrative organization within schools of medicine. This model has the potential advantage of unifying pediatric psychologists with other psychologists in the department of psychiatry and with child psychiatrists. Disadvan-tages include the difficulties involved in planning collaborative programs with pediatric colleagues who are based in another department and limits on the profes-sional autonomy of psychologists that can be placed by psychiatrists.

By far the least frequently used model of administrative organization of pediatric psychology in schools of medicine is the separate and independent department of psychology model, which has the clear advantage of professional autonomy. How-ever, this model is very difficult to fund and implement.

Irrespective of the specific administrative arrangement, the strong support of the departmental chairperson for pediatric psychology services and the quality of the relationship between the chief of psychology and the medical chairperson are, in my experience, crucial to program success. It is critical that the chairperson of the medical department value the services that are provided by the psychologists, especially so because such services are not likely to make the department a lot of money!

Professional Needs of Pediatric Psychology Service Providers

In order to respond most effectively to the strenuous demands of patient care, psychologists in pediatric settings need to be supported by an administration that meets their professional needs and facilitates their professional development. Meeting the professional needs of psychologists who provide services in pediatric settings presents a significant challenge, partially because medical settings are not organized to accomplish this. Psychologists are not physicians and have different needs for professional autonomy, training, and professional development.

In some medical settings, the development of adequate provisions to maintain professional autonomy and responsibility for psychologists (e.g., ensuring appropriate supervision for trainees and psychology assistants, credentialing, staff privileges) may lag behind the level of development of medical, clinical, teaching, or research programs (Enright, Resnick, Ludwigsen, & Deleon, 1993; Thompson, 1987, 1991). Hospital privileges constitute the permission to provide medical or other patient care services based on professional license, expertise, competence, ability, and judgments. The Joint Commission on the Accreditation of Health Care Organization (JCAHO, 1991) requires that there be a single organized staff, for example, physicians and other licensed individuals who are permitted by law to provide patient care services and who are responsible for the quality of professional services provided by those individuals with clinical privileges (JCAHO, 1991). Bases for membership in the medical staff include evidence of current licensure, training, experience, current competence, and documented experience in specific categories of treatment or procedures (e.g., psychotherapy, psychological testing, etc.). Clinical privileges are hospital specific and require a reappraisal for renewal based on current licensure, professional performance, and clinical technical skills as indicated by quality assurance activities and other indicators of continuing professional qualifications, such as peer and departmental recommendations (Thompson, 1987).

Quality Assurance

Quality assurance includes implementation of a planned and systematic process for monitoring and evaluating the quality and appropriateness of the treatment of patients and clinical performance of individuals with clinical privileges (Thompson, 1991). Pediatricians can certainly judge whether a psychologist fills the needs of their program, gets along with their staff, and provides prompt service and useful reports. On the other hand, pediatricians and hospital administrators cannot adequately judge the professional training and experience or delineate standards for privileges for psychologists, any more than psychologists can set such standards for pediatricians. Consequently, pediatric psychologists need to take a leadership role in developing and implementing their hospital's procedures regarding clinical privileges and quality assurance, including delineating specific clinical responsibilities for psychologists (e.g., assessment, behavioral therapy) and deciding who is qualified to carry them out (Thompson, 1991). In our setting, a separate credentialing committee made up of psychologists and chaired by the senior author oversees the credentialing of psychologists across the different departments within the school of medicine.

Practicing within Boundaries of Professional Competence

Clear and careful delineation of clinical privileges also helps to ensure that professionals, including pediatric psychologists, practice within the areas of their professional competence. In pediatric settings, the ethical requirement to practice within one's area of professional competence can be challenged by several pressures. For example, many pediatricians want to refer their patients to psychologists in their own department and are very reluctant to refer their patients to "outside" professionals, even those who are highly competent. In order to be perceived by one's colleagues as a responsive consultant, pediatric psychologists may be tempted to answer as many requests for service as possible, including some that may be outside of their sphere of competence. On the other hand, if psychologists define their professional competence too tightly, they run the risk of being insufficiently responsive to their pediatric colleagues. Moreover, it is not always easy to decide whether a particular problem is in one's area of competence or not (Drotar, 1995).

Meeting the Challenges of Service Delivery in Pediatric Settings: Some Examples from Real Life

Thus far, we have noted a broad array of problems that are involved in delivering and administering psychological services for children and families in pediatric settings. How can these challenges be met? Although there are no easy solutions, it may be instructive for readers to learn how we have tried to solve these problems in hopes that some of these strategies may be useful in other settings.

Administrative Structure and Organization

In our setting, services are organized within a division of behavioral pediatrics and psychology, which is housed administratively and physically within a department of pediatrics. This division is on equal administrative footing with the other pediatric divisions (e.g., oncology, neurology, etc.). All division chiefs participate equally in planning for clinical care, teaching, and research in the department. Comprising 14 full-time and 3 part-time faculty members and 2 master's-level psychologists, this interdisciplinary division includes 3 pediatricians, 10 pediatric psychologists, a speech pathologist, and 2 part-time child psychiatrists. This particular administrative structure was conceived by the current pediatric chairperson, who wanted to focus and integrate psychological services, behavioral and psychological research, and teaching in the department of pediatrics in a single division. As chief of this division, the senior author works closely with the chairperson to organize service, research, and teaching programs, all of which focus on pediatric populations.

Deployment of Staff

To fulfill our triple mission of research, clinical service delivery, and teaching, staff in our division engage in a wide range of activities that are tailored to their individual talents, experience, and interests. Three psychologists in our group are primarily engaged in research, five are primarily engaged in full-time clinical practice, and two are engaged in both research and clinical service. Two staff pediatricians are involved primarily in research and teaching, and one is primarily involved in teaching and clinical work. Staff who provide the majority of clinical care see patients at the central hospital campus, as well as in the satellite clinics.

In addition to general pediatric psychology services that are rendered to a broad range of children and adolescents, our division's clinical service programs include specialized service programs such as pediatric neuropsychology, which provides assessment and remediation services for children with learning and cognitive and developmental problems; a clinic that provides comprehensive medical and developmental services to families of children who are newly adopted, with consultation and management provided by behavioral pediatricians; and a coordination/referral service for children with ADHD.

Services to pediatric inpatients are delivered in a consultation-liaison program that includes two part-time psychiatrists who reside in offices in our setting during the days that they provide these services. Requests for consultation for inpatients are managed by our division's clinical services coordinator. Specific providers respond to consultation requests based on the call schedule and presenting problem. Psychiatrists respond to the majority of requests to evaluate depression, suicidal behavior, and acute mental status changes and to questions related to medication treatment, whereas psychologists respond to referral problems such as noncompliance with medical treatment, problematic adjustment to chronic physical illness, and so forth.

We have also integrated advanced (third-year and beyond) graduate students in pediatric psychology from Case Western Reserve University into our service program. The proximity of the campus to the pediatric hospital (a five-minute walk) gives students flexibility in managing their schedules and facilitates their availability. We have developed three supervised placements for our students (16–20 hours per week) that focus on general pediatric psychology services, consultation to pediatric subspecialties (e.g., oncology or pulmonary), or psychological consultation for children with chronic health conditions who are hospitalized on a specialized collaborative care unit. Owing to the talents of our students, services provided in these placements have been very well received by pediatric colleagues.

Strategies to Coordinate Psychological Services for Special Populations: The Example of ADHD

To address the significant challenge of coordinating care for children with behavior problems who are referred to us by pediatricians, parents, and other professionals, we have implemented various strategies. One of these is a coordination service for children with ADHD, which is a highly prevalent problem in pediatric primary care. Our staff have experienced frustrations in providing care for this heterogeneous population, frustrations which, we understand from discussions with our colleagues in other settings, are widely encountered. For example, there was little consistency in the approach to referral and management of ADHD taken by providers in our setting, who included pediatric psychologists, behaviorally trained pediatricians, neurologists, and child psychiatrists. Referrals were often stimulated by teachers who felt that a neurological evaluation was the most appropriate course of action to help a child with ADHD. Not surprisingly, pediatric neurologists in our setting were overwhelmed and frustrated by the volume and inappropriateness of such referrals. Moreover, child psychiatrists in our hospital who potentially could make productive contributions to the management of complicated cases of ADHD were not necessarily consulted for these problems. Moreover, some parents who requested services for their children were frustrated because they could not easily or quickly access the providers who were most appropriate for their children. In fact, it can be very difficult for parents to make informed judgments about which type of provider should see their child because their children's problems may resemble ADHD but actually reflect other psychological and/or medical problems that need to be addressed.

Based on a planning group's recommendations, a service was developed to coordinate care for children with ADHD across the disciplines of neurology, child psychiatry, pediatrics, and pediatric psychology. This service has several goals, including clarification of the presenting problems with parents, referral to providers, and parent education and support. For example, through this service, parents have access to an experienced person who is knowledgeable about ADHD and can talk with them about their concerns about their child. Such discussions serve to clarify the nature of the child's problem and are designed to identify a specific provider who best fits the child's needs. In this way, the coordinator helps parents navigate the loosely connected system of care for children with ADHD in our hospital and community. Depending on the nature of the problem, insurance considerations, and so forth, children may be seen by one of our division members or by someone else who is well qualified to manage the child's problems. In addition to the information about referral to specific providers, parents are given information about ADHD and other relevant services, such as parent groups.

Parents who contact this service are also helped to recognize and manage problems that they may have mislabeled as attention-deficit/hyperactivity disorder. For example, a mother called the center for an ADHD evaluation for her 13-year-old son. She had difficulty dealing with his aggressive behavior and needed help controlling him. As the conversation evolved, she expressed concern that over the past few months her son had become withdrawn and had difficulty eating and sleeping. She eventually informed us that she had recently found out he had been sexually assaulted by his cousin around this time. She had not considered therapy to help her son deal with this trauma. We explained to her that we felt he demonstrated symptoms of depression that should be considered and managed first before an evaluation of ADHD was considered. She was referred to a provider with experience in managing such problems.

In the course of providing this service to more than four hundred families and obtaining information concerning pediatricians' and parents' satisfaction with the service, we have found that both parents and physicians have been satisfied with the services they received. The coordination program has also convened providers from different disciplines who provide care for children with ADHD in our hospital to discuss clinical care dilemmas, the development of new services, such as groups for parents of children with ADHD or summer camp programs for children with ADHD, and research needs and collaborative research projects.

Coordination and Management of Patient Services: The Role of a Clinical Services Coordinator

As the preceding description indicates, coordination of care has been a critical theme in the development of psychological services in our division. To enhance service coordination at all levels, we have expanded the work of the clinical services coordinator into a full-time position that meets broader needs, such as managing communications with staff at managed care companies. Although such functions are critical to the management of psychological services in order to facilitate reimbursement, in our experience they cannot be accomplished effectively by secretaries or by providers who are already stretched to the limit. To meet this challenge, our clinical-services coordinator's responsibilities include contacting insurance companies and parents concerning the status of their patients' insurance and their accounts and facilitating the scheduling of patients to improve their access to care and efficiency of scheduling (e.g., finding the best match between the child's problem and our providers' expertise, handling calls from parents and pediatricians who make inquiries about the availability of services and providers, and coordinating and managing calls for requests for psychological and psychiatric consultation for pediatric inpatients). The coordinator's successful management of these many responsibilities has been a key ingredient in the success of our division's programs, as well as a valued source of support for our staff.

Meeting Needs for Ongoing Planning for Service Development and Coordination

To address the ongoing dilemmas of coordinating the psychological services for children in our setting, we have developed several overseeing groups that include our division's providers and those from other divisions (e.g., psychiatry and neurology). One of these is a clinical services review committee that meets bimonthly to consider issues in the administration of psychological services. These include billing and reimbursement issues, such as collection of copayments from parents at the time of their visit, obtaining accurate insurance reimbursement information, and giving this information to parents and service providers; improving family access to services by reducing time to the first appointment, enhancing relationships with community pediatric providers by giving prompt feedback concerning their patients, and planning visits to pediatric practices to discuss their needs for psychological services.

A second interdivisional planning group is made up of the chiefs of our division, child psychiatry, and pediatric neurology and other staff from these divisions. The work of this group has focused on planning and troubleshooting concerning the problems of coordinating care for patient populations who require the services of multiple providers (e.g., children with autism and/or pervasive developmental disorders) or for children with chronic physical health conditions who also have comorbid mental disorders (e.g., depression).

The needs to inform pediatricians about the range of services that are offered by mental health providers and to facilitate pediatrician and family access to such services have also been salient topics on the agenda for interdivisional planning meetings. To enhance community pediatricians' awareness of available psychological and psychiatric services, we have developed user-friendly brochures that list all of the mental health providers in the hospital, their office locations, and their areas of expertise.

Supporting Staff and Their Professional Development

The challenge of developing ways to support the professional development of faculty and staff who provide services to children and families in the fast-paced world of a pediatric setting has been a difficult one. Several strategies have been useful in this regard. One of these is to involve as many staff members as possible in planning activities, such as in the overseeing committee described previously. To the extent that they have actively participated in developing strategies to manage various service delivery problems, faculty and staff have felt more engaged in this process. Moreover, they have contributed useful ideas to solve continuing problems, such as improving access to care and collection of copayments.

Other strategies to enhance support and professional development include developing forums for staff and faculty to present their work and to update their colleagues on their latest projects and clinical research interests. Because the work settings and interests of our faculty are so diverse, it is important to facilitate their knowledge of one another's work and foster their collaborations on projects of mutual interest whenever possible. Some of these experiences also can enhance professional development through continuing education. For example, as part of our division's journal club, two faculty members presented an article on the treatment of anxiety disorders in children and led a productive discussion concerning dilemmas of clinical management of families of children with this problem.

Our faculty's involvement in teaching pediatricians about child behavior and development has also facilitated their collaboration. For example, our faculty have put on a lecture series for the pediatric faculty that featured our faculty's research interests (e.g., learning disabilities, mental health, interventions with children with chronic illness, interventions to promote children's literacy). Other collaborative teaching has included a well-received educational program for community pediatricians that focused on the management of common behavioral and developmental problems in primary care, such as encopresis, ADHD, and developmental delay, and featured didactic presentations to pediatric residents as a part of our division's rotation in behavioral pediatrics. We are now in the process of planning continuing education programs for community psychologists and other mental health service providers.

A final area of support for faculty concerns mentorship. In this regard, the senior author's role as division chief includes periodic reviews and discussions with faculty concerning their productivity and professional directions, and, where relevant, provides mentoring and feedback concerning the development of research protocols, grant proposals, and manuscripts.

Proactive Planning for Psychological Service Delivery

Psychologists and behavioral pediatricians who are engaged in service provision in medical settings are continually challenged to develop innovative, cost-effective, and consumer-friendly services in a managed care environment that continues to limit the payment for such services. Our setting is no exception. The continually changing health care environment requires pediatric psychologists to be entrepreneurial and tough minded yet continually vigilant concerning the quality of patient care. For this reason, psychologists in pediatric settings need to engage in proactive planning for psychological services in collaboration with departmental faculty and leadership. As departmental programs expand in response to new programs developed by pediatric faculty, new opportunities inevitably open up for expansion of psychological services. Consequently, we have found that it is critical for our division to be involved whenever pediatric faculty are planning new programs that could involve new psychological services. Otherwise, pediatric faculty may assume (erroneously) that psychological services for new programs can easily be provided by existing faculty and staff.

Another new frontier in managing and planning for psychological services in our and other pediatric settings is the need to develop proactive strategies of dialogue with managed care companies, such as informing companies about the efficacy of psychological services and advocating for reimbursement. In our setting, we worked with one insurer to inform them of the empirical support for the efficacy of biofeedback and hypnotherapy with children for conditions such as pain, stress-related symptoms, and so forth. Following several discussions with the medical board concerning the evidence for the efficacy of these treatments based on controlled studies, the insurer eventually agreed to pay for such services out of the company's medical benefit. Although this was but one small victory in a war that pediatric and other psychologists are not necessarily winning with managed care, it did establish a precedent for the kind of proactive planning and dialogue that could make a difference.

To remain competitive, pediatric psychologists also need to work closely with their hospital administrators and planners at the level of contracting with managed care companies. In many settings, including our own, psychological services are not generally considered when hospitals are contracting with managed care companies for medical services. However, if psychological services are to be truly integrated with medical care, especially for children with chronic illnesses and handicaps, they need to be funded as part of a comprehensive reimbursement package (see Walders & Drotar, 1999, for more extensive discussion of this issue).

Evaluating the Effectiveness of Psychological Services in Pediatric Settings

A final challenge in the delivery of psychological services in pediatric settings, including our own, is the development of data concerning the evaluation of such services. In recent years, psychological researchers have underscored the need to develop data concerning the "effectiveness" of interventions that are delivered in clinical settings by practitioners to heterogeneous populations as contrasted with studies of the "efficacy" of treatments that are provided to homogenous, nonclinical populations (Weisz & Hawley, 1998). Pediatric psychologists and behavioral pediatricians have an extraordinary opportunity to provide clinically relevant data concerning the effectiveness of psychological services that are delivered in pediatric settings (Drotar, 1997), especially to specialized populations such as children with chronic illness, recurrent pain, and so forth. Potentially important indicators of clinical effectiveness include reduction of the functional impact of symptoms on patient, family, and pediatric provider and family satisfaction. Models for such studies (Bickman et al., 1985; Charlop et al., 1987; Finney, Lemanek, Cataldo, Katz, & Fuqua, 1989; Finney, Riley, & Cataldo, 1991) should be considered by pediatric psychologists in developing studies of effectiveness of services. As one example, in developing and administering our coordination service for children with ADHD, we have found that provider and parent satisfaction data have informed us how the service was being received and helped us convince our department chairperson of the utility of our program.

Summary

What will the future bring for pediatric psychologists who provide services to children and families in pediatric settings? The good news is that our experience and that of our colleagues in other settings indicate that pediatric psychological services are very much in demand. The bad news is that the challenges of paying for and organizing such services effectively in a managed care environment are formidable. Meeting these challenges will take ingenuity, commitment, and, most certainly, hard work. This was true when the field of pediatric psychology was new in that halcyon time before anyone had ever heard of managed care. It is equally true now.

ACKNOWLEDGMENTS   The help of Kathy McGowan in processing this manuscript is gratefully acknowledged. Address correspondence to the authors at Rainbow Babies and Children's Hospital, Department of Pediatrics, 11100 Euclid Avenue, Cleveland, Ohio 44106.

REFERENCES

Bickman, L., Guthrie, P. R., Foster, E. M., Lambert, E. W., Summerfelt, W. T., Breda, C. S., & Heflinger, C. A. (1995). *Evaluating managed mental health services: The Fort Bragg experiment.* New York: Plenum Press.

Charlop, M. H., Parrish, J. M., Fenton, L. R., & Cataldo, M. D. (1987). Evaluation of hospital-based pediatric psychology services. *Journal of Pediatric Psychology, 12,* 485–503.

Drotar, D. (1977). Clinical psychological practice in the pediatric hospital. *Professional Psychology, 8,* 72–80.

Drotar, D. (1993). Influences on collaborative activities among psychologists and physicians: Implications for practice, research, and training. *Journal of Pediatric Psychology, 18,* 159–172.

Drotar, D. (1995). *Consulting with pediatricians: Psychological perspectives for research and practice.* New York: Plenum Press.

Drotar, D. (1997). Intervention research: Pushing back the frontiers of pediatric psychology. *Journal of Pediatric Psychology, 22,* 415–424.

Drotar, D., & Bush, M. (1985). Mental health issues and services. In N. Hobbs & J. M. Perrin (Eds.), *Issues in the care of children with chronic illness* (pp. 232–265). San Francisco: Jossey-Bass.

Drotar, D., & Sturm, L. (1996). Interdisciplinary collaboration in the practice of mental retardation. In J. W. Jacobsen & J. A. Mulick (Eds.), *Manual of diagnosis and professional practice in mental retardation* (pp. 393–402). Washington, DC: American Psychological Association.

Enright, M. F., Resnick, R. J., Ludwigsen, K. R., & Deleon, P. L. (1993). Hospital practice: Psychology's call to action. *Professional Psychology: Research and Practice, 24,* 135–141.

Finney, J. W., Lemanek, K. L., Cataldo, M. F., Katz, H. P., & Fuqua, R. W. (1989). Pediatric psychology in primary health care: Brief target therapy for recurrent abdominal pain. *Behavioral Therapy, 29,* 283–291.

Finney, J. W., Riley, A. W., & Cataldo, M. F. (1991). Psychology in primary care: Effects of brief target therapy on children's medical care utilization. *Journal of Pediatric Psychology, 16,* 447–462.

Joint Commission on the Accreditation of Hospitals (1991). *Accreditation Manual for Hospitals.* Chicago: Author.

Mullins, L. D., Gillman, J., & Harbeck, C. (1992). Multiple-level interventions in pediatric psychology setting: A behavioral systems perspective. In A. M. La Greca, L. J. Siegel, J. L. Wallander, & C. E. Walker (Eds.), *Stress and coping in child health* (pp. 371–399). New York: Guilford Press.

Olson, R. A., Holden, E. W., Friedman, A., Faust, J., Kenning, M., & Mason, P. J. (1989). Psychological consultation in a children's hospital: An evaluation of services. *Journal of Pediatric Psychology, 13,* 479–482.

Roberts, M. C., & Hurley, L. K. (1997). *Managing managed case.* New York: Plenum Press.

Schroeder, C. S., & Mann, J. (1991). A model for clinical child practice. In C. S. Schroeder & B. N. Gordon (Eds.), *Assessment and treatment of childhood problems: A clinician's guide* (pp. 375–398). New York: Guilford Press.

Singer, L., & Drotar, D. (1989). Psychological practice in a pediatric rehabilitation hospital. *Journal of Pediatric Psychology, 14,* 479–489.

Thompson, R. J., Jr. (1987). Psychologists in medical schools: Medical staff status and clinical privileges. *American Psychologist, 42,* 866–868.

Thompson, R. J., Jr. (1991). Psychology and the health care system: Characteristics and transactions. In J. J. Sweet, R. H. Rosensky, & S. M. Tovian (Eds.), *Handbook of clinical psychology in medi-*

cal settings (pp. 11–25). New York: Plenum Press.

Walders, N., & Drotar, D. (1999). Integrating mental health services in the care of children and adolescents with chronic health conditions: Assumptions, challenges, and opportunities. *Chil-*

dren's Services: Social Policy, Research, and Practice, 2, 117–138.

Weisz, J. R., & Hawley, K. M. (1998). Finding, evaluating, refining and applying empirically supported treatments for children and adolescents. *Journal of Clinical Child Psychology, 27,* 217–226.

PART III

Preventive
Interventions

6

VICTOR J. BERNSTEIN
SALLY CAMPBELL
ADRIENNE AKERS

Caring for the Caregivers

Supporting the Well-Being of At-Risk Parents and Children through Supporting the Well-Being of the Programs That Serve Them

In the study of children born at environmental risk, one of the most widely replicated findings is that a nurturing relationship between the child and his or her primary caretaker protects the child from the powerful negative influences of being born into concentrated poverty (Rutter, 1990; Werner & Smith, 1992). This finding holds for poverty and its many associated risk conditions, such as adolescent parenting and parental substance abuse. Strengthening the parent-child relationship is now a primary program goal of a wide variety of primary prevention and early intervention programs (Barnard, Morisset, & Spieker, 1993; Bernstein, Hans, & Percansky, 1991; Bromwich, 1997; Paulsen, 1993; Van Breman & Graziano, 1997; Weston, Ivins, Heffron, & Sweet, 1997). Increasingly, home visiting and family support program personnel are beginning to recognize that direct service staff (primarily home visitors) need to develop a positive, supportive relationship with the parents if they are to be of help to children (Barnard & Morisset, 1995; Bernstein, Percansky, & Weschler, 1996).

Developing such a relationship is easier said than done. Because poverty packs tremendous power, information and education programs targeting poor families often are ineffective (Mahoney, Boyce, Fewell, Spiker, & Wheeden, 1998; Seitz, 1990). Not surprisingly, just like many families, these programs may become swept up by many of the problems associated with poverty. Rather than keeping the focus on the well-being of the child and nurturing parent-child relationships, program staff become distracted by the families' immediate needs and lose sight of their priorities. Home visitors who try to help families cope with their multitude of problems gradually begin to resonate with these problems. This pattern typically evolves in the following manner. As one family problem gets resolved (e.g., getting emergency food stamps), another problem follows right behind (e.g., the family being evicted). Parents learn to expect that their interactions with program staff (i.e., their home visitors and their supervisors) will center on problems. This pattern follows the behavioral adage, "You get what you attend to." Not surprisingly, parents become predisposed to sharing problems with home visitors. Consequently, home visitors have more problems with which to deal. Although it is considered "best practice" in family support programs to focus on family strengths (Weissbourd, 1990), another serious consequence of adopting a crisis orientation and problem-solving approach is that staff and parents are drawn to what is wrong with the family rather than to what is going well. Problem solving and a crisis orientation can exhaust home visitors. A well-documented characteristic of preventive intervention programs is high staff turnover (Daro & Harding, 1999; Gomby, Culross, & Behrman, 1999). Whereas this characteristic is often thought to be the result of low salaries, exit interviews reveal that the primary cause of departure is stress-related burnout. Stress is the enemy of nurturing.

Just as some families raise children successfully while living in poverty, some programs seem to survive the day-to-day stresses of working with at-risk families better than others. In order to maintain more positive energy, programs must not lose sight of the importance of nurturing and of identifying and building on strengths. Given the forces of risk, how can this be accomplished? The same supportive, nurturing relationships (e.g., between home visitor and parent, social worker and parent, or teacher and parent) can support growth and change both in the parent and in the parent-child relationship. This multilevel modeling of nurturing is referred to as parallel process (Fenichel, 1992; Musick, Bernstein, Percansky, & Stott, 1987; Wall, 1994; Weston, Ivins, Heffron, & Sweet, 1997). Jeree Pawl described the parallel process as "Do unto others as you would have others do unto others" (Pawl & St. John, 1998, p. 7).

The purpose of this chapter is to describe the experiences of two training programs that support home visiting through on-site training and that create a nurturing supervisory environment by focusing on relationships and building on strengths. The training model is based on the Ounce of Prevention Fund Developmental Training and Support Program (DTSP; Bernstein, Percansky, & Weschler, 1996), which began in 1986 in Chicago, Illinois. Since that time, three trainers, Victor Bernstein, Candice Percansky, and Nick Weschler, have worked with 24 Ounce of Prevention Fund programs that annually serve more than two thousand teenage mothers and their children in Illinois. The DTSP has been adapted to primary prevention, early intervention, and drug treatment programs. For this chapter, we first describe the theoretical underpinnings of the DTSP and the initial training. Then we present two adaptations of the DTSP: (1) a training of trainers implemented in Utah and (2) a training of supervisors implemented in Washington, D.C. We present the work of the Utah State University Early Intervention Research Institute Promoting Resilient Outcomes program (in Logan, Utah) (PRO; Akers & Bernstein, 1998) and the Healthy Families America National Capital Area Consortium (DCHFA; Campbell, Gray, Earley, & Bernstein, 1999) in Washington, D.C.

This chapter is based on four premises:

1. The major source for growth and change in young children is the experience of nurturing relationships. This type of relationship makes the child feel special and valued rather than ignored, taken for granted, or burdensome to the parent.
2. Home visiting staff must enter into supportive, nurturing relationships with parents and their extended families if they are to support growth and change in the parent and in the parent-child relationship.
3. The experience of supportive nurturing relationships in the workplace enhances the ability of program staff to enter into supportive, nurturing relationships with families. Reflective supervision, peer support, and training provide the fuel to support and nurture home visitors.
4. Program supervisors and managers need to experience the same nurturing, supportive relationships if they are to be able to support and nurture their home visiting staff.

These premises make up the power of nurturing relationships in parallel. In the rest of this chapter, we describe the parallels between what happens during staff training and supervision and what happens when home visiting staff apply this model of nurturing and building on strengths in their work with families.

Risk and Resilience in the Parent-Child Relationship

Environmental risk factors associated with poverty, such as crime, unemployment, single parenting, poor education or intellectual ability, substance abuse, domestic violence, sexual abuse, child abuse and neglect, and poor health and prenatal care, have all been linked to an overall increase in developmental problems. In young children these poverty-related multiple risks have been associated with developmental delays and maladaptive insecure attachment to the primary caregiver (Halpern, 1993; Wallach & Caulfield, 1998). For school-aged children, multiple risks are linked to continued developmental delays, school failure, and juvenile delinquency (Meisels & Wasik, 1990; Wakschlag & Hans, 1999). By the time these children exposed to environmental risk reach adolescence, they are more likely to become high school dropouts and teenage parents, to have emotional and behavioral problems, and to be involved with the criminal justice system (Osofsky, 1990; Sameroff, Seifer, Baldwin, & Baldwin, 1993). As adults, many of these same problems continue, and others are added into the mix, such as welfare dependence and health problems (Rutter, 1990; Werner & Smith, 1992). In other words, many children born into poverty grow into adults who transform environmental risk factors into behavioral reality.

Environmental risk factors operate to limit the parent-child relationship by reducing the parent's and the child's capabilities to respond positively to one another (Bernstein, Hans, & Percansky, 1991). These early maladaptive patterns of interactions can prevent the child from developing a sense of self as effective, of being one who can make a difference in the world. A central goal of early intervention is to support the development of a nurturing relationship between the child and the primary caretaker, one in which the child is made to feel special.

How does the nurturing parent-child relationship protect the child from environmental risk? The importance of the parent-child relationship to development has come, in large part, from the study of attachment—the affectional tie with the caregiver that develops and becomes observable around the time of the infant's first birthday (Ainsworth, Blehar, Waters, & Wall, 1978). Secure attachment is the first step to social competence. Infants who develop secure attachments to their mothers in the first year of life are found to be more competent as toddlers and preschoolers in peer interaction, exploration, and play behavior and are more enthusiastic and persistent in approaching problem-solving tasks. They show higher levels of ego resilience and increased social competence through age 6. They are better able to form appropriate relationships with peers and to positively engage adults as young adolescents (Urban, Carlson, Egeland, & Sroufe, 1991). Furthermore, problematic, disorganized attachment in infancy and toddlerhood has been shown to be related to the manifestation of psychopathology during later adolescence (Carlson, 1998).

What kinds of child behaviors indicate that the child is becoming socially competent? A competent young child approaches the parent for relief from stress, and, after a brief refueling from the parent's attention, the child is able to resume play, exploration, and positive social interaction. When not upset, the child organizes play around the parent and initiates positive interaction with a look, smile, gesture, touch, or language. What are the kinds of parental behaviors that support the development of social competence? A parent's prompt and sensitive response to the child's needs is the critical factor that fosters secure attachment (Blehar, Lieberman, & Ainsworth, 1977; De Wolff & van Ijzendoorn, 1997). Additional parental characteristics, such as warmth, affection, and having accurate developmental expectations, also have been found to be associated with other positive developmental outcomes (Bernstein & Hans, 1994). Note that these are the same kinds of observable behaviors that characterize a nurturing relationship.

Through the consistency of the parent's caring involvement, the child learns that his or her behavior makes a difference, that is, the child experiences success in affecting the environment. These successes sharpen the child's behavior as he or she learns how to generate the desired response from the parent. The child learns to expect that the parent will respond in the desired way; this is the essence of trust (Erikson, 1963). As the child recognizes the parent's role in meeting his or her needs, the child begins to anticipate and initiate interaction. In this way, the parent can recognize that her or his efforts to respond to the child are on target. Just as the parent makes the child feel special through creating a sense of self-efficacy in the child, the child makes the parent feel special by showing that parental efforts made a difference. Parents gain confidence and develop in their role through their successes in communicating with and supporting their infant.

To support parent-child relationships, all program staff first need to know how to observe parent-child interaction. Based on the research cited here, Susan Goldberg's (1977) theoretical construct, mutual competence — the development of increasingly effective communication in the interaction between parent and infant — provides a useful lens for observing parent-child interaction (Figure 6.1). Mutual competence is defined as any interchange in which the parent and child (1) feel secure, (2) feel valued, (3) feel successful, (4) are happy, or (5) enjoy learning together. Such interactions are good for the development of both the child and the parent. Program

Question: What type of communication between parent and child is good for the development of the child and of the parent?

Answer: Any interaction which enables both the parent and child to feel secure, valued, successful, and happy or to enjoy learning.

	Behaviors observed that are supportive of mutual competence strengths	Behaviors we need to know more about: Those not observed or not consistent with the mutual development of mutual competence concerns	What could you say (or do)? Ask questions—Gather more information Make positive comments Do more observation
CHILD			
PARENT			

FIGURE 6.1   Mutual Competence Model for Parent-Child Interaction (after Susan Goldberg, 1977)

staff easily learn to observe parent-child interaction in an objective manner through the lens of mutual competence. This skill becomes essential for increasing the parents' recognition and realization of important aspects of their interaction and supports the development of a nurturing relationship. Home visiting staff record their observations on a 2 by 3 mutual competence grid. They write down actual behaviors that represent examples of a mutually competent, nurturing relationship for both the child and the parent (Column I). They then record their concerns about either the parent or child (Column II). Finally, they record what they might say to highlight this observation of strengths in the parent-child relationship (Column III). These forms are used in supervision and team meetings. Some home visitors find it helpful to use the grid with parents as they look at a "home movie" videotape together.

Building a Nurturing Program: Training and Supervision

This section is derived from the DTSP training experience and describes the initial training and supervisory model that is referred to as the mutual competence model.

For a program to support the growth and development of the parent-child relationship, home visitors must learn how to create a "safe place" for their work with the family where nurturing can occur, one that is not constantly bombarded by the family's problems associated with living in poverty. A program must be able to nurture its home visitors so they in turn can nurture the parents, who in turn become fortified to nurture their children in the face of multiple stresses. How does a program accomplish this feat? One does not learn to develop nurturing relationships with families through reading about them or going to a conference to hear a speaker talk about them. The way to learn about relationships is to experience them and to reflect on them.

Programs that build on strengths within the family and the parent-child relationship are characterized by three critical elements. The first is *ongoing relationship-based training* that must include staff from all levels of the program. All levels of personnel need to participate if the training is to be translated into new program activities that are sustained after training ends. Training provides the foundation for identifying the principles that underlie the relationship-based work with families and the experience of and insight into the nature of nurturing. The training also provides regular opportunities for all staff to take a step back, draw a deep breath, and reflect. Home visitors have the opportunity to share with one another what is most effective and to consider what other ideas and new approaches they would like to try next with a family. The second critical element is a *paradigm shift*, in which the program begins to evolve from a focus on family problems to a focus on strengths in the child, parent, mother, family, home visitors, supervisors, and program managers. The third critical element is *regular, reflective, relationship-based supervision* (Fenichel, 1992) throughout all levels of the program to help sustain home visitors in their work with families (Campbell, Gray, Earley, & Bernstein, 1999). All three of these elements are central to best practice for prevention and intervention programs (Gomby, Culross, & Behrman, 1999; Weissbourd, 1990).

Supervision is the necessary mechanism for ensuring that training becomes translated into practice. Supervision can take many forms, for example, individual or group, hierarchical or peer. But all program staff must experience supervision on a regular basis in order to limit the disorganizing power of stress that directs program staff toward problems and problem-solving and away from strengths in the family, in the parent-child relationship, and in the child. A supportive, nurturing supervisory relationship is as critical to the growth and change in home visitors as nurturing is for the parent and child. Training provides the initial element of the nurturing parallel process. It is a forum in which all staff interact as peers, support one another, reflect together on their work, and focus on strengths.

In the first training session participants are asked to consider the meaning of the word *nurturing*. A discussion ensues about how a nurturing relationship protects a child from environmental risk. Trainees are then instructed, "Think about a nurturing relationship in your own lives, one that makes you feel special. It can be with a parent, grandparent, spouse, partner, friend, teacher, or a child. It does not matter with whom you experienced this. It's about specialness. Think about a time you spent together." After a minute or two of silent meditation trainees are then asked, "What did it feel like to do that?" Most often we hear comments such as "peaceful," "happy," and "secure." They are asked for words to further describe that relationship. Typical responses included *affectionate touch, acceptance, encouragement, belief in me, confidence, support, unconditional love, respect, trust, marvel, wonder, one-on-one time, affirmation, safety, warmth, understanding, being listened to, fun, comfort, communication,* and *caring.*

Following this sharing, the trainer summarizes by saying, "This is what it means to focus on strengths." Then the trainer says, "But here's the punch line. *Please note that nobody said, 'Someone who told me what to do or someone who gave me advice.'"* We usually get a few chuckles or gasps following this exercise, which often evokes an "aha!" experience for many participants. In other words, a focus on problem solving does not feel nurturing. To nurture is to make ready and to support growth. The purpose of nurturing is not to direct, make, or force a person to do something. The person must be free to grow as he or she will from a base of support. Nurturing provides a "holding environment" for personal and professional growth.

One notion trainees find helpful is applying the parallel process to a discussion of the difference between nurturing and caretaking. When parents are asked, "What do you think it means to be a good parent?" they generally reply, "Keeping the child safe, well cared for, and healthy." In other words, they view attending to the child's basic needs as their central role. Nurturing, that is, attending to their child's social and emotional needs, is often not a central part of their view of their role as parents. When parents are asked about nurturing, they say, "Of course all parents love their children." But parents do not necessarily think it is important that the child experience love directly; the children will just know it is there. Similarly, any staff person's focus on problem solving is the parallel to a parent's focus on providing care. It is something concrete they know they can do for the parent, and home visitors are good at problem solving. During training, home visitors now want to learn more about how to nurture families. This is the beginning of the paradigm shift away from problem solving and to a clearer focus on the parent-child relationship, as well as on their relationship with the family. In supervision, the parallel continues. For example, caretaking has to do with memos, time sheets, vacations, paperwork, and so forth. A nurturing supervisory relationship is regular (i.e., not canceled), reflective, and collaborative rather than critical. It builds on the expertise of the home visitor, not the supervisor.

Two concepts are used in training to help home visitors and supervisors learn how to enter nurturing relationships with one another:

1. The stages of the helping relationship. The stages represent the parallel of a mutually competent, nurturing parent-child relationship. For a detailed discussion of these stages see Bernstein, Percansky, and Weschler (1996, pp. 121–123).
2. Observation and inquiry as intervention.

Stages of the Helping Relationship

Stage 1. *Recruitment and Orientation / Defining Expectations*   During training, home visitors learn the importance of explaining the goals and setting the expectations and rules for program participation to families. This stage defines what topics are legitimate for the program to address. We suggest that programs prepare a brochure to distribute during recruitment. For example, it could be titled "Our Program Helps Build Strong Parent-Child Relationships." This emphasis on parent-child relationships early on helps to legitimize the importance of focusing on this during home visits as opposed to a focus on problem solving.

Stage 2. *Acceptance*   If a particular belief, activity, or child-rearing practice has not been defined by the program as being unacceptable (such as selling drugs during a home visit), then program staff are obligated to accept what the family chooses to do. Acceptance becomes the foundation of nurturing, of mutual trust and respect, and of growth and change.

Stage 3. *Shared Understanding*   Through discussion of the home visitor's observations about the parent and child, both the parent and visitor will increase their understanding of both the child's and the parent's behavior. This task is accomplished by using "observation and inquiry as intervention," which is described in greater detail later in this chapter.

Stage 4. *The Family Service Plan*   Once the home visitor and the family have gone through the stages previously outlined, they will be ready to mutually agree on a plan of action. The plan includes agreed-upon goals and methods for supporting positive, mutually satisfying parent-child communication. The parent's goals must form the basis for the plan if it is to be successful.

Stage 5. *Accountability*   With the goal and plan from Stage 4 in place, home visitors are now in a position to follow up and monitor. There should be continuity from one visit to the next to review what the parent has identified as being important. The visitor needs to remember to inquire about progress. The goals should be regularly discussed, evaluated, and revised as needed.

In parallel, these same stages apply to the nurturing supervisory relationship. Consistent with the parallel process, simply substitute "home visitor" for "parent" and "supervisor" for "home visitor." There are subtle differences, but the process is the same. For example, home visitors need to be clearly oriented to the program's goals and expectations. Just as home visitors write anecdotal records after each visit, supervisors need to do the same after each supervisory session to ensure continuity from one supervision session to the next. Supervisors cannot allow themselves to be distracted by a discussion of a family's problems and must keep the focus on inquiring about the worker's observations and inquiries about strengths in parent-child relationships. Supervisors must remember to ask about parent-child interaction. If the home visitors know that they will be asked about this in supervision, they will learn to prepare for such questions. In a nurturing supervisory relationship, the supervisor encourages the worker to provide a clear description of what exactly transpired during a visit with the family. This provides a window into his or her work with families so both can see more clearly. Next the supervisor and home visitor compare what is working best with what is not going as well. By comparing the strength with a problem, they try to understand what makes something work, that is, the reason for the difference between what is working and what is not. The home visitor decides how to apply this understanding to the next encounter with the family. This is what is meant by building on strengths. As noted, in the next supervision session, they review how things went.

Observation and Inquiry as Intervention

This technique for discussion of observations applies to both focusing on strengths and exploring concerns. Through this technique of focusing on strengths, parents come to realize how important everyday nurturing interchanges are to the child's development. To focus on strengths, we begin by noticing something positive the child is doing. For example, the home visitor might say, "He sure quieted down fast when you picked him up. How did you know that was what he wanted?" Through discussion of this positive transaction, parents solidify their ownership of positive interchanges with the child and are less likely to take nurturing for granted. Notice that although a positive interchange is acknowledged, home visitors try not to praise parents for doing the right thing. If we can praise, we can also criticize. This type of communication puts home visitors in a position of being judgmental, which works against the parent's feeling accepted and nurtured. We want the parent to feel successful and believe the experience will be more powerful if the parent sees it on her own rather than because we point it out or praise it.

Sometimes home visitors observe something that concerns them. To accept parents does not mean that home visitors necessarily have to agree with what the parent chooses to do. Disagreement should stimulate "inquiry as intervention" rather than problem-solving "fix-it" behavior on the part of the home visitor. The following principle, based on the pioneering work of Rose Bromwich (1997), guides our work: If you hear or see something that concerns you, don't try to fix it. Instead, gather more information through observation, discussion, or questions. When observations are of concern to a home visitor, they learn to ask the family to help them understand what was happening. Home visitors learn to raise their concerns with families in the following ways: "I noticed. . . . Did you notice that too? What do you think your child was trying to tell you? . . . What did you mean when you said . . . ?" "What made you decide to. . . . ?" Thus the first reaction to a concern is to use inquiry as a springboard to further understanding. Over and over we have seen that using this process of inquiry causes parents to reflect on how they think and behave. Insight and new understanding often leads parents to consider what they might do instead and can be a harbinger of change. For inquiry as intervention to be effective, home visitors must be genuinely interested in the parent's point of view rather than trying to get them to do what the home visitor feels is best. Importantly, hearing the parent's point of view serves the same purpose for home visitors. Often workers, based on their values, beliefs, and experience, can misinterpret the parent's behavior. This approach is meant to put the parents in the role of expert on their own family.

After parents have shared their point of view, the home visitor is in a legitimate position to address his or her original concern. Having observed, discussed, and inquired about a particular subject of concern, it becomes natural — as part of conversation and follow-up to the parent's sharing — to present alternative points of view, that is, a home visitor may share his or her experiences, information, and expertise with families. Insight from gathering information thus provides home visitors with the opportunity to share knowledge, opinions, and expertise. This sharing happens sensitively and is delivered in context rather than by being didactic or judgmental. Similarly, supervisors will become more effective if they use observation (primarily of what the home visitor has to say) and inquiry (to help the supervisor understand exactly what was happening) before moving in the direction of a plan or solution. The best course of action in dealing with a concern usually comes from home visitors when supervision has provided them a clearer understanding of the family and the home visitor–family relationship.

Training of Trainers — Replicating the DTSP: The PRO Project

The following description provides an example of how two trainers, a physical therapist and a psychologist, both trained in the implementation of the DTSP, adapted and carried out the DTSP training at two programs serving families living in poverty in Utah. A federal grant, called Promoting Resilient Outcome (PRO), attempted to replicate the model of mutual competence within two existing home visiting programs in Utah. One of the major outcomes of the PRO intervention was the development of secure attachment between mothers and their infants. The PRO study used a mixed-methods, quasi-experimental design to examine the effects of training and home visiting intervention on the families being served. Preliminary process and outcome data are presented in the following pages.

One of the chapter authors (Bernstein) served as a consultant for the project staff throughout the grant period (1996–1999) to provide support for the local adaptation and application of the model. Briefly, the two Utah home visiting programs provided services and support for environmentally at-risk women and their infants. Generally, the home visitors were bachelor's-level staff or were experienced nondegreed community helpers. However, the two programs differed on several dimensions. For example, the programs were not affiliated with one another and had different funding patterns and different foci for children and families. One PRO staff trainer was assigned to each of the two programs. Each trainer had the responsibility for preparing the training sessions, overheads, and handouts for the specific site. The "site trainer" was also responsible for developing positive, mutually competent relationships with the program supervisor and home visitors over the course of the training sessions. At each site, three-hour monthly workshops were conducted for a period of one year.

The PRO trainers worked with master's-level program supervisors to support the parallel use of the model of mutual competence within supervisory and staff peer relationships, home visitor-parent relationships, and parent-infant relationships. Gradually, as the training progressed, the torch was passed from trainer to supervisor and home visitors. Following each workshop, trainees were asked to fill out a brief written evaluation, using the following questions:

1. What new ideas and/or concepts did you learn today?
2. What would have made today's session better?
3. What would you like to learn more about in future sessions?

Following the sessions, the trainer would review the comments and incorporate input from all the trainees, home visitors and supervisors, into the next workshop. The subsequent session began with a group review of both homework assignments and the comments from the written workshop evaluations. Gradually, staff began to learn that their input and participation was a valued part of the workshops in a parallel way to the way it is hoped that parents will come to understand that their input during home visits is important and valued.

To support the gradual incorporation of the model, trainees were asked to carry out simple homework assignments. For their initial assignments, home visitors were asked to begin with a family with whom they felt they already had a good relationship rather than picking a more problematic one. Supervisors were encouraged to follow up on the assignments with home visitors between workshops. This helped the supervisors develop their ability to focus on *what was going right* with their home visitors, just as they hope the visitors will do with their families. The purpose of the homework assignments was to gradually enlarge the home visitors' focus in the home to watch for and support mutually competent interactions between the parent and infant. The first homework assignment was simply to observe a parent and child and write down a few examples of interactions that were supportive of mutual competence and also those they may have had concerns about. For the second month, the assignment was to make at least one comment about the child's behavior that brought a smile to the parent's face. For example, when the newborn turned to his mother's voice, the home visitor might have said, "Did you see how he turned his head when he heard your voice? Oh, he really knows you!" For the third month, home visitors were asked to discuss some positive aspect of the child's behavior with the parent. For the fourth month, trainees were asked to encourage a parent to share a concern about the child and to make a plan together to address it. In the fifth month, the trainees were asked to carry out a joint developmental screening, such as the Denver II (Frankenburg & Dodds, 1990) or the Ages and Stages Questionnaire (Squires, Potter, & Bricker, 1995). The parent served as coadministrator in order to support both the parent's understanding of her child's development and her self-confidence.

In subsequent sessions, staff were encouraged to review the policies and procedures of their program to see how they could begin to build the model of mutual competence into all aspects of their program. During this process, the real transformation began to emerge, as supervisor and home visitors decided how to integrate the model within the components of their particular work setting. In the PRO project, one of the programs redesigned its brochure to describe the importance of building positive parent-child relationships as an overall goal of the program. Another site redesigned its home visiting forms to include a focus on *what was going right* within the parent-child relationship.

It is important to note that the exact order and focus of these assignments may vary, particularly when a program has additional constraints or staff requirements. An underlying goal of this type of training and supervision is that staff come to expect that they have something to share during the training sessions and that they begin to learn from sharing their experiences. In the PRO project, staff began to define what they as individuals needed to pay attention to in terms of positive aspects of parent-child communication, as well as to become more aware of their own biases. Trainers attempted to incorporate ideas generated in the discussion into the next homework assignment. Most assignments incorporated activities that required home visitors and supervisors to review their work as a group between training sessions. This practice of building peer supervision into team meetings created a program structure that paralleled the training and facilitated the program's focus on the mutual competence model. Prior to the initiation of the workshops, PRO staff sat in on team staffings at both sites. These sessions typically began with staff reports on the current crises in the families on their caseload. As the workshops progressed, the trainees realized that the model encouraged a format in which team staffings should begin with each person sharing a recent positive (i.e., mutually competent) experience he or she had with a family. Ideally, these staff experiences would have already been reviewed during supervision, which also begins with a review of what has been going right rather than what has been going wrong during home visits. The focus on positive home visiting experiences was intended to parallel how staff members can help parents focus on positive aspects of parent-child interaction, rather than on crises.

The training process and homework activities spanned a 12-month period. The first eight sessions, conducted over a minimum of six months, provided the informational and skill-building aspect of the training. The rest of the year was spent refining these skills and gradually implementing them into the program's practices. At first, home visitors were encouraged to implement the model with families with whom they felt most comfortable. Later, as new families entered services, home visitors began incorporating the mutual competence model when introducing their program, emphasizing its new focus during the orientation phase. Eventually, home visitors began to implement their refined practices with their newest participants. Only when home visitors felt that they had mastered specific skills discussed during workshop sessions and piloted with families with whom they had good relationships would they then try to implement the key program practices with families who had a more problematic history. Families who were enrolled in services before the training began, and who therefore were not oriented to the "new and improved" purpose of the program, were brought on board more gradually.

Home Visiting Tools

During training, home visitors learn to use two primary tools to help parents increase their insight into both their children's and their own behavior. The first is developmental demonstrations. It is important that parents develop empathy with and have accurate expectations of their children. We engage parents in being "codemonstrators." During the newborn period, the Family Administered Newborn Activities demonstration (FANA; Cardone & Gilkerson, 1989) is used to help parents recognize their infants' capabilities. Parents interact more when they realize their newborns can hear and see them. Parents of older children also participate in administering a developmental screening, such as the Denver Developmental Screening Test (Frankenburg & Dodds, 1990). This experience orients parents to the concept that development is sequential and that children learn through play. They become eager to help children master the next steps and become more involved in playing with them.

The second tool is the use of "home movies" (Bernstein, 1997). Home visitors learn to make videotapes of parents and children at least twice a year. Using the camera to *shine a light* on parent-child interaction, the program communicates that its goal of supporting the parent-child relationship is a program priority. Because most interaction between parents and children typically occurs during everyday routines, home visitors videotape everyday activities, such as mealtime or dressing, in contrast to asking the parent to play with the child. Home visitors refrain from talking while taping. The primary purpose of making home movies is to bring a smile to the parent's face when the tapes are viewed at a later time with the home visitor. Most important, the home movie is primarily for *fun and enjoyment*, rather than as an opportunity to scrutinize parent-child interaction. Watching the movie together during the next visit helps to underscore, for both the parent and home visitor, the parent's ability to understand and support the child's efforts. Most parents enjoy the results and appreciate being given a copy of the videotape as a remembrance. When home visitors and parents view the tapes together, the overall goal is for the parent to see the positive things the child is doing and to realize what an important contribution the parent is making to the child's development. This is accomplished by using "observation and inquiry," especially at times when the parent laughs—a signal that something enjoyable or positive has caught the parent's attention.

Outcomes: Progress and Problems

After 12 months of training, the two PRO sites differed in the degree to which each one was able to incorporate the training and technical assistance into its overall purpose and practices. One site successfully revamped its home visiting forms so that visits were begun by asking the parent to relate a positive experience she has had with her child since the last visit. This site has also restructured its team staffings to reflect the model's emphasis on building strong relationships. The supervisor at this site actively sought new ways to infuse the model in all aspects of the program and agreed to serve as a workshops facilitator at other programs interested in learning about the model. At the second site, the program brochure was rewritten to emphasize its focus on building positive relationships between parent and child, in addition to case management and resource referral. Almost all staff were initially enthusiastic about the model, but several programmatic challenges stymied future attempts by the supervisor to incorporate other aspects of the model into the program. Specifically, the program's funding was cut significantly, and several home visitors left to take other jobs. The program supervisor's time was drawn away from supervision to fixing the program's problems by trying to write grants to increase the program's funding base. The process of implementing other aspects of the model into the program was slowed down due to these unexpected challenges.

As part of its overall process evaluation, the PRO project used an independent researcher with strong ethnographic training as an outside evaluator to interview and summarize the impact of the training on the supervisors and home visitors at both sites. Focused interviews on the impact of the training were conducted with all staff members at both sites. The report (Eastmond, 1999) indicated that "the PRO Project effectively captured the loyalty of the majority of participants in the workshop series. The idea of the . . . model and accompanying practices appear to have been well internalized by most program site personnel." It was also noted that the site's underlying program philosophy had an impact on the depth of adoption of the model and on the relationships developed among program staff.

The project also collected longitudinal Time 1 and Time 2 child and family descriptive and outcome data to date, with Time 3 data to be completed in the later half of 2000. Preliminary analyses of outcomes have been disappointing. The results do not indicate more positive outcomes on attachment for the experimental group over the comparison group. Initial findings yielded a concern about the comparability of the groups in that the experimental group had a greater occurrence of multiple risk factors. It should be noted that the training phase of the grant put the site staff in the position of having to "hit the ground running"—that is, the children and families they served were being assessed at the same time the staff was being trained in the model. The possibility that this study was investigating an immature intervention cannot be discounted. Upon completion of the final round of data collection, more sophisticated analyses will be executed. The final results of the PRO study will be forthcoming on completion.

Supporting Supervisors—Washington, D.C., Area Healthy Families Consortium (DCHFA)

In more than four hundred programs across the United States, Healthy Families America (HFA)[1] programs work to strengthen the relationships between vulnerable parents and their young children. Based on the Healthy Start program, which originated in Hawaii in the early 1970s, and is now supported by public-private partnerships in many states, HFA uses degreed and nondegreed professional home visitors called Family Support Workers (FSWs) to assess the strengths and needs of families of newborns and provide ongoing comprehensive support services for up to five years. This national model has drawn from best practice standards for family support (e.g., being family centered and strength based) and from recent research findings from effective early intervention programs. Initial and ongoing training of staff and regular, consistent professional supervision are integral to the model and well defined in Healthy Families credentialing standards. HFA guidelines suggest two hours of individual supervision per week. Supervisors are master's-level personnel or experienced bachelor's-level personnel. In theory, supervision is designed to reflect a "parallel process" of the work that is being done in the home. As FSWs build trusting and nurturing relationships with families to support the growing relationship between the parent and child, program supervisors build supportive and trusting relationships with FSWs. It is this nurturing supervisory relationship which allows FSWs the foundation and experience from which to provide relationship-based direct service.

HFA's initial training is intensive and well designed. It provides a strong theoretical background for FSWs and supervisors that highlights the importance of parent-child interaction and of building resiliency in children at risk. It also stresses the limited effectiveness of a problem-solving, case management approach for families when program goals are to support parents to nurture healthy development in their young children.

Although the initial "core" training for FSWs was effective, HFA programs in the Washington, D.C., area had difficulty maintaining a focus on parent-child interaction in the months following the core training. The very real, everyday crises — such as a parent losing a job, being evicted from a home, using drugs and alcohol, or living with an abusive spouse — took precedence over plans to promote parent-child interaction on home visits. FSWs experienced minor victories in assisting families to stave off one crisis after another but struggled with a sense of inadequacy in the face of multiple problems. The forces of risk for families and for FSWs were too strong to allow the focus to remain on the parent-child relationship.

Similarly, supervisors struggled with supporting overwhelmed FSWs. Feeling overwhelmed themselves, supervisors felt most competent when they had helped resolve a crisis successfully. All wondered how to help FSWs find the time to work on the developmental curriculum and activities designed to strengthen parent-child interaction. Babies were often asleep when the home visitors arrived, their parents anxious to talk to the FSW about the latest developments in the problems facing the family. Home visitors were tired and struggled with burnout, their supervisors were frustrated and feeling inadequate. Home visiting rates were low, and FSWs found it difficult to complete developmental screenings on time. Occasional victories were not enough to sustain them and keep them motivated. Concern grew that the children were getting lost in the work. FSWs and supervisors remembered the importance of supporting parent-child interaction from the training, but they were unable to sustain it as part of their work.

Program Support for Supervisors

In January 1998, the Washington, D.C., Area Consortium of HFA programs had a unique opportunity to develop and implement a training and support program to help FSWs and supervisors aid families in staying focused on nurturing their young children. In designing this project, sites decided to focus the effort on supervisors. Whereas FSWs received a significant amount of ongoing training, supervisors were often left on their own following their initial training. With technical assistance from the Zero To Three Cornerstone Project and the generous support of a private donor, 10 Healthy Families programs in the Washington, D.C., metropolitan area worked with Victor Bernstein to train FSWs and develop an ongoing training and support system for supervisors. The mission of Zero to Three is to strengthen and support families, practitioners, and communities to promote the healthy development of young children.

The project began with full-day training (described previously) for all staff and six half-day sessions for program supervisors throughout the spring. The sessions have continued with monthly 2½-hour sessions for supervisors facilitated by Healthy Families Alexandria program manager Sally Campbell and Maryland-based child development specialist and psychologist Brenda Jones Harden (at the time of this writing, sessions have been ongoing for more than 2½ years).

A Developmental Process

The learning took place in stages. The goal of the first half-day sessions with supervisors was to develop skills in staying focused on parent-child interaction by creating an experience of mutual competence. Supervisors were excited about the process. The first two months of sessions with supervisors were given over primarily to their venting about their frustrations with the work. Although this stage was unexpected, it was crucial to the success of the project. Just like families in the programs, supervisors were struggling against the forces of risk. Although they strongly believed in the importance of focusing on what was working and of building on strengths, the supervisors were overwhelmed with the demands of too little time, too much to do, and too few resources. Supervision time was constantly interrupted by program demands; FSWs were tired and needy. Supervisors were overburdened with too many differing tasks, felt a lack of support, and looked forward to peer training sessions as an opportunity to vent frustrations. It was hard to change thinking from what the problem was to what was working (i.e., to make the paradigm shift). Learning a new model is difficult. It is time-consuming and feels awkward at first, like learning to write with the opposite hand. It took time for trusting relationships to develop and for supervisors to be willing to risk doing something that initially made everyone feel a little inept. But everyone kept coming. One supervisor said, "It was the first time I felt nurtured in a long time and it felt good. I realized that I was on to something powerful right from the start."

Bringing the Baby Back into the Work

The second stage was bringing the baby back into the work. This meant shifting the emphasis away from problem solving to focusing on the relationship between the parent and the child, both in home visits and in supervision. Although supervisors understood the importance of making this shift, it was hard to do given the real daily crises and other distractions in supervision. No one quite knew how to do it. One creative supervisor made a sign that read "THE BABY!! WHAT DID THE BABY DO?" and hung it on the wall in her office to remind herself to ask about the baby during supervision sessions.

After four months of working together, the real breakthrough came when sites purchased video equipment and visitors started to make videotapes of parent-child interaction on home visits. As each site started to use their cameras, the supervisors came back to monthly meetings beaming. It was fun! Fun to watch, fun for families, for home visitors, and for supervisors. It turned out that lurking among the families' problems were wonderful things that happened on home visits, wonderful moments between parents and children. Because they had a tool to observe them, FSWs learned how to identify the simple, everyday interactions between parents and children that constitute a nurturing relationship. The videotapes had an almost magical quality of making families' abilities to nurture their children more observable and concrete. They allowed parents an opportunity to see their children responding to them and gave FSWs and supervisors an opportunity to capture those moments and build on them. What they could observe, they could support. Sharing the good things, looking for competence instead of problems, resulted in everyone feeling more competent and hopeful. Program staff started to develop a new confidence and expertise in "observing" parent-child interaction.

Viewing home movies gave supervisors a real and tangible way to support parent-child interaction work in supervision, and over the next six months, the work started to shift from theory to practice. Supervisors began to use the mutual competence grid while viewing videos to help FSWs focus on families' competencies and plan for future home visits. Both supervisors and FSWs began to build skills in using "Inquiry as Intervention" as a tool to discuss areas of concern and build on parents' expertise with their children. Supervisors began to help FSWs understand the parent's perspective before offering their own expertise or information. This approach promoted a more strength-based, collaborative, family-centered relationship with program participants, a model that research shows to be most effective with at-risk families, a philosophy strongly supported by HFA (Dunst, Trivette, & Mott, 1994).

Everyone was excited. It was a relief to change the program focus from case management/crisis intervention to a consistent focus on parent-child interaction. Supervisors rewrote their introductory brochures to ensure that participants were clear about the goals of the program when they enrolled. (See Stage I, Orientation, in the section Stages of the Helping Relationship). Sites reclarified their roles with community providers. They no longer talked about the program as case management but focused instead on the goals of promoting child development and enhancing parent-child interaction. FSWs learned how to set boundaries in new ways and liked their redefined role. They still talked to families about concerns and made referrals to community partners, but problems were less often the primary focus of the relationship. When FSWs stopped problem solving, however, something new emerged. They were less sure what to do on home visits. They could not make home movies every week. They needed more tools to encourage child development and parent-child relationships during home visits.

Filling the Toolbox

Supervisors organized to build FSWs' knowledge of child development and skills in providing anticipatory guidance. They researched and purchased new activity-based curriculum materials that supported family strengths. They expanded toy lending libraries and worked with FSWs to develop catalogs of activities for home visits that supported child development and parent-child interactions. They provided additional training on developmental screening tools and early brain development. To ensure that families had the additional resources they needed, programs built new relationships with community providers to facilitate referrals for domestic violence, substance abuse, employment, and mental health.

As supervisors and FSWs became more skilled in how to support parent-child relationships, supervision increasingly became a time not to vent or solve problems but to plan for the next home visit. Home visiting rates went up from less than 70% each month to routinely over 80%.[2] Developmental screening completion rates went up from a 50% completion rate to over 85% during the 18-month period. Both rates have remained at these levels for the past 12 months.[3] Families who had been talking to FSWs about ongoing problems with domestic violence stopped talking to the FSW about the problem and entered counseling. They preferred to spend the visit focusing on their children.

The Parallel Process

The most unique learning experience of the project has been "sliding around in the parallel process." Paradoxically, as supervisors became increasingly skilled in the mutual competence model and had a vision of the experience they wanted to create for families, they became increasingly didactic with FSWs in an attempt to "teach" them the model. Supervisors typed out the "Inquiry as Intervention" questions and suggested FSWs use them as a tool to address concerns with families. They coached FSWs in how to plan for the next home visit and revised staff evaluations to include understanding the model and using videotape in home visits. Whereas some FSWs took to the model naturally, others resisted. Supervisors' well-intentioned attempts at getting staff to use the new tools left FSWs feeling judged and incompetent.

During the monthly meetings, supervisors tried to help one another figure out what was going wrong. Working together, they came to discover that mutual competence was not about teaching new methods. It was about creating the experience of a collaborative, nurturing relationship for FSWs, which resulted in their feeling competent and understood. In the same way in which supervisors wanted FSWs to build collaborative partnerships with parents, they needed to build a collaboration with the FSWs that acknowledged their unique skills and expertise and took into account their perspective on the family. Only then could supervisors effectively offer their own expertise.

Applying this insight to a particularly difficult supervision session, a supervisor exclaimed, "She (the FSW) was the expert on this family. I had never really listened to her thoughts, opinions, and experience with the family. I was too busy thinking about what I thought she should be doing. When I took time to have her tell me what was going on with the family, what she had tried and what had worked in the past, not only did my opinion of what was best for the family change, she came up with ideas that were far more effective than mine!"

Supporting Supervisors

As they developed expertise in the mutual competence model, supervisors shifted their emphasis from monitoring FSWs' performance and compliance to building expertise, from being "caretakers" to helping FSWs build skills and grow professionally. FSWs responded to the new sense of respect in supervision and took on new challenges. FSWs began to make home movies routinely in home visits. They reviewed the tapes with families to support parent-child interaction and shared them with supervisors. Together, supervisors and FSWs used the mutual competence grid to build skills and plan for home visits. Some FSWs began to make videotapes of themselves reviewing the videotapes with families in home visits. Supervisors used the FSWs' tapes in supervision so FSWs could observe and develop their interactions with parents. In the same way that videotape provided an opportunity to observe parent-child interaction, it also provided an opportunity for supervisors and FSWs to observe the parallel process at work.

Whereas some sites flourished with the new model, others struggled. The challenge became maintaining a strength-based, collaborative model of supervision while faced with the real and daily crises of operating a program. Families continued to have crises, monthly reports still had to be done, supervisors were pulled off the task with credentialing demands and personnel concerns. Supervisors struggled with integrating the daily "caretaking" aspects of the program with the new model of using supervision to "nurture" FSWs. The forces of risk are too strong for supervisors to hold at bay alone. Although the monthly meetings were a source of renewal for everyone, it became clear that program managers and administration had to be involved for the model to take root and prosper. Just as FSWs needed strength-based, collaborative supervision to offset the forces of risk, supervisors needed a consistent, nurturing relationship that built on their skills and expertise and helped refocus their work. Providing relationship-based supervision to supervisors was crucial to maintaining the model and remains the most difficult aspect of the project to put in place.

To build in support for supervisors, one site restructured its weekly meetings between supervisors and the program manager to parallel supervision for FSWs. "They threatened to go elsewhere for supervision if I didn't address their changing supervision needs," the program manager at this site laughed. One week the team of program manager and supervisors addressed the "caretaking" or administrative needs of the program. The meeting the subsequent week focused on "nurturing" supervisory skills. Together, program manager and supervisors used the mutual competence grid to identify strengths of the FSWs, to build on what was working, to gather information about areas of concern, and to plan for FSWs' growth. They watched videotapes of families, of FSWs viewing tapes with families, and tapes of supervisors watching tapes with FSWs. Paralleling the strength-based process in supervision, the role of the program manager shifted from expert to collaborator, from problem solver and taskmaster to colleague. The experience also gave both the program manager and the supervisors a new tool to solve problems. When faced with a question, they discovered they could move it up a notch or down a notch in the parallel process. Program managers and supervisors began to ask themselves, "How would I want my supervisor to handle this with me?" or, "How would I want a FSW to talk to a family about this?" Shifting the level of focus, or "sliding around in the parallel process," allowed supervisors to stay strength based and to avoid the all-too-familiar role of telling FSWs what to do.

Fortifying against the Forces of Risk: A Developmental Process

After 2½ years, no one would say they are experts in the model. Supervisors and home visitors are still learning, struggling, growing, just like the families with whom they work. They still battle against the forces of risk, but they are committed to the model. Supervisors come to training every month, they bring tapes of families, and they go back to their programs renewed and reenergized. Each site has developed its expertise in the mutual competence model at a different rate. Like the development of young children, each new stage builds on the mastery of the stage that proceeds it. The rate of development depends on the individual site, the access to tools that stimulate learning, and the nurturing environment created by the program administration. Some sites are up and toddling, others still working to sit alone. All are excited and energized by their successes and committed to maintaining the effort. Everyone is budgeting to pay for the costs of ongoing supervisory sessions when the pilot funding ends.

Preliminary data about program implementation are encouraging. A recent survey of consortium staff indicated both supervisors and FSWs felt that the quality of their work had been strengthened. The FSWs saw themselves as more effective helping parents understand their children's development and assisting parents in viewing themselves as the primary educators of their children. All staff felt the quality of supervision (e.g., supervision as an opportunity to reflect on one's own work, and on the needs of the families and the respect of supervisors and staff for one another) improved dramatically in the past 2½ years.

Lessons Learned and Implications for Implementation

1. Because the forces of risk work against the consistent implementation of strength-based practice, training is most effective if it takes place in stages, is regular, and is supported by consistent individual supervision sessions and monthly team meetings that emphasize peer supervision.
2. Nurturing, relationship-based supervision takes time. Supervisor-to-home-visitor ratio must be low enough to allow time for the process. (HFA best-practice guidelines suggest 1 : 5).
3. Sufficient video equipment is necessary. One camera per team of five FSWs was adequate for Healthy Families sites. FSWs also needed cables that allowed a camera to be used as a VCR or a viewer for families that did not have a VCR and sufficient

blank videotapes. Some sites found it useful to purchase an inexpensive, portable TV/VCR unit.

4. Supervisors should review videotapes with FSWs regularly, accompany staff on home visits, and be willing to make tapes of oneself in supervision.

5. Keep the work fun—fun for families, for FSWs, for supervisors, and for administration. Provide regular opportunities for everyone to get to experience the positive things that happen on home visits.

Summary

To strengthen families through strengthening relationships, programs must be able to nurture. As pointed out in this chapter, some family support programs are wracked by insecure funding and staff turnover. Just like parents, many programs do well on the caretaking level and are organized to respond to crisis and to manage cases. That is where they feel successful and comfortable. Unless these types of programs recognize a need to do their work differently and make a commitment to change their focus, the model presented here will not be successful. On various occasions, we have worked with eager home visitors and supervisors for up to a year only to have the model wither and die because ongoing support from the administrative level was not secured once the training was phased out. A program's ongoing commitment to the centrality of nurturing relationships is the only way to sustain the type of work described here in the face of poverty. With the program support for the staff in place, staff can turn their attention to supporting the nurturing relationships within the families.

Nurturing stems from the person in the supportive role responding to rather than directing the person receiving support. For each individual's role at every level (the parent for the child, the home visitor for the parent, the supervisor for the home visitor, the program manager for the supervisor, and all staff members for each other), the nurturing role means to facilitate understanding, recognize strengths, and encourage learning, but not to dictate. When the person being nurtured recognizes what is working and what his or her strengths are, the person begins to build on them. This is the natural course of growth and development. Acceptance, the foundation of nurturing, lies in the belief and in the trust that when a person understands and learns, that person will choose to do what is best. We must also believe that families have the right to choose to live their lives and raise their children in ways that may differ from ours. To be successful, we all need to have confidence in one another. To simplify the following discussion, we will not repeat each point for every level of the parallel process.

A recent report that summarized the results of several well-designed evaluations of home visiting programs called the effectiveness of home visiting programs into question (Gomby, Culross, & Behrman, 1999). Specifically, the authors took home visiting programs to task for problems with high staff turnover, high attrition of participants, and inconsistent program implementation:

> No matter what their skills level, close supervision is needed to help home visitors deal with the emotional stresses of the job and maintain objectivity, prevent drift from program protocols, and provide an opportunity for reflection and professional growth. Because

the connection between home visitors and families is the route through which change is hypothesized to occur, turnover among home visitors may be a serious problem for programs. Several of the programs [reviewed in the monograph] had significant turnover among home visitors. . . . there has been little investigation of this aspect of program implementation within home visiting programs, but if the fields are parallel, then programs might explore enhanced training of workers to increase the quality of services. (p. 18).

The training and supervision adaptations of the Developmental Training and Support Program described in this chapter addressed each of these concerns. We and other researchers caution against expecting too much from home visiting programs (Dunst & Trivette, 1997). Although the model presented by itself will not be sufficient to overcome the effects of concentrated poverty, the focus on strengths and nurturing relationships can begin to support families and programs in becoming more confident and resilient in coping with its effects.

We end with these basic principles that apply to all levels of the parallel process:

1. Parents want what is best for their children.
2. Parents can see what works and what doesn't — usually on their own and almost always with support.
3. Given the opportunity to really see, to realize (or, pardon the pun, to "real eyes"), parents will choose to do what is best.

ACKNOWLEDGMENTS   Many individuals played important roles in this collaborative effort. In Chicago, thanks go out to Irving Harris of the Harris Foundation and Judith Musick, founding director of the Ounce of Prevention Fund, for first encouraging and supporting the DTSP and to colleagues Candice Percansky and Nick Weschler for their original contributions as cofounders, trainers, and scribes of the work.

In the DCHFA, we would like to acknowledge all of the Healthy Families programs in the national capital area who have continued to work hard to make the Cornerstones Project successful: Melanie Gray and Nellie Earley for their creativity, vision, persistence, and editing assistance; the Family Support Workers in the Healthy Families Alexandria program for their patience, their professionalism, and their remarkable work; Emily Fenichel for having the idea in the first place and Elizabeth desCognets for making it possible. We would also especially like to thank Linda Dunphy and Northern Virginia Family Service for creating an environment which nurtures good ideas so they can take root and grow.

In Utah, we want to thank cotrainers Glenna Boyce and Mark Innocenti, whose experiences and insights strengthened our work, and Jim Akers, whose process evaluation clarified where we needed to concentrate our efforts. We would like to express our appreciation to the staff of the Utah State Early Intervention Research Institute, in particular director Richard Roberts, the research assistants, and support staff who made our work possible. Finally, we are most grateful to the children, parents, home visitors, supervisors, and program managers from all the programs for their hearty participation and for teaching us so much.

NOTES

1. An expanded description of the D.C. Area Healthy Families Consortium Cornerstones Project may be found in Campbell, S., Earley, W. & Gray, M. *Zero to Three*, 19(5), April/ May 1999, 27–33.

2. This statistic is for the Healthy Families Alexandria program only.
3. This statistic is for the Healthy Families Alexandria program only.
4. These figures are for the Healthy Families Alexandria program only.

REFERENCES

Akers, A., & Bernstein, V. J. (1998, December). Enhancing child development by supporting secure attachment. Poster session presented at the annual conference of the Council for Exceptional Children, Chicago, IL.

Ainsworth, M. D. S., Blehar, M., Waters, E., & Wall, S. (1978). *Patterns of attachment: A psychological study of the strange situation.* Hillsdale, NJ: Erlbaum.

Barnard, K. E., & Morisset, C. E. (1995). Preventive health and developmental care for children: Relationships as a primary factor in service delivery with at risk populations. In H. E. Fitzgerald & B. M. Lester (Eds.), *Children of poverty: Research, health, and policy issues* (pp. 167–195). New York: Garland.

Barnard, K. E., Morisset, C. E., & Spieker, S. (1993). Preventive interventions: Enhancing parent-infant relationships. In C. H. Zeanah, Jr. (Ed.), *Handbook of infant mental health* (pp. 386–401). New York: Guilford Press.

Bernstein, V. J. (1997, Winter). Using videotapes to strengthen the parent-child relationship. *IMPrint, Newsletter of the Infant Mental Health Promotion Project,* 20 (pp. 1–4). Toronto: Hospital for Sick Children.

Bernstein, V. J., & Hans, S. L. (1994). Predicting the developmental outcomes of two-year-old children born exposed to methadone: Impact of social-environmental risk factors. *Journal of Clinical Child Psychology,* 23, 349–359.

Bernstein, V. J., Hans, S. L., & Percansky, C. (1991). Advocating for the young child in need through strengthening the parent-child relationship. *Journal of Child Clinical Psychology,* 20(1), 28–41.

Bernstein, V. J., Percansky, C., & Weschler, N. (1996). Strengthening families through strengthening relationships: The Ounce of Prevention Fund developmental training and support program. In M. C. Roberts (Ed.), *Model programs in child and family mental health* (pp. 109–133). Mahwah, NJ: Erlbaum.

Blehar, M. C., Lieberman, A. F., & Ainsworth, M. D. S. (1977). Early face-to-face interaction and its relationship to infant attachment. *Child Development,* 48, 182–194.

Bromwich, R. (1997). *Working with families and their infants at risk.* Austin, TX: PRO-ED.

Campbell, S., Earley, N., & Gray, M. (1990). Fortifying families against the "forces of risk." *Zero to Three,* 19(5), April/May, 27–34.

Campbell, S., Gray, M., Earley, N. & Bernstein, V. J. (1999, March). Who cares for the caregivers? Supporting Healthy Families America managers and supervisors. Workshop presented at the Healthy Families America National Conference, Chicago, IL.

Cardone, I. A., & Gilkerson, L. (1989). Family administered neonatal activities. *Zero to Three,* 10, 23–28.

Carlson, E. A. (1998). A prospective longitudinal study of attachment disorganization/disorientation. *Child Development,* 69, 1107–1128.

Daro, D. A., & Harding, K. A. (1999). Healthy families America: Using research to enhance practice. *Future of Children,* 9(1), 152–176.

De Wolff, M. S., & van Ijzendoorn, M. H. (1997). Sensitivity and attachment: A meta-analysis on parental antecedents of infant attachment. *Child Development,* 68(4), 571–591.

Dunst, C., & Trivette, C. (1997). Early intervention with young children. In R. T. Ammerman & M. Hersen (Eds.), *Handbook of prevention and treatment with children and adolescents: Intervention in the real world context* (pp. 157–180). New York: Wiley.

Dunst, C., Trivette, C., & Mott, D. (1994). Strengths-based family centered intervention practices. In C. Dunst & C. Trivette (Eds.), *Supporting and strengthening families: Vol. 1. Methods, strategies, and practices* (pp. 115–131). Cambridge, MA: Brookline Books.

Eastmond, N. (1999). A qualitative inquiry into the PRO project. Instructional Technology Department. Utah State University, unpublished report.

Erikson, E. (1963). *Childhood and society* (2nd Ed.). New York: Norton.

Fenichel, E. (1992). *Learning through supervision and mentorship to support the development of infants and toddlers and their families: A sourcebook.* Washington, DC: Zero to Three.

Frankenburg, W. K., & Dodds, J. P. (1990). *The Denver II technical manual.* Denver, CO: Denver Developmental Materials.

Goldberg, S. (1977). Social competence in infancy: A model of parent-infant interaction. *Merrill-Palmer Quarterly, 23,* 163–178.

Gomby, D. S., Culross, P. L., & Behrman, R. E. (1999). Home visiting: Recent program evaluations — Analysis and recommendations. *Future of Children, 9*(1), 4–26.

Halpern, R. (1993). Poverty and infant development. In C. H. Zeanah (Ed.), *Handbook of infant mental health* (pp. 73–86). New York: Guilford Press.

Mahoney, G., Boyce, G., Fewell, R. R., Spiker, D., & Wheeden, A. (1998). The relationship of parent-child interaction to the effectiveness of early intervention services for at-risk children and children with disabilities. *Topics in Early Childhood Special Education, 18,* 5–17.

Meisels, S., & Wasik, B. (1990). Who should be served? Identifying children in need of early intervention. In S. J. Meisels & J. P. Shonkoff (Eds.), *Handbook of early childhood intervention* (pp. 605–632). New York: Cambridge University Press.

Musick, J., Bernstein, V., Percansky, C., & Stott, F. (1987). A chain of enablement: Using community-based programs to strengthen relationships between teen parents and their infants. *Zero to Three, 8*(2), 1–6.

Osofsky, J. (1990, Winter). Risk and protective factors for teenage mothers and their infants. *Newsletter of the Society for Research in Child Development,* Winter, pp. 1–2.

Paulsen, M. K. (1993). Strategies for building resilience in infants and young children at risk. *Infants and Young Children, 6*(2), 29–40.

Pawl, J. H., & St. John, M. (1998). *How you are is as important as what you do.* Washington, DC: Zero to Three.

Rutter, M. (1990). Psychosocial resilience and protective mechanisms. In J. Rolf, A. S. Masten, D. Cicchetti, K. H. Nuechterlein, & S. Weintraub (Eds.), *Risk and protective factors in the development of psychopathology* (pp. 181–214). Cambridge, England: Cambridge University Press.

Sameroff, A. J., Seifer, R., Baldwin, A., & Baldwin, C. (1993). Stability of intelligence from preschool to adolescence. *Child Development, 64,* 80–97.

Squires, J., Potter, L., & Bricker, D. (1995). *The ages and stages questionnaires: A parent-completed child-monitoring system.* Baltimore: Brookes.

Urban, J., Carlson, E. A., Egeland, B., & Sroufe, L. A. (1991). Patterns of individual adaptation across childhood. *Development and Psychopathology, 3*(4), 445–460.

Van Breman, J., & Graziano, D. (1997). Building on strengths: Recovery and parent-child relationships. *The Source: Newsletter of the National Abandoned Infants Resource Center, 7*(2), 1–3.

Wakschlag, Lauren S., & Hans, S. L. (1999). Relation of maternal responsiveness during infancy to the development of behavior problems in high-risk youths. *Developmental Psychology, 35*(2), 569–579.

Wall, J. C. (1994). Teaching termination to trainees through parallel processes in supervision. *Clinical Supervisor, 12*(2), 27–37.

Wallach, V., & Caulfield, R. (1998). Attachment and at-risk infants: Theoretical perspectives and clinical implications. *Early Childhood Education Journal, 26*(2), 125–129.

Weissbourd, B. (1990). Family resource and support programs. Changes and challenges in human services. *Prevention in Human Services, 9*(1), 69–85.

Werner, E. E., & Smith, R. S. (1992). *Overcoming the odds: High risk children from birth to adulthood.* Ithaca, NY: Cornell University Press.

Weston, D. R., Ivins, B., Heffron, M. C., & Sweet, N. (1997). Formulating the centrality of relationships in early intervention: An organizational perspective. *Infants and Young Children, 9*(3), 1–12.

7

TIMOTHY A. CAVELL
SUSAN T. ENNETT
BARBARA T. MEEHAN

Preventing Alcohol and Substance Abuse

The use and abuse of alcohol, tobacco, and other drugs (ATOD) remains a significant problem among the youth in our society. Although substance use among adolescents has declined since the 1970s, prevalence rates remain high based on findings from the Monitoring the Future (MTF) study, an annual survey of 8th-, 10th-, and 12th-grade students in the United States (Johnston, O'Malley, & Bachman, 1996). MTF data from 1995 revealed lifetime prevalence rates for adolescent alcohol use of 54.5% for 8th-grade students and 80.7% for high school seniors. Alcohol misuse was also high, as indicated by the fact that 20.8% of 10th-graders and 33.2% of 12th-graders reported being drunk during the preceding 30 days. Prevalence rates for lifetime marijuana use were 19.9% and 41.7% for 8th- and 12th-graders, respectively (Johnston et al., 1996).

Aside from the risk of developing substance abuse or substance dependence disorders, adolescents who are involved with ATOD also carry a greater risk for other negative outcomes (Hawkins, Kosterman, Maguin, Catalano, & Arthur, 1997). Maladaptive sequelae associated with substance abuse include motor vehicle accidents (Perrine, Peck, & Fell, 1988), suicide (Berman & Schwartz, 1990), HIV infection and unwanted pregnancies (Leigh & Stall, 1990), interpersonal violence (Fagan & Browne, 1994), criminal behavior (Miczek et al., 1994), diminished academic performance, school dropout (Newcomb, Maddahian, & Bentler, 1986), and occupational difficulties (Newcomb & Bentler, 1988).

When one considers both the level of ATOD use and the harm associated with use, the importance of early identification and prevention becomes clear. In this chapter, we describe several prevention programs that have undergone empirical scrutiny and that hold promise for future prevention efforts. We also provide an overview of a prevention project that is currently ongoing so that readers can better appreciate the challenges and opportunities that exist in this field. The chapter begins, however, with a review of the factors that appear to play an etiological role in adolescents' involvement with ATOD.

Etiology of Adolescent Substance Use

After more than two decades of research on the determinants and prevention of adolescent ATOD use, a consensus among prevention scientists is that there are multiple etiologic pathways by which youth begin and maintain their substance use. Borrowing a common epidemiologic heuristic, some researchers have assembled empirically identified correlates and predictors of adolescent substance use under the umbrella of risk and protective factors (Hawkins, Catalano, & Miller, 1992; Newcomb & Felix-Ortiz, 1992; Newcomb, Maddahian, & Bentler, 1986). Underlying this organizing schema, and in some ways departing from the usual traditions of epidemiology, research into why some adolescents use substances has been guided substantially by social science theory. Social science theory has also provided the underpinnings for an array of preventive interventions. That body of theory — principally, cognitive-affective, social learning, and social control theories — underscores the multicausal nature of adolescent substance use in that the theoretical constructs span a range of determinants from the intrapersonal to the societal.

A useful way to organize the numerous empirically and theoretically identified determinants of adolescent substance use is that based on spheres of influence (Brook, Nomura, & Cohen, 1989). These spheres begin with the inner world of the adolescent and move outward into concentric social contexts: family, peers, school, and neighborhood/community. These outer spheres represent primary social settings in which adolescents interact and develop, as well as interconnecting domains of influence on adolescent substance use. This conceptualization is rooted in the social ecological perspective on adolescent problem behavior, which postulates that the circumstances that promote ATOD use include aspects of both the adolescent and his or her social environment (Bronfenbrenner, 1979; Cassel, 1976). Fundamental to this perspective is a holistic understanding of individuals within their social context and a recognition that each sphere provides unique influences but that the effects of one sphere on another are also consequential in the development of youth ATOD use.

As the determinants of adolescent substance use move outward from the self and from substance-specific to more general social contextual constructs, different social theories can be brought to bear. At the center, cognitive-affective theories emphasize adolescents' substance-specific beliefs, attitudes, and intentions to use or not use drugs (Petraitis, Flay, & Miller, 1995). Moving to the primary socialization contexts of family and peers, explanations based on social learning theory are commonly invoked to explain the observed associations between peers' and family members' substance-use behavior and adolescents' level of use. Social learning theories focus on interactions with individuals who both model substance use behavior and provide reinforcement for use (Akers, Krohn, Lanza-Kaduce, & Radosevich, 1979; Bandura, 1977, 1986). Social control theory concepts have been used to understand family, school, and neighborhood-related variables that are not substance specific but are nevertheless linked to adolescent substance use. Control theories emphasize adolescents' attachment to conventional people and their commitment to and involvement in conventional activities, postulating that when social bonds are weak, adolescents are free to deviate from conventional behavior (Elliot, Huizinga, & Ageton, 1985; Hirschi, 1969).

Consistent with the social ecological perspective, some researchers have linked constructs from diverse theories and proposed integrative causal pathways. For example, weak societal, school, and family attachments may free adolescents to associate with substance-using peers who provide opportunities, incentives, and definitions favorable to use (Hawkins & Weis, 1985; Oetting & Donnermeyer, 1998; Skinner, Massey, Krohn, & Lauer, 1985). Others have linked social learning and cognitive-affective concepts to suggest that the effect of a substance-using environment is to enhance both the development of positive expectancies about the consequences of substance use and intentions favorable to engaging in substance use behavior (Flay et al., 1994). Such integrative approaches recognize the interplay of personal and social factors in adolescent substance use and highlight the etiologic role of multiple influences.

Inherent in this organization of spheres of influences and associated social science theories is the principle that substance-use determinants range from proximal to distal to ultimate influences (Petraitis et al., 1995). As described by Petraitis and colleagues, *proximal* influences are immediate precursors of substance use and are typically substance specific. *Distal* influences are steps removed from substance-use behavior and likely to work indirectly through more proximal factors to exert their influence. *Ultimate* influences are more removed still and refer to broader background factors that shape risk trajectories. Although proximal, distal, and ultimate levels of influence map loosely onto the spheres of self, family, peers, school, and neighborhood/community, it is also clear that within any one sphere, theoretical determinants may range from near to far in proximity to substance-use behavior. For example, within the sphere of self, adolescents' relative evaluations of the costs and benefits of using a specific substance are important proximal determinants of substance use, whereas biological and genetic factors that may predispose youth to use must be considered ultimate sources of influence.

Without putting too fine a point on organizational schemes, references to spheres and levels of influence emphasize the complex nature of adolescent substance use and help when deciding which factors and which contexts are to be targeted by preventionists. We refer to these organizing schemes in our review of key determinants of adolescent substance use. Our particular focus is on psychosocial antecedents of substance use and not on biogenetic factors; the former have been extensively studied, whereas empirical investigations of the latter have generally been restricted to special populations of youth, such as children of alcoholic parents (Sher, 1991). Also, we review the literature that addresses adolescents' initial and experimental use of ATOD rather than that on adolescent substance abuse and dependence. (See Weinberg, Rahdert, Colliver, & Glantz, 1998, for a review of recent research on adolescent substance abuse.) In this brief overview, we focus on determinants generally shared across substance-use behaviors rather than on identifying determinants of the use of specific substances or predictors of initial versus continued substance use.

Child Factors

Both substance-specific beliefs and attitudes and more general personality and behavioral characteristics have been implicated in adolescent substance use. Attitudes that reflect expectations about the costs and benefits of use, beliefs about self-efficacy in avoiding substance use, and intentions to take up the behavior have been linked with substance use (Ary & Biglan, 1988; Bauman, Fisher, Bryan, & Chenoweth, 1984, 1985; Chassin, Presson, Sherman, Corty, & Olshavsky, 1984; DeVries, Kok, & Dijkstra, 1990; Ellickson & Hays, 1992). As suggested earlier, these determinants reflect central constructs in the cognitive-affective theories of subjective expected utility (Bauman et al., 1984, 1985), theory of reasoned action (Ajzen & Fishbein, 1980), and theory of planned behavior (Ajzen, 1991). These theories posit that adolescents' expectations for positive and negative outcomes of substance use are proximal determinants of use behavior. When the balance tips toward greater expected benefits than costs associated with substance use, adolescents' decisions go in favor of engaging in substance-specific behavior. According to the theory of reasoned action, these evaluative beliefs contribute to the formation of adolescents' intention to use or not use drugs. Also contributing is youths' refusal self-efficacy, a key concept in the theory of planned behavior. Adolescents who doubt their efficacy to resist social pressures to use drugs are more likely to initiate and continue substance use.

According to the cognitive-affective theories, personality and behavioral characteristics are ultimate factors that act indirectly to influence adolescent substance use through their impact on substance-specific beliefs and attitudes. Personality and behavioral characteristics commonly implicated in the development of adolescent substance use are tendencies toward sensation seeking (Donohew, Helm, Lawrence, & Shatzer, 1990), early conduct problems and aggression (Brook, Brook, Gordon, Whiteman, & Cohen, 1990; Loeber, 1988), other deviant behaviors such as precocious sexual intercourse (Barnes & Welte, 1986; Donovan & Jessor, 1985; Jessor & Jessor, 1977), and prior substance use experience (Ellickson & Hays, 1992). Conversely, strong religious commitments have been shown to be protective against ATOD involvement (Cochran, Wood, & Arneklev, 1994; Jessor & Jessor, 1977; Webb, Baer, McLaughlin, McKelvey, & Caid, 1991). Interestingly, low self-esteem, commonly thought to be a precursor of adolescent substance use, has little empirical support for a direct role in the etiology of adolescent ATOD use (Conrad, Flay, & Hill, 1992).

Peer Factors

Peer factors, especially perceived peer substance use and perceived peer approval of substance use, have been shown to be among the strongest correlates and determinants of adolescent substance use (Brook et al., 1989; Conrad et al., 1992;

Hawkins et al., 1992; Newcomb et al., 1986). Adolescents who report that their best or close friends are substance users are more likely to report being users themselves, as are adolescents who overestimate the level of use among peers generally. Some researchers have used the term *normative expectations* to refer to adolescents' generalized expectations about the prevalence and approval of drug use among their peers (Botvin, Baker, Goldberg, Dusenbury, & Botvin, 1992; Hansen & Graham, 1991). Beliefs about the expectations others have for one's own behavior are a key construct of cognitive-affective theories. Peer effects are often explained in social learning theory terms: adolescents who interact with substance-using models and who anticipate positive consequences from substance use are more likely to initiate and continue ATOD use.

It should be noted that although the relation between adolescents' substance-use behavior and the substance-use behavior and attitudes attributed to close friends and peers has often been interpreted as evidence of peer socialization or influence, other factors contribute to this phenomenon (Bauman & Ennett, 1996). Longitudinal studies have demonstrated that concordance in the behavior of adolescents and their peers is also due to *selection*, the process whereby substance-using adolescents show a tendency to choose other substance users as friends (Cohen, 1977; Fisher & Bauman, 1988; Kandel, 1978; Urberg, Degirmencioglu, & Pilgrim, 1997). Because measures of peers' use are typically based on adolescents' perceptions, previous studies may be subject to the false consensus effect, whereby individuals perceive their own behavioral choices as relatively common and alternative choices as relatively uncommon (Marks & Miller, 1987; Ross, Greene, & House, 1977). Hence, adolescents who use substances compared with those who do not are more likely to perceive nonusing peers as users (Iannotti & Bush, 1992; Sherman, Presson, Chassin, Corty, & Olshavsky, 1983; Urberg, Shyu, & Liang, 1990). Studies that have not partialed out peer selection processes nor accounted for the false consensus effect have overestimated the extent to which peers socialize adolescents into using substances. Therefore, direct peer influence on adolescent substance use may be less significant than commonly thought.

Family Factors

Although orientation toward peers gains ascendency in adolescence, parents remain a primary socialization source and exert substantial influence on the substance-use behavior of their children (Douvan & Adelson, 1966; Glynn, 1981; Kandel & Andrews, 1987). Most family research has focused on parents, but some studies suggest that siblings also influence adolescent substance use. When parents or older siblings use tobacco, alcohol, or marijuana, adolescents are more likely to initiate use of these substances (Andrews, Hops, Ary, Tildesley, & Harris, 1993; Brook, Whiteman, Gordon, & Brook, 1985; Needle et al., 1986). Adolescents also are more likely to be substance users when they perceive less parental disapproval for use (Andrews et al., 1993; Brook, Whiteman, Gordon, & Cohen, 1986; Kandel & Andrews, 1987). As with the effects of peer substance use, these findings are usually interpreted within the context of social learning theory and as evidence of values transmission and observational learning through modeling.

More distal family factors that are not specific to substance use have also been linked to adolescent ATOD use. Among these are features of the parent-child relationship, such as quality of attachment between parent and child, the level of conflict in the family, and the effectiveness of parents' child-rearing practices (e.g., discipline and monitoring strategies). In general, adolescents are less likely to use substances when they are closely bonded with parents, when family relationships are not overly conflicted, and when parents provide clear and firm guidelines about coercive behavior and the use of substances (Brook et al., 1990; Dishion & Loeber, 1985; Hops, Tildesley, Lichtenstein, Ary, & Sherman, 1990; Hundleby & Mercer, 1987; Stice & Barrera, 1995). The combination of warmth and guidance, a parenting style termed authoritative parenting, may be particularly effective in insulating youth from substance use (Baumrind, 1985, 1991; Jackson, Henriksen, & Foshee, 1998). These parenting-related effects are usually understood in the context of social control theory in that the family is assumed to embody conventional values that influence the child toward conformity. Adolescents whose parents are effective socialization agents also acquire social competencies needed to withstand inducements to use substances (Jackson, Bee-Gates, & Henriksen, 1994).

School Factors

Poor school performance and low educational aspirations have been consistently linked with adolescent substance use (Bailey & Hubbard, 1990; Jessor & Jessor, 1977; Johnston, O'Malley, & Bachman, 1985; Kandel, Kessler, & Margulies, 1978; Smith & Fogg, 1978). Consistent with the general precept of social control theory, adolescents who are not involved in school activities and who have a low sense of commitment to school are more likely to engage in substance use (Ensminger, Brown, & Kellam, 1982; Krohn & Massey, 1980; Resnick et al., 1997). Academic performance, educational goals, and school involvement/attachment are typically construed as characteristics of individual adolescents, but these constructs can also reflect the more distal impact of the school environment. Very few studies have examined the extent to which the school context itself affects adolescent substance use. Several studies confirm, however, that the prevalence of substance use varies considerably across schools, suggesting that school environments systematically influence adolescent substance use (Ennett, Flewelling, Lindrooth, & Norton, 1997). Schools that are effectively organized, that foster commitment, and that are characterized by student attitudes opposed to substance use tend to have lower rates of use (Battistich & Hom, 1997; Ennett et al., 1997). Brook and colleagues (Brook et al., 1989) found that students' perceptions that school was disorganized and not oriented toward academic achievement were predictive of greater student involvement in ATOD. Battistich and Hom (1997) recently reported that student drug use was lower in schools in which students had a sense of community. Schools with a higher sense of community were characterized by caring and supportive interpersonal relationships, opportunities to participate in school activities and decision making, and shared norms, goals, and values. Theoretically, the findings suggest that when the school context promotes bonding, students are less likely to engage in deviant activities such as substance use.

Neighborhood/Community Factors

Like the school environment, neighborhood characteristics remain relatively unexplored with respect to their role in adolescent substance use. Several studies have linked neighborhood sociodemographic attributes with other adolescent problem behaviors, such as delinquency, sexual behavior, and low educational attainment (Mayer & Jencks, 1989; Kandel, Simcha-Fagan, & Davies, 1986; Simcha-Fagan & Schwartz, 1986). Rates of problem behaviors tend to be higher in neighborhoods that are disorganized and impoverished. These findings are usually explained in terms of social disorganization theory, which is a macrolevel control theory that posits that an absence of community-level social control mechanisms in declining neighborhoods contributes to the spread of delinquency (Bursick, 1988; Sampson & Groves, 1989; Shaw & McKay, 1942). The few studies that have investigated neighborhood characteristics as predictors of adolescent substance use have led to a mixed set of findings. In some studies, higher neighborhood risk was associated with drug involvement (Brook et al., 1989; Cochran & Bo, 1989; Newcomb & Felix-Ortiz, 1992), whereas other researchers found that economically advantaged neighborhoods had higher rates of substance use (Ennett et al., 1997; O'Malley, Bachman, & Johnston, 1988; Skager & Fisher, 1989). More research is clearly needed if we are to understand how the social contexts of neighborhoods and schools shape adolescent substance use.

Empirically Tested Prevention Programs

Without a doubt, efforts to prevent adolescent substance use and abuse are aided by the kind of empirical research just reviewed. Particularly helpful are conceptual models that help to organize the overwhelming laundry list of contributory variables (e.g., Petraitis et al., 1995). Additional research is needed, however, before we can fully understand how multiple factors operate, interact, and change over time (e.g., Smith, Goldman, Greenbaum, & Christiansen, 1995). Also needed are studies that explore the important shift from substance initiation to more regular use and abuse (e.g., Scheier, Botvin, & Baker, 1997). It is unlikely that the risk factors for the initiation of substance use are identical to the risk factors for problematic use. Nor is it likely that a given risk factor will have a uniform effect at all points in the developmental trajectory. Instead, the interplay among various risk and protective factors appears to be a complex, reciprocal, and dynamic process that can vary over time and across individuals (Scheier et al., 1997). Conceptual models that adopt a comprehensive perspective (e.g., Petratis et al., 1995) economize the thinking of prevention scientists and bring order to prevention programming.

Conceptual models of adolescent substance use must be tested, however, for these models can be inaccurate or incomplete despite being comprehensive and well conceived. Inadequacies in a theoretical model are often not apparent until the model is subjected to the empirical scrutiny of an experimental prevention trial (Coie et al., 1993). Prevention trials are invaluable in advancing our knowledge of the development and curtailment of adolescent ATOD involvement. Prevention trials also raise the bar for prevention scientists in that a model explaining the onset or continued use of a substance does not by itself guide the development and implementation of an effective prevention program. Despite tremendous advances in our understanding of the etiology of adolescent substance use, this understanding must eventually be translated into an effective technology of prevention.

We review here some of the more well-researched prevention programs that target adolescent substance use. These programs differ in a number of ways, but perhaps the most important distinction is in the population targeted. Included in our review are (1) *universal* prevention programs that target large nonselect populations (e.g., schools); (2) *selective* prevention programs that target specific groups known to have a heightened risk for a disorder (e.g., children of alcoholics); and (3) *indicated* prevention programs that target high-risk individuals identified as having detectable signs or symptoms of a currently subdiagnostic disorder (Munoz, Mrazek, & Haggerty, 1996). Reviewing the history of adolescent substance abuse prevention reveals a strong preference for universal prevention programs over those that are selective.

Universal Prevention Programs

Universal prevention programs differ based on both their content and process (Daugherty & Leukefeld, 1998; Tobler & Stratton, 1997). For example, *knowledge* about ATOD is often a part of the content of prevention programs that target entire school populations. Included here is information about the properties of different substances, the immediate and long-term effects of these substances, the laws regulating their use, and accurate normative information about the extent to which peers are using these substances. The role of *social influence* in the decision to use ATOD is also a common focus in universal prevention programs. The influence of both the mass media and one's peers is emphasized in these programs. *Affective education* is a term used to describe programs that assume the importance of *intra*personal constructs in the etiology of adolescent substance use. Note that the focus of affective education is not substance-use specific; rather, the tendency is to focus on broader affective issues such as self-esteem, awareness of feeling states, and insight into one's motives and values. Like the affective education programs, prevention efforts that address *generic interpersonal skills* also take a broad perspective that is not specific to substance use. The difference, however, is that the emphasis is on skills used within *inter*personal contexts. Among the skills covered are those that facilitate adolescent communication, problem solving, and coping. A final content category involves *refusal skills* designed to prepare youth for those occasions in which others may try to influence them to use substances. Included here are strategies and scripts for responding to specific situations, as well as efforts to elicit a more general and public commitment by youth against future substance use.

Aside from these important content distinctions, Tobler and Stratton (1997) also categorized programs on the basis of whether the group process was primarily interactive or noninteractive. The former refers to programs in which the target youth were coparticipants who interacted with one another, as well as with group leaders. The latter refers to programs in which the expert-led presentation was primarily didactic or experiential but with little or no give-and-take among participating youth. The relation between program content and process has not been random. Noninteractive programs typically place greater emphasis on intrapersonal content, including knowledge about ATOD, affective education, and the clarification of one's beliefs and values. Interactive programs, on the other hand, place greater emphasis on interpersonal competence, often paying particular attention to skills that enable youth to resist social influences to engage in ATOD use.

Recent reviews of the prevention literature reveal clear and important differences in the outcomes associated with these prevention efforts (Daugherty & Leukefeld, 1998; Tobler & Stratton, 1997). The most effective programs are those that combine an interactive group process with a goal of enhancing the skills by which youth can counter negative social influences to use ATOD. Programs that did not provide an interactive forum for participants were found to be generally ineffective, even when addressing content similar to that covered by successful interactive programs. Tobler and Stratton (1997) found a mean effect size of .04 for noninteractive programs. The mean effect size across interactive programs was .30, but Tobler and Stratton (1997) noted that such programs were not effective if the content was of a placebo nature. It should also be noted that in the majority of prevention trials, comparisons were made against a no-treatment condition.

Perhaps the most impressive outcome data has come from the Life Skills Training (LST) programs developed by Botvin and colleagues (Botvin, 1995, 1997). LST programs are more comprehensive than most other programs in that an interactive approach is used to enhance skills that have both broad applicability and direct relevance for substance-use resistance. Botvin (1997) identifies three main foci of the LST curriculum. The first is personal self-management skills, a blend of fairly generic intrapersonal skills designed to help with solving problems, coping with anxiety, promoting self-improvement and behavior change (e.g., goal setting), and understanding and resisting mass media influences. Second, LST attempts to enhance youth's interpersonal skills in the areas of conversation, communication, and assertiveness. The third LST component focuses on knowledge and skills that are specifically related to substance use. Included here is information designed to correct youths' misperceptions about the effects of various drugs and the actual level of substance use among age-mates. Also covered is information about the declining popularity and the immediate physiological effects of cigarette smoking. Knowledge and skills designed to make participants more aware of and resistant to the social influence of the media and substance-using peers is also an integral part of this third component of LST. It should be noted that LST programs administered to middle-school or junior-high youth are typically followed in subsequent years by one or two brief booster sessions.

Particularly impressive in the work of Botvin and colleagues is their systematic approach to planning, testing, and expanding their prevention program. LST has been shown to be effective across a variety of methods of selecting and training intervention providers. Both adult (usually teachers) and older peer leaders have been used with success. Proponents of LST have also examined the suitability of LST programs for minority populations. Their investigations have led to efforts to adapt the LST curriculum in ways that retain its integrity while making the materials, the language, and the examples more accessible to minority youth. One of the few research questions that may remain to be pursued by these researchers is the relative contribution of specific treatment components (e.g., changes in normative beliefs vs. training in peer refusal skills vs. inoculation against social influences) to the overall success of LST.

Compared with the LST approach to universal prevention, the program implemented in the Seattle Social Development Project (Hawkins et al., 1992) was quite different. Derived from the social developmental model of Hawkins, Catalano, and others (Catalano & Hawkins, 1996; Hawkins & Weis, 1985; O'Donnell, Hawkins, & Abbot, 1995), greater emphasis was given in this prevention program to variables that were predictive of but not immediately proximal to substance-use behavior (e.g., school disruptiveness, problem-solving skills, parenting practices). This program also targeted a much younger population of children, beginning when children entered the first grade and continuing through fourth grade.

The Seattle social development program involved three intervention components geared specifically for teachers, children, and parents, respectively. However, the emphasis in this program was clearly on assisting classroom teachers with their teaching practices. Teachers were trained (1) to use proactive classroom management techniques (e.g., clear expectations, contingent rewards), (2) to engage in interactive forms of teaching (frequent monitoring of students' performance, proceeding only when certain objectives are mastered), and (3) to foster an atmosphere of cooperative learning (i.e., students of differing abilities work together on a common project). Children received instruction and training in interpersonal problem-solving skills, but this curriculum was administered by teachers when children were in the first grade. For parents, brief programs (four to seven sessions) of parent training were offered, one focusing on responding contingently to children's behavior and the other designed to promote children's success in school. Unfortunately, the rate of participation in these voluntary parenting programs was predictably poor: only 43% of parents attended at least one session. Results showed that intervention was effective at improving many of the psychosocial variables (e.g., bonding to parents, commitment and attachment to school) thought to be predictive of later adolescent ATOD use (Hawkins et al., 1992; Hawkins, Kosterman, et al., 1997). Importantly, there was also evidence that treated children were less likely to have initiated alcohol use in fifth grade, though the findings in subsequent years were mixed regarding the impact on adolescent substance use.

There exist a host of other universal prevention programs that have been tested empirically (see Tobler & Stratton, 1997, for a review). Outcome data examining their impact on youth substance use are supportive for some programs (e.g., Hansen, Johnson, Flay, Graham, & Sobel, 1988; Pentz et al., 1989), are mixed for others (e.g., Shope, Dielman, Butchart, Campanelli, & Kloska, 1992), and are rather limited for still other programs (e.g., Battisch, Schaps, Watson, & Solomon, 1996; Cherry et al., 1998). Readers who wish to learn more about other universal prevention programs have available a number of excellent resources (Ammerman & Hersen, 1997; Botvin, Schinke, & Orlandi, 1995; Daugherty & Leukefeld, 1998; Durlak, 1997), including those provided through the National Institute on Drug Abuse.

Selective Prevention Programs

As mentioned previously, selective prevention programs target specific groups of children known to be at greater risk for a particular disorder. In the area of alcohol and substance abuse, one of the best examples of selective prevention is the Strengthening Families Program (SFP) developed by Kumpfer and her colleagues (Kumpfer, DeMarsh, & Child, 1989; Kumpfer, Molgaard, & Spoth, 1997). SFP has been used primarily with children of substance-abusing parents and thus differs significantly from universal programs that target nonselect school populations. Like many other programs, SFP involves skills training for both parents and children. What sets SFP apart is that it also entails family skills training (Kumpfer & Alvarado, 1995). With family skills training, parents and children are brought together to practice skills learned separately and to engage in fun family activities. The skills-training curricula in SFP is a mix of both general interpersonal skills and skills specific to issues of substance use and abuse. Compared to family-based prevention programs that target very young children, Kumpfer's SFP has been used with somewhat older children (ages 6–12 years), many of whom are at immediate risk for engaging in ATOD use. Results from the original investigation of SFP indicated that families who received all three treatment components fared better than families who received only parent training or only parent training and children's skill training. Analyses also suggested that gains were specific to the issues addressed by a particular intervention (i.e., parenting skills, children's interpersonal skills). It is significant that older children evinced reductions in their use of alcohol and tobacco and nonusing children reported a decrease in their expectations to use alcohol and tobacco in the future.

In addition to Kumpfer's SFP, there exist other selective prevention programs that target children at risk because of parental substance abuse or substance dependence. However, most of these programs target much younger children, and published outcome studies typically lack follow-up data on children's later involvement in ATOD (e.g., Catalano, Haggerty, Gainey, & Hoppe, 1997; Maguin, Zucker, & Fitzgerald, 1994; Miller-Heyl, MacPhee, & Fritz, 1998). Some also suffer from the use of nonexperimental designs (e.g., Atkin, Kumpfer, & Turner, 1996). Among the groups targeted are children whose parents are alcoholic (Maguin et al., 1994), opiate addicted (Catalano et al., 1997), or currently receiving substance abuse treatment (Atkin et al., 1996).

Another type of selective prevention program is one in which the target population is aggressive children. Extreme aggression exhibited by children, particularly boys, places them at risk for later delinquency and substance abuse. Common to these prevention programs is an emphasis on risk and protective factors that have been found to be important causes and correlates of aggression and later delinquency (e.g., parental monitoring, discipline, social cognitive skills). Typically these programs eschew treatment components that directly target behaviors and issues specific to substance use. Lochman's (1992) Anger Coping (AC) program is one example of this approach. Lochman compared his school-based, AC program to a no-treatment control condition. Participants were boys in fourth, fifth, and sixth grades who had been identified by teachers as aggressive and disruptive. Aggressive boys in the AC program received training designed to improve their ability to inhibit impulsive behavior and to engage in a more systematic social problem-solving process (e.g., identify the problem, generate solutions). Training was conducted in small groups that met for 12–18 sessions. Compared with untreated aggressive boys, those in the AC program had lower rates of drug and alcohol involvement at a three-year follow-up.

Encouraging results have also come from the Montreal Prevention Experiment (Tremblay, Masse, Pagani, & Vitaro, 1997). This selective prevention project also targeted aggressive boys, although these boys were in kindergarten when first identified and were 7 years old when the two-year intervention began. The prevention program combined parent training and social skills training. Outcome analyses revealed impressive treatment effects on posttreatment measures of aggression and on follow-up measures of delinquency. The investigators also found that fewer treated boys, compared with untreated boys, reported drinking to the point of being drunk at age 15. A similar pattern was found for self-reported drug use.

Indicated Prevention Programs

Alcohol and substance abuse prevention programs that fit the category of indicated prevention target youth whose behavior already suggests some movement toward substance abuse. These youth may be engaging in nonnormative but regular use of substances, they may have initiated their substance use much sooner than their peers, or they may have begun to show intermittent signs of high-risk use or evidence of substance abuse itself. One of the few empirically evaluated interventions designed to prevent problems associated with adolescent substance use is that developed by Szapocznik and his colleagues (Santisteban et al., 1997; Szapocznik et al., 1988; Szapocznik et al., 1989). These investigators have worked extensively with Cuban Hispanic families in which there is an adolescent suspected of engaging in the use of illegal drugs (typically marijuana or cocaine). Families were eligible for the study if the parent had direct evidence of the adolescent's drug use or if the parent endorsed at least four items on an adolescent problem behavior checklist. Items on this checklist included such behaviors as school dropout, contact with police, deviant friends, and frequent family arguments. For the purpose of this chapter, two points are significant about the work of Szapocznik and his colleagues. The first is that structural family therapy appears to hold promise as an intervention for adolescents already engaged in drug use. The second point is that Szapocznik and his team have made a significant contribution to our understanding of what is required to recruit and retain adolescent drug users and their families in therapy. Their program of research with these families led to the development of a therapeutic strategy for engaging resistant families in therapy (Szapocznik et al., 1988; Szapocznik, Kurtines, Santisteban, & Rio, 1990). Known as strategic structural-systems engagement (SSSE), this therapeutic approach involves first identifying the particular nature of a family's resistance. This could involve an unwilling but powerful adolescent, a distant father, or a highly ambivalent mother. Once the type of resistance is identified, therapists then follow strict therapeutic guidelines derived from a mix of strategic and structural family therapy techniques (e.g., bypassing a "weak" mother and meeting directly with the identified patient). Compared with families that did not receive SSSE, those who did showed a much greater likelihood of entering treatment (43% vs. 93%) and of completing treatment once it was begun (59% vs. 83%).

The Adolescent Transitions Program (ATP), developed by Dishion and Andrews (1995), is another example of an indicated prevention program. Participants in the ATP were older children and adolescents between the ages of 10 and 14 years of age. To be eligible for the study, parents had to endorse at least 4 out of 10 items on a measure of child risk. Among the 10 items were those related to child substance use, peer substance use, and family substance use history. Dishion and Andrews (1995) developed both a parent-focused and a teen-focused format to ATP. The parent-focused program was designed to improve parents' use of four techniques: monitoring, positive reinforcement, limit setting, and problem solving. The teen-focused intervention targeted the following skills: self-monitoring, prosocial goal setting, developing prosocial peer relationships, setting limits with friends, and problem solving and communication with peers and parents.

Dishion and Andrews (1995) tested the relative benefits of a parent-only, a teen-only, and a combined parent and teen intervention. Immediately following treatment, participants in all three ATP conditions were found to engage in less family conflict compared with control participants. The parent-only intervention also led to significant reductions in school behavior problems immediately following treatment and to a nonsignificant decrease in smoking at one-year follow-up. Intriguing and perhaps most important from the results of Dishion and Andrews (1995) were findings suggestive of iatrogenic effects associated with the teen-focused intervention. Specifically, adolescents participating in the teen treatment groups had higher teacher-rated externalizing scores and reported more frequent smoking than control participants at follow-up. A subsequent study by Dishion and his colleagues (Dishion, Spracklen, Andrews & Patterson, 1996) provided further support for the notion that aggregating deviant youth, as happened in the teen-focused treatment groups, may lead to the reinforcement and escalation of antisocial group norms.

Criticisms of Current Substance Abuse Prevention Programs

Daugherty and Leukefeld (1998), working from a life-span prevention perspective, have criticized current prevention programs that focus almost exclusively on low-risk child and adolescent populations and that adopt a single-minded focus on the goal of nonuse. They suggest that such programs do not carry forward into later adolescence and adulthood, when alcohol use is normative and when both alcohol and tobacco are both legal to use. Daugherty and Leukefeld (1998) argue that by adopting a position that all substance use should be considered abuse (Dupont, 1989), policy makers essentially derailed the prevention process from the more reasonable goal of reducing high-risk use of substances. An overemphasis on the goal of nonuse, as opposed to the goals of delaying use or reducing high-risk use, has resulted in too many prevention programs ignoring the rather obvious but critically important parameters of frequency and quantity of use. Attention has been given instead to ultimate and more distal antecedents of adolescent substance abuse. Daugherty and Leukefeld (1998) also criticize current no-use models of prevention for failing to recognize that reductions in the proportion of youth who use substances may have little or no impact on the proportion of youth who engage in high-risk substance use. Most substance-use problems are not manifested by low-risk youth, and high-risk youth may be the least likely to benefit from universal prevention programs given the greater number of risk factors they face.

Daugherty and Leukefeld's (1998) criticisms of current prevention programs are certainly provocative and should generate further debate and research. Their recommendation that prevention should emphasize the reduction of high-risk use appears sound, particularly if the substance in question is alcohol and if the individuals targeted are late adolescents or adults. However, when the target population involves children and early adolescents, the goals of no use and delayed initiation may make more sense given that training children, most of whom are nonusers, in the skills of low-risk use may be difficult to do, both practically and politically. Empirical support for the added goal of delayed use comes from a recent study by Hawkins, Graham, et al. (1997). These researchers found that children's age at initiation of alcohol use fully mediated virtually all other predictors of later misuse (e.g., parent drinking, proactive parenting, school bonding). The one exception to this finding was child gender. Daugherty and Leukefeld (1998) have urged caution, however, when interpreting the predictive power associated with the age of initial substance use. They review a number of studies that indicate that early users differ from the majority of users in a variety of important ways (e.g., greater psychosocial risk factors). Therefore, age at first use may be more an indicator of later problems than a cause of those problems.

The PrimeTime Approach to Preventing Adolescent Substance Use

In this part of the chapter we describe PrimeTime (Cavell & Hughes, 2000; Hughes & Cavell, 1996), a school-based prevention trial that is currently in progress and codirected by the first author. PrimeTime follows in the tradition of those programs based on models of risk and protective factors (e.g., Hawkins, Kosterman, et al., 1997). Recognizing the link between childhood aggression and adolescent substance use, Hughes and Cavell have developed a 17-month-long selective prevention program that targets aggressive children at risk for later substance abuse and delinquency. Two features of this program that are particularly innovative are highlighted here, although the real promise of the program will not be known until the intervention is completed and outcomes are examined.

Overview of the PrimeTime Model

In designing PrimeTime, we sought to develop a theoretically coherent intervention program that combined innovative and cost-effective treatment components. We assumed that both environmental and dispositional variables contribute to the development of childhood aggression, and we assumed that recurring transactions among these variables and reorganizations of children's internal structures conspire to shape the direction of subsequent development. This confluence of dispositional and environmental factors is often an obstacle to efforts at reversing the downward trajectory of aggressive children. However, from an organizational-developmental framework (e.g., Cicchetti & Richters, 1993; Stattin & Magnusson, 1996), future transactions and reorganizations also represent potential turning points (Rutter, 1996) in the lives of aggressive children — opportunities to introduce interventions, as well as contexts for amplifying the emergent ("sleeper") effects of earlier interventions (Coie et al., 1993; Yoshikawa, 1994).

The first rather innovative aspect of the PrimeTime model is that it is guided by both attachment and social learning theories of childhood aggression (Cavell & Hughes, in press). These two perspectives are used to understand the reciprocal contributions of both environmental factors and child effects to children's development. In keeping with this framework, the PrimeTime model assumes that interventions for aggressive children will be effective to the extent that therapeutic changes in children's internal working models and social cognitive skills promote positive transactions with the environment. Perhaps most unique to the PrimeTime model is the emphasis on providing children with the combination of problem-solving skills training and transforming relationships. In fact, the name of the project stems from the belief that specific skills training should follow therapeutic efforts to provide children with the kind of relationships that essentially *prime* them to be open to learning prosocial skills. We also make specific assumptions about the kind of relationship that is likely to be positively transforming for an aggressive child. These assumptions also reflect the integration of social learning and attachment theories in that the following conditions are considered essential: (1) accurate emotional understanding and acceptance, (2) strict limits on antisocial behavior, and (3) guidance and modeling of prosocial beliefs and behaviors (Cavell, 2000; Hughes & Cavell, 1996). Because parents and teachers of aggressive children often struggle to provide all three relationship conditions, the PrimeTime program combines consultation for parents and teachers with therapeutic mentoring for children.

Identifying and Recruiting Children

Children are identified for the program by second- and third-grade teachers who nominate children who fit the description of a physically or relationally aggressive child. Eligibility is based on the following criteria: (1) a T score of at least 60 (i.e., 1 SD) on the Aggressive Behavior subscale of Achenbach's (1991) Teacher Report Form (TRF) *and* a peer-rated aggression score above the mean, or (2) a score of at least 2 SDs above the mean on either the teacher- or peer-rated measure of aggression. Mean T scores on the TRF Aggression scale were above 70 for the first two cohorts of children in the study. Children are randomly assigned to PrimeTime or to a control condition.

Assessment

Variables used to assess the immediate effects of treatment are obtained at pre- and at posttreatment and at yearly follow-up periods. Primary outcome variables include level of aggression and delinquency, school achievement, and sociometric peer status. Variables that reflect specific mechanisms of treatment change are also assessed. Here the focus is on children's social cognitive skills, the quality of their mentoring relationships, and various facets of their self-systems, including the quality and accuracy of their views of self and others (Hughes, Cavell, & Grossman, 1997). The prevention impact of the PrimeTime program is assessed via measures of ATOD use and the proximal antecedents of use (e.g., perceptions of peers' use of substances, expectations about peers' and parents' attitudes regarding substance use, expectancies regarding alcohol use, and peer isolate status). Prior to children's participation in the program, a number of variables that could potentially moderate or limit the effects of treatment were assessed. Potential moderator variables included demographics, parents' level of substance use and their history of delinquency, mothers' level of depression and history of maternal acceptance or rejection, level of neighborhood violence and stressful life events, and children's intellectual ability and degree of psychopathic traits.

Treatment Components

The PrimeTime program involves four interrelated treatment components. Three of these components—parent consultation, teacher consultation, and problem-solving skills training—are provided directly by case managers. The fourth component is therapeutic mentoring, and it is provided by college students under the supervision of case managers. Case managers, who are doctoral-level students in school, clinical, or counseling psychology, are responsible for the dissemination of services to 8 to 10 families. The case management system allows for increased communication flow and reduced information loss among program personnel, parents, teachers, and children.

PARENT CONSULTATION   Parent consultation is designed to assist parents who have difficulty establishing and maintaining an effective socializing relationship with their aggressive child. Consultants meet with parents in the home and try to develop a strong working alliance before targeting specific domains of parenting (Cavell, 2000; Webster-Stratton & Herbert, 1994). For parents willing to engage in the consultative process, the emphasis is on enhancing parents' provision of the essential conditions of a socializing relationship—acceptance, containment, and prosocial values. Depending on parents' skill and motivation, case managers may provide skills training in these specific areas or they may focus on the broader themes of parenting goals, family structure, and parental self-care. For parents who are reluctant to engage in the consultative process, the emphasis is on children's success at school, academically and behaviorally. Case managers place less emphasis on issues of parenting and make fewer demands on parents; instead, consultation is cast as a means by which parents can assist case managers in pursuing these child-oriented goals.

TEACHER CONSULTATION   The principal goal of teacher consultation is to help teachers identify and promote the conditions that would give rise to more frequent positive teacher-student interactions. This may entail developing alternative classroom strategies to counter disruptive behavior (e.g., the Good Behavior Game), encouraging teachers to adopt techniques that promote accurate understanding and acceptance of the child, or devising competence-promoting opportunities for the child. When working with teachers, consultants rely on a collaborative problem-solving process in which areas of concern are jointly identified and assessed and in which classroom interventions are jointly developed (Hughes & DeForest, 1993). Case managers are also responsible for arranging and guiding conjoint meetings between parents and teachers (Hughes, 1997). The chief reason for conducting conjoint meetings is to increase the degree to which teachers and parents convey to target children a common set of prosocial expectations. Before these meetings can be productive, however, case managers often have to spend a great deal of time engaged in "shuttle diplomacy," meeting separately with parents and teachers to identify common ground and to establish realistic goals for the meeting.

THERAPEUTIC MENTORING   PrimeTime mentors are undergraduate psychology or education students who receive about 20 hours of training prior to the start of their mentoring. Training is intended to enhance their understanding of childhood aggression and to increase their capacity to develop and maintain a relationship that offers emotional acceptance, behavioral limits, and prosocial values (Cavell, 1997). Mentor visits take place outside of school hours at least once a week for the entire 17 months of the program, excluding vacations and holidays. Small-group supervision occurs weekly, and mentors maintain logs of each mentor contact. Mentors are free to pursue a variety of activities but are apprised of activities that are likely to promote significant emotional interactions (e.g., working on a scrapbook) versus activities that may preclude such interactions (e.g., going to the video arcade). During the last four months of the mentor relationship, supervision focuses extensively on termination issues, and at termination mentors give to their protégés a scrapbook documenting their time together.

PROBLEM SOLVING SKILLS TRAINING (PSST)   PSST is conducted in the school setting by case managers, often with the assistance of the school counselor. Training sessions last about an hour and occur weekly during the fall and spring semesters of the second year of intervention. PSST groups contain three to six children, with a ratio of two prosocial children to each aggressive child. Failure to include prosocial children in such groups may lead inadvertently to groups with antisocial norms and to iatrogenic effects (Cavell & Hughes, 2000; Dishion & Andrews, 1995). PSST is designed to enhance children's ability to use skills known to differentiate aggressive and nonaggressive children (e.g., empathy, attention to social cues, interpretation of intentions, generating competent solutions, anticipating outcomes of solutions). Various techniques (e.g., games, stories, role-play, videotaping) are used to teach targeted skills and beliefs. Leaders strive to maintain accepting relationships with each child and to provide high levels of praise and warmth. Children earn or lose points based on their compliance with group rules for behavior, and points are exchanged each week for small prizes. Case managers and counselors receive training prior to beginning PSST and follow a detailed manual (Hughes, 1998).

PrimeSquare: A Booster Intervention

The second innovative feature of the PrimeTime prevention model is a one-year booster intervention planned for target children entering sixth grade, the first year of middle school. Previous efforts to intervene with aggressive children have assessed the impact of treatment on later use of ATOD (Dishion & Andrews, 1995; Hawkins, Kosterman, et al., 1997; Lochman, 1992; Tremblay et al., 1997), but these programs have not directly targeted the more proximal antecedents of adolescent substance use. This booster intervention, which is called PrimeSquare, is designed to focus on these proximal antecedents, thereby providing an important complement to the heavy emphasis in earlier grades on factors thought to be ultimate or distal antecedents of adolescent substance use (Petraitis et al., 1995). Given that Prime-Time targets children in Grades 2 and 3, the emphasis on ultimate and distal factors is appropriate. However, as these children move forward developmentally, they begin to transact with a wider and potentially more deviant peer ecology (Dishion, Capaldi, Spracklen, & Li, 1995). Therefore, the value of addressing the more proximal antecedents of substance abuse and delinquency increases dramatically.

The purpose of PrimeSquare is to reduce children's access to substance-abusing peers and involvement in deviant activities, while also seeking to enhance school bonding and adult supervision. In line with the PrimeTime prevention model, PrimeSquare will use a case manager system of service delivery that combines therapeutic mentoring with parent and teacher consultation. However, Prime-Square mentors will have the added goals of monitoring children's nonschool activities, limiting their access to deviant peers, and promoting their engagement in nondeviant activities. Because of this more intensive role, PrimeSquare mentors will be required to maintain at least three contacts per week for a minimum of six contact hours per week. Beginning in the spring semester, PrimeSquare mentors will also assist case managers as they engage target children in skills training focusing on general social problem-solving skills and on issues specific to substance use (e.g., peer use norms, peer refusal skills). Also assisting case managers with this skills training component will be two peer leaders assigned to each target child. Peer leaders will be identified by teachers asked to nominate slightly older students (e.g., eighth-graders) who are socially competent and prosocial and who are ethnically matched to the target child. Our current plans are for these pairs to consist of one boy and one girl, based on the assumption that some training issues or tasks may be better suited to one sex or the other.

Implementation Issues for Practitioners

Knowledge of the empirical outcome literature is an important prerequisite for practitioners who wish to offer interventions that meet a minimum standard of care and that have a greater likelihood of being effective. This is true whether the goal is preventing alcohol and substance abuse or treating obsessive-compulsive disorder. But such knowledge is not enough. Practitioners also need guidelines for implementing interventions in real-world settings, where obstacles often arise unexpectedly. For example, Hawkins, Kosterman, et al. (1997) note that in some communities, substance use may be viewed as normative and prevention may be seen as futile. Lochman and Wells (1997) describe a number of challenges to implementing school-based prevention programs. Among these are inadequate teacher involvement, low parent engagement, and the negative effect that aggressive children can have on each other when brought together in treatment. Challenges such as these become increasingly likely as practitioners move from universal prevention to more selective and indicated types of prevention. A useful set of guidelines is that offered by Kumpfer and Alvarado (1995) based on their work with families:

1. *Provide programs of sufficient intensity.* Recognize that some families are quite needy and may require a great deal of services (e.g., 30–40 contact hours).
2. *Match the program to the family's needs.* Programming should follow assessment information that is accurate and representative for the family or community being served.
3. *Time programs for developmental appropriateness.* For younger children, the focus should be on the ultimate and distal antecedents of substance use; for older children and adolescents, the focus should include more proximal antecedents.
4. *Screen for parental dysfunction.* It is particularly important to screen for signs of depression and substance abuse.
5. *Pay sufficient attention to recruitment and retention.* As evidenced by the findings of Szapocznik et al. (1990), issues of recruitment and retention may be the most important factors in family intervention, given that comparison studies typically find few differences among various interventions.
6. *Provide other needed services.* The needs of some high-risk families go far beyond that of substance abuse prevention. Therefore, practitioners must be ready to respond to parents who need information, assistance, or referral because of other pressing demands and problems (Cavell, 2000).
7. *Review program materials for cultural relevance.* Often this means asking the families with whom one works about the relevance and usefulness of what is offered.
8. *Measure program effectiveness.* Implementing a program that has "proven" efficacy offers no guarantee of real-world effectiveness. Practitioners should routinely measure the impact of their efforts or run the risk of providing ineffective or possibly counterproductive services.

Summary

In our society, the emphasis in health care has long been on treatment and rehabilitation rather than on prevention. The difficulties associated with treating disorders of substance abuse and substance dependence argue strongly for a shift in the direction of prevention. Governmental policies to reduce the supply of illegal drugs and to increase the penalties associated with drug possession and sale have also not diminished the need for effective prevention programming. As we learn more about the prevention of alcohol and substance abuse, especially the importance of recognizing one's own level of risk and what can be done about it, the greater the need for practitioners who can implement prevention programs. The empirically tested programs described in this chapter hold the most promise for those practitioners whose goal is to prevent alcohol and substance abuse among our youth.

REFERENCES

Achenbach, T. M., & Edelbrock, C. S. (1991). Manual for the Child Behavior Checklist and Revised Child Behavior Profile. Burlington, VA: Author.

Ajzen, I. (1991). The theory of planned behavior. *Organizational Behavior and Human Decision Processes, 50,* 185–204.

Ajzen, I., & Fishbein, M. (1980). *Understanding attitudes and predicting social behavior.* Englewood Cliffs, NJ: Prentice-Hall.

Akers, R. L., Krohn, M. D., Lanza-Kaduce, L., & Radosevich, M. (1979). Social learning and deviant behavior: A specific test of a general theory. *American Sociological Review, 44,* 636–655.

Ammerman, R. T., & Hersen, M. (Eds.). (1997). *Handbook of prevention and treatment with children and adolescents: Intervention in the real world context.* New York: Wiley.

Andrews, J. A., Hops, H., Ary, D., Tildesley, E., & Harris, J. (1993). Parental influence on early adolescent substance use: Specific and nonspecific effects. *Journal of Early Adolescence, 13,* 285–310.

Atkan, G. B., Kumpfer, K. L., & Turner, C. W. (1996). Effectiveness of a family skills training program for substance use prevention with inner city African-American families. *Substance Use and Misuse, 31,* 157–175.

Ary, D. V., & Biglan, A. (1988). Longitudinal changes in adolescent cigarette smoking behavior: Onset and cessation. *Journal of Behavioral Medicine, 11,* 361–382.

Bailey, S. L., & Hubbard, R. L. (1990). Developmental variation in the context of marijuana initiation among adolescents. *Journal of Health and Social Behavior, 31,* 58–70.

Bandura, A. (1977). *Social learning theory.* Englewood Cliffs, NJ: Prentice-Hall.

Bandura, A. (1986). *Social foundations of thought and action: A social cognitive theory.* New York: Prentice-Hall.

Barnes, G. M., & Welte, J. W. (1986). Adolescent alcohol abuse: subgroup differences and relationships to other problem behaviors. *Journal of Adolescent Research, 1,* 79–94.

Battistich, V., & Hom, A. (1997). The relationship between students' sense of their school as a community and their involvement in problem behaviors. *American Journal of Public Health, 87,* 1997–2001.

Battistich, V., Schaps, E., Watson, M., & Solomon, D. (1996). Prevention effects of the Child Development Project: Early findings from an ongoing multisite demonstration trial. *Journal of Adolescent Research, 11,* 12–35.

Bauman, K. E., & Ennett, S. T. (1996). On the importance of peer influence for adolescent drug use: Commonly neglected considerations. *Addiction, 91,* 185–198.

Bauman, K. E., Fisher, L. A., Bryan, E. S., & Chenoweth, R. L. (1984). Antecedents, subjective expected utility, and behavior: A panel study of adolescent cigarette smoking. *Addictive Behaviors, 9,* 121–136.

Bauman, K. E., Fisher, L. A., Bryan, E. S., & Chenoweth, R. L. (1985). Relationship between subjective expected utility and behavior: A longitudinal study of adolescent drinking behavior. *Journal of Studies on Alcohol, 46,* 32–38.

Baumrind, D. (1985). Familial antecedents of adolescent drug use: A developmental perspective. In C. L. Jones & R. L. Battjes (Eds.), *Etiology of drug abuse: Implications for prevention* (NIDA Research Monograph No. 56, pp. 13–44). Rockville, MD: National Institute on Drug Abuse.

Baumrind, D. (1991). The influences of parenting style on adolescent competence and substance use. *Journal of Early Adolescence, 11,* 56–95.

Berman, A. L., & Schwartz, R. H. (1990). Suicide attempts among adolescent drug users. *American Journal of Diseases in Children, 144,* 310–314.

Botvin, G. J. (1995). Drug abuse prevention in school settings. In G. J. Botvin, S. Schinke, & M. A. Orlandi (Eds.), *Drug abuse prevention with multiethnic youth* (pp. 169–192). Thousand Oaks, CA: Sage.

Botvin, G. J. (1997). Substance abuse prevention through Life Skills Training. In R. D. Peters & R. J. McMahon (Eds.), *Preventing childhood disorders, substance abuse, and delinquency* (pp. 215–240). Thousand Oaks, CA: Sage.

Botvin, G. J., Baker, E., Goldberg, C. J., Dusenbury, L., & Botvin, E. M. (1992). Correlates and predictors of smoking among black adolescents. *Addictive Behaviors, 17,* 97–103.

Botvin, G. J., Schinke, S., & Orlandi, M. A. (1995). School-based health promotion: Substance abuse and sexual behavior. *Applied and Preventive Psychology, 4,* 167–184.

Bronfenbrenner, U. (1979). *The ecology of human development.* Cambridge, MA: Harvard University Press.

Brook, J. S., Brook, D. W., Gordon, A. S., Whiteman, M., & Cohen, P. (1990). The psychosocial etiology of adolescent drug use: A family interactional approach. *Genetic, Social, and General Psychology Monographs, 116,* 111–267.

Brook, J. S., Nomura, C., & Cohen, P. (1989). A network of influences on adolescent drug involvement: Neighborhood, school, peer, and family. *Genetic, Social, and General Psychology Monographs, 115,* 125–145.

Brook, J. S., Whiteman, M., Gordon, A. S., & Brook, D. W. (1985). The role of older brothers in younger brothers' drug use viewed in the context of parent and peer influences. *Journal of Genetic Psychology, 15,* 59–75.

Brook, J. S., Whiteman, M., Gordon, A. S., & Cohen, P. (1986). Dynamics of childhood and adolescent personality traits and adolescent drug use. *Developmental Psychology, 22,* 403–414.

Bursick, R. J. (1988). Social disorganization and theories of crime and delinquency: Problems and prospects. *Criminology, 26,* 519–551.

Cassel, J. (1976). The contribution of the social environment to host resistance. *American Journal of Epidemiology, 104,* 107–123.

Catalano, R. F., & Hawkins, J. D. (1996). The social development model: A theory of antisocial behavior. In D. J. Hawkins (Ed.), *Delinquency and crime: Current theories* (pp. 149–197). Cambridge Criminology Series. Cambridge: Cambridge University Press.

Catalano, R. F., Haggerty, K. P., Gainey, R. R., & Hoppe, M. J. (1997). Reducing parental risk factors for children's substance misuse: Preliminary outcomes with opiate-addicted parents. *Substance Use and Misuse, 32,* 699–721.

Cavell, T. A. (1997). PrimeTime mentor training manual. Unpublished manuscript. College Station: Texas A&M University.

Cavell, T. A. (2000). *Working with parents of aggressive children: A practitioner's guide.* Washington, DC: American Psychological Association.

Cavell, T. A., & Hughes, J. N. (2000). Secondary prevention as context for assessing change processes in aggressive children. *Journal of School Psychology, 38,* 199–235.

Chassin, L., Presson, C. C., Sherman, S. J., Corty, E., & Olshavsky, R. (1984).

Predicting the onset of cigarette smoking in adolescents: A longitudinal study. *Journal of Applied Social Psychology, 14,* 224–243.

Cherry, V. R., Belgrave, F. Z., Jones, V., Kennon, D. K., Gray, F. S., & Phillips, F. (1998). NTU: An Africentric approach to substance abuse prevention among African American youth. *Journal of Primary Prevention, 18,* 339.

Cicchetti, D., & Richters, J. E. (1993). Developmental considerations in the investigation of conduct disorder. *Development and Psychopathology, 5,* 331–344.

Cochran, J. K., Wood, P. B., & Arneklev, B. J. (1994). Is the religiosity-delinquency relationship spurious? A test of arousal and social control theories. *Journal of Research in Crime and Delinquency, 31,* 91–123.

Cochran, M., & Bo, I. (1989). The social networks, family involvement, and pro- and antisocial behavior of adolescent males in Norwood. *Journal of Youth and Adolescence, 18,* 377–398.

Cohen, J. M. (1977). Sources of peer group homogeneity. *Sociology of Education, 50*(4), 227–241.

Coie, J. D., Watt, N. F., West, S. G., Hawkins, J. D., Asarnow, J. R., Markman, H. J., Ramey, S. L., Shure, M. B., & Long, B. (1993). The science of prevention: A conceptual framework and some directions for a national research program. *American Psychologist, 48,* 1013–1022.

Conrad, K. M., Flay, B. R., & Hill, D. (1992). Why children start smoking cigarettes: Predictors of onset. *British Journal of Addiction, 87,* 1711–1724.

Daugherty, R. P., & Leukefeld, C. (1998). *Reducing the risks for substance abuse: A lifespan approach.* New York: Plenum.

DeVries, H., Kok, G., & Dijkstra, M. (1990). Self-efficacy as a determinant of the onset of smoking and interventions to prevent smoking in adolescents. *European Perspectives in Psychology, 2,* 209–222.

Dishion, T. J., & Andrews, D. W. (1995).

Preventing escalation in problem behaviors with high-risk young adolescents: Immediate and 1-year outcomes. *Journal of Consulting and Clinical Psychology, 63,* 538–548.

Dishion, T. J., & Loeber, R. (1985). Adolescent marijuana and alcohol use: The role of parents and peers revisited. *American Journal of Drug and Alcohol Abuse, 11,* 11–25.

Dishion, T. J., Capaldi, D., Spracklen, K. M., & Li, F. (1995). Peer ecology of male adolescent drug use. *Development and Psychopathology, 7,* 803–824.

Dishion, T. J., Spracklen, K. M., Andrews, D. W., & Patterson, G. R. (1996). Deviancy training in male adolescents friendships. *Behavior Therapy, 27,* 373–390.

Donohew, L., Helm, D. M., Lawrence, P., & Shatzer, M. J. (1990). Sensation seeking, marijuana use, and responses to prevention messages: Implications for public health campaigns. In R. R. Watson (Ed.), *Drug and alcohol abuse prevention: Drug and alcohol abuse reviews* (pp. 73–93). Clifton, NJ: Humana Press.

Donovan, J. E., & Jessor, R. (1985). Structure of problem behavior in adolescence and young adulthood. *Journal of Consulting and Clinical Psychology, 53,* 890–904.

Douvan, E., & Adelson, J. (1966). *The adolescent experience.* New York: Wiley.

Dupont, R. L. (1989). *Stopping alcohol and other drug abuse before its starts.* OSAP Prevention Monography No. 1. Washington, DC: U.S. Department of Health and Human Services.

Durlak, J. A. (1997). *Successful prevention programs for children and adolescents.* New York: Plenum.

Ellickson, P. L., & Hays, R. D. (1992). On becoming involved with drugs: Modeling adolescent drug use over time. *Health Psychology, 11*(6), 377–385.

Elliot, D. S., Huizinga, D., & Ageton, S. S. (1985). *Explaining delinquency and drug use.* Beverly Hills, CA: Sage.

Ennett, S. T., Flewelling, R. L., Lindrooth, R. C., & Norton, E. C. (1997). School and neighborhood characteristics associated with school rates of alcohol, cigarette, and marijuana use. *Journal of Health and Social Behavior, 38*(1), 55–71.

Ensminger, M. E., Brown, C. H., & Kellam, S. G. (1982). Sex differences in antecedents of substance use among adolescents. *Journal of Social Issues, 38,* 25–42.

Fagan, J., & Browne, A. (1994). Violence between spouses and intimates: Physical aggression between women and men in intimate relationships. In A. J. Reiss, Jr., & J. A. Roth (Eds.), *Understanding and preventing violence: Social influences* (pp. 115–292). Washington, DC: National Academy Press.

Fisher, L. A., & Bauman, K. E. (1988). Influence and selection in the friend-adolescent relationship: Findings from studies of adolescent smoking and drinking. *Journal of Applied Social Psychology, 18*(4), 289–314.

Flay, B. N., Hu, F. B., Siddiqui, O., Day, L. E., Hedeker, D., Petraitis, J., Richardson, J., & Sussman, S. (1994). Differential influence of parental smoking and friends' smoking on adolescent initiation and escalation of smoking. *Journal of Health and Social Behavior, 35,* 248–265.

Glynn, T. J. (1981). From family to peer: Transitions of influence among drug-using youth. In L. Lettieri & J. Ludford (Eds.), *Drug abuse and the American adolescent* (DHHS Publication No. ADM 81-1166). Washington, DC: U.S. Government Printing Office.

Hansen, W. B., & Graham, J. W. (1991). Preventing alcohol, marijuana, and cigarette use among adolescents: Peer pressure resistance training versus establishing conservative norms. *Preventive Medicine, 20,* 414–430.

Hansen, W. B., Johnson, C. A., Flay, B. R., Graham, J. W., & Sobel, J. (1988). Affective and social influences approaches to the prevention of multiple substance abuse among 7th grade students — Results from Project Smart. *Preventive Medicine, 17,* 135–154.

Hawkins, J. D., Catalano, R. F., & Miller, J. Y. (1992). Risk and protective factors for alcohol and other drug problems in adolescence and early adulthood: Implications for substance abuse prevention. *Psychological Bulletin, 112*(1), 64–105.

Hawkins, J. D., Graham, J. W., Maguin, E., Abbott, R., Hill, K. G., & Catalano, R. F. (1997). Exploring the effects of age of alcohol use initiation and psychosocial risk factors on subsequent alcohol misuse. *Journal of Studies on Alcohol, 58,* 280–290.

Hawkins, D. J., Kosterman, R., Maguin, E., Catalano, R. F., & Arthur, M. W. (1997). Substance use and abuse. In R. T. Ammerman & M. Hersen (Eds.), *Handbook of prevention and treatment with children and adolescents* (pp. 203–237). New York: Wiley.

Hawkins, J. D., & Weis, J. G. (1985). The social development model: An integrated approach to delinquency prevention. *Journal of Primary Prevention, 6*(2), 73–97.

Hirschi, T. (1969). *Causes of delinquency.* Berkeley, CA: University of California Press.

Hops, H., Tildesley, E., Lichtenstein, E., Ary, D., & Sherman, L. (1990). Parent-adolescent problem-solving interactions and drug use. *American Journal of Drug and Alcohol Abuse, 16,* 239–258.

Hughes, J. N. (1997, August). Responsive Systems Consultation: A developmental systems model for home-school consultation. Paper presented at annual meeting of the American Psychological Association, Chicago.

Hughes, J. N. (1998). LASO: Learning acceptance of self and others. Unpublished manuscript. College Station: Texas A&M University.

Hughes, J. N., & Cavell, T. A. (1996). *Preventing substance abuse in aggressive children* (Grant No. 5 R01 DA10037). Rockville, MD: National Institute on Drug Abuse.

Hughes, J. N., & DeForest, P. A. (1993). Consultant directiveness and support as predictors of consultation outcomes. *Journal of School Psychology, 31,* 355–373.

Hughes, J. N., Cavell, T. A., & Grossman, P. A. (1997). A positive view of self: Risk or protection for aggressive children? *Development and Psychopathology, 9,* 75–94.

Hundleby, J. D., & Mercer, G. W. (1987). Family and friends as social environments and their relationship to young adolescents' use of alcohol, tobacco, and marijuana. *Journal of Marriage and the Family, 49,* 151–164.

Iannotti, R. J., & Bush, P. J. (1992). Perceived vs. actual friends' use of alcohol, cigarettes, marijuana, and cocaine: Which has the most influence? *Journal of Youth and Adolescence, 21,* 375–389.

Jackson, C., Bee-Gates, D. J., & Henriksen, L. (1994). Authoritative parenting, child competencies, and initiation of cigarette smoking. *Health Education Quarterly, 21,* 103–116.

Jackson, C., Henriksen, L., & Foshee, V. A. (1998). The authoritative parenting index: Predicting health risk behaviors among children and adolescents. *Health Education and Behavior, 25(3),* 319–337.

Jencks, C., & Mayer, S. E. (1990). The social consequences of growing up in a poor neighborhood. In L. E. Lynn & M. G. H. McGeary (Eds.), *Inner-city poverty in the United States* (pp. 111–186). Washington, DC: National Academy Press.

Jessor, R., & Jessor, S. L. (1977). *Problem behavior and psychosocial development: A longitudinal study of youth.* New York: Academic Press.

Johnston, L., O'Malley, P. M., & Bachman, J. G. (1985). *Use of licit and illicit drugs by America's high school students: 1975–1984.* Rockville, MD: National Institute on Drug Abuse.

Johnston, L. D., O'Malley, P. M., & Bachman, J. G. (1996). *National survey results on drug use from the Monitoring the Future Study: 1975–1995.* Washington, DC: National Institute on Drug Abuse.

Kandel, D., Simcha-Fagan, O., & Davies, M. (1986). Risk factors for delinquency and illicit drug use from adolescence to young adulthood. *Journal of Drug Issues, 16,* 67–90.

Kandel, D. B. (1978). Homophily, selection, and socialization in adolescent friendships. *American Journal of Sociology, 84(2),* 427–436.

Kandel, D. B., & Andrews, K. (1987). Processes of adolescent socialization by parents and peers. *International Journal of the Addictions, 22(4),* 319–342.

Kandel, D. B., Kessler, R. C., & Margulies, R. Z. (1978). Antecedents of adolescent initiation into stages of drug use: A developmental analysis. In D. B. Kandel (Ed.), *Longitudinal research on drug use: Empirical findings and methodological issues* (pp. 73–99). Washington, DC: Hemisphere.

Krohn, M. D., & Massey, J. (1980). Social control and delinquent behavior: An examination of the elements of the social bond. *Sociological Quarterly, 21,* 529–543.

Kumpfer, K. L., & Alvarado, R. (1995). Strengthening families to prevent drug use in multiethnic youth. In G. J. Botvin, S. Schinke, & M. A. Orlandi (Eds.), *Drug abuse prevention with multiethnic youth* (pp. 225–294). Thousand Oaks, CA: Sage.

Kumpfer, K. L., DeMarsh, J. P., & Child, W. (1989). *Strengthening Families Program: Children's skills training curriculum manual, parent training manual, children's skill training manual, and family skills training manual.* Manuscript submitted for publication. Salt Lake City: University of Utah, Social Research Institute, Graduate School of Social Work.

Kumpfer, K. L., Molgaard, V., & Spoth, R. (1997). The Strengthening Families Program for the prevention of delinquency and drug use. In R. D. Peters & R. J. McMahon (Eds.), *Preventing childhood disorders, substance abuse, and delinquency* (pp. 241–267). Thousand Oaks, CA: Sage.

Leigh, B. C., & Stall, R. (1993). Substance use and risky sexual behavior for exposure to HIV: Issues in methodology, interpretation, and prevention. *American Psychologist, 48,* 1035–1045.

Lochman, J. E. (1992). Cognitive-behavioral intervention with aggressive boys: Three-year follow-up and preventive effects. *Journal of Consulting and Clinical Psychology, 60,* 426–432.

Lochman, J. E., & Wells, K. C. (1996). A social-cognitive intervention with aggressive children: Prevention effects and contextual implementation issues. In R. D. Peters & R. J. McMahon (Eds.), *Preventing childhood disorders, substance abuse, and delinquency. Banff international behavior science series: Vol.* 3 (pp. 111–143). Thousand Oaks, CA: Sage.

Loeber, R. (1988). Natural histories of conduct problems, delinquency, and associated substance use: Evidence for developmental progressions. In B. B. Lahey & A. E. Kazdin (Eds.), *Advances in clinical child psychology* (Vol. 11, pp. 73–124). New York: Plenum Press.

Maguin, E., Zucker, R. A., & Fitzgerald, H. W. (1994). The path to alcohol problems through conduct problems: A family-based approach to early intervention with risk. *Journal of Research on Adolescence, 4,* 249–269.

Marks, G., & Miller, N. (1987). Ten years of research on the false-consensus effect: An empirical and theoretical review. *Psychology Bulletin, 102,* 72–90.

Mayer, S. E., & Jencks, C. (1989). Growing up in poor neighborhoods: How much does it matter? *Science, 243,* 1441–1445.

Miczek. K. A., DeBold, J. F., Haney, M., Tidey, J., Vivian, J., & Weerts, E. M. (1994). Alcohol, drugs of abuse, aggression, and violence. In A. J. Reiss, Jr., & J. A. Roth (Eds.), *Understanding and preventing violence: Social influences* (pp. 115–292). Washington, DC: National Academy Press.

Miller-Heyl, J., MacPhee, D., & Fritz, J. J. (1998). DARE to be you: A family-support, early prevention program. *Journal of Primary Prevention, 18,* 257–285.

Munoz, R. F., Mrazek, P. J., & Haggerty, R. J. (1996). Institute of Medicine report on prevention of mental disorders: Summary and commentary. *American Psychologist, 51,* 1116–1122.

Needle, R., McCubbin, H., Wilson, M., Reineck, R., Lazar, A., & Mederer, H. (1986). Interpersonal influences in adolescent drug use: The role of older siblings, parents, and peers. *International Journal of the Addictions, 21,* 739–766.

Newcomb, M. D., & Bentler, P. M. (1988). *Consequences of adolescent drug use: Impact on the lives of young adults.* Newbury Park, CA: Sage.

Newcomb, M. D., & Felix-Ortiz, M. (1992). Multiple protective and risk factors for drug use and abuse: Cross-sectional and prospective findings. *Journal of Personality of Social Psychology, 63,* 280–296.

Newcomb, M. D., Maddahian, E., & Bentler, P. M. (1986). Risk factors for drug use among adolescents: Concurrent and longitudinal analyses. *American Journal of Public Health, 76,* 525–531.

O'Donnell, J., Hawkins, J. D., & Abbott, R. D. (1995). Predicting serious delinquency and substance use among aggressive boys. *Journal of Consulting and Clinical Psychology, 63,* 429–437.

O'Malley, P. M., Bachman, J. G., & Johnston, L. D. (1988). *Student drug use in America: Differences among high schools 1986–1987* (Monitoring the Future Occasional Paper 24). Unpublished manuscript, University of Michigan, Ann Arbor, Institute for Social Research.

Oetting, E. R., & Donnermeyer, J. F. (1998). Primary socialization theory: The etiology of drug use and deviance. *Substance Use and Misuse, 33*(4), 995–1026.

Pentz, M., Johnson, C. A., Dwyer, J. H.,
MacKinnon, D. M., Hansen, W. B., &
Flay, B. R. (1989). A comprehensive
community approach to adolescent
drug abuse prevention: Effects on cardiovascular disease risk behaviors. *An-
nals of Medicine, 21,* 219–222.

Perrine, M. W., Peck, R. C., & Fell, J. C.
(1988). Epidemiologic perspectives on
drunk driving. In U.S. Department of
Health and Human Services (Ed.),
*Background papers of Surgeon General's
workshop on drunk driving* (pp. 35–76).
Washington, DC: U.S. Department of
Health and Human Services.

Petraitis, J., Flay, B. R., & Miller, T. Q.
(1995). Reviewing theories of adolescent substance use: Organizing pieces
in the puzzle. *Psychological Bulletin,*
117(1), 67–86.

Resnick, M. D., Bearman, P. S., Blum,
R. W., Bauman, K. E., Harris, K. M.,
Jones, J., Tabor, J., Beuhring, T., Sieving, R. E., Shew, M., Ireland, M., Bear-
inger, L. H., & Udry, J. R. (1997). Protecting adolescents from harm:
Findings from the National Longitudinal Study on Adolescent Health. *Journal of the American Medical Association, 278,* 823–832.

Ross, L., Greene, D., & House, P. (1977).
The "false consensus effect": An egocentric bias in social perception and attribution processes. *Journal of Experimental
Social Psychology, 13,* 279–301.

Rutter, M. (1996). Transitions and turning
points in developmental psychopathology: As applied to the age span between
childhood and mid-adulthood. *International Journal of Behavioral Development, 19,* 603–626.

Sampson, R. J., & Groves W. B. (1989).
Community structure and crime: Testing social-disorganization theory. *American Journal of Sociology, 94,* 774–802.

Santisteban, D. A., Coatsworth, J. D., Perez-
Vidal, A., Mitrani, V., Jean-Gilles, M., &
Szapocznik, J. (1997). Brief structural/
strategic family therapy with African
American and Hispanic high-risk

youth. *Journal of Community Psychology, 25,* 453–471.

Scheier, L. M., Botvin, G. J., & Baker, E.
(1997). Risk and protective factors as
predictors of adolescent alcohol involvement and transitions in alcohol use: A
prospective analysis. *Journal of Studies
on Alcohol, 58,* 652–667.

Schope, J. T., Dielman, T. E., Butchart,
A. T., Campanelli, P. C., & Kloska,
D. D. (1992). An elementary school–
based alcohol misuse prevention pro-
gram: A follow-up evaluation. *Journal of
Studies on Alcohol, 53,* 106–121.

Shaw, C. D., & McKay, H. D. (1942). *Juvenile delinquency and urban areas.* Chicago, IL: University of Chicago Press.

Sher, K. J. (1991). *Children of alcoholics:
A critical appraisal of theory and research.* Chicago, IL: University of Chicago Press.

Sherman, S., Presson, C. C., Chassin, L.,
Corty, E., & Olshavsky, R. (1983). The
false consensus effect in estimates of
smoking prevalence: Underlying mechanisms. *Personality and Social Psychology
Bulletin, 9,* 197–207.

Simcha-Fagan, O., & Schwartz, J. E.
(1986). Neighborhood and delinquency: An assessment of contextual effects. *Criminology, 24,* 667–699.

Skager, R., & Fisher, D. G. (1989). Substance use among high school students
in relation to school characteristics. *Addictive Behaviors, 14,* 129–138.

Skinner, W. F., Massey, J. L., Krohn,
M. D., & Lauer, R. M. (1985). Social
influences and constraints on the initiation and cessation of adolescent tobacco use. *Journal of Behavioral Medicine, 8,* 353–375.

Smith, G. M., & Fogg, C. P. (1978). Psychological predictors of early use, late
use, and non-use of marijuana among
teenage students. In D. G. Kandel
(Ed.), *Longitudinal research on drug
use: Empirical findings and methodological issues* (pp. 101–113). Washington,
DC: Hemisphere-Wiley.

Smith, G. T., Goldman, M. S., Greenbaum, P. E., & Christiansen, B. A. (1995). Expectancy for social facilitation from drinking: The divergent paths of high-expectancy and low-expectancy adolescents. *Journal of Abnormal Psychology, 104,* 32–40.

Stattin, H., & Magnusson, D. (1996). Antisocial development: A holistic approach. *Development and Psychopathology, 8,* 617–645.

Stice, E., & Barrera, M. (1995). A longitudinal examination of the reciprocal relations between perceived parenting and adolescents' substance use and externalizing behaviors. *Developmental Psychology, 31,* 322–334.

Szapocznik, J., Kurtines, W., Santisteban, D. A., & Rio, A. T. (1990). Interplay of advances between theory, research, and application in treatment interventions aimed at behavior problem children and adolescents. *Journal of Consulting and Clinical Psychology, 58,* 696–703.

Szapocznik, J., Perez-Vidal, A., Brickman, A. L., & Foote, F. H. (1988). Engaging adolescent drug abusers and their families in treatment: A strategic structural systems approach. *Journal of Consulting and Clinical Psychology, 56,* 552–557.

Szapocznik, J., Santisteban, D., Rio, A. T., Perez-Vidal, A., Santisteban, D., & Kurtines, W. M. (1989). Family Effectiveness Training. An intervention to prevent drug abuse and problem behaviors in Hispanic adolescents. *Hispanic Journal of Behavioral Sciences, 11,* 4–27.

Tobler, N. S., & Stratton, H. H. (1997). Effectiveness of school-based drug prevention programs: A meta-analysis of the research. *Journal of Primary Prevention, 18,* 71–128.

Tremblay, R. E., Masse, L. C., Pagani, L., & Vitaro, F. (1997). From childhood physical aggression to adolescent maladjustment: The Montreal prevention experiment. In R. D. Peters & R. J. McMahon (Eds.), *Preventing childhood disorders, substance abuse, and delinquency* (pp. 268–298). Thousand Oaks, CA: Sage.

Urberg, K., Shyu, S., & Liang, J. (1990). Peer influence in adolescent cigarette smoking. *Addictive Behaviors, 15,* 247–255.

Urberg, K. A., Degirmencioglu, S. M., & Pilgrim, C. (1997). Close friend and group influence on adolescent cigarette smoking and alcohol use. *Developmental Psychology, 33,* 834–844.

Webb, J. A., Baer, P. E., McLaughlin, M. J., McKelvey, R. S., & Caid, C. D. (1991). Risk factors and their relation to initiation of alcohol use among early adolescents. *Journal of the American Academy of Child and Adolescent Psychiatry, 30,* 563–568.

Webster-Stratton, C., & Herbert, M. (1994). *Troubled families — problem children: Working with parents — A collaborative process.* Chichester, England: Wiley.

Weinberg, N. Z., Rahdert, E., Colliver, J. D., & Glantz, M. (1998). Adolescent substance abuse: A review of the past 10 years. *Journal of the American Academy of Child and Adolescent Psychiatry, 37,* 252–261.

Yoshikawa, H. (1994). Prevention as cumulative protection: Effects of early family support and education on chronic delinquency and its risk. *Psychological Bulletin, 115,* 28–54.

8

ARNOLD P. GOLDSTEIN

Low-Level Aggression

New Targets for Zero Tolerance

Whether via primarily direct or vicarious experience, it is now generally well established that aggression is primarily learned behavior (Bandura, 1973; Baron & Richardson, 1994; Huesmann, 1988). A distinction is usually made, however, between learning a behavior (i.e., acquisition) and actually carrying it out (i.e., performance).

Once one knows how to share, confront, cooperate, ignore, or aggress, whether or not one chooses to do so is largely a matter of rewards or punishments such behavior has received in the past and one's appraisal of how likely it is that the behavior will be rewarded or reinforced if used at a particular time. The core purpose of this chapter revolves around this key consequence of reinforced performance on the continued, and especially escalated, use of the behavior rewarded. If a young student curses a teacher and by that act believes he has grown in stature in the eyes of his classmates, continued cursing becomes all the more probable. If a boy in late adolescence deals with jealousy by slapping his girlfriend after seeing her talking to another boy, her subsequent obedience to his wishes makes further slapping more likely when, in his view, she has transgressed in other ways. So, too, for the adult who bullies at the workplace, the daughter or son who abuses or neglects an aged parent, the husband and wife who scream at each other, and the parent who disciplines with harsh spankings. Unfortunately, it is not only the continued use of cursing, slapping, bullying, abuse, neglect, or screaming that is made more likely by their perceived success but also their escalation to progressively higher levels of more serious and more injurious forms of aggression.

This chapter concerns escalation. Initial empirical support is developing for the idea that low-level aggression, when rewarded, grows (often rapidly) into those several forms of often intractable high-level aggression. Although schools, media, politicians, and social and behavioral scientists focus on murder, rape, assault, gangs, guns, and other forms and correlates of serious aggression, they ignore their precursors—aggressive behavior such as cursing, threats, insults and incivilities, vandalism, bullying, and harassment.

Chronology of Low-Level Aggression

Aggression is commonly defined as intentional physical or psychological injury to another person. Providing a companion definition for low-level aggression is less straightforward. Is it intentional physical or psychological injury that is only mildly or moderately injurious to another person? Whose perspective should be called on to provide such seriousness or severity ratings or rankings? What is the role of frequency or repetitiveness? Is a steady diet of cutting insults from peers a higher level of aggression than occasional hard slaps to the face?

The tracing of aggression pathways contributes to definition because, generally, less harmful (target's perspective) or less intense (perpetrator's perspective) aggressive behaviors precede its more harmful and/or intense expression. Loeber et al. (1993) have identified three common developmental pathways, from "less serious manifestations" to "more serious manifestations," followed by a large percentage of the boys they studied as they progressed from disruptiveness to delinquency.

The *authority conflict* pathway appears earliest. It begins with stubborn behavior; proceeds to defiance, such as refusal and disobedience; and is followed by authority avoidance, as concretized by truancy and running away from home. The *covert* pathway starts with frequent lying, shoplifting, and other "minor covert behaviors"; moves on to property damage as incurred by vandalism or firesetting; and culminates in moderate to serious covert delinquency, such as fraud or burglary. The *overt* pathway commences with minor overt behaviors such as annoying others or bullying; proceeds to individual or gang physical fighting; and reaches its extreme of severity in assault, rape, or other violent behavior.

Other pathway models have been offered to depict common routes of escalation from minor to serious levels of aggression or delinquency (Elliott, 1994; Farrington, 1991; LeBlanc, 1996; Moffitt, 1993; Nagin, Farrington & Moffitt, 1995). According to these models, the timing (age of onset) of aggressive acts, their variety, their rate of escalation, and their chronicity relate to the eventual seriousness of expression.

Low-level aggression may be further understood by examining the sequencing of behavior within the temporal confines of single aggressive incidents. The opening moves made by perpetrators toward targets in violent incidents occurring in school settings include unprovoked offensive touching, interfering with something owned by or being used by another, verbal insults and teasing, and rough physical play (National Institute of Justice, 1977). These authors concluded:

> Reducing the occurrence of opening moves appears to be the most promising approach to preventing escalation to violence. . . . One of the most frequent opening moves is offensive touching. The design of school-based violence prevention programs could

include policies and practices that strongly discourage this type of behavior, however minor some of its expressions may appear. The study findings reveal many instances in which these opening moves escalate to fierce combats, suggesting that efforts to reduce this behavior will reduce serious violent incidents. (pp. 5, 7)

When such policies and practices are not in place or are ineffective, aggressive opening moves are often followed by an escalating sequence some have termed "character contests." These are retaliatory progressions of verbal and eventually physical attempts to harm, to save face, and ultimately to defeat one's protagonist.

Felson (1978) has studied such character contests in his work on aggression as impression management. He comments:

An insult . . . places the target into an unfavorable situational identity by making the person appear weak, incompetent and cowardly. A successful counterattack is one effective way of nullifying the imputed negative identity by showing one's strength, competence, and courage. . . . Given the sacredness and vulnerability of the self, the ambiguous line between disagreement and disparagement, and the tendency for perceived attack to result in counterattack, small arguments readily escalate through a reciprocal process into aggressive encounters. (pp. 207, 211)

Ratings and Rankings of Antisocial Behaviors

Forgas, Brown, and Menyhart (1980) investigated the criteria employed when making judgments about the seriousness of antisocial behavior. They found probability of occurrence to be a significant influence on such ratings, along with the perceived justifiability of the act and the degree to which the act was sanctioned or not by those in authority.

In a seriousness rating study conducted by O'Connell and Whelan (1996), raters were asked to judge the seriousness of an array of offenses and apparently did so based on a joint reflection of harmfulness and wrongfulness. Five clusters of ratings emerged. The lowest in seriousness, the authors note, were crimes held by some to be "victimless," namely dealing in soft drugs and consensual underage sex. Those in the next cluster, dole fraud and fraud against business, do have victims, but "it is either diffuse or is an impersonal institution, so that the impact on any particular individual is diluted" (p. 308). In the third cluster (corruption in the police, fraud against the public), the researchers note, the victims are more concentrated, less diffuse groups of people who are harmed by the offense. The final two clusters (burglary, mugging, assault on police; and murder, respectively) show increasing levels of individualized violation and personal harmfulness.

Goldstein, Palumbo, Striepling, and Voutsinas (1995) took a complementary approach to defining aggression levels. Their national survey of American teachers yielded a pool of 1,000 descriptions of in-school aggressive incidents, along with the details of how each incident was resolved. These investigators grouped the 1,000 incident reports into 13 categories arrayed from low-level through moderate-level to high-level aggression, as depicted in Table 8.1.

What then is low-level aggression? We have examined a number of diverse operational definitions in aggression-seriousness research conducted both across and within incidents and employing either rating or ranking methodologies. Al-

TABLE 8.1   Schoolhouse Incident Categories,
in Order of Growing Severity

1. Horseplay
2. Rules violation
3. Disruptiveness
4. Refusal
5. Cursing
6. Bullying
7. Sexual harassment
8. Physical threats
9. Vandalism
10. Out-of-control behavior
11. Fights
12. Attacks on teachers
13. Group aggression

From Goldstein et al. (1995). Copyright 1995 by
Research Press. Used with permission.

though one can pull from this body of research a general consensus regarding which particular behaviors are deemed to be "low level," it must be quickly acknowledged that judgments about the level of intensity of an aggressive act must remain very much in the eyes of its target: different people will experience the same aggressive act quite differently. For example, Sparks, Genn, and Dodd (1977) found that given acts of aggression are perceived to be more serious with increasing age of the rater. Victims of aggressive behavior rate such actions as more serious than do the perpetrators of the behavior (Idisis, 1996; Wolf, Moav, & Silfen, 1991). Walker (1978) reported that men rate violent offenses more seriously than women do, and persons of higher social class also perceive violent offenses as significantly more serious than do raters from lower social class backgrounds. The reverse social class finding emerged in work by Sparks et al. (1977) for property offenses. Consistent ethnic differences in aggression-seriousness ratings have also been reported (Lubel, Wolf, & Krausz, 1992; Rossi, Waite, Bose, & Berk, 1974).

The Escalation of Low-Level Aggression: Research Findings

Insults, threats, teasing, and even many forms of bullying, harassment, and abuse are often merely unpleasant, annoying, or aversive, not seriously injurious. These several incarnations of low-level aggression are important because of their not-infrequent high-level aggressive sequelae. In the previous sections, pathway models and aggressive-incident chronologies were described. Research supporting escalation is described in the following section.

Laboratory Research

An initial series of investigations conducted by J. Goldstein and colleagues consistently found what these researchers termed a "trials effect" (Goldstein, Davis & Herman, 1975; Goldstein, Davis, Kernis, & Cohn, 1981). As several others have also reported, studies using the Buss (1961) aggression machine find that both experimental and control participants regularly increase, in both intensity and duration, the level of shock they believe they are administering to another person as the study's trials proceed. Examining alternative explanations for this consistent escalation result, the researchers found evidence in support of a process of disinhibition. As the researchers state, "once punishment is administered, it becomes increasingly easy to administer more intense punishment, regardless of the behavior of the learner [target]" (Goldstein et al., 1981, p. 167). Others have suggested that pain cues from the victim may be able to break into this process and halt the escalation by the aggressor, although under some circumstances such feedback has served as reinforcement for pain infliction and caused it to continue to escalate, not diminish (Suedfeld, 1990; Zimbardo, 1969).

Taylor, Shuntich, and Greenberg (1979) had their research participants engage in a short series of aggressive interactions in the form of competitive encounters in which, as discussed herein, progressively greater shock intensities were seemingly administered. The researchers then examined each participant's behavior in a subsequent session, one in which the other party did not behave in a provocative manner. In this session, too, participants continued to behave in a highly aggressive manner, a finding explained by the researchers as a trials or practice effect, as well as a response to anticipated counteraggression in the face of one's own aggressive provocation.

Yet another mechanism that apparently facilitates escalation in this paradigm is what Freedman and Fraser (1966) have termed the "foot-in-the-door" phenomenon. Willingness to engage in high levels of diverse negative behaviors has reliably been shown to be made more likely by prior compliance with requests to participate in low levels of such behaviors. Extending this effect to the realm of aggression, Gilbert (1981) made this observation:

> Milgram's (1963) incremental shock procedure for quantifying obedience may be partly responsible for the high levels of obedience obtained. The innocuous beginning of the shock sequence (low voltage, no negative feedback) may elicit compliance before the frightening implications of the procedure are clear, and the gradual escalation in shock intensity may deprive subjects of a qualitative breakpoint needed to justify changing obedience to disobedience. (p. 690)

In addition to disinhibition with practice, anticipated retaliation, and foot-in-the-door, a fourth explanation for the escalation of aggression rests on the concept of deindividuation. A construct first introduced by Festinger, Pepitone, and Newcombe (1952), deindividuation is the circumstance in which individuals, usually in groups, experience diminished self-awareness and self-regulation, lessened inner restraint, and heightened freedom to engage in aggressive or other deviant behaviors. Examples of deindividuation can be found in mob behavior, in group bullying, in gang violence, and in the thuglike behavior of fans at football or other athletic events. It is a process engendered by high levels of emotional arousal, by diffusion of personal responsibility, and by the anonymity of single persons in collectives and a process whose expression in aggressive behavior is further facilitated by modeling and contagion influences. Jaffe and Yinon (1979) and Jaffe, Shapir, and Yinon (1981) studied this phenomenon in a laboratory context and indeed found consistent outcomes when comparing individual- versus group-administered aggression, as measured by the pace and intensity of (apparent) shock administered. On both escalation criteria, persons in groups significantly exceeded individuals acting alone, thus strongly suggesting support for the role of deindividuation in the escalation of aggression, especially group aggression.

Whether and why escalation occurs is largely a function of the appraisals and behavior of the parties involved. But it is also a function of the physical and social context in which the character contest takes place. I have examined aggression and its growth as a "person-environment duet" elsewhere, in an exploration of the ecology of aggression (Goldstein, 1994). Its likelihood of escalation, to be sure, is influenced by qualities of the persons involved—their impulsiveness (Halperin et al., 1995), levels of self-esteem (Kernis, Granneman, & Barclay, 1989), cognitive biases (Dodge & Frame, 1982), temperamental difficulties (Kingston & Prior, 1995), school and family bonding (O'Donnell, Hawkins, & Abbott, 1995), values (McCarthy, 1994), dominance needs (Weisfeld, 1994), and more. However, these several person qualities take on their escalation potency as they interact as a duet with the qualities of the setting in which the event is based. Some of these qualities are physical. Aggression and its escalation in schools is more likely to take place on the playground, in the (boy's) bathrooms, in the cafeteria, and in the hallways between classes than in the classroom or other venues (Goldstein & Conoley, 1997). In the home, the bedroom is the deadliest room, the kitchen the second most dangerous, followed by the living room and other sites, with the safest room in the house being the bathroom (Gelles, 1972). Stores are most vulnerable to becoming violent crime sites when they are (1) close to major transportation routes, (2) on streets with small amounts of vehicular traffic, (3) next to vacant lots, and (4) in areas with few other stores or commercial activity (Duffalo, 1976). Alcohol intoxication, a person quality, certainly has been shown to prime character contests and their escalated aggressive responding (Pernanen, 1991), but the degree to which such escalation takes place has also been demonstrated to be a result of qualities of the bar or other drinking establishment itself (Felson, Baccaglini, & Gmelch, 1986; Leather & Lawrence, 1995). Neighborhoods, too, matter a great deal in determining whether or not aggression is likely and its escalation frequent.

The social environment plays an equally significant role in the escalation process. Audience effects have been shown to matter a great deal, especially in the context of character contests (Borden, 1975; Cratty, 1981). Perhaps most important, however, regarding the social ecology component of the person-environment duet is the behavior of the target person. Floyd (1985) is correct in asserting that "victimization needs to be understood in terms of the reciprocal behaviors in a relationship between an aggressor and a victim" (p. 9). With regard to bullying, for example, it is the behavior of both the bully and the victim that may make the bullying begin, continue, and at times escalate. Here, as with victims of rape, assault, murder, or other aggressive acts, one must be especially careful not to blame the target for his or her own victimization even while seeking to identify his or her contribution to the aggressive incident. Laboratory study of the aggression escalation process is modest in amount, interesting in result, and pregnant in potential.

Delinquency Research

Many delinquent youths' behavior progresses along the three pathways noted earlier that were posited by Loeber et al. (1993). Although there are exceptions, a great many youths do indeed follow one or another of the pathways quite as described. Loeber and Stouthamer-Loeber (1998) importantly observe that the model's fit is best when a distinction is made between youths whose antisocial behavior is a transient event (i.e., "experimenters") and those for whom aggression and criminal behavior continue over an extended period of time (i.e., "persisters"). It is these latter youths whom these investigators, as well as Elliott (1994), have most clearly shown to follow the pathway sequences proposed.

Related escalation outcomes have been reported by a number of investigators (Mitchell & Rosa, 1979; Roff & Wirt, 1984; Viemero, 1996). In each investigation, childhood aggression emerged as an antecedent of later frequency of often considerably more severe adolescent and adult criminal offending. Le Blanc (1990) describes this sequence well:

> We find that there are five stages in the development of offending and that they form a sequence. They are, in order, emergence, exploration, explosion, conflagration, and outburst. At first, usually between age 8 and 10, the delinquent activities are homogeneous and benign, almost always expressed in the form of petty larceny; this is the stage of emergence. This period is followed, generally between ages 10 and 12, by a diversification and escalation of the offenses, essentially comprising shoplifting and vandalism; this stage is one of exploration. Later, at about age 13, there is a substantial increase in the variety and seriousness of the crimes; and four new types of crime develop — common theft, public disorder, burglary, and personal theft; this is the stage of explosion. . . . Around age 15, variety and seriousness increase further as four more types of crime are added — drug trafficking, motor vehicle theft, armed robbery, and personal attack; this is the stage of conflagration. [There is] also a fifth stage which occurs only during adulthood; it is a progress toward more sophisticated or more violent forms of criminal behavior; it is called outburst. (pp. 11–12)

Tracking a large sample of youth from their adolescent years into adulthood, Stattin and Magnusson (1989) found that compared with youngsters who were low or average on aggression, highly aggressive youth were, as adults, (1) involved in more serious crimes, (2) involved in more frequent crimes, and (3) particularly more likely to engage in confrontive and destructive offenses.

Focusing on school-based predictors, Hamalainen and Pulkkinen (1996) found that serious crime at age 27 was accurately forecast by aggressive (verbal and physical) and norm-breaking (disobedience, truancy) behavior at age 8. Many investigators have shown that aggression is a remarkably stable behavior over the life span. The intensity or seriousness of such behavior, however, is far from stable and often shows substantial and predictable escalation of intensity.

Incivility Research

The escalation of aggression and kindred behaviors has also been well demonstrated in field studies that focus on the consequences of physical and social incivilities.

Physical incivilities are concrete ecological features that serve as both reflections of and impetus for neighborhood disuse, disdain, decay, and deterioration. They include trash and litter; graffiti; abandoned or burned-out stores, houses, and automobiles; dirt; vacant lots; broken windows and streetlights; ill-kept buildings; vandalism of diverse sorts; and similar expressions of a cycle of decline. Physical incivilities are accompanied by social incivilities in a display of person-environment reciprocal influence. Such social incivilities may include increased presence of aggressive gangs, drug users, prostitutes, "skid row" alcoholics, and bench or street sleepers; increased presence of drug purveyors; increased crime by offenders and increased fear of crime by neighborhood residents; and increased panhandling, harassment, chronic loitering, gambling, and drinking.

Does the level of incivility relate to and perhaps actually help cause the level of neighborhood crime? Taylor and Gottfredson (1986) reported a correlation of .63 between incivilities and crime rates.

Skogan's (1990) investigation in this domain gathered information regarding incivilities and their consequences from an average of 325 people in each of 40 different neighborhoods in the United States. In his appropriately titled report, *Disorder and Decline*, he found strong evidence that perceived crime, fear of crime, and actual level of crime victimization were each a function of neighborhood physical and social incivility.

Others have observed similar aggression-escalating consequences of disorder and incivility in school settings. J. Wilson and Petersilia (1995), for example, describe graffiti on school walls, debris in corridors, and students coming to school late and wandering the halls as the foundation on which more serious violence rests.

> [Low-level] disorder invites youngsters to test further and further the limits of acceptable behavior. One connection between the inability of school authorities to maintain order and an increasing rate of violence is that, among students with little faith in the usefulness of the education they are supposed to be getting, challenging rules is part of the fun. When they succeed in littering or writing on walls, they feel encouraged to challenge other, more sacred rules, like the prohibition against assaulting fellow students and even teachers. (p. 149)

A major step forward in both planning and evaluating a citywide incivility intervention program was reported by Kelling and Coles (1996) in their aptly titled book, *Fixing Broken Windows*. Enhanced police attention to an array of low-level infractions or quality-of-life crimes — panhandling, subway fare beating, graffiti, loitering — decreased not only these behaviors but also an extended series of more serious crimes.

Implications and Applications

What are the policy implications of such findings? In American schools today, for example, there is growing use of a zero-tolerance intervention toward high-level infractions such as weapons possession. Zero-tolerance contingencies to low-level infractions need not be severe, but they do need to be perceived by their recipients as unpleasant and to be administered in a consistent manner.

TABLE 8.2   Forms of Low-Level Aggression

Verbal Maltreatment
Verbal abuse
Teasing
Cursing
Gossip
Ostracism
Physical Maltreatment
Bullying
Sexual harassment
Criminal Maltreatment
Vandalism
Shoplifting
Sabotage
Animal cruelty
Stalking
Road rage
Minimal Maltreatment
Rough-and-tumble play
Hazing
Baiting
Booing
Tantrums

From Goldstein (1999). Copyright 1999 by Research Press. Used with permission.

Table 8.2 presents examples of low-level aggressive behaviors in need of such consistent consequences (Goldstein, 1999). Bullying and vandalism are two instances of behaviors that are often considered to be low-level violence but that are, in fact, very critical to confront in school settings. These behaviors are described in detail in the following sections.

Bullying

Bullying is behavior of a verbal and/or physical character that intends to harm and that is typically both unprovoked and repeated. Blevens (1993) has employed a definitional distinction between direct and indirect bullying. The former involves face-to-face confrontations, open physical attacks by bully on victim, and the use in such contexts of threats and intimidating gestures. Indirect bullying is exemplified by social exclusion and isolation, scapegoating, the spreading of rumors, and similar behaviors more akin to the verbal maltreatments examined earlier.

Bullying has received relatively little attention in the United States (Hoover & Hazler, 1991). Its early recognition and research examination occurred primarily in Scandinavian countries (Olweus, 1993) and in Great Britain (Elliott, 1997a, b; Smith & Sharp, 1994). In spite of its substantial frequency of occurrence, it is often the school's best kept secret. Teachers and administrators may be preoccupied with acts reflecting higher levels of aggression or they may simply ignore it because most victims elect not to call it to their attention. When it does occur, it is more likely to do so on the playground or in the school corridors between classes rather than in the classroom, so it usually does not disrupt the class. Further, even when its reality is acknowledged, it may still be ignored given the belief of many school personnel (and parents) that bullying is a "natural" part of growing up and perhaps even a positive contributor to the toughening up purported to be so useful in a competitive society. Thus school staff may be unaware that bullying is taking place or, if aware, may ignore it. Others, too, may be blind or mute to its occurrence. The bully won't tell; why should he or she volunteer to get in trouble? The victim won't tell for fear of bringing on further and perhaps more severe episodes of the very behavior he or she wishes to avoid. Other students often elect not to speak up out of concern for becoming targets themselves and out of reluctance to break the code of silence that prevails among students regarding such matters. The victim's parents are also likely to be unaware that bullying is taking place. They may wonder why their child comes home during the school day to use the bathroom or how his clothing gets torn or why she seems so hungry at supper time, unaware that the school bathroom was too scary, the clothing was ripped by a bully, or her lunch money was extorted earlier. Thus bullying in American schools is little studied, little spoken about, and infrequently thwarted.

As with all other forms of low-level aggression that are similarly ignored, the incidence of bullying continues and grows in frequency, and its sequelae emerge and escalate in intensity. Greenbaum, Turner, and Stephens (1989) report that adults who had been childhood bullies are five times more likely to have a serious criminal record by age 30 than are those who were not bullies. In a longitudinal study conducted by Olweus (1991), 60% of the boys who were identified as bullies in Grades 6 through 9 had at least one criminal conviction by age 24, and 40% of them had three or more arrests. Such was true for only 10% of boys who earlier were neither bullies nor victims. Eron, Huesmann, Dubow, Romanoff, and Yarmel (1987) found that youths who bullied at age 8 had a 1 in 4 chance of having a criminal record by age 30, as compared with the 1 in 20 chance that most children have. Early adult arrest record is not the only illustration of the escalation potential of physical maltreatment via bullying. Bullies also have greater potential for school dropout, spouse abuse, drug dealing, and vandalism (Eron & Huessman, 1987; Rigby & Cox, 1996). Findings on bullying escalation provide direct confirmation of the earlier-cited literature concerning developmental pathways begun with low-level aggression.

Beginning with the pioneering school bullying program developed by Olweus (1993) and progressing through the similarly comprehensive interventions offered by Elliott (1995); Garrity, Jens, Porter, Sager, and Short-Camilli (1994); Pepler, Craig, Ziegler, and Charach (1994); Roland (1989); and Stephenson and Smith (1995), it has become clear that the optimal intervention strategy for dealing effectively with bullying by and of students is a whole-school approach. All acts of aggression derive from a multiplicity of causes and thus will yield best when broached by an equally complex and comprehensive intervention program. Following Olweus (1993), program intervention components at the school, class, and individual levels can be identified. The training manuals *Bully-Proofing Your School*

(Garrity et al., 1994) and *Bullying at School* (Olweus, 1993) are especially helpful in understanding how to implement antibully programs (Table 8.3).

Whole-school, antibullying programs employing variable combinations of these several school-, class-, and individual-level components have been systematically evaluated by a number of investigators in widely dispersed locations. These studies have consistently yielded substantial reductions in bullying (Arora, 1994; Olweus, 1993; Pepler et al., 1994; Roland, 1989; Smith & Sharp, 1994).

TABLE 8.3   School-Based Interventions to Reduce Bullying

School-Level Interventions

Schoolwide survey to determine amount, frequency, and locus of bullying
Discussion of bullying (nature, sources, signs, prevention) at PTA/PTO meetings
Discussion of bullying (nature, sources, signs, prevention) at assemblies
Increased quantity and quality of student surveillance and supervision
Establishment of school antibullying policy concretized by mission statement distributed to all staff, students, and parents
Creation of a schoolwide "telling" climate that legitimizes informing about bullying, concretized by a phone hot line, an anonymous mail drop, or other means
Regular staff meetings to exchange relevant information about bullying and monitor intervention effectiveness
Development and dissemination of antibullying rules via posters, memos, and other means
Restructuring of school locations in which bullying frequently occurs
Separate break time for younger and older students

Class-Level Interventions

Discussions of bullying (nature, sources, signs, prevention) at class meetings
Regular role-playing of responses to bullying
Announcement of use of nonviolent sanctions in response to bullying behavior
Training of students as helpful bystanders/informers when bullying occurs
Formation of victim support groups
Increased use of cooperative learning for curriculum delivery
Use of student-run "bully courts" to adjudicate incidents
Avoidance of use of bullying behavior by teachers
Monitoring of student understanding of and compliance with schoolwide antibullying policy and rules
Contracting with students for compliance with antibullying rules
Use of stories, art, and activities to communicate and reinforce antibullying policy and rules
Announcement and use of positive consequences for following rules concerning bullying behavior

Individual-Level Interventions

Bullies	Victims
Social-skills training	Assertiveness training
Sanctions for bullying behavior	Martial arts training
Employment as a cross-age tutor	Social-skills training
Individual counseling	Change of class or school
Anger-control training	Encourage association with new peers
Empathy training	Individual counseling

Vandalism

Vandalism has been defined as:

> The willful or malicious destruction, injury, disfigurement, or defacement of property without the consent of the owner or person having custody or control by cutting, tearing, breaking, marking, painting, drawing, covering with filth, or any such means as may be specified by local law. (FBI, 1978, p. 217)

School (and other) vandalism is an expensive fact of U.S. life. Monetary cost estimates of vandalism illustrate that the expense of vandalism, like its incidence, is both absolutely high and increasing. In the approximately 84,000 schools in the United States, for example, cost estimates over the past 25 years show a near-linear upward trend, peaking in recent years at $600 million (Stoner, Shinn, & Walker, 1991).

Arson, a particularly dangerous form of vandalism, deserves special comment. Whereas window breaking is the most frequent single act of aggression toward property in schools, arson is clearly the most costly, typically accounting for approximately 40% of total vandalism costs annually (Mathie & Schmidt, 1977).

The costs of vandalism are not only monetary but social, as described by Vestermark and Blauvelt (1978) regarding its expensive impact in school settings:

> By limiting criteria of vandalism's impact to only monetary costs, we overlook those incidents which have low monetary cost but, nevertheless, tremendous impact upon the school. The impact of a seventy-nine cent can of spray paint, used to paint racial epithets on a hallway wall, far exceeds the monetary cost of removing the paint. A racial confrontation could result, which might force the closing of the school for an indefinite period. How does one calculate that type of expense: confrontation and subsequent closing of a school? (p. 138)

Intervention Strategies

Changing the Ecology of the School

An ecological perspective on vandalism control and reduction has appeared and reappeared under a variety of rubrics: "utilitarian prevention" (Cohen, 1973), "deopportunizing design" (Wiesenthal, 1990), "architectural determinism" (Zweig & Ducey, 1978), "crime prevention through environmental design" (Wood, 1991), "situational crime prevention" (Clarke, 1992), and "environmental criminology" (Brantingham & Brantingham, 1991). Person-oriented strategies seek to reduce the potential or actual vandal's motivation to perpetrate such behavior. In contrast, environment-oriented strategies seek to alter the physical setting, context, or situation in which vandalism might occur, so that the potential or actual vandal's opportunity to perpetrate such behavior is reduced. This ecological strategy, of altering the physical or social environment to prevent or reduce the occurrence of vandalism, has been an especially popular choice, particularly in the United States. Thus venues as diverse as school districts, mass transit systems, museums, shopping malls, national and state parks, and many others have time and again opted for hardening targets, controlling access, deflecting offenders, screening entry and exit, increasing surveillance, removing inducements, and similar environment-altering intervention strategies as their first and often only means of defense against vandalism (Goldstein, 1996).

Yet, paradoxically, very little other than anecdotal, impressionistic, or testimonial "evidence" exists for the actual effectiveness of these widely used strategies in controlling vandalism. Furthermore, the very scope of their implementation — in their most extreme form, the "Bastille response" (Ward, 1973) or the "crime-proof fortress" (Zweig & Ducey, 1978) — has in some settings had a negative impact on the very mission for which the setting was created in the first place. For example, "more and more high schools are becoming mechanical systems ruled by constraints on timing, location, and behavior. The similarity between schools and jails is becoming ever more pronounced" (Csikszentmihalyi & Larsen, 1978, p. 25).

Changing the Vandal

In contrast to intervention efforts directed toward the actual or potential vandal's physical or social environment, here the intervention target is the vandal himself or herself. Cohen (1974) suggests three such person-oriented strategies:

1. *Education.* Here the effort is made to increase the potential vandal's awareness of the costs and other consequences of vandalistic behavior. These interventions assume that once this awareness is increased, the person will consider the possible consequences and choose to refrain from perpetrating vandalism.
2. *Deterrence and retribution.* These strategies rely on threat, punishment, or forcing those committing vandalistic acts to make restitution. Punishment strategies are especially widely employed. Ward (1973) comments:

The most frequent public reaction to vandalism is "Hit them hard": all that is needed is better detection by the police and stiffer sentences by the court. The general tendency is to support heavier fines, custodial sentences. . . . Other, extra-legal sanctions include banning offenders from swimming baths, sports fields, youth clubs or play centers. Some local authorities have suggested the evicting of tenants whose children are responsible for vandalism. (p. 256)

3. *Deflection.* These strategies "attempt to understand and redirect the motivational causes of vandalism into non-damaging means of expression" (Cohen, 1974, p. 54). They include allowing controlled destruction, providing substitute targets, or furnishing alternative outlets for energetic activity. Koch (1975) describes a parallel array of person-oriented strategies employing either coercive controls, the indoctrination of information, legal regulations, or the substitution of functional equivalents.

Although punishment, as noted, appears to be an especially frequently used person-oriented strategy (Heller & White, 1975; Stoner et al., 1991), there is evidence that heavy reliance on it may often actually result in an increase, not a decrease, in the frequency of vandalism (Greenberg, 1969; Scrimger & Elder, 1981). These and other investigators report a substantial decrease in vandalism as punitiveness decreases (Mayer & Butterworth, 1979; Mayer, Butterworth, Nafpaktitis, & Sulzer-Azaroff, 1983; Mayer, Nafpaktitis, Butterworth, & Hollingsworth, 1987).

In contrast to the use of extrinsic processes (e.g., teacher approval) targeted toward altering vandal behavior, Csikszentmihalyi and Larsen (1978) focus more directly on a strategy calling for enhancement of intrinsic processes. Reliance on extrinsically provided rewards or reinforcement, they propose, is cumbersome and cost ineffective; most significantly in their view, it functions to diminish the individual's intrinsic motivation not to engage in vandalistic behavior. A second vandal-oriented strategy of which they are similarly critical on these very same grounds of diminished intrinsic motivation is that of "strengthening the means-ends connection between adherence to school constraints and achievement of desired future goals" (p. 29). This is a difficult strategy to implement, as it requires a considerably closer correspondence between school performance and future rewards. For many youths and in many schools, such a connection is not easy to perceive. And when it is perceived, it is yet a second instance of training youths to guide their behavior on the basis of extrinsic rather than intrinsic motivations. As their recommended alternative strategy, Csikszentmihalyi and Larsen (1978) suggest reorientation of school procedures and curricula in a manner designed to stimulate and respond to youths' intrinsic motivation for challenge, for extension of their skills, for mastery, for growth, and for (in the researchers' terms) the experience of "flow." In their view:

> the state of enjoyment occurs when a person is challenged at a level matched by his or her level of skill. . . . Ideally, learning should involve systemic involvement in sequences of challenges internalized by students. . . . In the absence of such opportunities, antisocial behavior provides an alternative framework of challenges for bored students. Disruption of classes, vandalism, and violence in schools are, in part, attempts of adolescents to obtain enjoyment in otherwise lifeless schools. Restructuring education in terms of intrinsic motivation would not only reduce school crime, but also accomplish the goal of teaching youth how to enjoy life in an affirmative way. (p. 1)

Vandalism is a domain of interest that has a remarkably meager research base. Mayer and colleagues' extrinsic-reward studies (Mayer & Butterworth, 1979; Mayer et al., 1983, 1987) and relevant intrinsic-motivation studies (deCharms, 1968, 1976; Deci, 1975) stand in support of the value of both orientations in enhancing vandals' prosocial motivation.

One final point needs to be offered regarding vandal-oriented intervention strategies. Ideally, both who the vandals are (Griffiths & Shapland, 1979) and what level their vandalistic behaviors have reached (Hauber, 1989) will, in part, determine the nature of the intervention implemented. Griffiths and Shapland (1979) correctly assert that the vandal's motives and the very meaning of the act itself change with age and context and that strategies need to vary accordingly:

The preventive measures that need to be taken to make any given environment vandal-proof may be different according to the nature of the vandal. . . . As an example of this, look at how a window in a deserted house may be broken. This may have been done by kids getting in to play; by older children as a game of skill; by adolescents or adults in order to remove the remaining furniture or fittings; by someone with a grudge against the person or previous landlord; by a pressure group to advertise the dereliction of empty property; or by [a vagrant] to gain attention or to [get in to spend] the night. (pp. 17–18)

Changing Person-Environment

Every act of vandalism springs from both person and environment sources — a dualism that must similarly characterize efforts at its prevention and remediation. The separate person-oriented and environment-oriented vandalism intervention strategies explored previously will optimally be implemented in diverse, prescriptively appropriate combinations. Casserly, Bass, and Garrett (1980), Cohen (1973), Geason and Wilson (1990), Kulka (1978), Vestermark and Blauvelt (1978), and Wilson (1979) are among the several vandalism theorists and researchers who also champion multilevel, multimodal person-environment intervention strategies. Several practitioners have already put in place such joint strategies and, at least impressionistically, report having done so to good advantage (Hendrick & Murfin, 1974; Jamieson, 1987; Levy-Leboyer, 1984; Mason, 1979; Panko, 1978; Scrimger & Elder, 1981; Stover, 1990; Weeks, 1976; White & Fallis, 1980). Vandalism, like all instances of aggression, is a complexly determined behavior. Every act of vandalism derives from several causes and therefore is best combated with equally complex interventions.

Here, I draw on the large pool of vandalism interventions I have presented elsewhere (Goldstein, 1996) in order to illustratively reorganize samples of these interventions into just such multilevel, multichannel configurations. In the absence of efficacy evaluations, no particular interventions or intervention configurations can be singled out for recommended use at this time. However, this emphasis on the selection and implementation of meaningful intervention combinations is likely to prove a major step toward truly effective vandalism prevention, control, and reduction.

Table 8.4 presents a level-by-mode intervention schema targeted at reducing vandalism in school contexts. Practitioners and evaluators of vandalism prevention/reduction efforts should ensure that interventions at all levels and through all channels are included in their packages of interventions. (See also Harootunian, 1986; Zweir & Vaughn, 1984.)

Low-level aggression has for too long been ignored by practitioner and researcher alike. Approaches to defining what behaviors constitute low-level aggression of necessity yield to idiographic definitions obtained from its targets. Such behavior is of interest in its own right but assumes its major significance via its demonstrated tendency to escalate as its rewards become apparent. I have enumerated its several forms and illustrated by means of a lengthier consideration of bullying and vandalism what I recommend as an effective comprehensive intervention strategy.

TABLE 8.4 A Multilevel, Multichannel Schema for the Reduction of School Vandalism

Level of Intervention	Mode of Intervention				
	Psychological	Educational	Administrative	Legal	Physical
Community	"Youth vacation vigil" program	Arson education programs	"Adopt-a-school" programs	Monetary fines	Citizen, police, parent controls
School	Conflict negotiation programs	Year-round education	Schools-within-a-school	Code of rights and responsibilities	Lighting, painting, paving programs
Teacher	School-home collaboration	Multicultural sensitivity training	Reduced teacher-student ratio	Property marking with school ID	Distribution of faculty offices throughout school
Students	Interpersonal skills training	Vandalism awareness walks	School detention, suspension	Restitution, vandalism accounts	Graffiti boards, mural walls

From A. B. Goldstein (1996), *The Psychology of Vandalism* (p. 76). New York: Plenum Press.

REFERENCES

Arora, C. M. J. (1994). Is there any point in trying to reduce bullying in secondary schools? *Educational Psychology in Practice, 10,* 155–162.

Bandura, A. (1973). *Aggression: A social learning analysis.* Englewood Cliffs, NJ: Prentice-Hall.

Baron, R. A., & Richardson, D. R. (1994). *Human aggression.* New York: Plenum Press.

Borden, R. J. (1975). Witnessed aggression: Influence of an observer's sex and values on aggressive responding. *Journal of Personality and Social Psychology, 31,* 567–573.

Brantingham, P. J., & Brantingham, P. L. (1991). *Environmental criminology.* Newbury Park, CA: Sage.

Buss, A. H. (1961). *The psychology of aggression.* New York: Wiley.

Casserly, M. D., Bass, S. A., & Garrett, J. R. (1980). *School vandalism: Strategies for prevention.* Lexington, MA: Lexington Books.

Clarke, R. V. (Ed.). (1992). *Situational crime prevention: Successful case studies.* New York: Harrow & Heston.

Cohen, S. (1973). Campaigning against vandalism. In C. Ward (Ed.), *Vandalism.* London: Architectural Press.

Cohen, S. (1974). Breaking out, smashing up and the social context of aspiration. *Working Papers in Cultural Studies, 5,* 37–63.

Cratty, B. J. (1981). *Social psychology in athletics.* Englewood Cliffs, NJ: Prentice-Hall.

Csikszentmihalyi, M., & Larsen, R. (1978). *Intrinsic rewards in school crime.* Hackensack, NJ: National Council on Crime and Delinquency.

deCharms, R. (1968). *Personal causation.* New York: Academic Press.

deCharms, R. (1976). *Enhancing motivation: Change in the classroom.* New York: Irvington.

Deci, E. L. (1975). *Intrinsic motivation.* New York: Plenum.

Dodge, K. A. & Frame, C. L. (1982). Social cognitive biases and deficits in aggressive boys. *Child Development, 53,* 620–635.

Duffalo, D. C. (1976). Convenience stores, armed robbery and physical environmental features. *American Behavioral Scientist, 20,* 227–246.

Elliott, D. S. (1994). Serious violent offenders: Onset, developmental course, and termination. *Criminology, 32,* 1–21.

Elliott, M. (1995). A whole-school approach to bullying. In M. Elliott (Ed.), *Bullying: A practical guide to coping for schools.* London: Pitman.

Elliott, M. (1997a). Bullies and victims. In M. Elliott (Ed.), *Bullying: A practical guide to coping for schools.* London: Pitman.

Elliott, M. (1997b). Bullying and the under fives. In M. Elliott (Ed.), *Bullying: A practical guide to coping for schools.* London: Pitman.

Eron, L. D., Huesmann, R., Dubow, E., Romanoff, R., & Yarmel, P. W. (1987). Aggression and its correlates over 22 years. In D. H. Crowell, I. M. Evans, & C. P. O'Connell (Eds.), *Childhood aggression and violence.* New York: Plenum.

Farrington, D. P. (1991). Childhood aggression and adult violence: Early precursors and later-life outcomes. In D. J. Pepler & K. H. Rubin (Eds.), *The development and treatment of childhood aggression.* Hillsdale, NJ: Erlbaum.

Federal Bureau of Investigation. (1978). *Crime in the United States.* Washington, D.C.: U. S. Government Printing Office.

Federal Bureau of Investigation. (1993). *Crime in the United States.* Washington, DC: U. S. Government Printing Office.

Felson, R. B. (1978). Aggression as impression management. *Social Psychology, 41,* 205–213.

Felson, R. B., Baccaglini, W., & Gmelch,

G. (1986). Bar-room brawls: Aggression and violence in Irish and American bars. In A. Campbell & J. J. Gibbs (Eds.), *Violent transactions: The limits of personality*. Oxford, England: Blackwell.

Festinger, L., Pepitone, A., & Newcombe, T. (1952). Some consequences of deindividuation in a group. *Journal of Abnormal and Social Psychology, 47*, 382–389.

Floyd, N. M. (1985). "Pick on somebody your own size": Controlling victimization. *Pointer, 29*, 9–17.

Forgas, J. P., Brown, L. B., & Menyhart, J. (1980). Dimensions of aggression: The perception of aggressive episodes. *British Journal of Social and Clinical Psychology, 19*, 215–227.

Freedman, J. L., & Fraser, C. C. (1966). Compliance without pressure: The foot-in-the-door technique. *Journal of Personality and Social Psychology, 4*, 195–202.

Garrity, C., Jens, K., Porter, W., Sager, N., & Short-Camilli, C. (1994). *Bully-proofing your school*. Longmont, CO: Sopris West.

Geason, S., & Wilson, P. R. (1990). *Preventing graffiti and vandalism*. Canberra, Australia: Australian Institute of Criminology.

Gelles, R. J. (1972). "It takes two": The roles of victim and offender. In R. J. Gelles (Ed.), *The violent home: A study of physical aggression between husband and wives*. Thousand Oaks, CA: Sage.

Gilbert, S. J. (1981). Another look at the Milgram obedience studies: The role of the graduated series of shock. *Personality and Social Psychology Bulletin, 7*, 690–695.

Goldstein, A. P. (1994). *The ecology of aggression*. New York: Plenum Press.

Goldstein, A. P. (1996). *Violence in America*. Palo Alto, CA: Davies-Black.

Goldstein, A. P. (1999). *Low-level aggression: First steps on the ladder to violence*. Champaign, IL: Research Press.

Goldstein, A. P., & Conoley, J. C. (1997). *School violence intervention: A practical handbook*. New York: Guilford Press.

Goldstein, A. P., Palumbo, J., Striepling, S. H., & Voutsinas, A. M. (1995). *Break it up*. Champaign, IL: Research Press.

Goldstein, J. H., Davis, R. W., & Herman, D. (1975). Escalation of aggression: Experimental studies. *Journal of Personality and Social Psychology, 31*, 162–170.

Goldstein, J. H., Davis, R. W., Kernis, M., & Cohn, E. S. (1981). Retarding the escalation of aggression. *Social Behaviors and Personality, 9*, 65–70.

Greenbaum, S., Turner, B., & Stephens, R. D. (1989). *Set straight on bullies*. Malibu, CA: National School Safety Center.

Greenberg, B. (1969). *School vandalism: A national dilemma*. Menlo Park, CA: Stanford Research Institute.

Griffiths, R., & Shapland, J. M. (1979). The vandal's perspective: Meanings and motives. In P. Bural (Ed.), *Designing against vandalism*. New York: Van Nostrand Reinhold.

Halperin, J. M., Newcorn, J. H., Matier, K., Bedi, S., Hall, S., & Sherma, V. (1995). Impulsivity and the initiation of fights in children with disruptive behavior disorders. *Journal of Child Psychology and Psychiatry, 36*, 1199–1211.

Hamalainen, M., & Pulkkinen, L. (1996). Problem behavior as a precursor of male criminality. *Development and Psychopathology, 8*, 443–455.

Harootunian, B. (1986). School violence and vandalism. In S. J. Apter & A. P. Goldstein (Eds.), *Youth violence: Programs and prospects*. New York: Pergamon Press.

Hauber, A. R. (1989). The social psychology of driving behavior and the traffic environment: Research on aggressive behavior in traffic. *International Review of Applied Psychology, 29*, 461–474.

Heller, M. C., & White, M. A. (1975). Rates of teacher verbal approval and disapproval to higher and lower ability classes. *Journal of Educational Psychology, 67*, 796–800.

Hendrick, C., & Murfin, M. (1974). Project library ripoff: A study of periodical mutilation in a university library. *College and Research Libraries, 35,* 402–411.

Hoover, J., & Hazler, R. J. (1991). Bullies and victims. *Elementary School Guidance and Counseling, 25,* 212–219.

Huesmann, L. R. (1988). An information processing model for the development of aggression. *Aggressive Behavior, 14,* 13–24.

Idisis, Y. (1996). Meta moral judgment among preschool children. Unpublished master's thesis, Bar-Illan University, Ramat Gan, Israel.

Jaffe, Y., Shapir, N., & Yinon, Y. (1981). Aggression and its escalation. *Journal of Cross-Cultural Psychology, 12,* 21–36.

Jaffe, Y., & Yinon, Y. (1979). Retaliatory aggression in individuals and groups. *European Journal of Social Psychology, 9,* 177–186.

Jamieson, B. (1987). Public telephone vandalism. In D. Challinger (Ed.), *Preventing property crime.* Canberra, Australia: Australian Institute of Criminology.

Kelling, G. L., & Coles, C. M. (1996). *Fixing broken windows.* New York: Free Press.

Kernis, M. H., Granneman, B. D., & Barclay, L. C. (1989). Stability and level of self-esteem as predictors of anger arousal and hostility. *Journal of Personality and Social Psychology, 56,* 1013–1022.

Kingston, L., & Prior, M. (1995). The development of patterns of stable, transient, and school-age onset aggressive behavior in young children. *Journal of the American Academy of Child and Adolescent Psychiatry, 34,* 348–358.

Koch, E. L. (1975). School vandalism and strategies of social control. *Urban Education, 10,* 54–72.

Kulka, R. A. (1978). School crime as a function of person-environment fit. *Theoretical Perspectives on School Crime, 1,* 17–24.

Leather, P., & Lawrence, C. (1995). Perceiving pub violence: The symbolic influence of social and environmental factors. *British Journal of Social Psychology, 34,* 395–407.

LeBlanc, M. (1990). Two processes of the development of persistent offending: Activation and escalation. In L. Robins & M. Rutter (Eds.), *Straight and devious pathways from childhood to adulthood.* Cambridge: Cambridge University Press.

LeBlanc, M. (1996). Changing patterns in the perpetration of offences over time: Trajectories from early adolescence to the early 30s. *Studies on Crime and Crime Prevention, 5,* 151–165.

Levy-Leboyer, C. (Ed.). (1984). *Vandalism: Behavior and motivations.* Amsterdam: North Holland.

Loeber, R., & Stouthamer-Loeber, M. S. (1998). Development of juvenile aggression and violence: Some common misconceptions and controversies. *American Psychologist, 53,* 242–259.

Loeber, R., Wung, P., Keenan, K., Giroux, B., Stouthamer-Loeber, M., Van Kammen, W. B., & Maughan, B. (1993). Developmental pathways in disruptive child behavior. *Development and Psychopathology, 5,* 103–133.

Lubel, S., Wolf, Y., & Krausz, E. (1992). Inter-ethnic differences in the judgment of filmed violence. *International Journal of Group Tensions, 23,* 314–319.

Mason, D. L. (1979). *Fine art of art security: Protecting public and private collections against theft, fire, and vandalism.* New York: Van Nostrand Reinhold.

Mathie, J. P., & Schmidt, R. E. (1977). Rehabilitation and one type of arsonist. *Fire and Arson Investigator, 28,* 53–56.

Mayer, G. R., & Butterworth, T. W. (1979). A preventive approach to school violence and vandalism: An experimental study. *Personnel and Guidance Journal, 57,* 436–441.

Mayer, G. R., Butterworth, T., Nafpaktitis, M., & Sulzer-Azaroff, B. (1983). Preventing school vandalism and improving discipline: A three-year study. *Journal of Applied Behavior Analysis, 16,* 355–369.

Mayer, G. R., Nafpaktitis, M., Butterworth, T., & Hollingsworth, P. (1987). A search for the elusive setting events of school vandalism: A correlational study. *Education and Treatment of Children, 10,* 259–270.

McCarthy, B. (1994). Warrior values: A socio-historical survey. In J. Archer (Ed.), *Male violence.* London: Routledge.

Milgram, S. (1963). Behavioral study of obedience. *Journal of Abnormal and Social Psychology, 67,* 371–378.

Mitchell, S., & Rosa, P. (1979). Boyhood behavior problems as precursors of criminality: A fifteen-year follow-up study. *Journal of Child Psychology and Psychiatry, 22,* 19–33.

Moffitt, T. E. (1993). Adolescence-limited and life-course-persistent antisocial behavior: A developmental taxonomy. *Psychological Review, 100,* 674–701.

Nagin, D. S., Farrington, D. P., & Moffitt, T. E. (1995). Life-course trajectories of different types of offenders. *Criminology, 33,* 111–139.

National Institute of Justice. (1997, October). *Research in brief.* Washington, DC: Author.

O'Connell, M., & Whelan, A. (1996). Taking wrongs seriously. *British Journal of Criminology, 36,* 299–318.

O'Donnell, J., Hawkins, J. D., & Abbott, R. D. (1995). Predicting serious delinquency and substance use among aggressive boys. *Journal of Consulting and Clinical Psychology, 63,* 529–537.

Olweus, D. (1991). Bully/victim problems among school children: Basic facts and effects of a school based intervention program. In D. Pepler & K. H. Rubin (Eds.), *The development and treatment of childhood aggression.* Hillsdale, NJ: Erlbaum.

Olweus, D. (1993). *Bullying at school: What we know and what we can do.* Oxford, England: Blackwell.

Panko, W. L. (1978). Taxonomy of school vandalism. Unpublished doctoral dissertation, University of Pittsburgh, PA.

Pepler, D. J., Craig, W. M., Ziegler, S., & Charach, A. (1994). An evaluation of an anti-bullying intervention in Toronto

schools. *Canadian Journal of Community Mental Health, 13,* 95–110.

Pernanen, K. (1991). *Alcohol in human violence.* New York: Guilford Press.

Rigby, K., & Cox, I. (1996). The contribution of bullying at school and low self-esteem to acts of delinquency among Australian teenagers. *Personality and Individual Differences, 2,* 609–612.

Roff, J. D., & Wirt, R. D. (1984). Childhood aggression and social adjustments as antecedents of delinquency. *Journal of Abnormal Child Psychology, 12,* 111–126.

Roland, E. (1989). A system oriented strategy against bullying. In E. Roland & E. Munthe (Eds.), *Bullying: An international perspective.* London: Fulton.

Roland, E. (1994). A system oriented strategy against bullying. In E. Roland & E. Munthe (Eds.), *Bullying: An international perspective.* London: Fulton.

Rossi, P. H., Waite, E., Bose, C. E., & Berk, R. E. (1974). The seriousness of crimes: Normative structure and individual differences. *American Sociological Review, 39,* 224–237.

Scrimger, G. C., & Elder, R. (1981). *Alternative to vandalism: "Cooperation or wreakreation."* Sacramento: California Office of the Attorney General School Safety Center.

Skogan, W. G. (1990). *Disorder and decline.* Berkeley: University of California Press.

Smith, P. K., & Sharp, S. (1994b). *School bullying: Insights and perspectives.* London: Routledge.

Sparks, R., Genn, H., & Dodd, D. (1977). *Surveying victims.* London: Wiley.

Stattin, H., & Magnusson, D.(1989). The role of early aggressive behavior in the frequency, seriousness, and types of later crimes. *Journal of Consulting and Clinical Psychology, 57,* 710–718.

Stephenson, P., & Smith, D. (1995). Why some schools don't have bullies. In M. Elliott (Ed.), *Bullying: A practical guide to coping for schools.* London: Pitman.

Stoner, G., Shinn, M. R., & Walker, H. M. (Eds.). (1991). *Intervention for achievement and behavior problems.* Silver Spring, MD: National Association of School Psychologists.

Stover, D. (1990, November). How to be safe and secure against school vandalism. *Executive Educator,* 20–30.

Suedfeld, P. (1990). *Psychology and torture.* New York: Hemisphere.

Taylor, R. B., & Gottfredson, S. (1986). Environmental design, crime, and prevention: An examination of community dynamics. In A. J. Reiss & M. Tonry (Eds.), *Communities and crime.* Chicago: University of Chicago Press.

Taylor, S. P., Shuntich, R. J., & Greenberg, A. (1979). The effects of repeated aggressive encounters on subsequent aggressive behavior. *Journal of Social Psychology, 107,* 199–208.

Vestermark, S. D., & Blauvelt, P. D. (1978). *Controlling crime in the school: A complete security handbook for administrators.* West Nyack, NY: Parker.

Viemero, V. (1996). Factors in childhood that predict later criminal behavior. *Aggressive Behavior, 22,* 87–97.

Walker, M. A. (1978). Measuring the seriousness of crimes. *British Journal of Criminology, 18,* 348–364.

Ward, C. (1973). *Vandalism.* New York: Van Nostrand.

Weeks, S. (1976). Security against vandalism: It takes facts, feelings and facilities. *American School and University, 48,* 36–46.

Weisfeld, G. (1994). Aggression and dominance in the social world of boys. In J. Archer (Ed.), *Male violence.* London: Routledge.

White, J., & Fallis, A. (1980). *Vandalism*

prevention programs used in Ontario schools. Toronto, Canada: Ontario Ministry of Education.

Wiesenthal, D. L. (1990). Psychological aspects of vandalism. In P. J. D. Drenth, J. A. Sergeant, & R. J. Takens (Eds.), *European perspectives in psychology* (Vol. 3). New York: Wiley.

Wilson, J. Q., & Petersilia, J. (1995). *Crime.* San Francisco: Institute for Contemporary Studies Press.

Wilson, S. (1979). Observations on the nature of vandalism. In P. Bural (Ed.), *Designing against vandalism.* New York: Van Nostrand Reinhold.

Wolf, Y., Moav, Y., & Silfen, P. (1991). Judgments of verbal and physical aggression: An integrative perspective. *Crime and Social Deviance, 18,* 39–62.

Wood, D. (1991). In defense of indefensible space. In P. J. Brantingham & P. L. Brantingham (Eds.), *Environmental criminology.* Prospect Heights, IL: Waveland Press.

Zimbardo, P. G. (1969). The human choice: Individuation, reason and order versus deindividuation, impulse and chaos. In W. J. Arnold & D. Levine (Eds.), *Nebraska Symposium on Motivation.* Lincoln: University of Nebraska Press.

Zweig, A., & Ducey, M. H. (1978). *A paradigmatic field: A review of research on school vandalism.* Hackensack, NJ: National Council on Crime and Delinquency.

Zweir, G., & Vaughn, G. M. (1984). Three ideological orientations in school vandalism research. *Review of Educational Research, 54,* 263–292.

9

LEADELLE PHELPS

Prenatal Drug Exposure

Psychoeducational Outcomes
and Prevention Models

Intrauterine exposure to drugs may result in a wide variety of negative outcomes having notable social consequences. Because drugs vary in their teratogenic qualities (i.e., capability of producing abnormal structures in the embryo), the consequential effects may range from severe mental retardation and physical abnormalities to only subtle neurological markers. Thus prenatal drug exposure can be a serious social and public health problem deserving of concerted prevention and early intervention efforts. Yet there is a paucity of such prevention and intervention programs, and none have been empirically validated. In order that we may better understand the necessity of prevention (i.e., in this case, before pregnancy) or early intervention (i.e., during pregnancy to limit neurological involvement), the biological bases and psychoeducational manifestations of prenatal drug exposure are reviewed in this chapter. Because the two primary sources of intrauterine exposure are alcohol and cocaine, and because each results in significantly different outcomes, the two drugs will be discussed independently.

Prenatal Alcohol Exposure

The development of a growing fetus's entire central nervous system can be altered when a sufficient amount of alcohol interferes with neurotransmitter production, cell development, cell migration, and brain growth throughout gestation (Kaufman, 1997; Kotch & Sulik, 1992). Considerable damage can occur before the mother is even aware of her pregnancy. For example, the human brain develops via neurons generated within the ventricles (the innermost brain cavity) that migrate to the outer rim of the brain. These immature neurons first appear around the 11th day after gestation, when the embryo is about the size of a grain of rice (Strobel, 1993). Researchers have documented that alcohol significantly affects the growth and differentiation of these neural cells, resulting in a significant reduction in the size of the basal ganglia (Mattson, Riley, Sowell, & Jernigan, 1997) and alterations in the EEG pattern (Kaneko, Philips, Riley, & Ehlers, 1996).

Diagnosis and Prevalence

The diagnosis of fetal alcohol syndrome (FAS) is given when there is: (1) prenatal and/or postnatal growth retardation, that is, weight, length, and/or head circumference below the 10th percentile when corrected for gestational age; (2) evidence of central nervous system involvement, for example, signs of neurological abnormality, developmental delay, or intellectual impairment; and (3) the characteristic facial dysmorphology, that is, microcephaly (small head), microphthalmia (small eyes with skin folds at the corners), poorly developed philtrum (vertical ridge between nose and mouth), thin upper lip, and flattening of the midfacial jawbone region. Less severe variations are termed fetal alcohol effects (FAE). Because FAS/FAE symptomatology may not be readily evident, underdiagnoses and misdiagnoses are common (for an excellent review on diagnostic pitfalls, refer to Aase, 1995).

The worldwide incidence rate of FAS is now estimated at 0.97 per 1,000 live births (Abel, 1995). This is a twofold increase over previous estimates, with the augmentation being related to significantly improved sampling procedures. The United States has one of the highest occurrences (1.95 per 1,000), compared with only 0.08 per 1,000 in Europe. Within the United States, lower socioeconomic status (SES) is a major factor, with low-SES African American and Native American populations having 10 times higher prevalence rates than middle-SES Caucasian samples (Abel, 1995). Given these rates, an estimated 2,000 children are born with FAS each year in the United States, with FAS-related expenditures per year exceeding $250 million (Abel & Sokol, 1991).

Psychoeducational Outcomes of Prenatal Alcohol Exposure

Data generally support the conclusion that intrauterine alcohol exposure results in a broad range of deficits, with chronicity, timing, and severity of the exposure being associated with a corresponding continuum of negative outcomes. Different profiles of alcohol-related birth defects are related to varying exposures at critical periods of fetal development. For example, numerous large human prospective studies have documented the following: (1) chronic heavy alcohol consumption (i.e., an average of three or more drinks a day throughout pregnancy) usually results in structural anomalies, growth retardation, and compromised central nervous system functioning (the entire constellation of FAS); (2) episodic binge drinking (i.e., six or more drinks in a single day) or chronic consumption restricted to the first and second trimesters of pregnancy significantly increase the probability of general fetal developmental deficits, delay in speech acquisition, and skeletal anomalies, whereas such episodes and abuse limited to the third trimester can negatively affect future intellectual and behavioral functioning; (3) frequent moderate "social" drinking during pregnancy may result in more subtle neurobehavioral effects (e.g., attention difficulties, slow processing speed, memory problems); and (4) definitive outcomes of light consumption are not conclusive (Aronson & Hagberg, 1998; Autti-Ramo et al., 1992; Jacobson et al., 1993; Sampson et al., 1997; Streissguth, Barr, & Sampson, 1990).

Further diversity in FAS/FAE symptomatology is attributed to maternal and fetal alcohol metabolic rates, as well as to the modulating influence of the genetic makeup of mother or fetus or both. For example, Streissguth and Dehaene (1993) compared the developmental outcomes of monozygotic (MZ) and dizygotic (DZ) twin pairs born to alcoholic mothers and reported that the teratogenic qualities of ethanol could be modified by genetic differences. Although the twin pairs received comparable levels of prenatal alcohol exposure, FAS/FAE symptomatology was more uniformly expressed in MZ than in DZ twins. The authors concluded that fetal genotype affects the susceptibility of the central nervous system to alcohol.

Researchers have found that as children age, children with FAS and FAE are impaired on tests of intelligence, attention, learning, memory, fine-motor speed, visual-motor integration, and academic competencies relative to controls (Mattson, Gramling, Delis, Jones, & Riley, 1997; Mattson, Riley, Gramling, Delis, & Jones, 1997; Uecker & Nadel, 1996). In fact, FAS is now accepted as the leading known cause of mental retardation in the Western world, surpassing even Down syndrome, cerebral palsy, and spina bifida (Streissguth et al., 1991). Even when matched for intellectual competencies, children with FAS show inadequate judgment and problem-solving abilities, significant social deficits, and impaired working memory (Kodituwakku, Handmaker, Cutler, & Weathersby, 1995; Thomas, Kelly, Mattson, & Riley, 1998). Finally, diagnoses of attention-deficit/hyperactivity disorder (ADHD) and oppositional defiant disorder (ODD), as well as subclinical levels of other behavior problems, are frequent (Janzen, Nanson, & Block, 1995). In fact, ADHD has been found in about 85% of such children, cutting across all IQ categories and varying in severity from mild attention deficits to severe management difficulties (Steinhausen, Willms, & Spohr, 1993). Specific difficulties in the social domain include an inability to respect personal boundaries, demanding attention, bragging, stubbornness, poor peer relations, and being overly tactile in social interactions (Steinhausen et al., 1993).

During adolescence, mental retardation or below-average IQ, behavior problems, ADHD symptomatology (i.e., inattention, distractibility, impulsivity), decreased social competence, and poor school performance continue (Olson, Feldman, Streissguth, Sampson, & Bookstein, 1998; Steinhausen & Spohr, 1998). In adulthood, alcohol or drug dependence, depression, and psychotic disorders are not uncommon (Famy, Streissguth, & Unis, 1998). Even when cognitive deficits are not severe (i.e., IQ scores in low-average to above-average range), difficulties in concentration, verbal learning, and executive functioning are evident (Kerns, Don, Mateer, & Streissguth, 1998; Kopera-Frye, Dehaene, & Streissguth, 1996).

Prenatal Cocaine Exposure

Beginning in the early 1990s, the popular press published reports, based largely on single case studies, suggesting that children exposed prenatally to cocaine exhibited severe and irreversible damage (for a review of the media coverage, refer to Lyons & Rittner, 1998). Yet there was little definitive evidence specifically linking intrauterine cocaine exposure to adverse long-term developmental outcomes. Serious methodological problems, such as inadequate control of confounding variables and lack of control groups, obscured any clear demarcation regarding causality. In a review of 99 data-based studies which evaluated prenatal exposure and child outcomes, Lester, Lagasse, and Brunner (1997) concluded that most of the early data were compromised and that multiple risk factors, such as concurrent use of other drugs, postnatal parenting characteristics, and environmental lifestyle issues (e.g., continued drug usage), were seldom taken into consideration.

Prevalence

Although cocaine in various forms has been in use for some 15 centuries, crack (a mixture of cocaine with water and baking soda) was introduced in the late 1980s. Selling for $5 to $20 a "hit," crack cocaine has resulted in the drug being more readily available to a multitude of consumers (Weiss, Mirin, & Bartel, 1994). Estimates suggest that approximately 375,000 infants are born every year with prenatal expose to cocaine (Kinnison, Sluder, & Cates, 1995). These figures are likely an underestimation, for data indicate that approximately 25–30% of pregnant women who deny cocaine use when interviewed at the time of delivery test positive via hair analyses conducted later during their hospitalization (Kline, Ng, Schittini, Levin, & Susser, 1997).

Psychoeducational Outcomes of Prenatal Cocaine Exposure

Recent research using multivariate analyses, careful matching of comparison groups with no drug use, single-drug use, or multidrug use, and meta-analyses generally confirm only marginal intrauterine growth retardation (e.g., lower birth weight, infant length, and smaller head circumference) and neurobehavioral abnormalities (e.g., tremors, irritability, sleep pattern disturbances, excessive crying, and diminished responsiveness) in newborns that can be linked specifically to chronic fetal cocaine exposure (Eyler, Behnke, Conlon, Woods, & Wobie, 1998a; Hulse, English, Milne, Holman, & Bower, 1997; Phillips, Sharma, Premachandra, Vaughn, & Reyeslee, 1996). Growth impediments are viewed primarily as a function of the concurrent polydrug use of alcohol, tobacco, and marijuana that is ubiquitous in cocaine users, as well as inadequate prenatal care (Eyler et al., 1998a). The neurobehavioral effects that are frequently present appear to be transitory and reflect the pharmacological actions of cocaine present in the infant's system (Espy, Riese, & Francis, 1997; Eyler, Behnke, Conlon, Woods, & Wobie, 1998b; Richardson, Hamel, Goldschmidt, & Day, 1996). It should be noted, however, that the more frequent the cocaine exposure (i.e., chronicity), and the heavier the usage (i.e., severity), the higher the relative risk (Delaneyblack et al., 1996; Eyler et al., 1998a; Hulse et al., 1997; Jacobson, Jacobson, Sokol, Martier, & Chiodo, 1996).

There is consensus in the literature that as the infant matures, general development and motor skills (as measured by the Bayley Scales of Infant Development) are not adversely affected by prenatal cocaine exposure (Alessandri, Bendersky, & Lewis, 1998; Chasnoff, Griffith, Freier, & Murray, 1992; Edmondson & Smith, 1994; Hurt et al., 1995). For example, Alessandri et al. (1998) compared the functioning of 37 infants with heavy prenatal cocaine exposure, 30 infants with light exposure, and 169 with no exposure. After controlling for such confounding variables as neonatal medical and environmental risk factors, as well as polydrug exposure, the researchers reported that the groups did not differ on the Bayley Psychomotor or Mental Development indices at either 8 months or 18 months of age. An earlier study (Chasnoff et al., 1992) reported similar nonsignificant findings on the Bayley when comparing 3-, 6-, 12-, 18-, and 24-month-old infants who were either cocaine exposed, drug free, or exposed only to marijuana or alcohol. Likewise, Hurt et al. (1995) and Edmondson and Smith (1994) found no noticeable differences between cocaine-exposed and nonexposed infants at 6, 12, 18, 24, and 30 months of age.

Recognizing the importance of postnatal confounding variables such as parenting skills, medical care, and continued parental drug usage is imperative. Evaluating only infants with documented prenatal cocaine exposure, Blackwell, Kirkhart, Schmitt, and Kaiser (1998) reported a significantly lower Bayley Mental Index mean score among infants whose mothers had returned to drug usage compared with the mean score of infants whose mothers remained drug free. Likewise, Phelps, Wallace, and Bontrager (1997) found that children with prenatal cocaine exposure who resided with their grandmothers or with adopted parents or who were placed in foster care performed far better on cognitive, language, social skills, and behavioral measures than did exposed children who continued to live with their biological mothers.

Although there are speculations regarding more subtle long-term developmental outcomes, few well-controlled studies have been published with preschoolers or older children. Only seven investigations evaluating young children (i.e., 3 through 9 years of age) and using appropriate research designs that controlled for covariate factors were located (Beckworth et al., 1994; Griffith, Azuma, & Chasnoff, 1994: Phelps & Cottone, 1998; Phelps et al., 1997; Richardson, Conroy, & Day, 1996; Wasserman et al., 1998; Yolton & Bolig, 1994). None of these studies indicated significant effects of prenatal cocaine exposure on cognitive functioning, academic performance, social skills, speech and language development, or behavioral competencies.

For example, in a longitudinal prospective study, Richardson et al. (1996) compared the offspring of 28 women who had reported light to moderate cocaine use during pregnancy with the children of 523 women who had reported no such usage. At 6 years of age, each child received a thorough developmental assessment. After controlling for demographic confounding variables (e.g., SES, race), the researchers reported that there were no significant differences between the two groups on physical growth, intellectual ability, academic achievement, or teacher-rated classroom behavior.

In another well-designed longitudinal prospective study, Wasserman et al. (1998) evaluated the intellectual functioning of 88 children who had a history of prenatal exposure compared with that of 96 children who did not. The children ranged from 6 to 9 years of age. There were no significant differences in the mean IQ scores of the two groups (82.9 and 82.4 respectively) before multivariate analysis; results remained unchanged when several confounding variables were controlled (e.g., caregiver IQ, home environment, head circumference at birth). Likewise, Phelps et al. (1997) and Phelps and Cottone (1998) reported no significant differences in IQ, social skill functioning, externalizing and internalizing behavioral symptomatology, adaptive skills, or language competencies among cocaine-exposed compared with nonexposed 3- to 6-year-olds when the possible confounding variables of age, race, sex, and socioeconomic status were controlled by a matched sample or a multivariate research design. Thus the findings from these various studies suggest that many developmental difficulties ascribed to prenatal cocaine exposure may well reflect the myriad prenatal, postnatal, socioeconomic, and environmental factors that place these children at considerable risk.

Prevention Models

Effective psychosocial programs to prevent prenatal drug exposure are dependent on the identification of specific risk and protective factors that significantly influence the onset of a particular disorder or disease. Risk and protective factors always precede the onset of illness and encompass both environmental ingredients and intrapsychic or personal variables. Risk catalysts are associated with higher probability of onset, greater severity, and longer duration of the disorder, whereas protective variables are affiliated with improved resistance and resilience. After successful identification of such factors, highly specific strategies can be developed with the prevailing intent to reduce risk factors while enhancing protective factors. It should be noted that the goals of decreasing risk while increasing protection are not mutually exclusive and, in fact, may be highly similar (Munoz, Mrazek, & Haggerty, 1996). Thus the broad aims of a risk/protective model of prevention research are (1) deterrence of a specific disorder, (2) reduction of risk status, and (3) mental health promotion (Reiss & Price, 1996).

In order to prevent prenatal drug exposure, we must not only identify such risk and protective factors but also distinguish which precursors are the strongest predictors, how such variables interact, and which populations are most vulnerable. Obviously, the population to target is females of childbearing age (i.e., in order to expose a fetus to drugs, one must first be able to conceive). The identification of variables predictive of alcohol/drug usage among females of childbearing age would aid significantly in the development of early prevention programs designed to intervene before any such exposure has occurred. Likewise, recall that there are three subcategories within the realm of prevention programming: (1) universal preclusion activities designed for general populations with no identified risk status; (2) selective programming targeted to meet the needs of individuals or subgroups who, due to biological, psychological, and/or social considerations, are at significantly higher risk than the general population; and (3) specific procedures intended for high-risk persons who have minimal but nonetheless detectable symptoms of the disorder (Mrazek & Haggerty, 1994). Therefore, targeting nonpregnant females of childbearing age who are at significant risk for drug/alcohol abuse or who are already evidencing such abuse would be appropriate. It is generally hypothesized that multilevel (i.e., primary, secondary, and tertiary prevention) comprehensive programs that target specific populations and focus on precise risk and protective factors would be most efficacious in the prevention of intrauterine drug exposure.

Prenatal Alcohol / Drug Prevention Programs

To date, no intervention programs directed at reducing or eliminating consumption by pregnant women who abuse alcohol or cocaine have been successful (for a review of this literature, refer to Abel, 1998, and Schorling, 1993). Furthermore, knowledge of the negative consequences of prenatal exposure among minority women of childbearing age whose household income is less than $50,000 is alarmingly poor (Dufour, Williams, Campbell, & Aitkens, 1994). It seems evident that prenatal prevention instruction may be more successful if directed toward adolescents and young adults who have yet, or who have only begun, to experiment with alcohol or cocaine or both.

Two significant limitations of previously published primary prevention efforts with adolescents and young adult populations are the reliance on didactic presentations of factual information and the exclusive focus on risk factors. For example, alcohol and drug abuse prevention programs have frequently relied on dissemination of factual information in an effort to increase knowledge, change attitudes, and effectuate behavior change. Often relying on arousal of fear, such didactic approaches have been shown to affect knowledge and attitudes but have little impact in reducing current use, altering projected intentions, or changing future actions (for two excellent reviews of this literature, refer to Burgess, 1997, and Kim, Crutchfield, Williams, & Hepler, 1998). As the old adage goes: "Insight seldom changes behavior."

More recent approaches have focused primarily on the social mores and psychological factors presumed to encourage alcohol and cocaine use. Such activities as increasing student awareness of peer norms that promote drug use (i.e., social influence model), providing specific skills and techniques to resist inappropriate use (i.e., cognitive-behavioral model), and enhancing general self-esteem (i.e., life skills model) have been implemented with limited success. (Only studies that provided longitudinal follow-up data and utilized a control/experimental group design are cited.) A good example of such a program is Project DARE (Drug Abuse Resistance Education), which was designed to affect 6th- through 12th-grade students' attitudes, beliefs, social skills, and drug use behaviors. Using multilevel analyses (i.e., random-effects ordinal regressions) conducted over six years, Rosenbaum and Hanson (1998) reported no long-term effects on a wide range of drug use measures and no lasting effects on hypothesized protective factors. Unfortunately, all the previously documented short-term effects had dissipated by the conclusion of the six-year follow-up.

Other longitudinal studies have had similar outcomes. For example, the Michigan Model for Comprehensive School Health Education utilized a social-pressures-resistance skills prevention model completed over a two-year time frame during the sixth and seventh grades. Using a repeated-measures ANOVA intervention/no intervention research design, Shope, Copeland, Kamp, and Lang (1998) reported that by the five-year follow-up (completed in the 12th grade), all significant effects on alcohol, cigarette, cocaine, and other drug use had dissipated. Likewise, Werch, Pappas, Carlson, and DiClemente (1998) completed a brief alcohol prevention program which focused on enhancing protective social and personal factors with sixth-grade children. Although a significant difference in alcohol use between the experimental and control groups was noted at one-month follow-up, no differences were evident by one-year posttreatment. In conclusion, the high hopes researchers had for the "new generation" of social and psychological protective variable models that were aimed at the general population (i.e., primary prevention) have been dashed. (For a more in-depth discussion, refer to Brown & Kreft, 1998, and Gorman, 1998.)

On the positive side, a large-scale drug abuse prevention program (Project Towards No Drug Abuse) involving youth who were at high risk for drug abuse did show significant preventive effects for alcohol and hard drug use at one-year follow-up (Sussman, Dent, Stacy, & Craig, 1998). Likewise, Chou et al. (1998) reported significant differences between experimental and control groups at 1 ½-year follow-up in the use of cigarettes, alcohol, and marijuana among sixth- and seventh-grade students who were active users of these substances at the time of pretesting. Thus, when efforts are targeted for individuals who are at significantly higher risk for alcohol or cocaine use or both, or who already evidence minimal but detectable symptoms of drug use or abuse (i.e., secondary and tertiary prevention), results are more positive. However, more longitudinal data (e.g., five to six years posttreatment) are necessary.

Directions for Further Programs

Although there is no "crystal ball" to guide continuing efforts, findings from past unsuccessful attempts would suggest that future prevention programs should move away from global attempts and shift toward more concerted efforts with specified at-risk populations. In fact, Ernest Abel (1998), a noted researcher in the area, went so far as to state that the focus must be on reducing abuse rather than on more generalized endeavors. The most successful programs appear to be those that focus on a select subset of the population (i.e., at-risk status) and incorporate a multitude of risk and protective factors in the curriculum. With this in mind, it is recommended that future efforts focus on the unique psychosocial needs of adolescent and young adult females who are experimenting with early drug usage and that the interventions be aimed at enhancing individual resilience. Such could be accomplished by facilitating a critical evaluation of the sociocultural mores of drinking and drug use and by encouraging personal values clarification. Interactive activities that include group discussions, problem solving, and cooperative exercises are suggested. Thus this proposed prevention model would utilize active individual participation and highlight strengthening specific personal attributes and adaptive coping skills that attenuate the sociocultural pressures that promote drug and alcohol usage. Such a prevention program could employ group discussions, modeling, behavioral rehearsal, homework assignments, and frequent feedback as techniques to influence current behaviors and future behavioral intentions. Finally, the active participation of parents and extended family members may be of benefit (Ma, Toubbeh, Cline, & Chisholm, 1998). Regardless of the specific program curriculum, sensitivity to local social mores and cultural awareness is imperative.

REFERENCES

Aase, J. M. (1995). Clinical recognition of FAS: Difficulties of detection and diagnosis. *Alcohol Health and Research World, 18,* 5–9.

Abel, E. L. (1995). An update on the incidence of FAS: FAS is not an equal opportunity birth defect. *Neurotoxicology and Teratology, 17,* 437–443.

Abel, E. L. (1998). Prevention of alcohol abuse-related birth effects: I. Public education efforts. *Alcohol and Alcoholism, 33,* 411–416.

Abel, E. L., & Sokol, R. J. (1991). A revised conservative estimate of the incidence of FAS and its economic impact. *Alcoholism, 15,* 514–524.

Alessandri, S. M., Bendersky, M., & Lewis, M. (1998). Cognitive functioning in 8- to 18-month-old drug exposed infants. *Developmental Psychology, 34,* 565–573.

Aronson, M., & Hagberg, B. (1998). Neuropsychological disorders in children exposed to alcohol during pregnancy: A follow-up study of 24 children born to alcoholic mothers in Goeteborg, Sweden. *Alcoholism, Clinical, and Experimental Research, 22,* 321–324.

Autti-Ramo, I., Korkman, M., Hilakivi-Clarke, L., Lehtonen, M., Halmesmaki, E., & Granstrom, M. L. (1992). Mental development of 2-year-old children exposed to alcohol in utero. *Journal of Pediatrics, 31,* 740–746.

Beckworth, L. A., Rodning, C., Norris, D., Phillipsen, L., Khandabi, P., & Howard, J. (1994). Spontaneous play in two-year-olds born to substance-abusing mothers. *Infant Mental Health Journal, 15,* 189–201.

Blackwell, P., Kirkhart, K., Schmitt, D., & Kaiser, M. (1998). Cocaine/polydrug affected dyads: Implications for infant cognitive development and mother-infant interaction during the first six postnatal months. *Journal of Applied Developmental Psychology, 19,* 235–248.

Brown, J. H., & Kreft, I. G. (1998). Zero effects of drug prevention programs: Issues and solutions. *Evaluation Review, 22,* 3–14.

Burgess. R. (1997). Deconstructing drug prevention: Towards an alternative purpose. *Drug Education Prevention and Policy, 4,* 271–283.

Chasnoff, I. J., Griffith, D. R., Freier, C., & Murray, J. (1992). Cocaine/polydrug use in pregnancy: Two year follow-up. *Pediatrics, 89,* 284–289.

Chou, D., Montgomery, S., Pentz, M., Rohrbach, L. A., Johnson, C., Andersen, F., Brian, R., & MacKinnon, D. P. (1998). Effects of community-based prevention program in decreasing drug use in high-risk students. *American Journal of Public Health, 88,* 944–948.

Delaneyblack, V., Covington, C., Ostrea, E., Romero, A., Baker, D., Tagle, M. T., Nordstromklee, B., Silverstre, M. A., Angelilli, M. L., Hack, C., & Long, J. (1996). Prenatal cocaine and neonatal outcome: Evaluation of dose-response relationship. *Pediatrics, 98,* 735–740.

Dufour, M. C., Williams, G. D., Campbell, K. E., & Aitkens, S. S. (1994). Knowledge of FAS and the risks of heavy drinking during pregnancy: 1985 and 1990. *Alcohol Health and Research World, 18,* 86–92.

Edmondson, R., & Smith, T. M. (1994).

Temperament and behavior of infants prenatally exposed to drugs: Clinical implications for the mother-infant dyad. *Infant Mental Health Journal, 15,* 368–379.

Espy, K. A., Riese, M. L., & Francis, D. J. (1997). Neurobehavior in preterm neonates exposed to cocaine. *Infant Behavior and Development, 20,* 297–309.

Eyler, F. D., Behnke, M., Conlon, M., Woods, N. S., & Wobie, K. (1998a). Birth outcome from a prospective, matched study of prenatal crack/cocaine use: I. Interactive and dose effects on neurobehavioral assessment. *Pediatrics, 101,* 229–237.

Eyler, F. D., Behnke, M., Conlon, M., Woods, N. S., & Wobie, K. (1998b). Birth outcome from a prospective, matched study of prenatal crack/cocaine use: II. Interactive and dose effects on neurobehavioral assessment. *Pediatrics, 101,* 237–241.

Famy, C., Streissguth, A. P., & Unis, A. S. (1998). Mental illness in adults with fetal alcohol syndrome or fetal alcohol effects. *American Journal of Psychiatry, 155,* 552–554.

Gorman, D. M. (1998). The irrelevance of evidence in the development of school-based drug prevention policy. *Evaluation Review, 22,* 118–146.

Griffith, D. R., Azuma, S. D., & Chasnoff, I. J. (1994). Three-year outcome of children exposed prenatally to drugs. *Journal of the American Academy of Child and Adolescent Psychiatry, 33,* 20–27.

Hulse, G. K., English, D. R., Milne, E., Holman, C. D., & Bower, C. I. (1997). Maternal cocaine use and low birth weight newborns: A meta-analysis. *Addiction, 92,* 1561–1570.

Hurt, H., Brodsky, N. L., Betancourt, L., Braitman, L. E., Malmud, E., & Giannetta, J. (1995). Cocaine-exposed children: Follow-up through 30 months. *Journal of Developmental and Behavioral Pediatrics, 16,* 29–35.

Jacobson, J. L., Jacobson, S. W., Sokol, R. J., Martier, S. S., Ager, J. W., &

Kaplan-Estrin, M. G. (1993). Teratogenic effects of alcohol on infant development. *Alcoholism, Clinical, and Experimental Research, 17,* 174–183.

Jacobson, S. W., Jacobson, J. L., Sokol, R. J., Martier, S. S., & Chiodo, L. M. (1996). New evidence of neurobehavioral effects of in utero cocaine exposure. *Journal of Pediatrics, 129,* 581–590.

Janzen, L. A., Nanson, J. L., & Block, G. W. (1995). Neuropsychological evaluation of preschoolers with fetal alcohol syndrome. *Neurotoxicology and Teratology, 17,* 273–279.

Kaneko, W. M., Philips, E. L., Riley, E. P., & Ehlers, C. L. (1996). EEG findings in fetal alcohol syndrome and Down syndrome children. *Electroencephalography and Clinical Neurophysiology, 98,* 20–28.

Kaufman, M. H. (1997). The teratogenic effects of alcohol following exposure during pregnancy, and its influence on the chromosome constitution of the pre-ovulatory egg. *Alcohol and Alcoholism, 32,* 113–128.

Kerns, K., Don, A., Mateer, C. A., & Streissguth, A. P. (1998). Cognitive deficits in nonretarded adults with fetal alcohol syndrome. *Journal of Learning Disabilities, 30,* 685–693.

Kim, S., Crutchfield, C., Williams, C., & Hepler, N. (1998). Toward a new paradigm in substance abuse and other problem behavior prevention for youth: Youth development and empowerment approach. *Journal of Drug Education, 28,* 1–17.

Kinnison, L. R., Sluder, L. C., & Cates, D. (1995). Prenatal drug exposure: Implications for teachers of young children. *Early Childhood Special Education, 13,* 35–37.

Kline, J., Ng, S. K., Schittini, M., Levin, B., & Susser, M. (1997). Cocaine use during pregnancy: Sensitive detection by hair assay. *American Journal of Public Health, 87,* 352–358.

Kodituwakku, P. W., Handmaker, N. S.,

Cutler, S. K., & Weathersby, E. K. (1995). Specific impairments in self-regulation in children exposed to alcohol prenatally. *Alcoholism: Clinical and Experimental Research, 19,* 1558–1564.

Kopera-Frye, K., Dehaene, S., & Streissguth, A. P. (1996). Impairments of number processing induced by prenatal alcohol exposure. *Neuropsychologia, 34,* 1187–1196.

Kotch, L. E., & Sulik, K. K. (1992). Experimental fetal alcohol syndrome: Proposed pathogenic basis for a variety of associated facial and brain anomalies. *American Journal of Medical Genetics, 44,* 168–172.

Lester, B. M., Lagasse, L., & Brunner, S. (1997). Data base of studies on prenatal cocaine exposure and child outcome. *Journal of Drug Issues, 27,* 487–499.

Lyons, P., & Rittner, B. (1998). The construction of the crack babies phenomenon as a social problem. *American Journal of Orthopsychiatry, 68,* 313–320.

Ma, G. X., Toubbeh, J., Cline, J., & Chisholm, A. (1998). Fetal alcohol syndrome among Native American adolescents: A model prevention program. *Journal of Primary Prevention, 19,* 43–55.

Mattson, S. N., Gramling, L., Delis, D. C., Jones, K. L., & Riley, E. P. (1997). Global-local processing in children prenatally exposed to alcohol. *Child Neuropsychology, 2,* 165–175.

Mattson, S. N., Riley, E. P., Gramling, L., Delis, D. C., & Jones, K. L. (1997). Neuropsychological comparison of alcohol-exposed children with or without physical features of fetal alcohol syndrome. *Neuropsychology, 12,* 146–153.

Mattson, S. N., Riley, E. P., Sowell, E. R., & Jernigan, T. L. (1997) A decrease in the size of the basal ganglia in children with fetal alcohol syndrome. *Alcoholism, Clinical, and Experimental Research, 20,* 1088–1093.

Mrazek, R. F., & Haggerty, R. J. (Eds.). (1994). *Reducing risk of mental disorders: Frontiers for preventive intervention research.* Washington, D.C.: National Academy Press.

Munoz, R. F., Mrazek, P. J., & Haggerty, R. J. (1996). Institute of medicine report on prevention of mental disorders: Summary and commentary. *American Psychologist, 51,* 1116–1122.

Olson, H. C., Feldman, J. J., Streissguth, A. P., Sampson, P. D., & Bookstein, F. L. (1998). Neuropsychological deficits in adolescents with fetal alcohol syndrome: Clinical findings. *Alcoholism, Clinical, and Experimental Research, 22,* 1998–2012.

Phelps, L., & Cottone, J. W. (1998). Long-term developmental outcomes of prenatal cocaine exposure. Manuscript submitted for publication.

Phelps, L., Wallace, N. V., & Bontrager, A. (1997). Risk factors in early child development: Is prenatal cocaine/polydrug exposure a key variable? *Psychology in the Schools, 34,* 245–252.

Phillips, B., Sharma, R., Premachandra, B. R., Vaughn, A. J., & Reyeslee, M. (1996). Intrauterine exposure to cocaine: Effect on neurobehavior of neonates. *Infant Behavior and Development, 19,* 71–81.

Reiss, D., & Price, R. H. (1996). National research agenda for prevention research: The National Institute of Mental Health report. *American Psychologist, 51,* 1109–1115.

Richardson, G. A., Conroy, M. L., & Day, N. L. (1996). Prenatal cocaine exposure: Effects on the development of school-age children. *Neurotoxicology and Teratology, 18,* 627–634.

Richardson, G. A., Hamel, S. C., Goldschmidt, L., & Day, N. L. (1996). The effects of prenatal cocaine use on neonatal neurobehavioral status. *Neurotoxicology and Teratology, 18,* 519–528.

Rosenbaum, D. P., & Hanson, G. S. (1998). Assessing the effects of school-based drug education: A six-year multilevel analysis of Project DARE. *Journal of Research in Crime and Delinquency, 35,* 381–412.

Sampson, P. D., Kerr, B., Olson, H. C., Streissguth, A. P., Hunt, E., Barr, H. M., Bookstein, F. L., & Thiede, K. (1997). The effects of prenatal alcohol exposure on adolescent cognitive processing: A speed-accuracy tradeoff. *Intelligence*, 24, 329–353.

Schorling, J. B. (1993). The prevention of prenatal alcohol use: A critical analysis of intervention studies. *Journal of Studies on Alcohol*, 54, 261–267.

Shope, J. T., Copeland, L. A., Kamp, M. E., & Lang, S. W. (1998). Twelfth grade follow-up of the effectiveness of a middle school-based substance abuse prevention program. *Journal of Drug Education*, 28, 185–197.

Steinhausen, H., & Spohr, H. (1998). Long-term outcomes of children with fetal alcohol syndrome: Psychopathology, behavior, and intelligence. *Alcoholism, Clinical, and Experimental Research*, 22, 334–338.

Steinhausen, H., Willms, J., & Spohr, H. (1993). Long-term psychopathological and cognitive outcome of children with fetal alcohol syndrome. *Journal of American Academy of Child and Adolescent Psychiatry*, 32, 990–994.

Streissguth, A. P., Aase, J. M., Clarren, S. K., Randels, S. P., LaDue, R. A., & Smith, D. F. (1991). Fetal alcohol syndrome in adolescents and adults. *Journal of the American Medical Association*, 265, 1961–1967.

Streissguth, A. P., Barr, H. M., & Sampson, P. D. (1990). Moderate prenatal alcohol exposure: Effects on child IQ and learning problems at age 7-1/2 years. *Alcoholism, Clinical, and Experimental Research*, 14, 662–669.

Streissguth, A. P., & Dehaene, P. (1993). Fetal alcohol syndrome in twins of alcoholic mothers: Concordance of diagnosis and IQ. *American Journal of Medical Genetics*, 47, 857–861.

Strobel, G. (1993, November 13). Tracing earliest neurons' migration. *Science News*, p. 308.

Sussman, S., Dent, C. W., Stacy, A. W., & Craig, S. (1998). One-year outcome of Project Towards No Drug Abuse. *Preventive Medicine*, 27, 632–642

Thomas, S. E., Kelly, S. J., Mattson, S. N., & Riley, E. P. (1998). Comparison of social abilities of children with fetal alcohol syndrome to those of children with similar IQ scores and normal controls. *Alcoholism, Clinical, and Experimental Research*, 22, 528–533.

Uecker, A., & Nadel, L. (1996). Spatial locations gone awry: Object and spatial deficits in children with fetal alcohol syndrome. *Neuropsychologia*, 34, 209–223.

Wasserman, G. A., Kline, J. M., Bateman, D. A., Chiriboga, C., Lumey, L. H., Friedlander, H., Melton, L., & Haggarty, M. C. (1998). Prenatal cocaine exposure and school-age intelligence. *Drug and Alcohol Dependence*, 50, 203–210.

Weiss, R. D., Mirin, S. M., & Bartel, R. L. (1994). *Cocaine*. Washington, DC: American Psychiatric Press.

Werch, C. E., Pappas, D. M., Carlson, J. M., & DiClemente, C. C. (1998). Short- and long-term effects of a pilot prevention program to reduce alcohol consumption. *Substance Use and Abuse*, 33, 2303–2321.

Yolton, K. A., & Bolig, R. (1994). Psychosocial, behavioral, and developmental characteristics of toddlers prenatally exposed to cocaine. *Child Study Journal*, 24, 49–68.

10

ANNETTE M. LA GRECA

Children Experiencing Disasters

Prevention and Intervention

In the wake of devastating natural disasters (hurricanes, earthquakes, flood, brush-fires), human-made disasters (plane crashes, ferry sinkings, nuclear waste accidents), as well as recent school shootings, bombings, and terrorist activities, tremendous concern has developed regarding the impact of disasters on children and adolescents. Media coverage of such activities has alerted us to the significant trauma that children can and do experience. In fact, it has become apparent that children's exposure to such traumatic events can lead to reactions that may interfere substantially with their day-to-day functioning and cause them and their families significant distress.

Specifically, exposure to natural and man-made disasters represent traumatic events that can result in the emergence of a specific set of symptom patterns — those of posttraumatic stress disorder (PTSD; e.g., Green et al., 1991; La Greca, Silverman, Vernberg, & Prinstein, 1996; Lonigan, Shannon, Finch, Daugherty, & Taylor, 1991; Shannon, Lonigan, Finch, & Taylor, 1994; Shaw et al., 1995; Vernberg, La Greca, Silverman, & Prinstein, 1996). Moreover, exposure to violence of a personal nature, such as through rape, kidnapping, physical and sexual abuse, and community violence, also precipitates symptoms of PTSD (e.g., Pynoos et al., 1987; Terr, 1983). This chapter describes the symptoms and prevalence of PTSD in children and adolescents, as well as other reactions that may result from exposure to disasters. This chapter also outlines factors that contribute to the development and course of posttraumatic stress and discusses the implications of these findings for prevention and intervention with children and adolescents.

How Do Disasters Affect Children and Adolescents?

Posttraumatic Stress Disorder (PTSD)

The diagnostic category of PTSD was introduced in the third edition of the American Psychiatric Association's (1980) *Diagnostic and Statistical Manual of Mental Disorders* (*DSM-III*). At that time, PTSD was primarily considered to be an adult disorder. However, in recent years, there has been a growing awareness that children and adolescents also experience symptoms of PTSD, and this is reflected in the most recent revision of the *DSM* (*DSM-IV*; American Psychiatric Association, 1994).

In fact, recent findings have shown that disasters represent traumatic events for children that can result in posttraumatic stress reactions (e.g., Green et al., 1991; La Greca et al., 1996; Lonigan et al., 1991). Furthermore, findings also reveal that children's reactions to disasters can be severe and are not merely fleeting, transitory events that quickly dissipate. Rather, children's reactions appear to linger and persist and are likely to cause much distress to children and their families (e.g., La Greca et al., 1996). Moreover, because some children and adolescents display severe and persistent reactions, efforts to provide effective services and interventions for children and adolescents following a disaster represent an important, but frequently overlooked, mental health need.

In *DSM-IV* (American Psychiatric Association, 1994), PTSD refers to a set of symptoms that develop following exposure to an unusually severe stressor or event. Typically, the event is one that causes or is capable of causing death, injury, or threat to the physical integrity of oneself or another person. In order to meet criteria for a diagnosis of PTSD, a child's reaction to the traumatic event must include intense fear, helplessness, or disorganized behavior (American Psychiatric Association, 1994). In addition, specific criteria for three additional symptom clusters must be met: reexperiencing, avoidance or numbing, and hyperarousal. (See Table 10.1.)

Reexperiencing includes symptoms such as recurrent or intrusive thoughts or dreams about the event and intense distress at cues or reminders of the event. For young children, reexperiencing also may be reflected in repetitive play with traumatic themes or by a reenactment of traumatic events in play, drawings, or verbalizations. Pynoos and Nader (1988) reported that, following a sniper shooting, children described a specific vivid image or sound that disturbed them or reported traumatic dreams with a strong feeling of life threat. Findings such as these may help to explain why some children are afraid to sleep alone after a traumatic event.

Avoidance or numbing includes symptoms such as efforts to avoid thoughts, feelings, or conversations about the traumatic event, avoiding reminders of the event, diminished interest in normal activities, and feeling detached or removed from others. For example, children may report a lessened interest in play (or in their usual activities, such as Nintendo), and may feel distant from parents and friends.

Hyperarousal symptoms include difficulty sleeping or concentrating, irritability, angry outbursts, hypervigilance, and an exaggerated startle response. These behaviors must be newly occurring since the traumatic event. After exposure to gunfire

TABLE 10.1   Examples of Primary Symptoms Clusters for Posttraumatic Stress Disorder Based on *DSM-IV* Criteria

DSM-IV Cluster	Symptoms
Reexperiencing	Bad dreams
	Repetitive thoughts of the event
	Repetitive images of the event
	Repetitive play with traumatic themes
	Upsetting thoughts about the event
	Distress at reminders of the event
Numbing/Avoidance	Behavioral avoidance of reminders of the event
	Emotional avoidance of reminders of the event
	Emotional numbing
	Emotional isolation; feeling of detachment or distance from others
	Loss of interest in usual activities
	Reckless behavior
Hyperarousal	Increased startle response
	Somatic complaints
	Sleep difficulties
	Concentration difficulties
	Memory difficulties
	Fear of reoccurrence
	Irritability

and shootings, for example, Pynoos and Nader (1988) report that startle reactions seem to be especially persistent.

For a diagnosis of PTSD, the cited symptoms must be manifest for at least one month and be accompanied by significant impairment in the child's functioning (e.g., problems in school, social, or family relations).

Prevalence of Disorder and of Symptom Clusters

It is difficult to estimate the prevalence of PTSD in children and adolescents because studies have been extremely diverse with respect to the type of trauma evaluated, assessment methods and sampling procedures used, and the length of time passed since the traumatic event occurred. Community studies suggest that approximately 24% to 39% of children and adolescents exposed to trauma (such as community violence or a natural disaster) meet criteria for a PTSD diagnosis in the first weeks or months following the trauma (Berman, Kurtines, Silverman, & Serafini, 1996; Vernberg et al., 1996). When subclinical levels of PTSD are considered, more than 50% of the children in large community samples have reported at least moderate levels of PTSD during the first three to four months following a traumatic event (Shaw et al., 1995; Vernberg et al., 1996). Thus symptoms of PTSD appear to be common among children and adolescents exposed to trauma, although fewer children and youth will meet criteria for a full PTSD diagnosis.

Of the various PTSD symptom clusters, community studies of children suggest that symptoms of reexperiencing are most commonly reported by trauma victims.

For example, up to 90% of children exposed to a catastrophic hurricane reported symptoms of reexperiencing three months after the disaster (Vernberg et al., 1996). In contrast, symptoms of avoidance and numbing are much less commonly reported by children. However, because of this, the presence of symptoms of avoidance and numbing may be good markers for the presence of a PTSD diagnosis (e.g., Lonigan, Anthony, & Shannon, 1998).

Developmental Course

Very little is known about the course of PTSD symptoms in children over time. However, it does appear that PTSD symptoms may emerge in the days or weeks following a traumatic event and can take months or years for the symptoms to dissipate in some children and adolescents (e.g., Green et al., 1994; La Greca et al., 1996; McFarlane, 1987; Shaw, Applegate, & Schorr, 1996; Vincent, 1997). In the absence of reexposure to trauma or of the occurrence of other traumatic events, the typical developmental course of symptoms appears to be one of lessening frequency and intensity over time. For example, three months after a devastating and highly destructive natural disaster (Hurricane Andrew), 39% of the children informally met criteria for PTSD, but this number was reduced to 24% at 7 months postdisaster and to 18% by 10 months postdisaster (La Greca et al., 1996). A subgroup of children reporting moderate to severe PTSD symptoms was followed 42 months postdisaster into early adolescence (Vincent, 1997). Findings revealed that 40% of these "high-risk" youth continued to report moderate to severe levels of PTSD symptoms, as well as impairment in their day-to-day functioning; yet almost none of the children who reported mild or no symptoms at 10 months postdisaster reported any symptoms later on.

These data suggest a steady reduction in the frequency and severity of PTSD symptoms over time (with no further exposure to similar disasters), although a significant minority — approximately 7% to 10% of the full sample — did not recover and continued to report substantial difficulties almost four years postdisaster. These findings also indicate that it is highly unusual for children to report significant PTSD symptomatology a year or more after a traumatic event if they had not previously experienced symptoms closer to the event — despite occasional media reports that children's PTSD symptoms do not emerge for several months following a traumatic event. Although there may be a brief period of "shock" or numbing or sometimes even elation and relief at being alive, it is unusual to find children or adolescents reporting high levels of PTSD symptoms a year after the trauma if no signs of distress had been evident within the first few months.

Assessing Symptoms of PTSD in Children and Adolescents

Evaluating the presence of symptoms of PTSD in children can be a challenge and depends, to some extent, on the age or developmental level of the child. Due to their limited verbal capacity, the diagnosis of PTSD is especially difficult in very young children, such as infants, toddlers, and early preschoolers (see American Academy of Child and Adolescent Psychiatry, 1998; Scheeringa, Zeanah, Drell, &

Larrieu, 1995). In such cases, generalized anxiety and fears, avoidance of situations that may be linked to the traumatic event, and sleep disturbances may be useful indicators of PTSD (see Drell, Siegel, & Gaensbauer, 1993). Assessing symptoms of PTSD in children of preschool age and younger typically requires the input of the parent or primary caretaker. Parent versions of structured interviews would be the desired format for assessment. Alternatively, there are parent-completed questionnaires that report on children's PTSD symptoms, such as the Checklist of Child Distress Symptoms-Parent Report (Richters & Martinez, 1990) or the PTSD Checklist/Parent Report (Ford et al., 1996). For young children, observations of behavior, especially signs of distress, arousal, fear, and avoidance of trauma-related objects or events, can be important in evaluating reactions (American Academy of Child and Adolescent Psychiatry, 1998; Scheeringa et al., 1995).

Children of school age and older are themselves likely to be the best informants. Research suggests that parents often underestimate PTSD symptoms in their children (e.g., Earls, Smith, Reich, & Jung, 1988; Handford et al., 1986; La Greca et al., 1996). For children and adolescents, the most desirable method for assessing PTSD reactions is through structured interviews. Several structured interviews contain items pertinent to the PTSD diagnosis, such as the Anxiety Disorders Interview Schedule for Children (Silverman & Nelles, 1988), the Schedule for Affective Disorders and Schizophrenia for School-Age Children (Kaufman et al., 1997) or the Diagnostic Interview Schedule for Children (Shaffer et al., 1996). Child-oriented self-report measures, such as the PTSD Reaction Index (Frederick, 1985), the Children's PTSD Inventory (Saigh, 1989), and the Impact of Events Scale (Yule & Williams, 1990), have been found to be extremely useful for screening or research purposes — especially when a large number of children or adolescents are being evaluated or when personnel constraints preclude the use of individual interviews. (See McNally, 1996, for a detailed review of procedures used in the assessment of PTSD in children.)

Other Types of Postdisaster Reactions

Although recent work has focused on symptoms of PTSD, other reactions to trauma have been described in children and adolescents (see Vogel & Vernberg, 1993), and often symptoms of PTSD coexist with other psychological problems. Specifically, children or adolescents with high levels of PTSD symptoms have also reported significant symptoms of anxiety (e.g., Goenjian et al., 1995; Lonigan et al., 1994; Yule & Udwin, 1991) and depression (e.g., Goenjian et al., 1995; Kinzie, Sack, Angell, Manson, & Rath, 1986; Singer, Anglin, Song, & Lunghofer, 1995; Yule & Udwin, 1991). Depressive reactions are especially common following disasters that involve loss of loved ones (Amaya-Jackson & March, 1995). For the most part, it is difficult to determine whether affective or anxiety disorders preceded the disaster or constitute reactions to the trauma. Nevertheless, in most clinical situations it would be desirable to obtain a comprehensive assessment of youngsters' functioning following disasters that is not limited to PTSD symptoms.

Regardless of whether PTSD symptoms are present, children's anxiety levels appear to be affected by exposure to trauma. Certainly, traumatic events have long been viewed as a potential pathway to the development of phobias and other anxiety-based disorders in youth (see Silverman & Ginsburg, 1995). Evidence also indicates that exposure to disasters can increase anxiety levels in otherwise "normal" youth. For example, children in a community sample with high levels of exposure to a natural disaster displayed significant increases in their anxiety levels at three and seven months postdisaster compared with their predisaster levels (La Greca, Silverman, & Wasserstein, 1998).

Problems with academic achievement may also result from exposure to trauma (Shannon et al., 1994; Vincent, La Greca, Silverman, Wasserstein, & Prinstein, 1994; Yule, 1994). For example, significant declines in children's achievement levels over the year following a disaster have been noted among children with high levels of exposure to disasters (Shannon et al., 1994; Vincent et al., 1994). These findings make sense when one considers that disasters can seriously disrupt children's everyday routine and may also precipitate problems with sleep and concentration.

Safety and security concerns have also been frequently reported as common reactions to trauma and disasters (Yule, 1994). In young children, these concerns may be manifested by fear of separation from parents or loved ones. For example, Robin Gurwitch (1999) reported high levels of children's separation fears (e.g., clinging to parents) following the bombing of the Federal Building in Oklahoma City. She also reported that, following the bombing, children had a heightened sense of vigilance and a decreased sense of safety and security; and, because someone was responsible for the bombing, "revenge" fantasies appear to have been more common than in other disasters. With sniper shootings, bombings, and other "unpredictable" acts of violence, fears of reoccurrence (without warning), ongoing security concerns, and preoccupation with revenge may be evident (Pynoos & Nader, 1988).

Increased fears following a traumatic event or disaster may also be present in some children and adolescents (Yule, 1992; Yule, Udwin, & Murdoch, 1990). Usually (but not always) these fears are directly linked to the kind of trauma that is experienced. For example, fears of water, thunder, and rainstorms have been reported following natural disasters such as hurricanes (Vogel & Vernberg, 1993). Exaggerated startle responses to loud noises have also been reported following sniper shootings (Pynoos & Nader, 1988).

Factors That Predict Children's Postdisaster Reactions

Conceptual Model to Organize Factors That Predict PTSD Reactions

Although it is important to document the effects of disasters on children and adolescents, there is a critical need for information regarding the factors that put youth at risk for serious PTSD reactions and the ones that predict recovery. Such information is essential for identifying those children and adolescents most in need of psychological assistance and for designing empirically supported interventions. Thus, from a practical perspective, it is essential that the psychological literature move beyond a description of children's reactions to disasters to predicting and understanding who is most at risk and why.

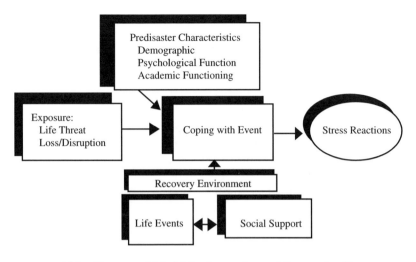

FIGURE 10.1   Conceptual Model for Integrating and Sequencing Treatments

Building on a conceptual model that was initially developed by Korol (1990) and Green et al. (1991), La Greca and colleagues (La Greca et al., 1996; Vernberg et al., 1996) described a framework for understanding factors that predict children's postdisaster reactions. According to the model, these predictive factors are multiple and complex and include: (1) level of exposure to the trauma (e.g., life threat, loss, or disruption), (2) preexisting characteristics of the child (e.g., demographic characteristics, predisaster functioning), (3) characteristics of the postdisaster recovery environment (e.g., availability of social support, occurrence of major stressors, family functioning), and (4) the youngster's efforts to process and cope with disaster-related distress. (See Figure 10.1.) Each of the factors in the model has accounted for significant variance in PTSD levels in studies of children following Hurricane Andrew (La Greca et al., 1996; Vernberg et al., 1996).

Exposure to Trauma

Exposure to the traumatic event is considered to be the primary and most critical factor for the emergence of posttraumatic stress symptoms (e.g., American Psychiatric Association, 1994; Eth & Pynoos, 1985; Green et al., 1991). Two key aspects of exposure contribute to children's reactions: the presence or perception of life threat and personal loss or disruption of everyday events. These aspects of exposure predict children's initial reactions to disasters (e.g., Lonigan, Shannon, Taylor, Finch, & Sallee, 1994; Nader, Pynoos, Fairbanks, & Frederick, 1990; Shannon et al., 1994; Vernberg et al., 1996), as well as persistent stress reactions (e.g., La Greca et al., 1996).

The presence or perception of life threat is thought to be essential for the emergence of PTSD symptoms (Green et al., 1991). It is easy to understand why children who witness or are exposed to acts of violence, such as sniper shootings or severe physical abuse by a caretaker, would feel that their lives are in danger.

However, it is also the case that catastrophic natural disasters or personal disasters (such as residential fires or motor vehicle accidents) can elicit perceptions of life threat in children, even if no one is injured or hurt. For example, although no lives were lost in South Florida as a result of Hurricane Andrew, the extensive destruction of homes and property that occurred during the storm was terrifying to many children and adults. Thousands of children and families spent up to six hours huddled in dark closets or bathrooms, without electricity, listening to intense winds (in excess of 160 miles per hour) as their homes and belongings were seriously damaged or destroyed. One study of nearly 600 children who resided in southern Dade County at the time of Hurricane Andrew reported that 60% of the children interviewed "thought that they were going to die" during the storm (Vernberg et al., 1996). Thus perceptions of life threat can and do occur in the absence of actual loss of life or serious injury.

Recent evidence also underscores the importance of loss (of family and friends, of pets, of personal property) and disruption of everyday life (displacement from home, school, community) as contributing to PTSD symptoms in children (e.g., La Greca et al., 1996; Vernberg et al., 1996). Following many natural disasters, for example, children and adolescents have to cope with a cascading series of life stressors that were set into motion by the disaster, including loss of home and/or personal property, a change of schools, loss of friends and of pets, altered leisure activities, and so on. These stressors may last for many weeks and months following the event and challenge children's and families' coping abilities. Not surprisingly, then, the life changes that result from this aspect of exposure to a disaster also predict PTSD symptoms in children (e.g., La Greca et al., 1996, 1998; Vernberg et al., 1996).

Predisaster Functioning

Certain aspects of children's functioning prior to a disaster may put them at risk for greater postdisaster reactions. In the conceptual model, child characteristics are considered after exposure to the disaster because they are preexisting factors and usually cannot be affected by the disaster. Considering child characteristics after exposure also provides statistical control for the possibility that exposure is not distributed equally across all levels of child characteristics (e.g., Lonigan et al., 1991; see Vernberg et al., 1996, for details).

The most widely (and easily) studied predisaster child characteristics are demographic factors, such as age, gender, and ethnicity. A few studies have examined whether predisaster psychological or academic functioning can predict PTSD reactions, although such studies are relatively rare and are often limited by retrospective reporting of predisaster adjustment. Nevertheless, they point to certain characteristics that may sensitize children to the effects of disasters, as described in the following discussion.

GENDER. Several studies find that PTSD symptoms appear more frequently among girls than boys (Green et al., 1991; Khoury et al., 1997; Lonigan et al., 1991; March, Amaya-Jackson, Terry, & Costanzo, 1997; Shannon et al., 1994;

Vernberg et al., 1996), although this has not consistently been the case (Earls et al., 1988; Handford et al., 1986; La Greca et al., 1996, 1998). Gender differences in postdisaster reactions may depend on the type of stress reaction that is studied. Girls tend to report more anxiety-related problems than boys (e.g., Anderson et al., 1987); thus, given the overlap between symptoms of anxiety and of PTSD (Amaya-Jackson & March, 1995), it would not be surprising to find that girls report more PTSD symptoms than boys. On the other hand, compared with girls, boys are typically elevated on externalizing symptoms, including conduct and attention problems; thus it might be the case that boys would display more signs of aggression, inattention, or other behavior problems following disasters. Of interest along these lines were the findings of Garbarino and Kostelny (1996); in this study, boys exposed to political violence in Palestine evidenced significantly more behavior problems than girls. In general, studies have not systematically examined gender in relation to the type of posttraumatic reaction studied. However, it is noteworthy that, even when gender differences have been found, their magnitude is relatively modest (Vernberg et al., 1996) and may dissipate over time (La Greca et al., 1996).

AGE. It is extremely difficult to draw generalizations regarding children's vulnerability to postdisaster stress reactions at different ages. For the most part, findings on age-related differences have been inconsistent, and few investigators have included sufficiently large samples of youth at different ages to adequately test developmental differences. In one study of children aged 2 to 15 years who were exposed to the Buffalo Creek dam collapse in 1972 (Green et al., 1994), fewer symptoms of PTSD were found among the youngest age group (2 to 7 years). However, such findings need to be tempered by the fact that evaluations of youngsters' postdisaster reactions are influenced by the diverse manifestations of PTSD disorder at different ages (American Academy of Child and Adolescent Psychiatry, 1998).

ETHNICITY. Children and adolescents from minority ethnic and cultural groups appear to be vulnerable to symptoms of PTSD following disasters or exposure to violence. Community studies suggest that minority youth (especially Blacks) exposed to severe natural disasters report more PTSD symptoms and have a more difficult time recovering from such events than nonminority youth (La Greca et al., 1996, 1998; Lonigan et al., 1998; March et al., 1997). In fact, following Hurricane Hugo, African American children reported more PTSD symptoms in comparison with White or other minority children (Shannon et al., 1994). African American and Hispanic American youth also reported more persistent levels of PTSD symptoms over the school year following Hurricane Andrew (La Greca et al., 1996) relative to White students. In studies of exposure to community violence, rates of PTSD symptoms appear to be highest in Black males (Berton & Stabb, 1996).

The reasons for these ethnic differences are not clear. Following destructive natural disasters, it is possible that socioeconomic factors might partially account for such findings in that families from minority backgrounds may have fewer financial resources or less adequate insurance to deal efficiently with the rebuilding and recovery process. This, in turn, could prolong the period of life disruption and loss of personal possessions that typically ensues after destructive natural disasters.

It is also possible that children from minority backgrounds have higher levels of predisaster exposure to trauma, which may "sensitize" them to the effects of a disaster or community violence. Consistent with this perspective, Berton and Stabb (1996) found that minority males were exposed to more violent crime than other adolescents in their neighborhoods; in turn, adolescents' exposure to domestic or community violence was the best predictor of PTSD symptoms among this sample of urban adolescents. Overall, the role of sociodemographic characteristics and their associated factors in predicting youngsters' responses to traumatic events are not well understood and should be examined more closely.

PRIOR PSYCHOLOGICAL FUNCTIONING. Although available evidence is scant, some findings suggest that predisaster psychiatric problems predict postdisaster stress reactions in children and adolescents (Earls et al., 1988). A recent prospective study revealed that children with preexisting psychological problems, especially anxiety, may be more vulnerable to PTSD reactions following disasters (La Greca et al., 1998). Children's anxiety levels 15 months before a devastating hurricane predicted their levels of PTSD symptoms 3 and 7 months postdisaster, even when their exposure to the event was controlled for (La Greca et al., 1998). In addition, children who had greater exposure to the disaster showed an increase in anxiety symptoms following the disaster. Studies with adults have similarly found that preexisting anxiety is a significant risk factor for the development of posttraumatic stress (Breslau, Davis, Andreski, & Peterson, 1991).

These findings are interesting in view of the current conceptualization of PTSD, reflected in *DSM-IV* (American Psychiatric Association, 1994), which suggests that trauma must be present for PTSD to emerge. However, anxious children and adults may have a vulnerability to developing PTSD reactions, even if their degree of exposure to trauma is relatively low.

Some other work points to predisaster depression levels and ruminative coping styles as potential risk factors for postdisaster stress. In an investigation of the 1989 Loma Prieta earthquake, Nolen-Hoeksema and Morrow (1991) evaluated 137 students 2 weeks before, 10 days after, and 7 weeks after the disaster. Youth who, before the earthquake, had elevated levels of depression and stress symptoms and a ruminative style of coping with symptoms had more depression and stress symptoms at both follow-up periods.

PREDISASTER ACADEMIC FUNCTIONING. Some research suggests that children with preexisting academic difficulties may exhibit greater postdisaster problems (Vogel & Vernberg, 1993). For example, child survivors of a ferry sinking were reported to exhibit fewer posttraumatic stress symptoms if they had higher levels of academic achievement (see Yule, 1994). Moreover, Vincent and colleagues (1994) found that elementary school students with low levels of academic achievement three-months prior to Hurricane Andrew reported significantly higher levels of PTSD symptoms seven months following the disaster, even when children's level of exposure to the hurricane was controlled for. Other work has identified low achievement and high levels of attention problems as risk factors for PTSD symptoms during the first three months postdisaster (La Greca et al., 1998). Such findings strongly suggest that children with academic difficulties may need careful monitoring and assistance following exposure to disasters.

Aspects of the Recovery Environment

After the initial impact of the disaster, various aspects of the recovery environment may either magnify or attenuate youngsters' subsequent reactions. Most notable among these aspects are the availability of social support, the occurrence of additional life events, and parental reactions to the disaster.

Given the numerous stressors that accompany a disaster, access to social support from a variety of sources should help to minimize youngsters' postdisaster distress. In fact, social support from family, friends, classmates, and teachers has been found to mitigate the impact of disasters on children and adolescents (La Greca et al., 1996; Vernberg et al., 1996). Such findings suggest that enhancing children's social support following disasters is an important mental health goal. However, this can also be a challenge following community-based disasters, as there is a high likelihood that support providers (e.g., parents, friends, and teachers) are also disaster victims themselves.

In contrast to social support, major life events (e.g., death or hospitalization of a family member, parental divorce or separation) that occur in the months following a disaster appear to significantly impede children's postdisaster recovery and are linked with greater persistence of PTSD symptoms in children over time (La Greca et al., 1996). Children and adolescents who encounter major life events following a disaster, in addition to the typical cascading series of disaster-related life stressors, appear to represent a high-risk group for severe and persistent posttraumatic stress reactions; they bear close monitoring. Similarly, youngsters who have multiple exposures to traumatic events appear to be at greater risk for PTSD symptoms following disasters (e.g., Robin, Chester, Rasmussen, Jaranson, & Goldman, 1997).

Another aspect of the recovery environment that may adversely affect children's functioning is the presence of parental psychopathology or adjustment problems. Green et al. (1991) found that parental psychopathology predicted higher levels of PTSD symptoms in children and adolescents following the Buffalo Creek dam collapse, and, in the case of a nuclear waste disaster, the psychological health of the parents was found to be a potent predictor of children's disaster reactions (Korol, Green, & Gleser, 1999). Similarly, Delamater (1999) reported that parents with high levels of PTSD following Hurricane Andrew had children with higher levels of PTSD symptoms, and Swenson et al. (1996) found that mothers' distress in the aftermath of Hurricane Hugo was associated with the persistence of their children's postdisaster emotional and behavioral difficulties. Moreover, other research has supported a linkage between children's symptoms of PTSD and parents' trauma-related symptoms (Foy, Madvig, Pynoos, & Camilleri, 1996). In all likelihood, parents who are having adjustment difficulties are less able to provide needed support and comfort to their children following disasters; such parents may also model trauma-related symptoms for their children. Thus families in distress bear close monitoring following disasters, as they may be at high risk for ongoing difficulties.

Coping with the Traumatic Event

Children's coping ability is the fourth and last component of the conceptual model, as coping is typically viewed as the product of the level of trauma suffered, child characteristics, and situational characteristics (i.e., access to social support from others). Several community studies have found that children and adolescents with more negative coping strategies for dealing with stress (e.g., anger, blaming others) show higher levels of PTSD symptoms in response to natural disasters (La Greca et al., 1996; Vernberg et al., 1996) and to community violence (Berman et al., 1996). Moreover, children with negative coping strategies evidence greater persistence in their PTSD symptoms over time (La Greca et al., 1996). Because of these findings, efforts to encourage problem-solving and adaptive coping skills may be useful for interventions with children following traumatic events (e.g., La Greca, Vernberg, Silverman, & Prinstein, 1994, 1995).

Summary of Descriptive Research

Recent research on children's and adolescents' reactions to disasters is beginning to move away from simple description of postdisaster reactions and is instead focusing to a greater extent on factors that predict which youngsters will have more severe and persistent postdisaster reactions. The conceptual model outlined in this section is a useful framework for organizing such findings and represents an important "first step" toward theory building in this area. Based on existing literature, we can begin to identify factors that put children and adolescents at risk for psychological difficulties following disasters; these characteristics are summarized in Table 10.2. The ability of professionals to identify high-risk children and youth early on will be critical to prevention and intervention efforts.

TABLE 10.2   Characteristics of Youth At Risk for Severe or Persistent Symptoms of Posttraumatic Stress Following Disasters

Characteristic	Specific Risk Factor
Demographic	Female gender
	Ethnic minority
Predisaster functioning	High levels of anxiety
	Poor academic achievement
	Attention problems
	Depressive symptoms
Level of exposure to the disaster	High reported "life threat" or perceived life threat
	High level of life disruption (changing schools, moving)
	High level of personal loss (family, friends, pets)
	High level of property loss (home, clothes, toys)
Recovery factors	Low levels of support from family, friends, classmates
	Presence of intervening life events (loss or illness in family)
	Poor family/parental functioning; parental PTSD
Child characteristics	Problems coping with events (e.g., blame, anger)
	High levels of PTSD symptoms (e.g., reexperiencing, hyperarousal, numbing/disinterest, etc.)

In reviewing the conceptual model (Figure 10.1), it is interesting to note that, to a large extent, the risk and protective factors identified as predictive of children's posttraumatic stress levels are similar to factors that have been predictive of other negative adjustment outcomes in children in the absence of traumatic events. For example, research has highlighted the role of major life events, lack of social support, the presence of family pathology, and problematic coping styles (e.g., cognitive distortions, withdrawal) in the development of depression in adolescents (e.g., Petersen, Compas, Brooks-Gunn, Stemmler, Ey, & Grant, 1993). To some extent, our understanding of psychopathology in children and adolescents might profit from the development of transactional models that incorporate key risk and protective factors within a developmental context and cut across various negative developmental trajectories. It is likely that the study of youngsters' reactions to trauma will provide a unique and important context for examining the role of particular risk and protective factors in the development of negative developmental trajectories in youth.

Helping Children Cope: Translating Research into Prevention and Intervention Strategies

There are several obstacles to implementing interventions following disasters, but the most critical one is that there is a dearth of outcome studies on the effectiveness of various postdisaster interventions (Vernberg & Vogel, 1993). Basically, we do not know when and how to best intervene. However, there are some promising models and "leads" based on the growing literature on disasters' effects (as reviewed herein). Current trends in and ideas about how to help children and adolescents following disasters are reviewed in this section. Most of the suggested interventions focus on efforts to process the event, to increase social support levels, and to improve problem solving and coping with the event and its aftermath.

Another major difficulty in helping children cope with disasters is that the significant persons in their lives — parents, teachers, and close friends — may also be affected by the disaster. It is often the case that the adults in children's lives are not sufficiently aware of their children's distress, perhaps because they are also affected by and preoccupied with the trauma. Moreover, supports from outside the community that are available shortly after a disaster dissipate quickly over time. Even the media loses interest in disaster coverage well before the "recovery" has been completed. Adding to this difficulty, parents and teachers may even minimize children's distress following disasters. For example, in our own work following Hurricane Andrew, several school principals declined to participate in a school-based community program to help children's coping and adjustment, stating that their students were "fine." Yet our subsequent evaluations in comparable schools revealed that 55% of the students had moderate to very severe levels of PTSD symptoms three months after the disaster and that nearly 90% of the children were reporting frequent symptoms of reexperiencing the event (Vernberg et al., 1996). In fact, when we notified parents of "high risk" youth that their son or daughter was showing signs of continuing distress, many called to thank us, indicating that they were unaware that their son or daughter was still bothered by the hurricane.

Even from a prevention standpoint, obstacles to providing services are difficult to surmount. Disaster preparedness constitutes an important aspect of prevention efforts. Yet many communities do not perceive themselves to be vulnerable to disasters and therefore have done little to develop disaster plans. Communities in the United States vary tremendously in terms of their risk for disasters and their degree of preparedness (Baum, 1987; Vernberg & Vogel, 1993). Planning is typically more advanced for natural disasters than for man-made disasters or terrorist activities (Vernberg & Vogel, 1993), although even high-risk areas for natural disasters have not developed disaster plans. For example, at the time that Hurricane Andrew struck South Florida, there was no formal disaster plan in place for dealing with children's mental health needs in the local public schools. Psychologists can be instrumental in helping schools and communities to develop disaster-preparedness plans that include mental health components.

The following sections of this chapter review interventions for children and adolescents following disasters, organized by the length of time since the disaster event. Disaster events vary in duration and may range from a few minutes (e.g., earthquakes, tornadoes, motor vehicle crashes) to hours or days (e.g., hurricanes, floods, fires, hostage taking; Vernberg & Vogel, 1993). However, in most cases, the recovery period is likely to ensue for months or even years following the disaster, and intervention efforts may be appropriate at varying points during the recovery period. In general, interventions closer in time to the event are more likely to be brief, universal, and community based. Interventions that extend past the initial, acute recovery phase (approximately three months) focus increasingly on high-risk youth or those who demonstrate persistent adjustment difficulties.

Short-Term Recovery Period

The short-term recovery period extends from the "event" through the first three months of recovery. The initial impact phase of a disaster begins with the onset of the disaster event (hurricane, earthquake, school shooting), extends through the end of the event, and concludes when an initial assessment of casualties and other loss is communicated to people directly affected by the disaster (Vernberg & Vogel, 1993). During this brief period, efforts to restore children's sense of personal safety and security are paramount.

A common time for initial interventions occurs during the short-term adaptation phase (24 hours or so until approximately three months after the event). Community or school-based interventions that target all youth in affected areas have generally been recommended (Vernberg & Vogel, 1993); this is also a good time to identify and monitor youth who are most severely affected by the disaster. As Vernberg and Vogel (1993) indicate, interventions might include classroom and small group activities, family approaches, and individual treatment. The purpose of these interventions is: (1) to provide information and help to normalize individual's reactions to the disaster, (2) to provide a sense of safety and security, and (3) to return to a sense of routine and normalcy. During the same time period, efforts to provide information to helping professionals and the general public (e.g., via fact sheets, Web sites, telephone, mass media) are also useful (Vernberg & Vogel, 1993). Table

TABLE 10.3 Helping Children Cope with Disasters: Selected Resources for Fact Sheets, Brochures, or Manuals

Web Materials[a]	Brief Description
www.fema.gov/kids/	Child-oriented Web site on disasters, developed by the Federal Emergency Management Association. It contains information on different types of disasters, how to prepare for them, and how to cope.
www.redcross.org/disaster/safety/guide.html	Brochure developed by the American Red Cross, *A Guide to Talking About Disasters*. Check the main Web site (www.redcross.org) for additional and news-breaking information on disasters.
www.apa.org/practice/kids.html	Web site developed by the American Psychological Association. Contains a fact sheet on "Helping Children Cope: A Guide to Helping Children Cope with the Stress of the Oklahoma City Explosion." Useful for a wide range of disasters. Check the main web site for additional and news-breaking information: www.apa.org.
www.aacap.org	Web site of the American Academy of Child and Adolescent Psychiatry. Contains many "fact sheets" for children and families, including how to help children cope with disasters.
www.jmu.edu/psychologydept/4kids.htm	Contains disaster-related information for children.
disastertraining.org	Site provides adults with information to help children cope with natural disasters and with violence.
Selected Manuals[b]	**Request Single Copies in Writing From:**
Helping Children Prepare and Cope with Natural Disasters (La Greca et al., 1994)	Annette M. La Greca, University of Miami, P.O. Box 249229, Coral Gables, FL 33124
The Bushfire and Me (Storm et al., 1994)	VBD Publications, P.O. Box 741, Newtown NSW 2042, Australia
Healing After Trauma: Skills Manual for Helping Children (Gurwitch & Messenbaugh, 1998)	Robin H. Gurwitch, Child Study Center, 1100 NE 13th Street, Oklahoma City, OK 73117

a. Web addresses begin with: http://
b. All contain activities for adults (parent, school personnel, or counselors) to use with children.

10.3 lists several resources for fact sheets and brochures that may be especially useful to children, parents, teachers, and mental health professionals in the aftermath of a disaster.

The types of short-term interventions that have been evaluated during this initial recovery phase primarily have been limited to "debriefing" efforts. Debriefing, also referred to as Critical Incident Stress Debriefing (CISD), is a crisis intervention that is designed to relieve and prevent trauma-related distress in normal individuals who are experiencing abnormally stressful events or disasters (e.g., Chemtob, Tomas, Law, & Cremniter, 1997; Mitchell, 1983). Such interventions provide opportunities for children (or adults) to ventilate feelings, normalize their responses to the disaster, and learn about common psychological reactions to the disaster in the context of a supportive group (Chemtob et al., 1997). At this point in time, however, little empirical support exists for the effectiveness of debriefing with children and adolescents. In fact, a review of controlled studies of CISD with adults (Rose & Bisson, 1998) suggests that, due to methodological flaws in existing studies, the effectiveness of this procedure remains in question. It has also been suggested that multiple applications of CISD may be required for it to be effective (Horowitz & Schreiber, 1999). Although it is likely that CISD may be beneficial to some youth, these brief, one-shot interventions are probably insufficient in length and scope to begin to address some of the multiple, complex, and cascading stressors that result from major disasters and that may last for months or years for some children and adolescents.

Similar to debriefing, several authors have described "psychological first aid" that can be implemented in schools or community crisis centers to help children cope initially with the postdisaster crises (Amaya-Jackson & March, 1995; Eth, Silverstein, & Pynoos, 1985; Pynoos & Nader, 1988). These first-aid efforts provide children with an opportunity to express their feelings (e.g., through drawings or storytelling), clarify confusion, and identify areas of need (Amaya-Jackson & March, 1995). Such efforts also can help professionals identify children who are having severe reactions so that they may receive more intensive interventions. Table 10.2 lists several characteristics of high-risk youth, based on the empirical literature reviewed earlier in this chapter; it might serve as a guide for professionals to identify children early on who are likely to have continuing problems.

As an alternative to debriefing and "first aid" efforts, one study reported that the use of massage therapy was beneficial in reducing symptoms of anxiety and depression among schoolchildren (Grades 1 to 5; mean age = 7.5 years) following a natural disaster (Field, Seligman, Scafidi, & Schanberg, 1996). Specifically, 60 children who displayed behavior problems and reported severe levels of PTSD symptoms following Hurricane Andrew were randomly assigned to either a massage therapy or a video–attention control condition one month after the hurricane. The massage group received twice-weekly back massages (30 minutes per session). Compared with the controls, children receiving massage reported less anxiety and depression, evidenced lower salivary cortisol levels (a physiological measure of stress), and were observed to be more relaxed following treatment. Although further replication with follow-up would be desirable, the authors suggest that teaching parents to administer massage to their children might be useful in reducing children's distress following a traumatic disaster (Field et al., 1996).

Aside from formal interventions, literature from the American Red Cross (1992) and other sources (Corder & Haizlip, n.d.; Farberow & Frederick, 1978; Federal Emergency Management Agency, 1989; National Organization for Victim Assistance, 1991) suggests that, following a disaster, parents, teachers, and mental health professionals should encourage children and adolescents to express their feelings in developmentally appropriate ways (e.g., through discussion, drawings, storytelling, or journal writing) and should be sensitive to fears, worries, and concerns that children may have. In addition, efforts to return children and youth to their "normal" roles and routines may help youngsters to renormalize their lives following disasters (Prinstein, La Greca, Vernberg, & Silverman, 1996). In fact, Prinstein et al. (1996) found that children who reported high levels of assistance from parents, friends, and teachers in resuming their normal roles and routines during the first few months after Hurricane Andrew reported significantly lower levels of PTSD symptoms seven months postdisaster. Consistent with this finding, in our clinical experiences, several elementary school teachers told us that some students did not want to return home after the school day because things felt "normal" at school, whereas at home they still encountered considerable hurricane-related damage and destruction in their neighborhoods. These informal observations speak to the value of helping children and youth to normalize their lives following a disaster.

Medium to Long-Term Recovery Period

The medium to long-term recovery period extends three months or longer after the disaster. Few controlled investigations of interventions for children and adolescents following disasters exist, even though a significant proportion of youngsters have moderate to severe levels of posttraumatic stress that persist for a year or more following a disaster (e.g., Green et al., 1994; McFarlane, 1987; Shaw et al., 1996; Vincent, 1997; Yule, 1992). The existing treatment literature is reviewed here; it may be especially pertinent for clinicians who are working with children and adolescents with persistent and severe posttraumatic stress following a disaster.

Also discussed are some promising intervention ideas based on community-based studies that have linked certain coping strategies and coping assistance with better child adjustment following disasters. The community-based studies suggest avenues that could be explored by teachers, school counselors, or other mental health professionals to enhance children's and adolescents' adjustment following large-scale, community-wide disasters (e.g., hurricanes, tornadoes, floods, bombings); they may be especially appropriate for primary and secondary prevention efforts.

CONTROLLED OUTCOME STUDIES OF CHILDREN AND YOUTH FOLLOWING DISASTERS: HELPING YOUTH WITH MODERATE TO SEVERE PTSD. To date, only three controlled studies of child treatment following disasters or single-incident stressors could be found (Goenjian et al., 1997; March, Amaya-Jackson, Murray, & Schulte, 1998; Yule & Canterbury, 1994). Two used cognitive-behavioral therapy (CBT) as an approach to dealing with postdisaster distress (March et al., 1998; Yule & Canterbury, 1994), and one developed a model of trauma and grief-focused psychotherapy (Goenjian et al., 1997). However, one theme that is central to both therapeutic approaches is the notion that trauma victims need to be gradually "reexposed" to the traumatic event and allowed to "emotionally process" the event in a safe, controlled setting. The reprocessing allows the therapist to correct any distortions or misattributions the child may have developed concerning the traumatic event. Moreover, the safe, controlled setting, sometimes paired with relaxation (e.g., March et al., 1998), helps the youngster to gradually extinguish high levels of arousal to the traumatic events and trauma-related cues.

Brief trauma and grief-focused psychotherapy was used by Goenjian and colleagues (1997) to treat symptoms of PTSD and depression among early adolescents who were exposed to the 1988 Armenian earthquake. This particular earthquake devastated four cities and 350 villages in Armenia, killing at least 25,000 people; in the city of Gumri, where the intervention took place, at least 18,000 people (7%

of the population) were killed and about 50% of the buildings were destroyed (Goenjian et al., 1997). At 18 months postdisaster, 64 early adolescents (average age = 11 to 12 years) participated in the intervention; 35 were treated and 29 served as controls. After another 18 months (3 years postdisaster), the adolescents were reevaluated for PTSD and depressive symptoms. The school-based treatment was conducted in classroom groups (four half-hour sessions) and individually (two one-hour sessions) over a three-week period. The most symptomatic adolescents received two additional individual treatment sessions, and in all cases, treatment was completed within a six-week period. The trauma and grief-focused psychotherapy included: (1) reconstructing and reprocessing the traumatic event, in part by clarifying distortions and misattributions, and addressing resulting avoidance and maladaptations; (2) identifying traumatic reminders and assisting youth to develop tolerance and increase social support during and after the reminders; (3) coping with stresses and adversities by encouraging proactive measures to assist in coping with changes and losses that resulted from the disaster; (4) handling bereavement by helping the bereaved reconstitute a nontraumatic mental image of the deceased person; and (5) assessing developmental impact by identifying missed developmental opportunities (due to avoidance, loss, or life disruption) and promoting normal developmental tasks (see Goenjian et al., 1997, for more details). Results indicated that by three years postdisaster, the treated adolescents showed a significant decline in PTSD symptom scores relative to pretreatment levels, whereas controls showed a significant increase over the same time period. Similarly, over the 18-month period since treatment began, the rates of "likely" PTSD cases decreased from 60% to 28% among treated adolescents but increased from 52% to 69% for the control adolescents. With regard to depressive symptoms, treated adolescents showed no significant change in symptoms over the 18-month period, whereas control adolescents evidence a significant increase. Despite these positive findings, the authors caution that, until further studies are conducted, it is not known whether the results would generalize to youth with less severe trauma exposures (Goenjian et al., 1997).

In another approach to treating trauma in children, March and colleagues (1998) evaluated the efficacy of group-administered CBT with 17 youth (aged 10 to 15 years) who had experienced one or more stressors of sufficient magnitude to produce PTSD (e.g., car accidents, severe storms, accidental injury, gunshot injury, and fires). In some cases, the stressors happened to a loved one (e.g., death by assault, illness, car accident, fire). Prior to treatment, participants reported mild to moderately severe PTSD, anxiety, and depression, and the average duration of PTSD symptoms was 1.5 to 2.5 years; youngsters with high levels of disruptive behaviors were excluded from participation. Using an experimental design of a single case across time and setting, participants entered an 18-week treatment program. The multimodality trauma treatment (MMTT) protocol was an adaptation of CBT protocols designed for treating PTSD in adults (Foa, Rothbaum, Riggs, & Murdock, 1991) and for treating anxiety in children (Kendall, 1994). MMTT included several elements: anxiety management training; relaxation training; anger coping; cognitive training, especially for dealing with PTSD intrusions; developing a stimulus hierarchy based on traumatic reminders; and narrative, gradual "exposure" to the trauma with corrective information regarding distortions and misattributions (see March et al., 1998, for more details). Homework was provided to promote treatment generalization and relapse prevention. Of the 14 youngsters who completed treatment, 8 (57%) no longer met *DSM-IV* criteria for PTSD following treatment, and 12 (86%) no longer met criteria at the six-month follow-up. Similar improvements were observed for symptoms of depression, anxiety, and anger; moreover, youngsters' locus of control had changed from external to internal by the time of the follow-up assessment.

These two key studies (Goenjian et al., 1997; March et al., 1998) are promising and suggest that gradual exposure to traumatic events, with opportunity to reprocess the event in a reparative manner, is a critical component of treating youth with severe levels of PTSD following disaster (see also Amaya-Jackson & March, 1995; Saigh et al., 1996). In conducting exposure-based treatments, it is essential that the professional understands the child's "perception of the event, subjective meaning, level of exposure, and attributions of cause" (Amaya-Jackson & March, 1995, p. 291), and does not "cut off" the reprocessing until the child's arousal level has been returned to normal. Other associated treatment strategies (e.g., grief management, anger management) also may be appropriate depending on the nature of the trauma (e.g., involving death or loss of loved ones) and the types of secondary or concurrent difficulties that are present (e.g., anxiety, depression, anger, behavior problems).

Aside from these few studies conducted with children or adolescents following disasters, there has been considerable discussion regarding how to treat youth with PTSD that results from other types of trauma (e.g., rape, sexual abuse, motor vehicle accidents.). Saigh, Yule, and Imandar (1996) reviewed studies of treatment outcome for PTSD, with an emphasis on exposure-based intervention techniques. They emphasized that what we know about the treatment of PTSD in children is drawn primarily from single-case research designs. On the positive side, such studies typically involve real clients who experienced tremendous trauma and who were treated in the natural environment with tailor-made treatment protocols that featured flooding therapies. Nevertheless, there is a clear need for more large-scale controlled outcome studies of the efficacy and effectiveness of exposure-based (and other) treatments.

Although behavioral-psychological interventions have been the primary focus of attention, there is some suggestion that pharmacologic treatments also may be useful for youngsters who develop serious symptoms of PTSD following a disaster. Drug treatment of PTSD may be especially useful when anxiety or depression are comorbid conditions, and it could be used as an adjunct to exposure-based therapy. Potential drugs to consider include propranolol, clonidine, and benzodiazepines (Botteron & Geller, 1993).

One final area of concern is how to deal with children and adolescents who are exposed to multiple or chronic traumatic events. Much of the existing work has been conducted with youth exposed to "single incident" trauma. As the treatment literature develops further, much more attention is needed to developing effective programs for children exposed to multiple traumatic events.

COMMUNITY STUDIES AND IDEAS FOR PREVENTION. Community-based interventions with children following disasters have not been evaluated systematically; however, there is a reasonable empirical literature on factors that play a critical role in the persistence of children's distress following disasters. The interventions described in this section of the chapter meet the criteria of being "consistent with" empirical research on factors that have been linked with youngsters' stress levels and their recovery following disasters.

Specific treatment and prevention manuals. As reviewed earlier, certain factors that may be present during the recovery period have been found to be predictive of children's PTSD symptoms over several months following disasters. Specifically, higher levels of social support (from family, friends, and teachers), lower levels of stressors and life events, and more positive (or less negative) coping strategies have been associated with less severe levels of posttraumatic stress for children and adolescents (e.g., La Greca et al., 1996; Vernberg et al., 1996). These findings suggest that efforts to enhance children's social support networks, to reduce stress, and to cope effectively with ongoing stressors might be extremely valuable following disasters.

Building on these empirically based factors, La Greca and colleagues (1994, 1995) developed a school-based intervention for elementary school children following Hurricane Andrew. (See Table 10.3 for information on how to obtain the manual.) The program included "lessons" that teachers, school counselors, or psychologists could use with children in disaster-affected areas to: (1) increase children's level of social support, especially from teachers and peers, (2) identify stressors or ongoing problems that resulted from the hurricane and that were affecting children's everyday lives, and (3) promote positive methods for coping with ongoing stressors (or at least avoid negative ones). Some lessons focused on how to help children cope with holidays (e.g., Thanksgiving) that are "different" because of the disaster (e.g., loss of home, possessions, friends, etc.); others dealt with identifying ongoing stressors that bothered the children and that they wanted to "fix." Children worked on classroom activities in small groups of four children each to facilitate peer interactions and friendship development among classmates (i.e., increase social support). In addition to activities that can be used with children in the weeks and months following a disaster, the manual also reviews "risk factors" to help teachers, school counselors, or psychologists identify children with severe stress reactions and contains some "preparation" activities so that children can feel prepared should another disaster strike. Although the school-based program has not been evaluated systematically, the manual has been distributed to thousands of schools, American Red Cross centers, and psychologists across the United States and abroad and has received very favorable reviews from mental health professionals. In fact, the manual was translated into Japanese (La Greca et al., 1995) and used to help children in Kobe, Japan, cope with the aftermath of a devastating earthquake in 1995. The manual has also been reported to be useful for psychologists and other mental health workers in identifying "at risk" youth and in facilitating school-based discussions during the weeks following the bombing of the Federal Building in Oklahoma City in April of 1995 (J. Gonzalez, personal communication, May 1995).

Other clinical investigators also have developed manuals to help children cope with large-scale disasters (see Table 10.3). Most notable among these are *The*

Bushfire and Me (Storm, McDermott, & Finlayson, 1994) and a manual developed for helping youth cope with the aftermath of the bombing of the Federal Building in Oklahoma City (Gurwitch & Messenbaugh, 1998). What these various materials and manuals share in common are efforts to help children talk about or otherwise process the traumatic events in a structured manner, deal with ongoing problems that develop as a result of the trauma, and prepare for other "predictable" disasters (e.g., fires, hurricanes, etc.).

Other community-based research and suggestions. Almost no research has examined what children and families actually do to cope with disasters and how their coping relates to their recovery. However, one study by Prinstein et al. (1996) of more than five hundred children in Grades 3 through 5 attempted to identify the kinds of "coping assistance" children received from parents, friends, and teachers following Hurricane Andrew and linked the frequency and type of "coping assistance" with children's level of PTSD symptoms. Coping assistance was defined as the specific ways that significant others helped children to cope with the trauma. Based on a review of disaster-related mental health materials, three types of coping assistance were identified and evaluated: (1) emotional processing of the event (i.e., controlled and repeated exposure to reminders of the traumatic event); (2) resuming normal roles and routines; and (3) distraction. Of the three types of coping assistance, resuming normal roles and routine was reported to be the most frequent, followed by distraction, and then by emotional processing. In addition, children reported receiving the most coping assistance from parents, followed by friends, and last by teachers, although when it came to emotionally processing the event (e.g., talking about it), children reported doing this significantly more with friends than with parents or teachers. Of most interest was the linkage between different types and sources of coping assistance and children's PTSD symptoms seven months postdisaster. Specifically, children with moderate to very severe levels of PTSD symptoms reported more emotional processing and distraction than children with doubtful to mild levels of symptoms; in contrast, resuming normal roles and routines was significantly more frequent among children with low levels of PTSD symptoms. Moreover, resuming normal roles and routines significantly predicted declines in children's PTSD levels from 7 to 10 months postdisaster (Prinstein & La Greca, 1999). Although further work of a prospective nature would be desirable, the findings of these two studies highlight the importance of friends as well as family in helping children cope with the aftermath of a disaster. They also suggest that efforts to resume normal roles and routines (e.g., return to playing sports, sharing activities with friends, maintaining a similar home and school routine) may be especially beneficial to children following disasters.

Other suggestions that have been offered for helping children and their families cope with the long-term aftermath of disasters include having public ceremonies, memorials, or other disaster-related rituals that provide an opportunity for disaster survivors to remember the event and place it in context (Vernberg & Vogel, 1993). According to Vernberg and Vogel (1993), rituals may serve several important psychological functions, including public expression of shared grief and support, reassurance that disaster victims are remembered, review and interpretation of disaster experiences, and obtaining closure on a difficult life event. The anniversary of an event is an especially common time for community-based ceremonies or rituals. For example, a special ceremony was held in Oklahoma City on the first anniversary of the bombing of the Federal Building. In South Florida, the local media highlighted the one-year anniversary of Hurricane Andrew with special TV programs and newspaper articles that reviewed the disaster and the recovery period, with emphasis on the rebuilding and recovery process. Group meetings for families of disaster victims have also been arranged by mental health professionals on the anniversary of the event (Yule & Williams, 1990). As Vernberg and Vogel (1993) point out, although there is little research on value of rituals, "the timelessness of human rites to mark deaths and tragedies bears witness to their appeal" (p. 496). Rituals and commemorative activities are especially appealing for disasters that affect large numbers of children and families.

Although, at present, there are little "hard data" on the efficacy or effectiveness of various efforts to help child disaster victims, the current literature suggests several important directions to pursue. In the immediate aftermath, efforts to reassure children, provide information, and "normalize" their reactions may be helpful. Parents, teachers, and clinicians might focus on identifying children with the most severe reactions, so that they can talk with them and provide additional help; the materials gleaned from Web sites of various professional organizations (see Table 10.3) contain resources (e.g., fact sheets, activities, information) for parents, children, and mental health professionals that should facilitate this process. For large-scale community-wide disasters, efforts to deal with children and families in the community may be most productive from a preventive standpoint; however, it is also desirable to target those with more severe reactions for additional services. For youth who are severely traumatized, the use of exposure-based cognitive-behavioral therapy appears to hold promise for reducing levels of posttraumatic stress in children and adolescents exposed to trauma, especially when combined with other strategies for dealing with ancillary and comorbid problems such as loss of a loved one.

Summary

This chapter highlights children's and adolescents' reactions to disasters, with a special focus on symptoms of posttraumatic stress disorder. It also reviews community-based strategies for helping children cope following disasters, as well as initial treatment efforts for children with more severe or persistent posttrauma reactions.

The reader should keep in mind that this area of child mental health is relatively new and should expect considerable developments to emerge in the near future. In particular, given the commonly reported linkage between children's and parents' postdisaster adjustment, especially for young children (e.g., Delamater, 1999; Green et al., 1991), greater attention to helping children and their families cope with disasters and to developing family-based strategies for those who are severely affected represent important clinical directions for the future. Moreover, it is critical that consideration be given to developing disaster interventions that are developmentally and culturally sensitive and that take into account the particular phase of the recovery period (i.e., immediate, short-term, long-term) and the type of disaster that has occurred (e.g., with or without mass casualty). Given that disasters are unexpected and serendipitous events and that most individuals are unprepared for the event and its aftermath, efforts to develop networks of disaster mental health "experts" (both researchers and clinicians) would be useful. Such experts could provide consultation following disasters and might help to further the quality of assessment and treatment outcome research on disasters.

REFERENCES

Amaya-Jackson, L., & March, J. S. (1995). Posttraumatic stress disorder. In J. S. March (Ed.), *Anxiety disorders in children and adolescents* (pp. 276–300). New York: Guilford Press.

American Academy of Child and Adolescent Psychiatry (1998). AACAP Official Action: Practice parameters for the assessment and treatment of children and adolescents with posttraumatic stress disorder. *Journal of the American Academy of Child and Adolescent Psychiatry, 37* (Suppl.), 4S–26S.

American Psychiatric Association (1994). *Diagnostic and statistical manual of mental disorders* (4th Ed.). Washington, DC: Author.

American Psychiatric Association (1980). *Diagnostic and statistical manual of mental disorders* (3rd ed.). Washington, DC: Author.

American Red Cross (1992). *Helping children cope with disaster.* ARC Publication No. 4499. Baltimore, MD: Author.

Anderson, J. C., Williams, S., McGee, R., & Silva, P. A. (1987). DSM-III disorders in preadolescent children: Prevalence in a large sample from the general population. *Archives of General Psychiatry, 44,* 69–76.

Baum, A. (1987). Toxins, technology, and natural disasters. In G. R. VandenBos & B. K. Bryant (Eds.), *Cataclysms, crises, and catastrophes: Psychology in action* (pp. 7–53). Washington, DC: American Psychological Association.

Berman, S. L., Kurtines, W. M., Silverman, W. K., & Serafini, L. T. (1996). The impact of exposure to crime and violence on urban youth. *American Journal of Orthopsychiatry, 66,* 329–336.

Berton, M. W., & Stabb, S. D. (1996). Exposure to violence and post-traumatic stress disorder in urban adolescents. *Adolescence, 31,* 489–498.

Botteron, K., & Geller, B. (1993). Disorders, symptoms, and their pharmacotherapy. In J. S. Werry & M. G. Aman (Eds.), *Practitioner's guide to psychoactive drugs for children and adolescents* (pp. 179–201). New York: Plenum Press.

Breslau, N., Davis, G. C., Andreski, P., & Peterson, E. (1991). Traumatic events and posttraumatic stress disorder in an urban population of young adults. *Archives of General Psychiatry, 48,* 216–222.

Chemtob, C. M., Tomas, S., Law, W., & Cremniter, D. (1997). Postdisaster psychosocial intervention: A field study of the impact of debriefing on psychological distress. *American Journal of Psychiatry, 154,* 415–417.

Corder, B. F., & Haizlip, T. (n.d.). *A coloring book after the hurricane for children and their parents or helpers.* Author.

Delamater, A. M. (1999, February). PTSD

in Head Start children after exposure to Hurricane Andrew. Paper presented at the Rocky Mountain Region Disaster Mental Health Conference, Laramie, WY.

Drell, M. J., Siegel, C. H., & Gaensbauer, T. J. (1993). Posttraumatic stress disorder. In C. H. Zeanah (Ed.), *Handbook of infant mental health.* New York: Guilford Press.

Earls, F., Smith, E., Reich, W., & Jung, K. G. (1988). Investigating the psychopathological consequence of disaster in children: A pilot study incorporating a structured diagnostic interview. *Journal of the American Academy of Child and Adolescent Psychiatry, 27,* 90–95.

Eth, S., & Pynoos, R. S. (Eds.) (1985). *Posttraumatic stress disorder in children.* Washington, DC: American Psychiatric Press.

Eth, S., Silverstein, S., & Pynoos, R. S. (1985). Mental health consultation to a preschool following the murder of a mother and child. *Hospital and Community Psychiatry, 36,* 73–76.

Farberow, N., & Frederick, C. (1978). *Field manual for field service workers in disasters.* Rockville, MD: National Institute of Mental Health.

Federal Emergency Management Agency (1989). *Coping with children's reactions to hurricanes and other disasters* (Document No. 1989 0-941-901). Washington, DC: U.S. Government Printing Office.

Field, T., Seligman, S., Scafidi, F., & Schanberg, S. (1996). Alleviating posttraumatic stress in children following Hurricane Andrew. *Journal of Applied Developmental Psychology, 17,* 37–50.

Foa, E. B., Rothbaum, B. O., Riggs, D. S., & Murdock, T. B. (1991). Treatment of posttraumatic stress disorder in rape victims: A comparison between cognitive-behavioral procedures and counseling. *Journal of Consulting and Clinical Psychology, 59,* 715–723.

Ford, J. D., Thomas, J. E., Rogers, K. C. et al. (1996, November). *Assessment of*

children's PTSD following abuse or accidental trauma. Paper presented at the annual meeting of the International Society for Traumatic Stress Studies, San Francisco, CA.

Foy, D. W., Madvig, B. T., Pynoos, R. S., & Camilleri, A. J. (1996). Etiologic factors in the development of posttraumatic stress disorder in children and adolescents. *Journal of School Psychology, 34,* 133–145.

Frederick, C. J. (1985). Children traumatized by catastrophic situations. In S. Eth & R. S. Pynoos (Eds.), *Posttraumatic stress disorders in children* (pp. 71–100). Washington, DC: American Psychiatric Press.

Garbarino, J., & Kostelny, K. (1996). The effects of political violence on Palestinian children's behavior problems: A risk accumulation model. *Child Development, 67,* 33–45.

Goenjian, A. K., Karayan, I., Pynoos, R. S., Minassian, D., Najarian, L. M., Steinberg, A. M., & Fairbanks, L. A. (1997). Outcome of psychotherapy among early adolescents after trauma. *American Journal of Psychiatry, 154,* 536–542.

Goenjian, A. K., Pynoos, R. S., Steinberg, A. M., Najarian, L. M., Asarnow, J. R., Karayan, I., Ghurabi, M., & Fairbanks, L. A. (1995). Psychiatric comorbidity in children after the 1988 earthquake in Armenia. *Journal of the American Academy of Child and Adolescent Psychiatry, 34,* 1174–1184.

Green, B. L., Korol, M. S., Grace, M. C., Vary, M. G., Kramer, T. L., Gleser, G. C., & Leonard, A. C. (1994). Children of disaster in the second decade: A 17-year follow-up of Buffalo Creek survivors. *Journal of the American Academy of Child and Adolescent Psychiatry, 33,* 71–79.

Green, B. L., Korol, M. S., Grace, M. C., Vary, M. G., Leonard, A. C., Gleser, G. C., & Smitson-Cohen, S. (1991). Children and disaster: Gender and parental effects on PTSD symptoms. *Journal of the American Academy of*

Child and Adolescent Psychiatry, 30, 945–951.

Gurwitch, R. H. (1999, February). *Children and trauma: Lessons from the Oklahoma City bombing.* Paper presented at the Rocky Mountain Region Disaster Mental Health Conference, Laramie, WY.

Gurwitch, R. H., & Messenbaugh, A. K. (1998). *Healing after trauma: Skills manual for helping children.* (Available from Robin H. Gurwitch, Child Study Center, 1100 NE 13th Street, Oklahoma City, OK 73117)

Handford, H. A., Mayers, S. D., Mattison, R. E., Humphrey, F. J., Bagnato, S., Bixler, E. O., & Kales, J. D. (1986). Child and parent reactions to the Three Mile Island nuclear accident. *Journal of the American Academy of Child Psychiatry, 25,* 346–356.

Horowitz, L., & Schreiber, M. (1999). *Psychological and behavioral aspects of emergency medical services for children.* Washington, DC: American Psychological Association.

Kaufman, J., Birmaher, B., Brent, D., Rao, U., Flynn, C., Moreci, P., Williamson, D., & Ryan, N. (1997). Schedule for Affective Disorders and Schizophrenia for School-Age Children — Present and Lifetime Version (K-SADS-PL): Initial reliability and validity data. *Journal of the American Academy of Child and Adolescent Psychiatry, 36,* 980–988.

Kendall, P. C. (1994). Treating anxiety disorders in children: Results of a randomized clinical trial. *Journal of Consulting and Clinical Psychology, 62,* 100–110.

Khoury, E. L., Warheit, G. J., Hargrove, M. C., Zimmerman, R. S., Vega, W. A., & Gil, A. G. (1997). The impact of Hurricane Andrew on deviant behavior among a multi-racial/ethnic sample of adolescents in Dade County, Florida: A longitudinal analysis. *Journal of Traumatic Stress, 10,* 71–91.

Kinzie, J. D., Sack. W. H., Angell, R. H., Manson. S., & Rath, B. (1986). The psychiatric effects of massive trauma on Cambodian children: I. The children. *Journal of the American Academy of Child and Adolescent Psychiatry, 25,* 370–376.

Korol, M. S. (1990). *Children's psychological responses to a nuclear waste disaster in Fernald, Ohio.* Unpublished doctoral dissertation, University of Cincinnati, Ohio.

Korol, M. S., Green, B. L., & Gleser, G. C. (1999). Children's response to a nuclear waste disaster: PTSD symptoms and outcome prediction. *Journal of the American Academy of Child and Adolescent Psychiatry, 38,* 368–375.

La Greca, A. M., Silverman, W. K., Vernberg, E. M., & Prinstein, M. (1996).Symptoms of posttraumatic stress after Hurricane Andrew: A prospective study. *Journal of Consulting and Clinical Psychology, 64,* 712–723.

La Greca, A. M., Silverman, W. K., & Wasserstein, S. B. (1998). Children's predisaster functioning as a predictor of posttraumatic stress following Hurricane Andrew. *Journal of Consulting and Clinical Psychology, 66,* 883–892.

La Greca, A. M., Vernberg, E. M., Silverman, W. K., & Prinstein, M. (1994). *Helping children prepare and cope with natural disasters: A manual for school personnel.* (Available from Annette M. La Greca, University of Miami, P. O. Box 249229, Coral Gables, FL 33124)

La Greca, A. M., Vernberg, E. M., Silverman, W. K., & Prinstein, M. (1995). *Helping children* [in Japanese]. Tokyo, Japan: Ashi.

Lonigan, C. J., Anthony, J. L., & Shannon, M. P. (1998). Diagnostic efficacy of posttraumatic symptoms in children exposed to disaster. *Journal of Clinical Child Psychology, 27,* 255–267.

Lonigan, C. J., Shannon, M. P., Finch, A. J., Daugherty, T. K., & Taylor, C. M. (1991). Children's reactions to a natural disaster: Symptom severity and degree of exposure. *Advances in Behaviour Research and Therapy, 13,* 135–154.

Lonigan, C. J., Shannon, M. P., Taylor, C. M., Finch, A. J., & Sallee, F. R. (1994). Children exposed to disaster: II. Risk factors for the development of post-traumatic symptomatology. *Journal of the American Academy of child Psychiatry, 33,* 94–105.

March, J. S., Amaya-Jackson, L., Murray, M. C., & Schulte, A. (1998). Cognitive-behavioral psychotherapy for children and adolescents with posttraumatic stress disorder after a single-incident stressor. *Journal of the American Academy of Child and Adolescent Psychiatry, 37,* 585–593.

March, J. S., Amaya-Jackson, L., Terry, R., & Costanzo, P. (1997). Posttraumatic symptomatology in children and adolescents after an industrial fire. *Journal of the American Academy of Child and Adolescent Psychiatry, 37,* 1080–1088.

McFarlane, A. C. (1987). Posttraumatic phenomena in a longitudinal study of children following a natural disaster. *Journal of the American Academy of Child and Adolescent Psychiatry, 26,* 764–769.

McNally, R. J. (1996). Assessment of post-traumatic stress disorder in children. *Journal of School Psychology, 34,* 107–131.

Mitchell, J. (1983). When disaster strikes: The critical incident stress debriefing process. *Journal of Emergency Medical Services, 8,* 36–39.

Nader, K., Pynoos, R. S., Fairbanks, L., & Frederick, C. (1990). Children's post-traumatic stress disorder reactions one year after a sniper attack at their school. *American Journal of Psychiatry, 147,* 1526–1530.

National Organization for Victim Assistance. (1991). *Hurricane! Issues unique to hurricane disasters.* Washington, DC: Author.

Nolen-Hoeksema, S., & Morrow, J. (1991). A prospective study of depression and posttraumatic stress symptoms after a natural disaster: The 1989 Loma Prieta earthquake. *Journal of Personality and Social Psychology, 61,* 115–121.

Petersen, A. C., Compas, B. E., Brooks-Gunn, J., Stemmler, M., Ey, S., & Grant, K. E. (1993). Depression in adolescence. *American Psychologist, 48,* 155–168.

Prinstein, M. J., & La Greca, A. M. (1999). *Children's coping assistance after a natural disaster: What predicts subsequent adjustment?* Manuscript in preparation.

Prinstein, M. J., La Greca, A. M., Vernberg, E. M., & Silverman, W. K. (1996). Children's coping assistance after a natural disaster. *Journal of Clinical Child Psychology, 25,* 463–475.

Pynoos, R. S., Frederick, C., Nader, K., Arroyo, W., Steinberg, A., Eth, S., Nunez, F., & Fairbanks, L. (1987). Life threat and posttraumatic stress in school-age children. *Archives of General Psychiatry, 44,* 1057–1063.

Pynoos, R. S., & Nader, K. (1988). Psychological first aid and treatment approach to children exposed to community violence: Research implications. *Journal of Traumatic Stress, 1,* 445–473.

Richters, J. E., & Martinez, P. (1990). *Checklist of Child Distress Symptoms: Parent Report.* Washington, DC: National Institute of Mental Health.

Robin, R. W., Chester, B., Rasmussen, J. K., Jaranson, J. M., & Goldman, D. (1997). Prevalence and characteristics of trauma and posttraumatic stress disorder in a southwestern American Indian community. *American Journal of Psychiatry, 154,* 1582–1588.

Rose, S., & Bisson, J. (1998). Brief early psychological interventions following trauma: A systematic review of the literature. *Journal of Traumatic Stress, 11,* 697–709.

Saigh, P. (1989). The development and validation of the Children's Post-traumatic Stress Disorder Inventory. *International Journal of Special Education, 4,* 75–84.

Saigh, P., Yule, W., & Imandar, S. C. (1996). Imaginal flooding of traumatized children and adolescents. *Journal of School Psychology, 34,* 163–183.

Scheeringa, M. S., Zeanah, C. H., Drell, M. J., & Larrieu, J. A. (1995). Two approaches to the diagnosis of posttraumatic stress disorder in infancy and early childhood. *Journal of the American Academy of Child Psychiatry, 34,* 191–200.

Shaffer, D., Fisher, P., Dulcan, M. K., Davies, M., Piacentini, J., Schwab-Stone, M. E., Lahey, B. B., Bourdon, K., Jensen, P. S., Bird, H. R., Canino, G., & Regier, D. A. (1996). The NIMH Diagnostic Interview Schedule for Children version 2.3 (DISC-2.3): Description, acceptability, prevalence rates, and performance in the MECA study. *Journal of the American Academy of Child and Adolescent Psychiatry, 35,* 865–877.

Shannon, M. P., Lonigan, C. J., Finch, A. J., & Taylor, C. M. (1994). Children exposed to disaster: I. Epidemiology of post-traumatic symptoms and symptom profiles. *Journal of the American Academy of Child Psychiatry, 33,* 80–93.

Shaw, J. A., Applegate, B., & Schorr, C. (1996). Twenty-one-month follow-up study of school-age children exposed to Hurricane Andrew. *Journal of the American Academy of Child and Adolescent Psychiatry, 35,* 359–364.

Shaw, J. A., Applegate, B., Tanner, S., Perez, D., Rothe, E., Campo-Bowen, A. E., & Lahey, B. L. (1995). Psychological effects of Hurricane Andrew on an elementary school population. *Journal of the American Academy of Child and Adolescent Psychiatry, 34,* 1185–1192.

Silverman, W. K., & Ginsburg, G. S. (1995). Specific phobia and generalized anxiety disorder. In J. S. March (Ed.), *Anxiety disorders in children and adolescents* (pp. 276–300). New York: Guilford Press.

Silverman, W. K., & Nelles, W. B. (1988). The Anxiety Disorders Interview Schedule for Children. *Journal of the American Academy of Child and Adolescent Psychiatry, 27,* 772–778.

Singer, M. I., Anglin, T., Song, L., & Lunghofer, L. (1995). Adolescents' exposure to violence and associated symptoms of psychological trauma. *Journal of the American Medical Association, 273,* 477–482.

Storm, V., McDermott, B., & Finlayson, D. (1994). *The bushfire and me: A story of what happened to me and my family.* Newtown, Australia: VBD.

Swenson, C. C., Saylor, C. F., Powell, M. P., Stokes, S. J., Foster, K. Y., & Belter, R. W. (1996). Impact of a natural disaster on preschool children: Adjustment 14 months after a hurricane. *American Journal of Orthopsychiatry, 66,* 122–130.

Terr, L. C. (1983). Chowchilla revisted: The effect of psychic trauma four years after a school bus kidnapping. *American Journal of Psychiatry, 140,* 1543–1550.

Vernberg, E. M., La Greca, A. M., Silverman, W. K., & Prinstein, M. (1996). Predictors of children's post-disaster functioning following Hurricane Andrew. *Journal of Abnormal Psychology, 105,* 237–248.

Vernberg, E. M., & Vogel, J. M. (1993). Interventions with children after disasters. *Journal of Clinical Child Psychology, 22,* 485–498.

Vincent, N. R. (1997). A follow-up to Hurricane Andrew: Children's reactions 42 months post-disaster. Unpublished doctoral dissertation, University of Miami, FL.

Vincent, N. R., La Greca, A. M., Silverman, W. K., Wasserstein, S., & Prinstein, M. (1994, August). Predicting children's responses to natural disasters: Role of academic achievement. Paper presented at the meeting of the American Psychological Association, Los Angeles, CA.

Vogel, J., & Vernberg, E. M. (1993). Children's psychological responses to disaster. *Journal of Clinical Child Psychology, 22,* 464–484.

Yule, W. (1992). Post-traumatic stress disorder in child survivors of shipping disasters: The sinking of the "Jupiter." *Psychotherapy and Psychosomatics, 57,* 200–205.

Yule, W. (1994). Posttraumatic stress disorder. In T. H. Ollendick, N. J. King, & W. Yule (Eds.), *International handbook of phobic and anxiety disorders in children and adolescents* (pp. 223–240). New York: Plenum.

Yule, W., & Canterbury, R. (1994). The treatment of posttraumatic stress disorder in children and adolescents. *International Review of Psychiatry, 6,* 141–151.

Yule, W., & Udwin, O. (1991). Screening child survivors for post-traumatic stress disorders: Experiences from the "Jupiter" sinking. *British Journal of Clinical Psychology, 30,* 131–138.

Yule, W., Udwin, O., & Murdoch, K. (1990). The "Jupiter" sinking: Effects on children's fears, depression, and anxiety. *Journal of Child Psychology and Psychiatry, 31,* 1051–1061.

Yule, W., & Williams, R. (1990). Posttraumatic stress reactions in children. *Journal of Traumatic Stress, 3,* 279–295.

PART IV

*Treatments
with Specific
Populations*

11

WENDY K. SILVERMAN
WILLIAM M. KURTINES

Anxiety Disorders

In the current climate in the United States of managed care, HMOs, and problems in obtaining third party payments, practitioners are under increasing pressure to provide psychological services to children and adolescents that are time limited, problem focused, and evidence based. In light of this pressure, this volume is particularly timely. This chapter focuses on the treatment of anxiety disorders in children. We begin with a brief summary of the prevalence, developmental precursors, and consequences of anxiety disorders in children. This is followed by a presentation of evidence-based or empirically supported interventions for anxiety disorders in children. Specifically, a conceptualization for interventions for anxiety disorders in children is presented. Next we describe the "basic" intervention and note studies that provide evidence of efficacy. The final part of the chapter discusses issues involved in integrating and adapting interventions in nonresearch-based settings.

Prevalence of Anxiety Disorders in Youth

The anxiety disorders specified in the fourth edition of the *Diagnostic and Statistical Manual of Mental Disorders* (DSM-IV; American Psychiatric Association, 1994) include separation anxiety disorder, generalized anxiety disorder, panic disorder without agoraphobia, panic disorder with agoraphobia, agoraphobia without history of panic disorder, specific phobia, social phobia (social anxiety disorder), obsessive-compulsive disorder, posttraumatic stress disorder, acute stress disorder, anxiety disorder due to a general medical condition, and substance-induced anxiety disorder.[1] To warrant an anxiety disorder diagnosis, the child must meet the criteria for at least one of these disorders; in addition, it is important to ascertain the level or extent of impairment that results from the disorder(s), in the areas of school, peer relationships, family life, or undue distress in the child.

Prevalence of anxiety disorders in youth has been found to vary considerably due to methodological differences across studies. These differences include the informant, the assessment method, the type of sample, the age of the participants, the specific disorder assessed, and whether an impairment index was included as part of the definition. These differences notwithstanding, estimated prevalence rates of "any anxiety disorder" appear to range between 5.78% and 17.7%, with overanxious/generalized anxiety disorder, separation anxiety disorder, and specific phobia being most prevalent.

Studies of prevalence using diverse ethnic or racial groups are rare. Bird et al. (1988) conducted a community study of behavioral and emotional problems in youth aged 4 to 16 years in Puerto Rico and found that prevalence rates for the most common anxiety disorders were 2.6% for specific phobia and 4.7% for separation anxiety disorder. Two studies conducted in childhood anxiety disorder specialty clinics (Ginsburg & Silverman, 1996; Last & Perrin, 1993) found no differences in rates of anxiety diagnoses between Hispanic American and Caucasian youth and African American and Caucasian youth, respectively. In terms of gender, although findings in the adult area document that anxiety disorders are more predominant in women than in men (Kessler et al., 1994), no clear and consistent pattern has emerged with children (see Costello & Angold, 1995). In terms of age, several studies have found that, with the exception of separation anxiety disorder, the prevalence of anxiety disorders generally increases with age. Inconsistencies have been reported, however, and appear to depend on the specific disorder (e.g., Anderson, Williams, McGee, & Silva, 1987; Cohen, Cohen, & Brook, 1993; McGee, Feehan, Williams, & Anderson, 1992).

Developmental Precursors

Several developmental precursors have been identified. These include, but are not limited to, genetic and neurobiological factors, behavioral/learning and cognitive factors, and familial precursors.

Genetic and Neurobiological Precursors

Findings from studies that have evaluated the offspring of patients with anxiety disorders (e.g., Fyer et al., 1990; Silverman, Cerny, Nelles, & Burke, 1988; Turner, Beidel, & Costello, 1987; Weissman, Leckman, Merikangas, Gammon, & Prusoff, 1984) and findings from studies that have evaluated the parents of children with anxiety disorders (e.g., Kashani et al., 1990; Last, Hersen, Kazdin, Francis, & Grubb, 1987; Last, Hersen, Kazdin, Orvaschel, & Perrin, 1991; Messer & Beidel, 1994) generally reveal familial aggregation for the anxiety disorders (see Ginsburg, Silverman, & Kurtines, 1995a). Although family studies demonstrate familiality, not heritability, recent studies in behavioral genetics document a genetic influence on anxiety in childhood, which accounts for about one third of the variance in most cases. Further, heritability appears to be greater for girls than for boys. Behavioral genetic methods also show, however, that shared environment (i.e., that which leads family members to resemble one another) is a significant influence for anxiety (but not for depression; e.g., see Eley, 1999).

Behavioral inhibition, a temperament style that predisposes infants to irritability, toddlers to shyness and fearfulness, and school-aged children to cautiousness and introversion, has received a great deal of recent research attention as a potential neurobiological precursor (Kagan, Reznick, & Snidman, 1987; Rosenbaum et al., 1988). Children with behavioral inhibition display many of the same behavioral, affective, and physiological characteristics (e.g., increased heart rate) as children with anxiety disorders when exposed to unfamiliar settings, people, and objects (e.g., Kagan, 1989; Kagan et al., 1987). In addition, significantly more children whose parents present with an anxiety disorder (i.e., panic disorder/agoraphobia) display behavioral inhibition than children whose parents present with a psychiatric disorder other than anxiety or depression (Rosenbaum et al., 1988), suggesting that behavioral inhibition may be a risk factor for later anxiety disorders in childhood. However, because not all children with early behavioral inhibition develop an anxiety disorder (approximately 70% do not), further research on behavioral inhibition and its interaction(s) with other developmental precursors is needed.

Behavioral/Learning and Cognitive Precursors

Research findings for a Pavlovian (conditioning) account of fear/anxiety acquisition have been inconsistent, leading to questions about its adequacy (see Menzies & Clarke, 1995). This has led to extensions of conditioning theory (e.g., Davey, 1992; Rescorla, 1988), including extensions of Mowrer's (1939) two-factor theory (e.g., Eysenck, 1979; Seligman, 1971; Solomon & Wynne, 1954). Rachman (1977) discussed the importance of additional pathways in "indirect" fear acquisition, namely, vicarious exposure and the transmission of information or instruction. Support for these pathways has been provided in the subclinical fears of adults (e.g., Ost, 1985), and in the fears of non–clinic-referred children (Ollendick & King, 1991). Overall, though, more research is needed, as the findings on behavioral/learning factors as specific precursors to anxiety disorders are inconsistent across laboratories, disorders, and samples.

With respect to cognitive precursors, there is controversy about whether the cognitions of children with anxiety disorders are developmental precursors or consequences of the fear/anxiety response. Nevertheless, there is evidence that anxiety-disordered children display distorted and maladaptive thoughts (e.g., Kendall & Chansky, 1991; Weems, Berman, Silverman, & Saavedra, in press). An individual-difference cognitive variable that also has been implicated in the development of anxiety disorders in children is anxiety sensitivity, that is, thinking that the experience of anxiety symptoms has harmful or aversive consequences (see Silverman & Weems, 1999). Additional factors that appear to influence the thinking of anxious children include causal attributions (see Bell-Dolan & Wessler, 1994) and information processing (Vasey, Daleiden, Williams, & Brown, 1995).

Familial Precursors

As noted, shared environment has been found to play a significant role in anxiety disorders in childhood. Shared environment influences are likely to consist of shared familial experiences during childhood (Eley, 1999). Retrospective reports of adults who suffer from anxiety disorders show that these adults view their parents and their relationship with them as overcontrolling and low in affection (see Rapee, 1997). Direct observations of parent-child interactions have provided further evidence that there may be family processes that are specific to families of children with anxiety disorders and that these processes might serve to bring out and/or maintain these disorders in children (e.g., Chorpita, Albano, & Barlow, 1996; Dadds, Barrett, Rapee, & Ryan, 1996; see Ginsburg et al., 1995a). For example, Dadds et al. (1996) have shown that following a family discussion, children with anxiety disorders were more likely to generate avoidant solutions than children with oppositional defiant disorder or normal controls. Undesirable parenting, such as inconsistent or restrictive patterns of behavior, is also associated with anxiety in children (Krohne & Hock, 1991).

Consequences

Relatively little research has been conducted on the consequences of having one or more anxiety disorders during childhood and adolescence. This is partly due to the challenges inherent in examining the "natural" course and outcome of childhood psychopathology in general (e.g., in community samples some children might receive treatment over time, some might not; in clinic-referred samples, most receive treatment). The small number of studies that have been conducted have several additional methodological constraints, including small sample sizes, lack of specificity regarding the specific diagnoses, and often lack of comparison control groups (see Silverman & Ginsburg, 1998).

With these constraints in mind, the main conclusion to be drawn about the consequences of having an anxiety disorder during childhood and adolescence is that a proportion of initial anxiety disorder diagnoses in youth remits, but a proportion does not remit. The range of remission is 34% to 54% (or, 46% to 66% do not remit). However, even when there is remission, oftentimes other disorders develop, particularly another anxiety disorder, a new depressive disorder, or a new externalizing behavior disorder (e.g., Last et al., 1996, found that 15.5% of the original sample developed another anxiety disorder, 13.1% a depressive disorder, and 7.1% an externalizing behavior disorder). One explanation for such findings is that the expression of anxiety disorders changes in accordance with the level of socioemotional development. Another explanation, not incompatible with the latter, is that the presence of an anxiety disorder forms a risk for the development of other disorders.

Little is known about the functioning or adjustment of children with anxiety disorders. In an eight-year follow-up study, Last et al. (1997) reported that adjustment was considerably worse for children who had anxiety comorbid with depressive disorder relative to children with anxiety only or to controls who were never psychiatrically ill. The comorbid group, for example, were less likely to be working or attending school and more likely to utilize mental health services. As noted, however, the research on this matter is sparse, and a great deal more research is needed before firm conclusions about consequences can be made.

Evidence-Based Interventions

Two main characteristics of the evidence-based or empirically supported interventions described in this chapter are that they are time limited and problem focused. Time limited means that the interventions are of relatively short duration, and it is generally known to the client and therapist when treatment will terminate. That is, both the client and the clinician are aware from the beginning that their "work together" will last a certain, general amount of time (e.g., 10 to 12 weeks; 16 to 18 weeks). This serves to keep the interventions focused on the main target problem, that is, impairing anxiety.

This brings up the second characteristic of the interventions, namely, being problem focused. Being problem focused is rooted, more generally, in a general attitude described elsewhere as pragmatic (Silverman & Kurtines, 1996a, 1997), which, in essence, is a problem-solving orientation or attitude. Within a pragmatic frame, priority is placed on using knowledge (e.g., knowledge about fear and anxiety reduction) to develop and implement interventions that help solve concrete and specific problems (e.g., excessive fears and anxiety and the resulting impairment).

Conceptualization of Intervention

Silverman and Kurtines (1996a, 1996b, 1997) have provided a conceptualization for interventions for anxiety disorders in children, including cognitive-behavioral interventions, which are the interventions that show most efficacy for reducing anxiety disorders in children. This conceptualization, referred to as a *transfer-of-control* approach, provides a general conceptual frame with respect both to why certain treatment strategies make sense to use to reduce anxiety disorders in children and to the sequence in which various treatment strategies should be implemented. Although empirical verification of the validity of the transfer-of-control approach is needed (and this work is currently under way), thinking about interventions, particularly cognitive-behavioral interventions, in terms of a transfer-of-control approach is a useful clinical heuristic, as illustrated in the following section. It should be emphasized, though, that this is a heuristic only, and we do not imply that this is the only way that one might view interventions for anxiety disorders in children.

TRANSFER OF CONTROL. The transfer-of-control approach explicitly recognizes that anxiety disorders in children are complex, multifaceted, and multidetermined, and it draws on the major theoretical traditions for its conceptualization of the basic, interrelated types of processes — behavioral, cognitive, and affective — that are at the core of the approach. In addition, the transfer-of-control approach focuses on delineating the links between the types of interrelated maladaptive processes or symptoms that provide the basis for a diagnosis of an anxiety disorder and the types of interventions (therapeutic procedures and strategies) that can be used to modify those processes or symptoms.

The transfer-of-control approach holds that effective long-term psychotherapeutic change in children involves a gradual "transfer of control" in which the sequence is generally from therapist to parent to child. The therapist is viewed as a consultant who "transfers" his or her knowledge about the skills and methods necessary to produce therapeutic change to the parent, and subsequently the parent transfers this knowledge to the child. In treating children with anxiety disorders, the primary focus of the transfer of control is on "controlling" the occurrence and successful implementation of a key change-producing procedure: exposure.

KEY CHANGE-PRODUCING PROCEDURE: EXPOSURE.   Exposure is the key therapeutic ingredient or change-producing procedure in the childhood anxiety interventions. There is a large body of research evidence showing that exposure to the feared situations and objects is important for effective reduction in phobic and anxious symptomatology (Barlow, 1988). The forms of direct therapeutic exposure particularly useful with children involve gradual or graduated exposures (in vivo and imaginal).[2]

Although exposure is merely a description of what occurs in treatment and is not an explanation of the process of change, the various theoretical accounts that have been suggested (but not sufficiently empirically confirmed) involve the modification of behavioral, cognitive, or affective processes or a combination thereof (see Barlow, 1988). For example, a cognitive explanation of exposure procedures would state that through direct experience with fear- or anxiety-provoking situations children's mastery expectations are raised (Bandura, 1977). Once strong expectations have been developed through repeated success, the child can tolerate the negative impact of the occasional failure.

Behavioral explanations involve the processes of habituation and extinction (Rachman, 1978). Habituation refers to the decline of the unlearned responses after repeated presentations of the fear- or anxiety-provoking stimulus. Extinction refers to the repeated presentation of the phobic or anxiety-provoking stimulus (conditioned stimulus) in the absence of the aversive stimulus (unconditioned stimulus) with a decrement in the strength of the conditioned response. Rachman (1978) has discussed the varying roles of habituation and extinction in decreasing phobic or anxious responses. Briefly, Rachman suggested that the former is most important for reducing the physiological component; that the latter is most important for reducing the behavioral component, that is, avoidance; and that both are important for reducing the subjective component.

At this juncture it also would be worthwhile to mention the link between exposure and diagnosis. Although treatment of all the anxiety disorders requires that children gradually expose themselves to fear- or anxiety-provoking situations, or to "face their fears," what varies across the anxiety disorder subcategories is content. That is, the content of a child's anxiety is different for a child with a diagnosis of separation anxiety disorder than for a child with a diagnosis of social phobia. Knowing, therefore, that a child has a social phobia or separation anxiety disorder simplifies the process of designing appropriate and effective exposure tasks.

FACILITATIVE STRATEGIES: CONTINGENCY MANAGEMENT AND SELF-CONTROL. Behavioral and cognitive strategies for facilitating the occurrence of exposure are contingency management and self-control, respectively. Both of these strategies are described in further detail subsequently. Briefly, however, based on behavioral processes of change, contingency management emphasizes the training of parents in the use of appropriate contingencies to facilitate the child's exposure or approach behavior toward feared objects or situations. A key element of contingency management is contingency contracting. In these contracts, the specific exposure task that the child is to attempt is indicated, as well as the specific consequence (i.e., reward) that the child is to receive for successfully attempting the exposure.

Based on cognitive processes of change, self-control emphasizes the training of the child in the use of appropriate cognitive strategies to facilitate exposure or approach behavior toward feared objects or situations. A key element of self-control training is cognitive restructuring and self-reward. Emphasis is placed on identifying one's anxious thoughts and ways either *not* to think these anxious thoughts or to think more positive, coping thoughts.

USING A TRANSFER-OF-CONTROL APPROACH FOR IMPLEMENTING AN EXPOSURE-BASED INTERVENTION. The transfer-of-control approach provides guidelines to the general sequence for administering the behavioral and cognitive strategies that are used. It is built on the links that exist between key maladaptive processes of anxiety disorders (i.e., behavioral, cognitive, affective), related contextual processes (e.g., relational, institutional) that give rise to or maintain these processes or both, and the key change-producing procedure (i.e., exposure) and related therapeutic facilitative strategies (e.g., contingency management and self-control training) that have an impact on these maladaptive processes. Hence, the transfer of control involves first the training of parents in contingency management and in using these skills to encourage the child's exposure (parent control). This is followed by a gradual fading of parental control while the child is taught to use self-control strategies to encourage his or her own exposure (child control). Consequently, parental (or external) control is gradually reduced while the child learns cognitive self-control strategies in contexts specific to his or her anxiety or fear problem.

Description of "Basic" Intervention

Individual, Group, or Conjoint Sessions

The intervention can be conducted using either an individual or group treatment format. The children and parents can be seen either in separate sessions (i.e., child, parent) or in sessions together. The treatment is time limited, as already noted. The range of the number of sessions is anywhere from 10 to 15 sessions. The beginning sessions make up the education phase, the middle sessions make up the application phase, and the final sessions constitute the relapse prevention phase, with participants still applying what they have learned.

Phases Overview

During the education phase, focus is on providing the information and the skills necessary for children and parents to control or manage the child's anxious behaviors. In the application phase of the program, the focus is on implementing the transfer of control. As noted, this phase specifically focuses on "controlling" the occurrence and on successful use of the key change-producing procedure, namely, child exposure or approach behavior. In the application phase, the parents and the children use the methods that were explained to them in the education phase. Specifically, contingency management, followed by self-control procedures, are used to facilitate the child's exposures.

In the relapse prevention phase, strategies are presented to handle and prevent the recurrence of the child's avoidant behaviors. This phase is important to help ensure a complete and final transfer of control so that in the event of relapse both the child and parent will be able to successfully manage the event, especially if they are no longer being seen by the therapist. A more detailed description of various aspects of the education, application, and relapse prevention phases of the program, as they relate specifically to exposure, contingency management, and self-control, follows (see Silverman, Ginsburg, & Kurtines, 1995; Silverman & Kurtines, 1996a, b).

EDUCATION PHASE

Fear hierarchy. Both children and parents are informed early on that the child will learn how to handle his or her anxiety or fears through exposure — "facing your fear." The gradual exposure tasks are designed along a fear hierarchy. Each hierarchy consists of 10 to 15 specific situations or objects that range from only slightly to extremely fear-provoking. Although the expectation is conveyed that the child is to progress up the hierarchy, it is made clear that the child ultimately determines the rate of progress. It also is explained that as the child progresses up the hierarchy and conducts exposures, the child should ensure that he or she experiences elevated levels of arousal or discomfort. The importance of facing this arousal and discomfort and of not leaving the situation until these feelings are reduced is stressed.

It is not uncommon that initial exposure tasks do not result in reduced feelings of arousal or discomfort. That is, the child may "do" an exposure, for example, a "high" one on the hierarchy, and may rate that exposure as eliciting a fear rating of 8, (on a 0- to 8-point fear thermometer). After 15 minutes, the rating drops, but only to a 7. In such instances, the child is encouraged to repeat the exposure again the following week and to remain even longer in that situation — hours, if necessary — to obtain a decrement. It is explained that unless the exposure is repeated (and repeated and repeated, as necessary!), it is difficult to continue up the fear hierarchy; that is, to do something that is even more anxiety-provoking than the current task. Reassuring the child that anxiety reduction will occur, if she or he stays in that situation and with that "experience," is important. Also, as described later, cognitive strategies are taught to help facilitate exposures and a decrement in the child's fear or anxiety response.

Principles of contingency management. Basic principles of learning, with an emphasis on contingency management training, are explained to the children and parents. Emphasis is placed on explaining the concept and the proper delivery of reinforcement. It is helpful to differentiate between different types of rewards (i.e., social, tangible, activity) and to encourage the use of social and activity rewards. Rewards are to be provided contingent on the child's completion of desired behaviors, namely, exposures. The importance of consistency and follow through also is explained to parents, as well as potential difficulties that parents encounter that prevent effective follow through. The advantages of using contracts that explicate the specific rewards that are to be delivered contingent on the emittance of specific behaviors also are provided.

Principles of self-control. Basic principles of cognitive self-control are explained to the children and parents following the explanation of the contingency management procedures. Emphasis is placed on explaining the concepts of self-observation, self-evaluation, and self-reward. The importance of parental support and encouragement for children's appropriate use of cognitive self-control procedures is explained to parents, along with potential difficulties that prevent effective parental delivery of support and encouragement.

APPLICATION PHASE

In-session and out-of-session activities. The main in-session and out-of-session activities that are implemented during the application phase are the exposure tasks. The exposure tasks represent the various steps that were listed on the fear hierarchy during the education phase. For example, a hierarchy for a child who presents with social phobia may begin with first saying hello to another child in school, then asking a child a question, holding a conversation for at least one minute, then three minutes, followed by calling a child up on the telephone and asking a question about schoolwork. A child with a specific phobia of dogs may begin by first looking at photographs of dogs, looking at a puppy at a pet shop, holding a puppy at a pet shop, visiting relatives or friends with a dog when the dog is leashed, visiting relatives or friends with a dog when the dog is unleashed, playing with a dog at a relative's or friend's house, and so forth. In all instances, it is emphasized to the child that in implementing the exposures, the emphasis is on trying and in doing one's best. The importance of "staying with the experience," as discussed earlier, is stressed once again.

Graduated exposure tasks also are implemented in-session in the presence of the therapist. This allows for additional exposure opportunities, as well as for the therapist to provide corrective feedback, to display appropriate adaptive responses for modeling, and to serve as a source of encouragement and positive reinforcement.

Contingency management procedures. As noted, contingency management is used to help in initially obtaining parental control of the child's avoidant behaviors. An important aspect of contingency management is the use of contingency contracts. Specifically, in each session a detailed contract is written between the child and parent, with the assistance of the therapist. The contract explicitly states the specific exposure task that the child is to attempt, in-session and out-of-session exposure (e.g., what to do, when to do it, how long to do it), and the consequence that follows for successful attempt or completion of the task (e.g., specific reward, when it is to be delivered).

Self-control procedures. After some degree of parental control of a child's exposure behavior has been obtained via contingency management procedures, the child's control is initiated through self-control procedures. As noted, the main focus of the self-control procedures is to help the child to identify his or her anxious thoughts and self-statements and their role in producing/maintaining anxiety and its disorders, including inhibiting the child's exposures to the situation. More specifically, it might be explained to the child that of course he or she is scared or uncomfortable to do a particular exposure in light of the terrible things that he or she is thinking about in terms of the situation itself or of the child's responses that result from being in that situation. This then leads into a discussion about "automatic thoughts" and how the child probably did not even realize that such thoughts occurred when he or she was faced with particular situations or events.

To further explain and also to help apply self-control strategies, the *STOP* acronym is taught: *S* stands for "Scared," *T* stands for "Thoughts," *O* stands for "Other thoughts" or "Other things I can do to handle my fear," and *P* stands for "Praise myself for successful handling of my fear and exposure." Hence, for example, a child with a phobia of attending school learned to recognize that he became *Scared (S)* as soon as the school bus pulled in the circular drive of the school building and that he began to feel "butterflies in his stomach" and began feeling really "sick." He identified his *Thoughts (T)* as "I hate this school. The teachers are terrible. I wish I did not have to go here." His *Other thoughts or other things he could do (O)* were: "Even though this is a crappy school, I did learn some things and at least three of the six teachers I have are actually pretty good. So that is one half." (This also involved a discussion about whether to view the glass as half empty or half full.) *Other things he did* included using a rubber band that he snapped on his wrist whenever the negative thoughts emerged, so that he would not have to "think these negative thoughts." Finally, when he successfully managed his responses and successfully entered and stayed in the school building, he *Praised himself (P)* for a "job well done," saying, for example, "I did it! I managed to stay in school!"

RELAPSE PREVENTION PHASE

Importance of continued exposure. The therapist explains that the more the child continues to engage in continued exposure, the less likely it is that he or she will have a relapse. It is explained that much of what the child has accomplished is due largely to the exposure exercises, and, like any accomplishment, "if you don't use it, you lose it." Examples are provided from other skills that the child may have learned in his or her life, such as playing a sport or an instrument, and how if the child did not continue to practice, or expose him or herself to this sport or instrument, the child lost the skill needed to successfully perform that sport or instrument.

Interpreting slips. The therapist explains that no matter how much the child may practice and continue to engage in exposure, it is likely, nevertheless, that a relapse or a "slip" will occur. It is emphasized that this is a common occurrence. The therapist may use the analogy of a person on a weight loss program who may have successfully lost 20 pounds but then eats a piece of cake at a party and who may have different ways of interpreting the "slip." This case is analyzed in detail with the child and the parent. Via this analysis, it becomes evident that the most adaptive interpretation is that "this is a single event. It does not mean that everything is blown or ruined. I need to pick myself back up and get back on the positive track I was on." Emphasis is placed on the parents' role in handling slips and how many children will look to the parents and take cues from them in interpreting the slips.

Evidence of Efficacy

As noted, research is under way to examine whether therapy outcome is mediated via a transfer of control, as articulated in the previous section. Research also is needed that examines the role of other variables and processes as potential mediators and moderators of outcome. In the meantime, the evidence that currently exists pertains to the efficacy of cognitive-behavioral interventions. This evidence comes from case study reports (e.g., Chiodos & Maddux, 1985; Eisen & Silverman, 1991), controlled single-case designs (e.g., Eisen & Silverman, 1998; Kane & Kendall, 1989; Ollendick, 1995), and randomized controlled clinical trials (e.g., Barrett, 1998; Barrett, Dadds, & Rapee, 1996; Cobham, Dadds, & Spence, 1998; Flannery-Schroeder & Kendall, in press; Kendall, 1994; Kendall et al., 1997; Silverman, Kurtines, Ginsburg, Weems, Lumpkin, & Carmichael, in press; Silverman, Kurtines, Ginsburg, Weems, Rabian, & Serafini, in press). Most of the controlled studies used rigorous methodological procedures, including the use of multisource assessments, structured diagnostic interviews, manualized treatments, treatment integrity checks, and systematic follow-up procedures (see Silverman & Ginsburg, 1998). In addition, there is evidence for not only child-focused, individual treatment formats (e.g., Kendall, 1994; Kendall et al., 1997; Silverman, Kurtines, Ginsburg, Weems, Rabian, & Serafini, 1999) but also for treatments that involve parents (e.g., Barrett et al., 1996; Cobham et al., 1998; Silverman, Kurtines, Ginsburg, Weems, Rabian, & Serafini, 1999) and use group formats (e.g., Barrett, 1998; Flannery-Schroeder & Kendall, 2000; Silverman, Kurtines, Ginsburg, Weems, Lumpkin, & Carmichael, in press).

It has been pointed out in the literature that the evidence of efficacy for most psychosocial interventions, including cognitive-behavioral interventions for anxiety disorders in children, comes from university-based research clinics, not from community clinics; and differences between research and community clinics have been noted (e.g., conditions, clients, therapists; Weisz, Donenberg, Han, & Weiss, 1995). Although questions have been raised about the actual extensiveness of the differences noted (e.g., there is pervasive pathology in the research clinic samples; see Barlow, 1994; Silverman, 1991), the fact is that many clinicians have been reluctant to jump on the "evidence- or empirically based treatment bandwagon" (more is said on this point in the subsequent section).

Nevertheless, it is important to further note that the available evidence suggests that psychological services received in community clinics are not effective (e.g., Weiss, Catron, Harris, & Phung, 1999). (We are not aware of studies that have examined this issue in other settings.) As a consequence, it has been argued that evidence-based treatments should be used in community clinics, as this might improve the outcomes of clinic-referred youth (Weisz et al., 1995). Research is currently under way at the University of California at Los Angeles (M. Southham-Gerow and J. Weisz, personal communication, May 26, 1999) to test the validity of this argument.

The final section of this chapter is based on the assumption that there is value in trying to integrate and adapt the previously described "basic" efficacious intervention to other psychological service delivery settings. Because it is not possible to provide an exhaustive discussion of the full range of challenges that might arise in trying to do so, particular challenges associated with conditions, clients, and therapists, respectively, are provided.

Integrating and Adapting the "Basic" Intervention

Conditions

A primary "condition" of research clinics is that they exist not only to help children and families but also to create and extend knowledge for the field as a whole. A primary way that knowledge is created and extended is by obtaining specific types of information from the presenting children and their families in ways that are deemed acceptable by the scientific community. "Specific types of information" implies information that has been empirically found useful (i.e., that can be directly applied to help solve problems, such as those associated with excessive anxiety). "Acceptable" implies ways or methods that will yield information that is reliable (i.e., consistent) and valid (i.e., accurate).

Although a wide variety of information is obtained in research clinics, one thing that is obtained in all of them (because it is useful) is a complete diagnostic picture of the child. This includes a complete picture of the nature and history of the child's problems, family members' reactions to the problems, and family history with respect to medical and psychological problems. Similarly, although all types of methods are used in research clinics, to obtain a complete diagnostic picture of the child, some type of structured data gathering procedure (i.e., a structured or semistructured interview schedule) is always used. The reason for obtaining diagnostic information with structured or semistructured interview schedules (and not with unstructured, clinical interviews) is that these schedules have been found to yield more reliable and valid information.

One could argue that it is this condition (i.e., the use of structured or semistructured information-gathering procedures such as interview schedules) that contributes, in part, to the positive findings obtained in research clinics. For example, given the high rates of comorbid (co-occurring) disorders in youth, it is not so simple to determine and prioritize all the various problems children display. Interview schedules can assist with making such determination and prioritization, reliably and accurately. By having this type of reliable and valid information, the clinician can have increased confidence that anxiety is a primary and impairing problem for the child and his or her family and thus that the targeting of anxiety is warranted. Also, as noted earlier, an accurate differential diagnosis (e.g., knowing that a child has a social phobia, not separation anxiety disorder) simplifies the process of designing appropriate and effective exposure tasks. In addition, some of the interview schedules are useful in obtaining information about the functional relations, or motivating conditions, with respect to anxiety problems.

In light of these findings, it would seem important to have this "condition" of research settings in place in other settings. At a minimum, this would mean that the intake session with the children and families would involve the administration of a semistructured interview schedule. One of the most widely used schedules for diagnosing anxiety and other internalizing and externalizing disorders in youth is the Anxiety Disorders Interview Schedule for Children-IV-Child and Parent Versions (ADIS-IV-C/P; Silverman & Albano, 1996; Silverman & Nelles, 1988). Semistructured in nature, the ADIS-IV-C/P contains specific questions that cover the diagnostic criteria for the anxiety disorders, as well as other internalizing and externalizing childhood disorders, described in the *DSM-IV*. The ADIS-IV-C/P also contains screening questions for other, less prevalent childhood disorders (e.g., sleep terror disorder).

Because of its extensive coverage, the ADIS-IV-C/P assists in determining primary, secondary, tertiary, and so on, diagnoses and thus helps to prioritize targets for treatment. Specifically, children's multiple or comorbid problems are prioritized by obtaining child and parent ratings of severity and interference via the ADIS-IV-C/P. These ratings are then used to determine a ranking of the symptoms that should be targeted in treatment. To the extent that the primary target symptoms are those other than anxiety, such as depression or attention deficit, it may become necessary to ascertain which of these symptoms, if any, may interfere with the anxiety treatment program. Symptoms that are deemed as interfering may deserve primary attention using modified methods of treatment (see, for example, Kendall, Kortlander, Chansky, & Brady, 1992).

The ADIS-IV-C/P also contains questions that can assist in providing a functional analysis (e.g., antecedents and consequence of various problems). Additional information that can be gathered via the ADIS-IV-C/P include questions about history of the problem(s), family members' reactions to the problem(s), family history with respect to medical and psychological problems, and so forth. All of this information is helpful not only in ascertaining diagnoses but also in case conceptualization and formulation.

Overall, it is useful to think of the interview schedules as templates that can guide clinicians' questioning (Silverman & Kurtines, 1996a). When viewed in this way, the interviews serve mainly as a tool to ensure that accurate and complete questioning occurs for the various disorders, not as rigid, inflexible scripts.

Despite the apparent importance of administering some type of diagnostic interview prior to treating children, in some settings (e.g., schools) it is usually not possible to administer a full diagnostic interview. Because research has found that child self-report measures, such as the Test Anxiety Scale for Children (Sarason, Davidson, Lighthall, Waite, & Ruebush, 1960), the Revised Children's Manifest Anxiety Scale (Reynolds & Richmond, 1978), and The Fear Survey Schedule for Children-Revised (Ollendick, 1983), can serve as screens for clinically diagnosable phobic and anxiety disorders (see, respectively, Beidel & Turner, 1988; Dadds, Spence, Holland, Barrett, & Laurens, 1997; Weems, Silverman, Saavedra, Pina, & Lumpkin, 1999), one of these questionnaires could be administered. Children with "high" scores (e.g., at least one to two standard deviations above the group's mean) could be followed up for further diagnostic interviewing, either in that setting or an alternative setting.

Clients

In research clinics, a part of the informed consent procedure is a description of who is expected to participate in, and be involved with, the treatment. In the basic intervention described in this chapter, as in all the efficacious cognitive-behavioral treatments, both child and parental involvement is expected. If either the child or parents are unwilling to participate, then the family is excluded from participating in the study and frequently are referred to another service agency.

In some settings, however, such as schools, parents are not readily available to participate in child interventions. In other settings, such as psychiatric or community settings, parents may be too impaired themselves to be of therapeutic help in the child's treatment. Unlike in research settings, treatment can (and should) not be withheld because of the absence of parental involvement.

The evidence suggests that either contingency management strategies or self-control strategies are efficacious when used alone to facilitate exposure (Silverman et al., 1999). In other words, one can think of a transfer from therapist to parent (contingency management) as one that will be efficacious. One also can think of a transfer from therapist to child (self-control) as one that will be efficacious. In addition, as already noted, there exists evidence that a group treatment format is efficacious (e.g., Barrett, 1998; Silverman et al., 1999).

What are the implications of this evidence in terms of working with children with anxiety disorders in settings in which parents are not available (physically or psychologically) to be involved in the treatment? One main implication is that it suggests that, as useful as it is to have parental involvement, and it is (Barrett et al., 1996; Barrett, 1998), if parental involvement is not possible, there are alternative things that can be done. The most obvious thing is to rely on the peer group, rather than parents, to help transfer control. For example, when a child in the group observes a peer perform a successful exposure task, it provides the opportunity for positive modeling to occur. The child's subsequent successful completion of his or her own exposure task, in turn, results in peer reinforcement for the child. The group format also provides a context for corrective or instructive feedback (e.g., when children share with each other their methods for doing exposure tasks). In addition, the group process itself provides support for the children. A group treatment format also is a time- and cost-effective approach, and thus offers many additional practical advantages for use in many types of institutional settings (see Ginsburg, Silverman, & Kurtines, 1995b).

Therapists

In research clinics, therapists are provided with a manual, and the importance of adhering to the main features of the treatment as outlined in the manual is emphasized. The fact that most treatment sessions are videotaped and that therapists are aware that a proportion of these tapes will be selected for treatment integrity checks undoubtedly increases therapists' adherence to the main aspects of the manualized therapy. Moreover, in many of the efficacy studies, the therapists are graduate students who typically do not possess excessively strong and long allegiances to a particular type of treatment or theoretical orientation.

Can these qualities of efficacy studies associated with therapists be transported to other settings? The answer would seem to be "yes," or at least, "partly yes." That is, therapists could use manualized treatments that have founded efficacy in research clinics. As with the interview schedules, adhering to a manual does not mean that therapists must use it as a script. It also does not mean that the only thing that can be discussed in sessions is anxiety. It merely means that the basic features of the intervention are implemented. But precisely when, and even how, they are implemented can be flexible and tailored to meet the particular circumstances of a case. Also likely to be transportable, though to a lesser extent in some settings than in others, would be the conducting of random checks on clinicians' adherence to the manuals, if this is thought to be necessary.

So why the "partly yes"? Because the main challenge in transporting evidence-based treatments to practitioners in other settings would seem not to be tangible things, such as the adopting of treatment manuals, having random spot checks, and so forth; rather, the challenge is something that is far less tangible and more difficult to change — it is a matter of attitude.

Why attitude? Because one can reasonably speculate that it is this that largely holds back the adoption of evidence-based treatments. In particular, many mental health professionals, when called on to make decisions about the treatment of childhood problems, including anxiety, likely fall into a pattern of routinely relying on a particular treatment method. Relying on a particular method — perhaps the one with which one has become most familiar or the one that is most consistent with one's theoretical approach — is a strategy that may work well in many or most of the contexts in which one needs to make decisions. The problem that arises from this strategy, however, is that sometimes these assumptions about treatment get in the way of choosing and using other treatments — treatments that might be more evidence based. When this occurs, we may no longer be providing optimal care to children and their families.

What can be done about this? It would seem important not to let one's assumptions get in the way of choosing and using treatments. This would require a reorientation of the ways many clinicians have been trained to think, particularly when it comes to helping children. That is, it would require that clinicians suspend their assumptions and judgments and adopt an attitude that is problem solving or, as mentioned earlier in the chapter, that is pragmatic (Silverman & Kurtines, 1996a).

Disseminating such information as that contained in this volume is an important step toward introducing mental health professionals to a variety of evidence-based interventions for youth. Hopefully, this chapter also serves toward reorienting clinicians with respect to how they think about helping children and adolescents who suffer from anxiety disorders.

NOTES

1. All of these disorders can be treated using the "basic" intervention described in this chapter. However, each disorder has its own set of particular issues that need to be considered in treatment, such as the use of additional therapeutic strategies (e.g., possible medication when treating obsessive-compulsive disorders). It is beyond the scope of this chapter to consider all the various issues that arise in working with each particular anxiety disorder.

2. Interestingly, two recently completed clinical trials (Last, Hansen, & Franco, 1998; Silverman, Kurtines, Ginsburg, Weems, Rabian, & Serafini, in press) showed that "school phobia" and other phobic disorders could be reduced by an education support condition, which did not involve the type of detailed therapists' prescriptions for exposures, as described in this chapter. Further research is needed to examine the robustness of these findings, including their generalizability to other anxiety disorders in children, as well as to examine the possibility that children and families engaged in self-directed exposures during the course of receiving education support.

REFERENCES

American Psychiatric Association. (1994). *Diagnostic and statistical manual of mental disorders* (4th ed.). Washington, DC: Author.

Anderson, J. C., Williams, S., McGee, R., & Silva, P. A. (1987). *DSM-III* disorders in preadolescent children. *Archives of General Psychiatry, 44,* 69–76.

Bandura, A. (1977). Self-efficacy: Towards a unifying theory of behavioral change. *Psychological Review, 84,* 191–215.

Barlow, D. H. (1988). *Anxiety and its disorders: The nature and treatment of anxiety and panic.* New York: Guilford Press.

Barlow, D. H. (1994). Psychological interventions in the era of managed competition. *Clinical Psychology: Science and Practice, 1,* 109–122.

Barrett, P. M. (1998). Evaluation of cognitive-behavioral group treatment for childhood anxiety disorders. *Journal of Clinical Child Psychology, 27,* 459–468.

Barrett, P. M., Dadds, M. R., & Rapee, R. M. (1996). Family treatment of childhood anxiety: A controlled trial. *Journal of Consulting and Clinical Psychology, 64,* 333–342.

Beidel, D. C., & Turner, S. M. (1988). Comorbidity of test anxiety and other anxiety disorders in children. *Journal of Abnormal Child Psychology, 16,* 275–287.

Bell-Dolan, D., & Wessler, A. E. (1994). Attributional style of anxious children: Extensions from cognitive theory and research on adult anxiety. *Journal of Anxiety Disorders, 8,* 79–97.

Bird, H. R., Canino, G., Rubin-Stipec, M., Gould, M., Ribera, J., Sesman, M., Woodbury, M., Huertas-Goldman, S., Pagen, A., Sanchez-Lacay, A., & Moscoso, M. (1988). Estimates of the prevalence of childhood maladjustment in a community survey in Puerto Rico. *Archives of General Psychiatry, 45,* 1120–1126.

Chiodos, J., & Maddux, J. E. (1985). A cognitive and behavioral approach to anxiety management of retarded individuals: Two case studies. *Journal of Child and Adolescent Psychotherapy, 2,* 16–20.

Chorpita, B. F., Albano, A. M., & Barlow, D. H. (1996). Cognitive processing in children: Relationship to anxiety and family influences. *Journal of Clinical Child Psychology, 25,* 170–176.

Cobham, V. E., Dadds, M. R., & Spence, S. H. (1998). The role of parental anxiety in the treatment of childhood anxiety. *Journal of Consulting and Clinical Psychology, 66,* 893–905.

Cohen, P., Cohen, J., & Brook, J. S. (1993). An epidemiological study of disorders in late childhood and adolescence: II. Persistence of disorders. *Journal of Child Psychology and Psychiatry, 34,* 867–875.

Costello, E. J., & Angold, A. (1995). Epidemiology. In J. S. March (Ed.), *Anxiety disorders in children and adolescents* (pp. 109–122). New York: Guilford Press.

Dadds, M. R., Barrett, P. M., Rapee, R. M., & Ryan, S. (1996). Family process and child anxiety and aggression: An observational analysis. *Journal of Abnormal Child Psychology, 24,* 715–734.

Dadds, M. R., Spence, S. H., Holland, D. E., Barrett, P. M., & Laurens, K. R. (1997). Prevention and early intervention for anxiety disorders: A controlled trial. *Journal of Consulting and Clinical Psychology, 65,* 627–635.

Davey, G. C. L. (1992). Classical conditioning and the acquisition of human fears and phobias: A review and synthesis of the literature. *Advances in Behaviour Research and Therapy, 14,* 29–66.

Eisen, A. R., & Silverman, W. K. (1991). Treatment of an adolescent with bowel movement phobia using self-control therapy. *Journal of Behavior Therapy and Experimental Psychiatry, 22,* 45–51.

Eisen, A. R., & Silverman, W. K. (1998). Prescriptive treatment for generalized anxiety disorder in children. *Behavior Therapy, 29,* 105–121.

Eley, T. C. (1999). Behavioral genetics as a tool for developmental psychology: Anxiety and depression in children and adolescents. *Clinical Child and Family Psychology Review, 2,* 21–36.

Eysenck, H. J. (1979). The conditioning model of neurosis. *Behavioral and Brain Sciences, 2,* 155–199.

Flannery-Schroeder, E., & Kendall, P. C. (2000). Group and individual cognitive behavioral treatment for youth with anxiety disorders: A randomized clinical trial. *Cognitive Therapy and Research, 24,* 327–344.

Fyer, A. J., Mannuzza, S., Gallops, M. P., Martin, L. Y., Aaronson, C., Gorman, J. M., Liebowitz, M. R., & Klein, D. F. (1990). Familial transmission of simple phobias and fears. *Archives of General Psychiatry, 47,* 252–256.

Ginsburg, G. S., & Silverman, W. K. (1996). Phobic and anxiety disorders in Hispanic and Caucasian youth. *Journal of Anxiety Disorders, 10,* 517–528.

Ginsburg, G. S., Silverman, W. K. & Kurtines, W. M. (1995a). Family involvement in treating children with phobic and anxiety disorders: A look ahead. *Clinical Psychology Review, 15,* 457–473.

Ginsburg, G. S., Silverman, W. K., & Kurtines, W. M. (1995b). Cognitive-behavioral group therapy. In A. R. Eisen,

C. A. Kearney, & C. E. Schaefer (Eds.), *Clinical handbook of anxiety disorders in children* (pp. 521–549). Northvale, NJ: Jason Aronson.

Kagan, J. (1989). Temperamental contributions to social behavior. *American Psychologist, 44,* 668–674.

Kagan, J., Reznick, J. S., & Snidman, N. (1987). The physiology and psychology of behavioral inhibition. *Child Development, 58,* 1459–1473.

Kane, M. T., & Kendall, P. C. (1989). Anxiety disorders in children: A multiple baseline evaluation of a cognitive behavioral treatment. *Behavior Therapy, 20,* 499–508.

Kashani, J. H., Vaidya, A. F., Soltys, S. M., Dandoy, A. C., Katz, L. M., & Reid, J. C. (1990). Correlates of anxiety in psychiatrically hospitalized children and their parents. *Journal of Psychiatry, 143,* 319–323.

Kendall, P. C. (1994). Treating anxiety disorders in children: Results of a randomized clinical trial. *Journal of Consulting and Clinical Psychology, 62,* 100–110.

Kendall, P. C., & Chansky, T. E. (1991). Considering cognition in anxiety-disordered children. *Journal of Anxiety Disorders, 5,* 167–185.

Kendall, P. C., Flannery-Schroeder, E., Panichelli-Mindel, S. M., Southam-Gerow, M., Henin, A., & Warman, M. (1997). Therapy for youths with anxiety disorders: A second randomized clinical trial. *Journal of Consulting and Clinical Psychology, 65,* 366–380.

Kendall, P. C., Kortlander, E., Chansky, T. E., & Brady, E. U. (1992). Comorbidity of anxiety and depression in youth: Treatment implications. *Journal of Consulting and Clinical Psychology, 60,* 869–880.

Kessler, R. C., McGonagle, K. A., Zhao, S., Nelson, C. B., Hughes, M., Eshleman, S., Wittchen, H. U., & Kendler, K. S. (1994). Lifetime and 12-month prevalence of *DSM-III-R* psychiatric disorders in the United States. *Archives of General Psychiatry, 51,* 8–19.

Krohine, H. W., & Hock, M. (1991). Relationships between restrictive mother-child interactions and anxiety of the child. *Anxiety Research, 4,* 109–124.

Last, C. G., Hansen, C., & Franco, N. (1997). Anxious children in adulthood: A prospective study of adjustment. *Journal of the American Academy of Child and Adolescent Psychiatry, 36,* 645–652.

Last, C. G., Hansen, C., & Franco, N. (1998). Cognitive-behavioral treatment of school phobia. *Journal of the American Academy of Child and Adolescent Psychiatry, 37,* 404–411.

Last, C. G., Hersen, M., Kazdin, A. E., Francis, G., & Grubb, H. J. (1987). Psychiatric illness in the mothers of anxious children. *American Journal of Psychiatry, 144,* 1580–1583.

Last, C. G., Hersen, M., Kazdin, A. E., Orvaschel, H., & Perrin, S. (1991). Anxiety disorders in children and their families. *Archives of General Psychiatry, 48,* 928–934.

Last, C. G., & Perrin, S. (1993). Anxiety disorders in African-American and white children. *Journal of Abnormal Child Psychology, 2,* 153–164.

Last, C. G., Perrin, S., Hersen, M., & Kazdin, A. E. (1996). A prospective study of childhood anxiety disorders. *Journal of the American Academy of Child and Adolescent Psychiatry, 35,* 1502–1510.

McGee, R., Feehan, M., Williams, S., & Anderson, J. (1992). *DSM-III* disorders from age 11 to age 15 years. *Journal of the American Academy of Child and Adolescent Psychiatry, 31,* 50–59.

Menzies, R. G., & Clarke, J. C. (1995). The etiology of phobias: A nonassociative account. *Clinical Psychology Review, 15,* 23–48.

Messer, S. C., & Beidel, D. C. (1994). Psychosocial correlates of childhood anxiety disorders. *Journal of the American Academy of Child and Adolescent Psychiatry, 33,* 975–983.

Mowrer, O. H. (1939). A stimulus-response theory of anxiety and its role as reinforcing agent. *Psychological Review, 46,* 553–565.

Ollendick, T. H. (1983). Reliability and validity of the revised Fear Survey Schedule for Children (FSSC-R). *Behaviour Research and Therapy, 21,* 685–692.

Ollendick, T. H. (1995). Cognitive behavioral treatment of panic disorder with agoraphobia in adolescents: A multiple baseline design analysis. *Behavior Therapy, 26,* 517–531.

Ollendick, T. H., & King, N. J. (1991). Origins of childhood fears: An evaluation of Rachman's theory of fear acquisition. *Behaviour Research and Therapy, 29,* 117–123.

Ost, L. G. (1985). Ways of acquiring phobias and outcome of behavioral treatments. *Behaviour Research and Therapy, 23,* 683–689.

Rachman, S. (1977). The conditioning therapy of fear acquisition: A critical examination. *Behaviour Research and Therapy, 15,* 375–387.

Rachman, S. (1978). *Fear and courage.* San Francisco, CA: Freeman.

Rapee, R. M. (1997). Potential role of childrearing practices in the development of anxiety and depression. *Clinical Psychology Review, 17,* 47–67.

Rescorla, R. A. (1988). Pavlovian conditioning: It's not what you think it is. *American Psychologist, 43,* 151–160.

Reynolds, C. R., & Richmond, B. O. (1978). What I think and feel: A revised measure of children's manifest anxiety. *Journal of Abnormal Child Psychology, 6,* 271–280.

Rosenbaum, J. F., Biederman, J., Gersten, M., Hirshfeld, D. R., Meminger, S. R., Herman, J. B., Kagan, J., Reznick, J. S., & Snidman, N. (1988). Behavioral inhibition in children of parents with panic disorder and agoraphobia: A controlled study. *Archives of General Psychiatry, 45,* 463–470.

Sarason, S. B., Davidson, K. S., Lighthall, F. F., Waite, R. R., & Ruebush, B. K. (1960). *Anxiety in elementary school children.* New York: Wiley.

Seligman, M. E. P. (1971). Phobias and preparedness. *Behavior Therapy, 2,* 307–320.

Silverman, W. K. (1991). Persons' description of psychotherapy outcome studies does not accurately represent psychotherapy outcome studies. *American Psychologist, 46,* 1351–1352.

Silverman, W. K., & Albano, A. M. (1996). *The Anxiety Disorders Interview Schedule for Children-IV (Child and Parent Versions).* San Antonio, TX: Psychological Corporation.

Silverman, W. K., Cerny, J. A., Nelles, W. B., & Burke, A. E. (1988). Behavior problems in children of parents with anxiety disorders. *Journal of the American Academy of Child and Adolescent Psychiatry, 27,* 779–784.

Silverman, W. K., & Ginsburg, G. S. (1998). Anxiety disorders. In T. H. Ollendick & M. Hersen (Eds.), *Handbook of child psychopathology* (3rd ed., pp. 239–268). New York: Plenum Press.

Silverman, W. K., Ginsburg, G. S., & Kurtines, W. M. (1995). Clinical issues in the treatment of children with anxiety and phobic disorders. *Cognitive and Behavioral Practice, 2,* 93–117.

Silverman, W. K., & Kurtines, W. M. (1996a). *Anxiety and phobic disorders: A pragmatic approach.* New York: Plenum Press.

Silverman, W. K., & Kurtines, W. M. (1996b). Transfer of control: A psychosocial intervention model for internalizing disorders in youth. In E. D. Hibbs & P. S. Jensen (Eds.), *Psychosocial treatment of child and adolescent disorders: Empirically based strategies for clinical practice* (pp. 63–82). Washington, DC: American Psychological Association.

Silverman, W. K., & Kurtines, W. M. (1997). Theory in child psychosocial treatment research: Have it or had it? A pragmatic alternative. *Journal of Abnormal Child Psychology, 25,* 359–367.

Silverman, W. K., Kurtines, W. M., Ginsburg, G. S., Weems, C. F., Lumpkin,

P. W., & Carmichael, D. H. (1999). Treating anxiety disorders in children with group cognitive behavior therapy: A randomized clinical trial. *Journal of Consulting and Clinical Psychology, 67,* 995–1003.

Silverman, W. K., Kurtines, W. M., Ginsburg, G. S., Weems, C. F., Rabian, B., & Serafini, L. T. (1999). Contingency management, self control, and education support in the treatment of childhood phobic disorders: A randomized clinical trial. *Journal of Consulting and Clinical Psychology, 67,* 675–687.

Silverman, W. K., & Nelles, W. B. (1988). The Anxiety Disorders Interview Schedule for Children. *Journal of the American Academy of Child and Adolescent Psychiatry, 27,* 772–778.

Silverman, W. K., & Weems, C. F. (1999). Anxiety sensitivity in children. In S. Taylor (Ed.), *Anxiety sensitivity: Theory, research and the treatment of the fear of anxiety.* (pp. 239–268). Mahwah, NJ: Erlbaum.

Solomon, R. T., & Wynne, L. T. (1954). Traumatic avoidance learning: The principles of anxiety conservation and partial irreversibility. *Psychological Review, 61,* 358–385.

Turner, S. M., Beidel, D. C., & Costello, A. (1987). Psychopathology in the offspring of anxiety disorders patients. *Journal of Consulting and Clinical Psychology, 55,* 229–235.

Vasey, M. W., Daleiden, E. L., Williams, L. L., & Brown, L. (1995). Biased attention in childhood anxiety disorders: A preliminary study. *Journal of Abnormal Child Psychology, 23,* 267–279.

Weems, C. F., Berman, S. L., Silverman, W. K., & Saavedra, L. S. (in press). Cognitive errors in youth with anxiety disorders: The linkages between negative cognitive errors and anxious symptoms. *Cognitive Therapy and Research.*

Weems, C. F., Silverman, W. K., Saavedra, L. S., Pina, A. A., & Lumpkin, P. W. (1999). The discrimination of children's phobias using the Revised Fear Survey for Children. *Journal of Child Psychology and Psychiatry and Allied Disciplines, 40,* 941–952.

Weiss, B., Catron, T., Harris, V., & Phung, T. M. (1999). The effectiveness of traditional child psychotherapy. *Journal of Consulting and Clinical Psychology, 67,* 82–94.

Weissman, M. M., Leckman, J. F., Merikangas, K. R., Gammon, G. D., & Prusoff, B. A. (1984). Depression and anxiety disorders in parents and children. *Archives of General Psychiatry, 41,* 845–852.

Weisz, J. R., Donenberg, G. R., Han, S. S., & Weiss, B. (1995). Bridging the gap between lab and clinic in child and adolescent psychotherapy. *Journal of Consulting and Clinical Psychology, 63,* 688–701.

12

ARTHUR D. ANASTOPOULOS
ERIKA E. KLINGER
E. PAIGE TEMPLE

Treating Children and Adolescents with Attention-Deficit/Hyperactivity Disorder

Attention-deficit/hyperactivity disorder (AD/HD; American Psychiatric Association, 1994) is a condition characterized by developmentally inappropriate levels of inattention and/or hyperactivity-impulsivity. Due to its pervasiveness across settings and its chronicity across development, AD/HD is one of the most common reasons why children and adolescents are referred to health care professionals for services. Unfortunately, the type of treatment that a child or adolescent with AD/HD might receive can be highly variable from one professional to the next. Such inconsistencies very often stem from differences in professional training, different levels of experience in working with AD/HD populations, and different beliefs about how child and adolescent psychopathology is conceptualized. Further complicating matters is that many clinicians do not routinely keep up with the research literature and therefore are unaware of which treatments have been empirically validated and which have not.

Given this state of affairs, the purpose of this chapter is to provide a critical review of the various treatments that are available for addressing AD/HD and its associated features. In order to make this review more meaningful, it is first necessary to provide some background information about AD/HD. Thus this chapter begins with a description of its defining features and of the criteria that are currently used to establish an AD/HD diagnosis. This is followed by a discussion of its prevalence, its developmental course, its clinical presentation, its impact on psychosocial functioning, and its associated features. Attention is then directed to recently proposed etiological conceptualizations. Against this background, many of the commonly used treatments for AD/HD are reviewed. Throughout this review, every effort is made to help bridge the gap between research and clinical practice. In particular, attention is directed to the many obstacles that practitioners face when providing clinical services to children and adolescents whose life circumstances are dysfunctional or at the very least nonsupportive. By including such a perspective, it is our intent to provide readers with an overview of AD/HD treatments that is not only comprehensive in scope but also practical and clinically useful.

Diagnostic Criteria

Children with AD/HD frequently display symptoms of inattention, including not listening to directions, not finishing assigned work, daydreaming, becoming bored easily, and so on. Common to all these referral concerns is a diminished capacity for vigilance; that is, difficulties sustaining attention to task (Douglas, 1983). Children with AD/HD may also exhibit impulsivity. This may be evident in terms of interrupting others, not being able to wait for their turn in game situations, beginning tasks before directions are completed, taking unnecessary risks, talking out of turn, or making indiscreet remarks without regard for social consequences. When hyperactivity is present, it is most often displayed through physical activity, but it can sometimes be expressed through verbalizations as well. In extreme cases, children who are hyperactive may appear to be in constant motion, unable to sit still, and so forth. Although most people think of hyperactivity in this way, it can also present itself in less severe forms, such as fidgeting when seated or talking excessively.

The currently accepted criteria for making an AD/HD diagnosis appear in the fourth edition of the *Diagnostic and Statistical Manual of Mental Disorders* (*DSM-IV*; American Psychiatric Association, 1994). At the heart of this decision-making process are two nine-item symptom listings — one pertaining to inattention symptoms, the other to hyperactivity-impulsivity concerns. Parents or teachers must report the presence of at least six of nine problem behaviors from either list to warrant consideration of an AD/HD diagnosis. Such behaviors must have an onset prior to 7 years of age, a duration of at least six months, and a frequency above and beyond that expected of children of the same mental age. Furthermore, they must be evident in two or more settings, have a clear impact on psychosocial functioning, and not be due to other types of mental health or learning disorders that might better explain their presence.

As is evident from these criteria, the manner in which AD/HD presents itself clinically can vary from child to child. For some children with AD/HD, symptoms of inattention may be of relatively greater concern than impulsivity or hyperactivity problems. For others, impulsivity and hyperactivity difficulties may be more prominent. Reflecting these possible differences in clinical presentation, the new *DSM-IV* criteria not only allow for but require, AD/HD subtyping. For example, when more than six symptoms are present from both lists and all other criteria are met, a diagnosis of AD/HD, Combined Type, is in order. If six or more inattention symptoms are present but fewer than six hyperactive-impulsive symptoms are evident, and all other criteria are met, the proper diagnosis would be AD/HD, Predominantly Inattentive Type. Those familiar with prior diagnostic classification schemes will quickly recognize these *DSM-IV* categories as similar but not exact counterparts to what previously was known as Attention-Deficit/Hyperactivity Disorder and Undifferentiated Attention Deficit Disorder in *DSM-III-R* (American Psychiatric Association, 1987) and Attention Deficit Disorder with or without Hyperactivity in *DSM-III* (American Psychiatric Association, 1980). Appearing for the first time in *DSM-IV*, however, is the subtyping condition known as AD/HD, Predominantly Hyperactive-Impulsive Type, which is the appropriate diagnosis whenever six or more hyperactive-impulsive symptoms arise, fewer than six inattention concerns are evident, and all other criteria are met. Along with these major subtyping categories, *DSM-IV* also makes available two additional classifications that have primary bearing on adolescents and adults. For example, a diagnosis of AD/HD, In Partial Remission, may be given to individuals who have clinical problems resulting from AD/HD symptoms that currently do not meet criteria for any of the above subtypes but nonetheless were part of a documented AD/HD diagnosis at an earlier point in time. In similar cases in which an earlier history of AD/HD cannot be established with any degree of certainty, a diagnosis of AD/HD, Not Otherwise Specified, would instead be made.

Prevalence

According to the *DSM-IV* itself, the overall prevalence of AD/HD among children — that is, the sum total of all subtyping categories — is 3–5% (APA, 1994). Higher global estimates have been reported for community samples, ranging from 7.5% to 21.6% for both parent- and teacher-generated samples (Baumgaertel, Wolraich, & Dietrich, 1995; DuPaul, Anastopoulos, et al., 1998; Gaub & Carlson, 1997). That these would be higher than the 3–5% prevalence described in *DSM-IV* is not at all surprising, given that the community rates were derived primarily on the basis of the AD/HD symptom frequency requirement alone. Thus such estimates very likely represent upper limits on the true prevalence of AD/HD within the general population.

Among clinic samples, the Combined type would appear to be the most commonly encountered subtype category (Lahey et al., 1994), whereas the Inattentive type occurs most often in community samples (DuPaul, Power, et al., 1997). According to teachers, younger children display the Combined subtype most often, whereas older children and adolescents are much more likely to be identified with the Inattentive classification. Similar findings have emerged from parent ratings of older children and adolescents, but parents are much more likely to identify very young children as having the Hyperactive-Impulsive subtype (DuPaul, Anastopoulos et al., 1998). Of additional interest is that the overall prevalence of *DSM-IV*-defined AD/HD — that is, the total for all three major subtypes — seems to decline with age. In terms of gender issues, boys outnumber girls across all subtypes, with ratios ranging from 1.3 : 1 to 3.3 : 1, depending on the informant and subtype under consideration (APA, 1994). Because mixed results have emerged with respect to the moderating influence of ethnicity, few conclusions can be drawn about this matter. Likewise, not much can be said about the impact of socioeconomic factors, due to the dearth of research on this topic.

Onset and Developmental Course

Most individuals with AD/HD begin to display their symptoms in early childhood, with hyperactive-impulsive difficulties typically preceding inattention (Green, Loeber, & Lahey, 1991). Most often such symptoms appear around 3 to 4 years of age, but they can also surface during infancy or on school entrance (McGee, Williams, & Feehan, 1992). The question of whether or not AD/HD symptoms can have onset after 7 years of age is a matter now being debated (Barkley & Biederman, 1997). In trying to clarify this issue, future researchers must clearly define symptom onset, recognizing that there may be an important distinction between the time when symptoms first appear versus when they begin to cause clinically significant impairment.

Upon reaching late childhood and early adolescence, many children with AD/HD begin to display significantly fewer hyperactive-impulsive symptoms (Hart, Lahey, Loeber, Applegate, & Frick, 1995). Some may also show a reduction in their overall level of inattention, but to a much lesser degree. Little is known about the course that AD/HD symptoms follow from adolescence into adulthood. Potentially complicating this situation is that childhood estimates are based on parent and teacher reports, whereas adult estimates stem from self-report. What evidence is available suggests that adults display fewer AD/HD symptoms than do children or adolescents (Shaffer, 1994). Moreover, the overall frequency of AD/HD symptoms seems to decline gradually across adulthood (Murphy & Barkley, 1996). Unlike what has been observed in children and adolescents, such declines are evident for both hyperactive-impulsive and inattention symptoms.

Clinical Presentation

Developmental Considerations

The exact manner in which AD/HD is expressed can vary a great deal, in part as a function of the child's age. Descriptions of inattention during infancy typically involve such comments as, "He could never entertain himself . . . somebody always had to be there keeping him busy." According to one mother, her infant daughter had on many occasions impulsively jumped out of her crib in a daredevil fashion, long before she even knew how to walk. Another distressed parent once lamented that "all hell broke loose" when her hyperactive infant son learned how to walk, because he was into everything, and he required constant monitoring.

One of the most frequently mentioned ways in which toddlers might exhibit inattentiveness is through their inability to watch more than a few minutes of a television program or videotape, even when it is of some interest. When something desirable captures a toddler's attention, he or she may impulsively go after it with little regard for what might be in the way, many times leading to injuries from bumping into tables, chairs, or other objects. Hyperactive toddlers have also been known to climb on top of dressers, tables, and kitchen counters.

Preschoolers with AD/HD very often display inattentiveness through their excessive shifting from one activity center to another in day care or preschool settings.

Preschoolers with AD/HD are also prone to take a toy away from another child, not so much from a desire to be aggressive or hurtful but more from being unable to wait for the other child to finish using it. Hyperactivity problems may also be evident in day care or preschool settings, where young children with AD/HD very often cannot sit in a circle for very long, lie down on a mat for the duration of rest time, or refrain from running when asked to walk in line.

Entrance into kindergarten and the early elementary grades typically brings with it a variety of new demands for self-regulation, thereby greatly increasing the number of opportunities in which AD/HD symptoms can occur. For a child with AD/HD, this might mean doing tasks incorrectly because of not listening to teacher instructions or forgetting to bring teacher notes home. Elementary school-aged children with AD/HD may also cut in front of other children in line, begin tasks before directions are completed, make careless mistakes, or interrupt a parent who is on the phone or otherwise busy. Walking slowly in line and remaining seated at a desk or at the dinner table can also pose major challenges during this developmental period.

During adolescence, many students with AD/HD have a great deal of difficulty remembering to bring books home or turning in homework assignments. Other inattention problems include forgetting to show up for work and getting into automobile accidents (Barkley, Guevremont, Anastopoulos, DuPaul, & Shelton, 1993). Teens with AD/HD may also fail to think through the consequences of their actions, resulting in sexual indiscretions and reckless experimentation with alcohol or illicit drugs (Mannuzza, Klein, Bessler, Malloy, & LaPadula, 1993). When hyperactivity symptoms are present, they typically appear in the form of restless leg movements, finger tapping, or incessant talking. Even when there are no outward signs of overactivity, some teens may still experience subjective feelings of restlessness, often described in terms of racing thoughts.

Situational Variability

Contrary to the belief of many individuals, AD/HD is not an all-or-none phenomenon, either always present or never present. Instead, it is a condition whose primary symptoms show significant fluctuations in response to different situational demands (Zentall, 1985). AD/HD symptoms are much more likely to occur in situations that are highly repetitive, boring, or familiar than in those that are novel or stimulating (Barkley, 1977). Significant AD/HD problems are also much more likely to arise when others place demands or set rules for behavior than in free-play situations (Luk, 1985). Group settings pose far more problems for children with AD/HD than would be the case in one-to-one situations. There is also an increased likelihood for AD/HD symptoms to arise in situations in which feedback is dispensed infrequently, on a delayed basis, or both (Douglas, 1983).

In view of this tendency for AD/HD symptoms to be subject to situational variability, it should come as no great surprise that children with AD/HD often display tremendous inconsistency in their task performance, both in terms of their productivity and their accuracy (Douglas, 1972). Although it may be argued that all children display a certain amount of variability in these areas, it is clear from clinical experience and research findings that children with AD/HD exhibit this to a much greater degree. Thus, instead of reflecting "laziness" as some might contend, the inconsistent performance of children with AD/HD may represent yet another manifestation of this disorder.

Psychosocial Impact and Comorbidity

Having AD/HD places individuals at risk for a multitude of psychosocial difficulties across the life span. The exact nature of these complications is determined in large part by a consideration of what is considered typical or normal at any given stage of development. Preschoolers with AD/HD place enormous caretaking demands on their parents and frequently display aggressive behavior when interacting with siblings or peers (Campbell, 1990, 1995). Difficulties acquiring academic readiness skills may be evident as well (McIntosh & Cole-Love, 1996), but these tend to be of less clinical concern than the family or peer problems that preschoolers present. As children with AD/HD move into the elementary school years, academic problems take on increasing importance (DuPaul & Stoner, 1994). Together with their ongoing family and peer relationship problems (Cunningham & Siegel, 1987), such school-based difficulties set the stage for the development of low self-esteem and other emotional concerns. Similar problems persist into adolescence but on a much more intense level (Klein & Mannuzza, 1991). New problems may develop as well (e.g., traffic violations, experimentation with alcohol and drugs), stemming from the increased demands for independence, self-regulation, and self-control that teenagers with AD/HD face (Barkley et al., 1990). AD/HD can also make the transition into adulthood very difficult. Particularly noteworthy in this regard are the obstacles that AD/HD imposes on adults in their efforts to establish and maintain a family or career.

In addition to being affected by its primary symptoms, individuals with AD/HD are at increased risk for having secondary or comorbid diagnoses. Preschoolers with AD/HD frequently display oppositional defiant disorder (ODD; Barkley, 1998). Oppositional-defiant disorder is also quite common among elementary school-aged children with AD/HD, as are secondary mood and anxiety disorders (August, Realmuto, MacDonald, Nugent, & Crosby, 1996). Among adolescents with AD/HD, conduct disorder is quite common (Barkley, Anastopoulos, Guevremont, & Fletcher, 1991). Antisocial personality disorder, major depression, and substance abuse are just a few of the many comorbid problems that may be found among older adolescents and young adults with AD/HD (Milberger et al., 1997). In combination with AD/HD, such comorbid conditions very often increase the severity of an individual's overall psychosocial impairment, thereby making the prognosis for such individuals less favorable.

Theoretical Considerations

Despite widespread interest in the topic, relatively little research has actually addressed the question of what might cause AD/HD. Among the small number of studies that have examined this matter, inconsistent findings have emerged, presumably due to cross-study differences in defining AD/HD samples, small sample sizes, and other methodological limitations. As a result of such circumstances, what we know about the etiology of AD/HD might best be described as theoretical rather than factual.

Biological Conceptualizations

Several lines of evidence point toward biological factors being involved. In particular, research has suggested that abnormalities in brain chemistry (e.g., dopamine, norepinephrine), structure (e.g., caudate nucleus, prefrontostriatal areas), function (e.g., diminished prefrontal glucose metabolism), or all of these may play an important role (Arnsten, Steere, & Hunt, 1996; Castellanos et al., 1996; Levy, Hay, McStephen, Wood, & Waldman, 1997; Pliszka, McCracken, & Maas, 1996; Zametkin et al., 1990). Multiple pathways presumably lead to these abnormalities. Among these, hereditary mechanisms (Gilger, Pennington, & DeFries, 1992; Levy et al., 1997) and certain pregnancy complications, such as excessive maternal consumption of alcohol, nicotine, or both (Milberger, Biederman, Faraone, Chen, & Jones, 1996; Streissguth, Bookstein, Sampson, & Barr, 1995), very likely account for the largest percentage of children who have AD/HD. For some children, AD/HD may be acquired after birth, resulting from head injury (Heilman & Valenstein, 1979), elevated lead levels (Gittelman & Eskinazi, 1983), and other biological complications. Despite their widespread public appeal, there is little support for the assertions of Feingold (1975) and others that the ingestion of sugar or other food substances directly causes AD/HD (Wolraich, Wilson, & White, 1995).

Although the exact manner in which these biological pieces fit together is far from clear, recent findings have offered some interesting leads. Particularly promising is the possibility that recently identified dopamine gene defects (Cook et al., 1995) may be a precursor to the dopamine deficiencies that have been reported in the neurochemical literature (Pliszka et al., 1996). These deficiencies in turn may be linked to some of the structural and functional abnormalities that have been observed, particularly in the frontostriatal region (Castellanos et al., 1996), where dopamine systems are known to be at work.

Psychological Conceptualizations

Building on what is now known about the biology of AD/HD, more recent theories have taken on a very distinctive neuropsychological flavor, emphasizing the impulsivity features of this disorder. Quay (1997), for example, has proposed that AD/HD stems from an impairment in a neurologically based behavioral inhibition system. In an extensive elaboration of this same theme, Barkley (1997) has also contended that a deficit in behavioral inhibition is central to understanding the cognitive, behavioral, and social deficits observed within AD/HD populations. Many others in the field share the view that deficits in behavioral inhibition lie at the core of many AD/HD problems (Schachar, Tannock, & Logan, 1993; Sergeant, 1995).

Psychosocial Conceptualizations

Although a few environmental theories have been proposed to explain AD/HD (Block, 1977; Jacobvitz & Sroufe, 1987; Willis & Lovaas, 1977), there is little empirical justification for claiming that poor parenting, chaotic home environments, or poverty cause AD/HD. The results of twin studies in particular have highlighted this limited role by showing that less than 5% of the variance in AD/HD symptomatology can be accounted for by environmental factors (Levy et al., 1997; Sherman, McGue, & Iacono, 1997; Silberg et al., 1996).

Treatment Approaches

What should be readily apparent from the preceding discussion is that many factors, both clinical and theoretical, need to be taken into account when providing treatment services to children and adolescents with AD/HD. Foremost among these are the cross-situational pervasiveness of primary AD/HD symptoms and the relatively high incidence of co-occurring or comorbid conditions. Such circumstances make it highly unlikely that any singular treatment approach can satisfactorily meet all of the clinical management needs of children with AD/HD. For this reason, clinicians must often employ multiple treatment strategies in combination, each of which addresses a different aspect of the child's psychosocial difficulties.

Among those treatments that have received adequate, or at the very least preliminary, empirical support are pharmacotherapy, parent training/counseling, classroom applications of contingency management techniques, and cognitive-behavioral training (Pelham, Wheeler, & Chronis, 1998). Despite such support, these interventions should not be viewed as curative of AD/HD. Instead, their value lies in their temporary reduction of AD/HD symptom levels and in their reduction of related behavioral or emotional difficulties. When these treatments are removed, AD/HD symptoms very often return to pretreatment levels of deviance. Thus their effectiveness in improving prognosis presumably rests on their being maintained over long periods of time.

Pharmacotherapy

For many years clinicians and researchers have employed medications in their management of children with AD/HD. The rationale for doing so rests on the assumption that neurochemical imbalances are involved in the etiology of this disorder. Although the exact neurochemical mechanisms that underlie their therapeutic action remain unclear, research has shown that at least two classes of medication — namely, stimulants and antidepressants — can be helpful in reducing AD/HD symptomatology.

Numerous studies have consistently demonstrated that stimulant medications are highly effective in the management of AD/HD symptoms in a large percentage of the children and adolescents who take them (Greenhill, Halperin, & Abikoff, 1999). According to some estimates, as many as 80–90% will respond favorably, with a majority of these displaying behavior that is relatively normalized (Rapport,

Denney, DuPaul, & Gardner, 1994). Somewhat lower response rates have been reported for preschoolers. In addition to bringing about improvements in primary AD/HD symptomatology, these medications very often can lead to increased child compliance and decreased aggressive behavior (Hinshaw, Henker, & Whalen, 1984). Although certain side effects can arise from their use (e.g., decreased appetite), these tend to be mild in nature, and most children tolerate them without great difficulty, even over extended periods of time (Zeiner, 1995). For reasons such as these, many child health care professionals have incorporated stimulant regimens into their clinical practices.

Historically, Ritalin, Dexedrine, and Cylert have been the most commonly prescribed stimulants. Of these, Ritalin has most often been the medication of choice. In its standard form, Ritalin acts rapidly, producing effects on behavior within 30 to 45 minutes after oral ingestion and peaking in its therapeutic impact within 2 to 4 hours. Its utility in managing behavior, however, typically dissipates within 3 to 7 hours, even though minuscule amounts of the medication may remain in the blood for up to 24 hours (Cantwell & Carlson, 1978). More often than not, it is prescribed in twice-daily doses, but recent research has suggested that adding a third dose to the daily regimen can be tolerated fairly well by most children. Although many children take this medication exclusively on school days, it can also be used on weekends and during school vacations, especially in cases in which AD/HD symptoms seriously interfere with home functioning.

A major disadvantage of using Ritalin in its standard form is that it must be administered several times over the course of a day. Although a sustained-release version of Ritalin has been available for many years, its use has not been adopted widely, primarily due to concerns about its failure to deliver therapeutic benefits for a full six- to eight-hour duration, as intended. Partially in response to this situation, a new stimulant medication, Adderall, was recently put on the market. Preliminary research findings have suggested that Adderall delivers therapeutic benefits evenly over the course of its six- to eight-hour duration (Swanson et al., 1998). An additional advantage to using this medication is that it comes in a variety of doses, thereby allowing physicians the opportunity to tailor medication regimens more precisely to the needs of individual children and adolescents.

Despite their overall utility, stimulants may not be appropriate for some children with AD/HD, who nevertheless require a medication component in their overall clinical management. As a way of meeting the needs of such children, child health care professionals have recently turned to the use of tricyclic antidepressants, such as imipramine and Wellbutrin. Most often, these medications are employed in situations in which certain side effects (e.g., motor tics), known to be exacerbated by stimulants, are present or in which significant mood disturbances accompany AD/HD symptomatology (Pliszka, 1987). As a rule, antidepressants are given twice daily, usually in the morning and evening. Because they are longer acting than stimulants, it takes more time to evaluate the therapeutic value of any given dose (Rapoport & Mikkelsen, 1978). Despite this limitation, recent research has suggested that low doses of these medications can produce increased vigilance and decreased impulsivity, as well as reductions in disruptive and aggressive behavior. Mood elevation may also occur, especially in children with significant pretreatment levels of depression or anxiety (Pliszka, 1987). Such treatment effects, however, can diminish over time. Thus antidepressants frequently are not the medication of choice for long-term management of AD/HD.

Parent Training

As was discussed earlier, AD/HD is now conceptualized as a condition characterized by deficiencies in behavioral inhibition (Barkley, 1997; Quay, 1997). Stated somewhat differently, children with AD/HD have difficulty regulating their behavior in response to situational demands. Such "demands" include not only the stimulus properties of the settings in which children function but also the consequences for their behavior. To the extent that these situational parameters can be modified, one might reasonably anticipate corresponding changes in AD/HD symptomatology. Assuming this to be valid, it provides ample justification for utilizing various behavior therapy techniques in the clinical management of children with AD/HD.

Despite the plethora of research on parent training in behavior modification, very few studies have examined the efficacy of this approach with children specifically identified as having AD/HD. What few studies exist can be interpreted with cautious optimism as supporting the use of behavioral parent training with such children (Anastopoulos, Shelton, DuPaul, & Guevremont, 1993; Pelham et al., 1988; Pisterman, McGrath, Firestone, & Goodman, 1989). Most of these interventions involved training parents in general contingency management tactics, such as positive reinforcement, response cost, time out strategies, or all of these. Some, however, combined contingency management training with didactic counseling, aimed at increasing parental knowledge and understanding of AD/HD (Anastopoulos et al., 1993). In addition to producing changes in child behavior, parent training interventions have also led to improvements in various aspects of parental and family functioning, including decreased parenting stress and increased parenting self-esteem (Anastopoulos et al., 1993; Pisterman et al., 1989).

Classroom Modifications

For reasons similar to the rationale that was given for parent training, another clinically appropriate method for treating children and adolescents with AD/HD is through classroom modifications. In comparison with the parent training literature, relatively more research has addressed the use of behavior management methods for children with AD/HD in the classroom. Such studies suggest that the contingent use of positive reinforcement alone can produce immediate, short-term improvements in classroom behavior, productivity, and accuracy (DuPaul & Stoner, 1994). For most children with AD/HD, secondary or tangible reinforcers would seem to be more effective in improving their behavior and academic performance than would teacher attention or other types of social reinforcement (Pfiffner, Rosen, & O'Leary, 1985). The combination of positive reinforcement with various punishment strategies, such as response cost, typically leads to even greater improvements in behavior than either one alone (Pfiffner & O'Leary, 1987).

Despite the promising nature of such findings, many of these reported treatment gains subside when treatment is withdrawn (Barkley, Copeland, & Sivage, 1980). Of additional concern is that these improvements in behavior and performance seldom generalize to settings in which treatment is not in effect. In response to this situation, researchers recently have directed their attention to the development of interventions that have greater potential for generalization. In an elaboration of the preceding behavioral themes, Barkley (1990) noted that children with AD/HD usually respond well to daily report card systems, which involve having teachers rate two or three target behaviors at various times throughout the day and then having parents convert these ratings into tangible reinforcers. Zentall (1985) has also found benefits to altering the properties of educational stimuli presented to children, such as when written instructions are highlighted with color. Recognizing that it is not always possible to make classroom modifications for only one child, DuPaul, Ervin, Hook, and McGoey (1998) recently demonstrated that classwide peer tutoring is an effective, nondisruptive way to bring about academic and behavioral improvements in children with AD/HD.

Cognitive-Behavioral Therapy

Over the past 20 years, clinicians and researchers have employed a large number and variety of cognitive-behavioral interventions with children who manifest AD/HD symptomatology. Included among these are various self-monitoring, self-reinforcement, and self-instructional techniques. Much of the appeal for their clinical application stems from their apparent focus on some of the primary deficits of AD/HD, including impulsivity, poor organizational skills, and difficulties with rules and instructions. Also contributing to their popularity is their presumed potential for enhancing treatment generalization, above and beyond that achieved through more traditional contingency management programs.

Research on self-monitoring has shown that it can improve on-task behavior and academic productivity in some children with AD/HD (Shapiro & Cole, 1994). The combination of self-monitoring and self-reinforcement can also lead to improvements in on-task behavior and academic accuracy, as well as in peer relations (Hinshaw, Henker, & Whalen, 1984). As for self-instructional training, the picture is less clear, with many recent studies (Abikoff & Gittelman, 1985) failing to replicate earlier reported successes (Bornstein & Quevillon, 1976; Meichenbaum & Goodman, 1971).

Readily apparent in these recent studies are several potential limitations. For example, in order to achieve desired treatment effects in the classroom, children with AD/HD must be reinforced for utilizing self-instructional strategies. Hence, contrary to initial expectations, this form of treatment apparently does not free children from control by the social environment. Instead, what it seems to accomplish is to shift such external control to a slightly less direct form. Another limitation is that treatment effects seldom generalize to settings in which self-instructional training is not in effect or to academic tasks that are not specifically part of the training process (Barkley et al., 1980). In this regard, self-instructional training apparently does not, as had been hoped, circumvent the problem of situation

specificity of treatment effects, which has plagued the use of contingency management methods for many years.

Combined Interventions

What should be evident from the preceding discussion is that singular treatment
approaches — whether they be pharmacological, behavioral, or cognitive-behavioral — are not, by themselves, sufficient to meet all of the clinical management
needs of children with AD/HD. In response to this situation, many child health
care professionals have recently begun to employ multiple AD/HD treatments in
combination.

Despite the intuitive appeal of this clinical practice, there presently exists little
empirical justification for utilizing such combinations. Although limited in number,
studies generally have shown that, regardless of which combination is used, the
therapeutic impact of the combined treatment package typically does not exceed
that of either treatment alone. This would certainly seem to be the case when
stimulant medication therapy is combined with classroom contingency management (Gadow, 1985). Similar findings have emerged from studies that have examined the use of stimulant regimens in combination with cognitive-behavioral interventions (Hinshaw et al., 1984). From a somewhat different perspective, there have
been attempts to evaluate, retrospectively, the long-term effects of individualized
multimodality intervention on AD/HD outcome (Satterfield, Satterfield, & Cantwell, 1980). Such multimodal interventions included medication, parent training,
individual counseling, special education, family therapy, and other treatments as
needed by the individual. The obtained results suggested that an individualized
program of combined treatments, when continued over a period of several years,
can produce improvements in the social adjustment of children with AD/HD, in
their rates of antisocial behavior, and in their academic achievement. Similar
prospective multimodal intervention research is currently nearing completion under
the sponsorship of the Child and Adolescent Branch of the National Institute of
Mental Health. Thus, in the not too distant future, additional light will be shed
on this matter.

Adjunctive Procedures

In the preceding sections we discussed numerous treatment strategies that directly
target the needs of children with AD/HD. What was not covered was the manner
in which various comorbid features are typically addressed. When certain types of
comorbid features, such as aggression, are present, very often they too will diminish
in frequency and severity when targeted AD/HD symptoms come under the control
of various interventions. This does not always occur, however. Moreover, there
are numerous occasions when secondary emotional or behavioral features arise
independent of the primary AD/HD diagnosis and therefore are unresponsive to
AD/HD interventions. In situations such as these, it becomes necessary to consider
the use of adjunctive intervention strategies. For example, individual therapy may

be appropriate for children or adolescents to assist them in their adjustment to parental divorce.

Due to the increased incidence of various psychosocial difficulties among the parents of such children, clinicians must sometimes recommend that they too receive therapy services, such as individual or marital counseling. In addition to providing therapeutic benefits for the parents themselves, these adjunctive procedures can produce indirect benefits for their children. For example, when parental distress is reduced, parents very often become better able to implement recommended treatment strategies, such as parent training, on behalf of their child. Although intuitively appealing and sound on the basis of clinical experience, the use of such adjunctive procedures within an AD/HD population has yet to be addressed empirically. Thus this would seem to be a fertile area for further clinically meaningful research.

Integrating and Adapting Interventions in Real World Settings

What should be evident from the preceding discussion is that much progress has been made in the development of treatments for AD/HD. What may not be so readily apparent is the degree to which clinicians have incorporated these findings into their practices. To date, there have been no published reports on how practitioners put together and implement treatment plans for children and adolescents with AD/HD. Thus much of what is known about typical clinical practice might best be described as speculation or conjecture.

Clinical experience would seem to suggest that a surprisingly large number of practitioners are simply not aware of the recent scientific advances that have been made in the treatment of AD/HD. This would certainly help to explain why some children with AD/HD continue to be placed on dietary regimens (e.g., food additive restrictions) for which there is no empirical validation. This would also help to explain why some children and their parents expend a great deal of time, energy, and money pursuing neurobiofeedback training, for which there is, at best, weak empirical justification. Even when using types of treatments for which there is some empirical justification (e.g., medication), some clinicians surprisingly opt for variations of these treatments (e.g., Prozac) that have been shown to work well for populations with other problems but not for children and adolescents with AD/HD.

For those who employ empirically validated approaches, uncertainties remain because of the large gap that seems to exist in bridging research to clinical practice. One factor contributing to this gap is the fact that treatment outcome studies generally assign participants to a certain type of treatment, whereas in real life, parents and children have some choice over the type of treatment they receive. Of additional significance is that most of the AD/HD treatment research that has been conducted to date has examined singular treatment approaches rather than combinations of treatment. In real life, multiple treatments are typically used in combination. Even among those treatment outcome studies that have employed combinations of interventions, little regard has been paid to the timing and sequential ordering of treatments (e.g., starting medication before psychosocial treatment).

Moreover, almost no research has addressed the question of which treatments work best for which children, under what conditions, for which target behaviors, and so forth. Thus the moderating influence of age, gender, socioeconomic status, and cultural diversity, among many other factors, remains unclear.

Given this state of affairs, how do clinicians implement treatment strategies on behalf of children and adolescents with AD/HD? Although there is no "correct" way of doing this, a good starting point is to conduct a comprehensive, multimethod assessment (Barkley, 1998). To the extent that clinicians are able to gather detailed information about a child's performance in school, at home, and with friends, they are in an excellent position to make an accurate determination not only about the presence or absence of AD/HD but also about its severity and cross-situational pervasiveness. Information gleaned from multimethod assessments can also shed much light on the presence and severity of various comorbid features (e.g., oppositional defiant disorder) that have a high probability of accompanying AD/HD. Multimethod assessments also generate important information about the child's family, which affords clinicians an opportunity for assessing a parent's capacity to implement home-based treatment strategies. Taken together, such assessment data make it possible to get a more complete picture not only of the child's diagnostic status but also of the settings in which the child's problems occur and of the factors that serve to exacerbate or maintain them. This information may then be used to put together the child's treatment plan.

What shape should this treatment plan take? Contrary to what is all too often encountered in clinical practice, a "one-size-fits-all" approach (e.g., always treat with medication) cannot and should not be used for treating children and adolescents with AD/HD. Simply stated, what works for one child may not work at all for another. Another factor limiting therapeutic success is a reliance on single treatments. Whether in the form of medication, classroom modifications, or parent training, treatment plans limited to single treatments have little chance of bringing about desired changes in all the areas of a child's life affected by AD/HD and its associated features. Successful intervention, therefore, requires a multimodal approach.

Therein lies the challenge for clinicians, as there are relatively few empirically established guidelines for putting together multimodal interventions. Until such guidelines are available, clinicians would be well advised to consider the following advice: unless there is a compelling reason to do otherwise, start with treatments that might be viewed as conservative in nature (e.g., psychosocial interventions), then gradually introduce treatments thought to be more aggressive (e.g., medications). This is by no means a novel concept, as this is the very same approach that most physicians utilize in their treatment of medical problems. To underscore this point, consider the following example. If a person has a sore shoulder, it is not automatically the case that surgery is recommended. Surgery may be required if an MRI reveals severe damage. However, if no serious damage is evident, then it may be best to allow an injured shoulder to heal through rest or inactivity or to treat it conservatively through the use of physical therapy, anti-inflammatory medication, or both. Only after such treatments have been tried and shown to be ineffective should consideration be given to surgery.

Using this same reasoning, it may be overkill to begin treating mild inattention symptoms in the classroom with stimulant medication when a less invasive approach, such as a daily report card system or other types of classroom modifications, might be just as effective. The needs of children whose AD/HD symptoms are somewhat severe but occur almost exclusively in school might best be met by an initial treatment plan that includes a stimulant medication component combined with classroom modifications. For children who have mild AD/HD symptoms that occur both in school and at home, a combination of classroom modifications and parent training may be all that is necessary. But if a child has severe AD/HD in combination with ODD, is failing at school, is causing extremely high levels of parental stress at home, is having major problems getting along with other children, and constantly verbalizes negative self-statements, a more aggressive treatment approach would be appropriate from the outset. This approach might include, for example, a combination of stimulant medication and classroom modifications for AD/HD symptoms in school, along with parent training to address AD/HD and ODD symptoms that occur at home, individual child therapy to deal with self-esteem issues secondary to the long-standing failure and frustration that many children and adolescents with AD/HD experience, and group social skills training to address peer relationship difficulties.

Regardless of the starting point, it is important to keep in mind that initial treatment plans are just an approximation of what is likely to be in effect at a later point in time. Thus, in a manner not dissimilar to that used in research, clinicians must systematically collect clinical data to test their "hypotheses," which in this case concern the effectiveness of the treatments that they have put into place. Such data then serve as a basis for deciding whether to adjust an ongoing treatment, to add a new treatment to the overall plan, or to remove a treatment whose effectiveness is highly questionable.

An excellent example of how to employ this empirical approach may be found in numerous pharmacotherapy studies. Such investigations typically assess the efficacy of different doses of medications in the context of highly controlled, double-blind, drug-placebo trials, in which objective measures are used to assess not only therapeutic benefits but also potential side effects. Unfortunately, most clinicians who recommend medication as a treatment for AD/HD do not follow this research lead. Instead, what many are inclined to do is to recommend medication with very little systematic assessment of its initial effectiveness or of its sustained effectiveness over time. It is certainly understandable why a clinician might not be able to conduct such a trial in its entirety, due to limited access to placebo preparations and other obstacles. Nevertheless, there remains little justification for not making some attempt to assess a medication's effectiveness. If a clinician cannot access placebos, he or she can still conduct a reasonably objective medication assessment by systematically introducing different doses of the same medication over equal time intervals. To approximate blind conditions in the assessment of school performance, parents can inform teachers that a trial is under way but not inform them of which dose is in effect at any given time. At the end of each dosage interval, relevant clinical data may then be obtained in the form of parent and teacher ratings of the child's behavior and potential side effects. Although not up to the standard of a formal double-blind, drug-placebo trial, data collected in this way can nevertheless provide a relatively objective assessment of a medication's efficacy at the outset of treatment. Once treatment is under way, trials of this sort can also be used periodically (e.g., annually) to help determine whether a child should be taken off medication or perhaps switched to a therapeutically more effective dose.

Although it is intuitively appealing, trying to treat AD/HD in the manner that has been described thus far is not always smooth sailing. Many obstacles can get in the way. One such obstacle is managed health care. Some managed health care plans specifically list AD/HD as one of the conditions for which they do not provide coverage. When AD/HD is accompanied by comorbid conditions for which coverage is allowed, clinicians must make these comorbid conditions the focus of their treatment plans in order to reduce the financial burden on families and to receive reimbursement for their services. An ethical and clinical dilemma arises, however, when there are no comorbid conditions accompanying AD/HD. Some clinicians may be tempted to list a comorbid diagnosis for symptoms that are present but subclinical in nature. Other clinicians may opt for reducing their fees to make it easier for a family to receive services. Still others may not have the luxury of making such a fee adjustment, in which case they are forced to refer the child and his or her family to another practitioner.

Even when coverage is available, many managed health care plans place major restrictions on the number of visits that can occur in a given year or over the course of a lifetime. Not uncommonly, the number of contacts allowed falls far short of what most children with AD/HD require. Once again, this places clinicians in the uncomfortable position of having to decide between drastically reducing their fees in order to continue working with a child and his or her family versus referring them elsewhere for services that are more affordable.

For families with no insurance and very limited financial resources, getting to a clinic to have a child or adolescent treated for AD/HD just may not be feasible. Even if they have the means to transport themselves to such a facility, they very likely may not have the necessary out-of-pocket monies to pay for the overall cost of a long-term clinical management plan. To the extent that highly specialized treatments can be streamlined to reduce their cost or can be delivered in community settings, higher percentages of economically disadvantaged children and adolescents may then have access to such services.

For those families who can get such services for their child or adolescent, additional obstacles may arise. Parents with limited education may have a great deal of difficulty adhering to a child's medication regimen or reading and understanding all of the materials that so often serve as handouts or as between-session homework assignments in parent training programs. Similar comprehension difficulties may occur among parents for whom English is not their primary language. When such situations arise, clinicians must then try to identify family friends or relatives who are willing to provide assistance as translators or interpreters. This, of course, introduces the possibility that something may "get lost in the translation," thereby complicating the treatment process. To address such problems, additional research is needed, focusing on the development of treatment guidelines and handout materials that have appropriate readability levels, as well as alternate forms written in languages other than English.

Dysfunctional home settings pose additional challenges to the treatment process. Not uncommonly, a decision must be made as to the appropriateness of putting a child or adolescent with AD/HD on a stimulant medication regimen, when the clinician knows full well that his or her parent has a history of substance abuse and therefore may abuse what was legally prescribed for their child. Completing 10 sessions of parent training can also be rather costly for families without health insurance. Even when cost is not an issue, many parents are unable to comply with the demands of the program for the very same reasons that they are unable to keep their personal and family lives under satisfactory control. Little research is available to guide such clinical decisions, which instead rest on the intuition and creativity of the practitioner.

Another commonly encountered situation is that of children and adolescents who are not living with their biological parents. When such a situation arises, obtaining clinically relevant historical information can be next to impossible. More often than not, whatever information is obtained tends to be scanty and limited at best. This type of problem is exacerbated even further when children and adolescents move about from one foster care placement to the next. Those currently responsible for their caretaking may have limited or no knowledge of their recent functioning, due to the typically brief and temporary nature of their contact. Such circumstances seriously complicate clinician efforts to provide ongoing treatment, thereby greatly reducing the chances for successful therapeutic outcome.

Summary

AD/HD is a chronic and pervasive condition characterized by developmentally inappropriate levels of inattention, hyperactivity-impulsivity, or both. Contrary to popular belief, AD/HD symptoms are highly subject to situational variability, occurring most often under low- and delayed-feedback conditions that are boring, repetitive, or familiar. Although the exact details of what causes AD/HD are not well understood, there has been a recent convergence of theory and empirical findings that point toward a combination of genetic, neurochemical, and other neurobiological factors being involved. Due to the highly variable manner in which epidemiological research has been conducted, the exact prevalence of AD/HD has been difficult to determine. What is relatively clear, however, is that AD/HD occurs more often among boys and among younger children. AD/HD symptoms typically arise in early childhood and persist across the life span, with hyperactivity-impulsivity symptoms diminishing somewhat over time. AD/HD is often accompanied, at least in clinic-referred populations, by secondary behavioral, academic, social, emotional, and family complications, which increase the overall severity of psychosocial impairment and increase the risk for negative outcomes.

Given the complexity of AD/HD in its clinical presentation, multiple treatments must be used in combination to bring about optimal therapeutic benefits. Unfortunately, little research has been conducted to date to address the question of which combinations of treatments should be used for which children. Until such research is conducted, clinicians must rely on their own clinical judgment to guide them in putting together multimodal treatment plans to meet the needs of individual children and their families. When doing so, clinicians should also make every effort to include in their multimodal interventions treatments for which there is at least some modicum of empirical validation. Among the many treatments that are available for dealing with this disorder, stimulant medication therapy is perhaps the one used most often and most effectively. Although it is not yet empirically validated, combining stimulant medication therapy with other types of treatments, such as parent training or classroom modifications, is regarded to be acceptable and desirable clinical practice.

As is the case for other types of child mental health difficulties, economic disadvantage, family dysfunction, and cultural diversity are factors that potentially complicate the treatment of AD/HD. Until further research is conducted to clarify such matters, practitioners must once again rely on their creativity and intuition to guide them in their clinical management of children and adolescents with AD/HD who come from such diverse backgrounds.

REFERENCES

Abikoff, M., & Gittelman, R. (1985). Hyperactive children treated with stimulants: Is cognitive training a useful adjunct? *Archives of General Psychiatry, 42*, 953–961.

American Psychiatric Association. (1980). *Diagnostic and statistical manual of mental disorders* (3rd ed.). Washington, DC: Author.

American Psychiatric Association (1987). *Diagnostic and statistical manual of mental disorders* (3rd ed., rev.). Washington, DC: Author.

American Psychiatric Association (1994). *Diagnostic and statistical manual of mental disorders* (4th ed.). Washington, DC: Author.

Anastopoulos, A. D., Shelton, T., DuPaul, G. J., & Guevremont, D. C. (1993). Parent training for Attention Deficit Hyperactivity Disorder: Its impact on parent functioning. *Journal of Abnormal Child Psychology, 21*, 581–596.

Arnsten, A. F. T., Steere, J. C., & Hunt, R. D. (1996). The contribution of alpha2 Noradrenergic mechanism to prefrontal cortical cognitive function. *Archives of General Psychiatry, 53*, 448–455.

August, G. J., Realmuto, G. M., MacDonald, A. W., Nugent, S. M., & Crosby, R. (1996). Prevalence of ADHD and comorbid disorders among elementary school children screened for disruptive behavior. *Journal of Abnormal Child Psychology, 24*, 571–595.

Barkley, R. A. (1977). The effects of methylphenidate on various measures of activity level and attention in hyperkinetic children. *Journal of Abnormal Child Psychology, 5*, 351–369.

Barkley, R. A. (1990). *Attention deficit hyperactivity disorder: A handbook for diagnosis and treatment.* New York: Guilford Press.

Barkley, R. A. (1997). *ADHD and the nature of self-control.* New York: Guilford Press.

Barkley, R. A. (1998). *Attention-Deficit Hyperactivity Disorder—A handbook for diagnosis and treatment* (2nd ed.). NY: Guilford Press.

Barkley, R. A., Anastopoulos, A. D., Guevremont, D. C., & Fletcher, K. E. (1991). Adolescents with AD/HD: Patterns of behavioral adjustment, academic functioning, and treatment utilization. *Journal of the American Academy of Child and Adolescent Psychiatry, 30*, 752–761.

Barkley, R. A., & Biederman, J. (1997). Towards a broader definition of the age of onset criterion for attention deficit hyperactivity disorder. *Journal of the American Academy of Child and Adolescent Psychiatry, 36*, 1204–1210.

Barkley, R. A., Copeland, A. P., & Sivage, C. (1980). A self-control classroom for hyperactive children. *Journal of Autism and Developmental Disorders, 10*, 75–89.

Barkley, R. A., Fischer, M., Edelbrock, C. S., & Smallish, L. (1990). The adolescent outcome of hyperactive children diagnosed by research criteria: I. An 8-year prospective follow-up study. *Journal of the American Academy of Child and Adolescent Psychiatry, 29*, 546–557.

Barkley, R. A., Guevremont, D. C., Anastopoulos, A. D., DuPaul, G. D., & Shelton, T. L. (1993). Driving-related risks and outcomes of Attention Deficit Hyperactivity Disorder in adolescents and young adults: A 3- to 5-year follow-up survey. *Pediatrics, 92*, 212–218.

Baumgaertel, A., Wolraich, M. L., & Dietrich, M. (1995). Attention deficit disorders in a German elementary school-aged sample. *Journal of the American Academy of Child and Adolescent Psychiatry, 34*, 629–638

Block, G. H. (1977). Hyperactivity: A cultural perspective. *Journal of Learning Disabilities, 110*, 236–240.

Bornstein, P. H., & Quevillon, R. P. (1976). The effects of a self-instructional package on overactive preschool boys. *Journal of Applied Behavior Analysis, 9*, 179–188.

Campbell, S. B. (1990). *Behavior problems in preschoolers: Clinical and develop*

mental issues. New York: Guilford Press.

Campbell, S. B. (1995). Behavior problems in preschool children: A review of recent research. *Journal of Child Psychology and Psychiatry, 36*, 113–149.

Castellanos, F. X., Giedd, J. N., Marsh, W. L., Hamburger, S. D., Vaituzis, A. D., Dickstein, D. P., Sarfatti, S. E., Vauss, Y. C., Snell, J. W., Lange, N., Kaysen, D., Krain, A. L., Ritchhie, G. F., Rajapakse, J. C., & Rapoport, J. L. (1996). Quantitative brain magnetic resonance imaging in attention-deficit hyperactivity disorder. *Archives of General Psychiatry, 53*, 607–616.

Cook, E. H., Stein, M. A., Krasowski M. D., Cox, N. J., Olkon, D. M., Kieffer, J. E., & Leventhal, B. L. (1995). Association of attention deficit disorder and the dopamine transporter gene. *American Journal of Human Genetics, 56*, 993–998.

Cunningham, C. E., & Siegel, L. S. (1987). Peer interactions of normal and attention-deficit disordered boys during free-play, cooperative task, and simulated classroom situations. *Journal of Abnormal Child Psychology, 15*, 247–268.

Douglas, V. I. (1972). Stop, look, and listen: The problem of sustained attention and impulse control in hyperactive and normal children. *Canadian Journal of Behavioural Science, 4*, 259–282.

Douglas, V. I. (1983). Attention and cognitive problems. In M. Rutter (Ed.), *Developmental neuropsychiatry* (pp. 280–329). New York: Guilford Press.

DuPaul, G. J., Anastopoulos, A. D., Power, T. J., Reid, R., Ikeda, M. J., & McGoey, K. E. (1998). Parent ratings of attention-deficit/hyperactivity disorder symptoms: Factor structure and normative data. *Journal of Psychopathology and Behavioral Assessment, 20*, 83–102.

DuPaul, G. J., Ervin, R. A., Hook, C. L., & McGoey, K. E. (1998). Peer tutoring for children with attention deficit hyperactivity disorder: Effects on classroom behavior and academic performance. *Journal of Applied Behavior Analysis, 31,* 579–592.

DuPaul, G. J., Power, T. J., Anastopoulos, A. D., Reid, R., McGoey, K. E., & Ikeda, M. J. (1997). Teacher ratings of attention-deficit/hyperactivity disorder symptoms: Factor structure and normative data. *Psychological Assessment, 9,* 436–444.

DuPaul, G. J., & Stoner, G. (1994). *ADHD in the schools: Assessment and intervention strategies.* New York: Guilford Press.

Feingold, B. (1975). *Why your child is hyperactive.* New York: Random House.

Gadow, K. D. (1985). Relative efficacy of pharmacological, behavioral, and combination treatments for enhancing academic performance. *Clinical Psychology Review, 5,* 513–533.

Gaub, M., & Carlson, C. (1997). Behavioral characteristics of *DSM-IV* AD/HD subtypes in a school-based population. *Journal of Abnormal Child Psychology, 25,* 103–111.

Gilger, J. W., Pennington, B. F., & DeFries, J. C. (1992). A twin study of the etiology of comorbidity: Attention-deficit hyperactivity disorder and dyslexia. *Journal of the American Academy of Child and Adolescent Psychiatry, 31,* 343–348.

Gittelman, R., & Eskinazi, B. (1983). Lead and hyperactivity revisited. *Archives of General Psychiatry, 40,* 827–833.

Green, S. M., Loeber, R., & Lahey, B. B. (1991). Stability of mothers' recall of the age of onset of their child's attention and hyperactivity problems. *Journal of the American Academy of Child and Adolescent Psychiatry, 30,* 131–137.

Greenhill, L. L., Halperin, J. M., & Abikoff, H. (1999). Stimulant medications. *Journal of the American Academy of Child and Adolescent Psychiatry, 38,* 503–512.

Hart, E. L., Lahey, B. B., Loeber, R., Applegate, B., & Frick, P. J. (1995). Developmental changes in attention-deficit hyperactivity disorder in boys: A four-year longitudinal study. *Journal of Abnormal Child Psychology, 23,* 729–750.

Heilman, K. M., & Valenstein, E. (1979). *Clinical neuropsychology.* New York: Oxford University Press.

Hinshaw, S. P., Henker, B., & Whalen, C. K. (1984). Self-control in hyperactive boys in anger-inducing situations: Effects of cognitive-behavioral training and of methylphenidate. *Journal of Abnormal Child Psychology, 12,* 55–77.

Jacobvitz, D., & Sroufe, L. A. (1987). The early caregiver-child relationship and attention-deficit disorder with hyperactivity in kindergarten: A prospective study. *Child Development, 58,* 1488–1495.

Klein, R. G., & Mannuzza, S. (1991). Long-term outcome of hyperactive children: A review. *Journal of the American Academy of Child and Adolescent Psychiatry, 30,* 383–387.

Lahey, B. B., Applegate, B., McBurnett, K., Biederman, J., Greenhill, L., Hynd, G. W., Barkley, R. A., Newcorn, J., Jensen, P., Richters, J. Garfinkel, B., Kerdyk, L., Frick, P. J., Ollendick, T., Perez, D., Hart, E. L., Waldman, I., & Shaffer, D. (1994). *DSM-IV* field trials for attention deficit/hyperactivity disorder in children and adolescents. *American Journal of Psychiatry, 151,* 1673–1685.

Levy, F., Hay, D. A., McStephen, M., Wood, C., & Waldman, I. (1997). Attention-deficit hyperactivity disorder: A category or a continuum? Genetic analysis of a large-scale twin study.*Journal of the American Academy of Child and Adolescent Psychiatry, 36,* 737–744.

Luk, S. (1985). Direct observations studies of hyperactive behaviors. *Journal of the American Academy of Child Psychiatry, 24,* 338–344.

Mannuzza, S., Klein, R. G., Bessler, A., Malloy, P., & LaPadula, M. (1993). Adult outcome of hyperactive boys: Educational achievement, occupational rank, and psychiatric status. *Archives of General Psychiatry, 45,* 13–18.

McGee, R., Williams, S., & Feehan, M. (1992). Attention deficit disorder and age of onset of problem behaviors. *Journal of Abnormal Child Psychology, 20,* 487–502.

McIntosh, D. E., & Cole-Love, A. S. (1996). Profile comparisons between ADHD and non-ADHD children on the Temperament Assessment Battery for Children. *Journal of Psychoeducational Assessment, 14,* 362–372.

Meichenbaum, D., & Goodman, J. (1971). Training impulsive children to talk to themselves: A means of developing self-control. *Journal of Abnormal Psychology, 77,* 115–126.

Milberger, S., Biederman, J., Faraone, S. V., Chen, L., & Jones, J. (1996). Is maternal smoking during pregnancy a risk factor of attention deficit hyperactivity disorder in children? *American Journal of Psychiatry, 153,* 1138–1142.

Milberger, S., Beiderman, J., Faraone, S. V., Chen, L., & Jones, J. (1997). Further evidence of an association between attention-deficit/hyperactivity disorder and cigarette smoking: Findings from a high-risk sample of siblings. *American Journal on Addictions, 6,* 205–217.

Murphy, K., & Barkley, R. A. (1996). Prevalence of *DSM-IV* symptoms of ADHD in adult licensed drivers: Implication for clinical diagnosis. *Journal of Attention Disorders, 1,* 147–161.

Pelham, W. W., Schnedler, R. W., Bender, M. E., Nilsson, D. E., Miller, J., Budrow, M. S., Ronnel, M., Paluchowski, C., & Marks, D. A. (1988). The combination of behavior therapy and methylphenidate in the treatment of attention deficit disorders: A therapy outcome study. In L. Bloomingdale (Ed.), *Attention deficit disorders* (Vol. 3, pp. 29–48). New York: Spectrum.

Pelham, W., Wheeler, T., & Chronis, A. (1998). Empirically supported psychosocial treatments for attention deficit hyperactivity disorder. *Journal of Clinical Child Psychology, 27,* 190–205.

Pfiffner, L. J., & O'Leary, S. G. (1987). The efficacy of all-positive management as a function of the prior use of negative consequences. *Journal of Applied Behavior Analysis, 20,* 265–271.

Pfiffner, L. J., Rosen, L. A., & O'Leary, S. G. (1985). The efficacy of an all-positive approach to classroom management. *Journal of Applied Behavior Analysis, 18,* 257–261.

Pisterman, S., McGrath, P., Firestone, P., & Goodman, J. T. (1989). Outcome of parent-mediated treatment of preschoolers with attention deficit disorder with hyperactivity. *Journal of Consulting and Clinical Psychology, 57,* 636–643.

Pliszka, S. R. (1987). Tricyclic antidepressants in the treatment of children with attention deficit disorder. *Journal of the American Academy of Child and Adolescent Psychiatry, 26,* 127–132.

Pliszka, S. R., McCracken, J. T., & Maas, J. W. (1996). Catecholamines in attention-deficit hyperactivity disorder: Current perspectives. *Journal of the American Academy of Child and Adolescent Psychiatry, 35,* 264–272.

Quay, H. C. (1997). Inhibition and attention deficit hyperactivity disorder. *Journal of Abnormal Child Psychology, 25,* 7–13.

Rapoport, J., & Mikkelsen, E. (1978). Antidepressants. In J. Werry (Ed.), *Pediatric psychopharmacology* (pp. 208–233). New York: Brunner/Mazel.

Rapport, M. D., Denney, C., DuPaul, G. J., & Gardner, M. J. (1994). Attention deficit disorder and methylphenidate: Normalization rates, clinical effectiveness, and response prediction in 76 children. *Journal of the American Academy of Child and Adolescent Psychiatry, 33,* 882–893.

Satterfield, J. H., Satterfield, B. T., & Cantwell, D. P. (1980). Three-year multimodality treatment study of 100 hyperactive boys. *Journal of Pediatrics, 98,* 650–655.

Schachar, R. J., Tannock, R., & Logan, G. (1993). Deficient inhibitory control in attention deficit hyperactivity disorder. *Journal of Abnormal Child Psychology, 23*, 411–438.

Sergeant, J. A. (1995). Hyperkinetic disorder revisited. In J. A. Sergeant (Ed.), *Eunnethydis: European approaches to hyperkinetic disorder* (pp. 7–17). Amsterdam: Author.

Shaffer, D. (1994). Attention deficit hyperactivity disorder in adults. *American Journal of Psychiatry, 151*, 633–638.

Shapiro, E. S., & Cole, C. L. (1994). *Behavior change in the classroom: Self-management interventions.* New York: Guilford Press.

Sherman, D. K., McGue, M. K., & Iacono, W. G. (1997). Twin concordance for attention deficit hyperactivity disorder: A comparison of teachers' and mothers' reports. *American Journal of Psychiatry, 154*, 532–535.

Silberg, J., Rutter, M., Meyer, J., Maes, H., Hewitt, J., Simonoff, E., Pickles, A., Loeber, R., & Eaves, L. (1996). Genetic and environmental influences on the covariation between hyperactivity and conduct disturbance in juvenile twins. *Journal of Child Psychology and Psychiatry, 37*, 803–816.

Streissguth, A. P., Bookstein, F. L., Sampson, P. D., & Barr, H. M. (1995). Attention: Prenatal alcohol and continuities of vigilance and attentional problems from 4 through 14 years. *Development and Psychopathology, 7*, 419–446.

Swanson, J., Wigal, S., Greenhill, L., Browne, R., Waslick, B., Lerner, M.,

Williams, L., Flynn, D., Agler, D., Crowley, K., Fineberg, E., Baren, M., & Cantwell, D. (1998). Analog classroom assessment of Adderall (R) in children with ADHD. *Journal of the American Academy of Child and Adolescent Psychiatry, 37*, 519–526.

Willis, T. J., & Lovaas, I. (1977). A behavioral approach to treating hyperactive children: The parent's role. In J. B. Millichap (Ed.), *Learning disabilities and related disorders* (pp. 119–140). Chicago: Yearbook Medical Publications.

Wolraich, M. L., Wilson, D. B., & White, J. W. (1995). The effect of sugar on behavior or cognition in children: A meta-analysis. *Journal of the American Medical Association, 274*, 1617–1621.

Zametkin, A. J., Nordahl, T. E., Gross, M., King, A. C., Semple, W. E., Rumsey, J., Hamburger, S., & Coher, R. M. (1990). Cerebral glucose metabolism in adults with hyperactivity of childhood onset. *New England Journal of Medicine, 323*, 1361–1366.

Zeiner, P. (1995). Body growth and cardiovascular function after extended (1.75 years) with methylphenidate in boys with attention-deficit hyperactivity disorder. *Journal of Child and Adolescent Psychopharmacology, 5*, 129–138.

Zentall, S. S. (1985). A context for hyperactivity. In K. D. Gadow & I. Bialer (Eds.), *Advances in learning and behavioral disabilities* (Vol. 4, pp. 273–343). Greenwich, CT: JAI Press.

13

STEPHEN R. HOOPER
CHRISTOPHER BAGLIO

Children and Adolescents Experiencing Traumatic Brain Injury

Traumatic brain injury (TBI) is the leading cause of death or permanent disability in children and adolescents (Guyer & Ellers, 1990). The sheer magnitude of this problem is complicated by the fact that most TBIs are mild in severity and that many likely go unreported or undetected. In the spirit of this text, what kinds of empirically validated treatments and services are available for work with children and adolescents who have sustained a TBI? Do these interventions work in specific situations and with particular clients having a particular profile of abilities? How long should the interventions be implemented? What about issues of maintenance and generalization of functioning? Can functions really return following a TBI? How does the communication between the various systems in the child's life contribute to facilitating or hindering treatment efforts? How can intervention strategies be utilized in the day-to-day practice of clinicians in communities across the country?

Although this chapter does not attempt to address all of these questions, a number of issues are discussed in relationship to the treatment of children and adolescents who have sustained a TBI. Following an overview of TBI, which includes a discussion of definitional issues, prevalence, precursors and risk factors, major causes, and general outcomes, several key intervention strategies that have been implemented for children and adolescents with TBI are presented. A third section describes the issues of integrating these interventions into real-world settings. In this fashion, several ongoing programs are described, along with selected problems and pitfalls.

Traumatic Brain Injury: An Overview

Definition

The National Head Injury Foundation (NHIF; 1985) defines a TBI as "an insult to the brain, not of a degenerative or congenital nature, but caused by an external force, that may produce a diminished or altered state of consciousness." This definition of TBI includes individuals with brain injury resulting from external causes (e.g., closed head injuries, open head injuries, rotational injuries) and, of particular importance, addresses the issue of change in functioning when compared with preinjury status. Although other brain injuries, such as strokes, tumors, and infections (e.g., meningitis), certainly are traumatic, they do not result from "external" causes and are excluded from this definition of TBI. Further, there are at least three key variables that appear pertinent to the diagnosis of TBI: (1) an alteration in the level of consciousness, (2) the severity of the injury, as defined by coma ratings and/or posttraumatic amnesia (PTA), and (3) the presence of neurophysiological, neuroanatomical, and/or some other type of physical damage (Bigler, 1990).

Incidence and Prevalence

TBI represents one of the most frequent neurological conditions that results in hospitalization of children and adolescents under 19 years of age (Frankowski, 1985). Approximately 150,000 to 200,000 children and adolescents are hospitalized annually in the Unites States with head injuries (Eiben et al., 1984). Prevalence of TBI varies across age, with men aged 15 to 24 years having the highest frequency, at around 400 to 600 per 100,000 (Annegers, Grabow, Kurland, & Laws, 1980), and gender, with TBI being two to three times more frequent in males than in females. More specifically, males show a heightened rate from ages 5 to 25 years, whereas females demonstrate a decline from age 3 years through 15 years. The cumulative risk of TBI from birth through age 15 is around 4% for boys and 2.5% for girls (Rivara & Mueller, 1986).

When taken together, Goldstein and Levin (1987) and Frankowski (1985) reported incidence rates of 150/100,000 for ages birth to 4 years; 550/100,000 for ages 15–19; 160/100,000 around age 50; and 200/100,000 for age 65 and beyond. Kraus, Rock, and Hemyari (1990) also reported different incidence rates for different degrees of TBI severity for individuals ranging in age from birth to age 15 years. These rates indicated that about 5% of TBIs are fatal, whereas 6%, 8%, and 81% were described as severe, moderate, and mild, respectively. From a treatment perspective, these cumulative findings suggest critical developmental periods on which to focus prevention efforts (e.g., middle to late adolescence) and highlight the fact that many neurobehavioral sequelae may go undetected or untreated because of their relatively mild manifestation.

Precursors and Risk Factors

Unlike many of the disorders described in this book, TBI does not "develop"; rather, it is the result of a traumatic event. In this regard, there are some sociodemographic and developmental factors that can contribute to someone sustaining a TBI.

Information has begun to emerge with respect to the impact of race and socioeconomic status on the incidence of TBI. Studies conducted by Kraus (1987), Rivara and Mueller (1986), and Cooper et al. (1983) showed a higher rate of TBI in minority populations when compared with Caucasians. As Fennell and Mickle (1992) noted, however, these studies generally failed to take into account the effects of socioeconomic status on the incidence rates. In fact, Kraus (1987) reported that the highest rates of TBI were observed in sociocultural groups with the lowest median income, suggesting that socioeconomic factors should be considered when examining incidence rates of TBI. Further, it has been speculated that children from more affluent backgrounds may show better improvement following an injury, in large part because of their ability to receive and sustain necessary intervention services (Hooper, 1998).

Craft, Shaw, and Cartlidge (1972) found an increased rate of teacher-reported problems, including hyperactivity, depression, and antisocial behaviors, that predated the brain injury. Premorbid developmental difficulties and specific learning problems (Klonoff & Paris, 1974), language problems (Mahoney et al., 1983), and lower academic achievement (Chadwick, Rutter, Brown, Shaffer, & Traub, 1981) also have been reported for pediatric TBI samples. Preinjury difficulties, particularly in the psychiatric domain, have proven to be predictive of later problems as well (Brown, Chadwick, Shaffer, Rutter, & Traub, 1981). These findings suggest the importance of gaining a comprehensive preinjury history when working with individuals who have sustained a TBI.

Finally, recent evidence does suggest that an individual who sustains a TBI is at increased risk, perhaps because of the sequelae incurred from the first TBI, for sustaining a second brain injury. Annegers et al. (1980) reported that this risk was age related, with risk being increased twofold under age 14 years, threefold between the ages of 15 and 24 years, and fivefold after age 25 years. Males also had twice the likelihood of sustaining a second TBI as females.

Major Causes of Traumatic Brain Injury

There are two broad types of TBI that can be seen: penetrating and nonpenetrating brain injuries. Penetrating brain injuries occur either through skull fragments tearing the dura or causing a brain laceration following a blow to the head or from an object penetrating the skull (e.g., a bullet). In general, it has been estimated that only about 2% to 5% of all head injuries brought to medical attention are penetrating types of injuries (Kampen & Grafman, 1989), and this figure is usually lower for children and adolescents. Nonpenetrating brain injuries typically cause brain contusions (i.e., bruising) or hematomas (i.e., bleeding), and account for over 90% of major pediatric head injuries (Menkes, 1990). Primary damage occurs to structures at the point of impact, as the brain is pushed against the interior of the skull, but damage also can occur at the point opposite the impact point (i.e., contrecoup injury). Even in its least severe form, a nonpenetrating head injury can produce a brief alteration of consciousness, or a concussion. Although a head injury can occur at any time in life, infants and young children are at particular risk for nonpenetrating closed head injuries because of specific skull-brain interface factors (Hooper, 1998).

Accidents in the home account for the major number of head injuries in preschool children, although child abuse is rapidly gaining in this age band (Christ-offel, 1990). Rivara (1984) observed that infants and preschoolers may be at greater risk for head than for trunk and extremity injuries due to the disproportionate size of the child's head at these ages and the associated higher center of gravity. Falls, pedestrian–motor vehicle accidents, bicycle–motor vehicle accidents, sporting ac-tivities, and playground accidents make up the majority of TBIs in school-aged children (Frankowski, 1985). Similar to adult epidemiological findings, motor vehicle accidents constitute the majority of severe TBI cases for older adolescents (Rutter, Chadwick, Shaffer, & Brown, 1980). It should be noted that these age-related findings appear across cultures in industrialized countries (Engberg, 1995).

Recovery and Outcomes

For adults and children, it seems that the major portion of recovery occurs during the first year or two following injury (Jaffe, Polissar, Fay, & Liao, 1995), perhaps due to spontaneous remission, the specific interventions employed, or both. There also are a variety of factors that may contribute to the recovery process and, ulti-mately, to outcomes. In particular, the severity of the injury appears to hold the most weight with respect to prognosis for recovery. Another key factor appears to be chronological age at the time of injury. Until recently, it was widely assumed that age at time of injury was inversely related to outcome due to a certain degree of plasticity in the brain of young children (Ylvisaker & Szekeres, 1996). It is now clear, however, that this idea is no longer tenable. A TBI may disrupt new learning, along with a variety of related neurocognitive functions. It has been speculated that younger children may be at greater risk for learning difficulties following a TBI in that most of their learning, even basic skills, will represent new information. In general, these difficulties are likely to be related to the physiological maturity of the developing brain and to the functional status of the brain at the time of the injury (Thompson et al., 1994). In fact, persistent cognitive deficits have been documented in preschool children who sustained a TBI (Ewing-Cobbs et al., 1997).

Given these recovery factors, a myriad of outcomes can occur following an injury to the brain. Ylvisaker and Szekeres (1996) indicated that the following broadband characteristics have been associated with a TBI that occurs after a substantial period of normal development:

- Neurological change over an extended period of time after the injury (usually improve-ment, but possibly delayed deterioration)
- An unusual profile of strengths and needs, based on the juxtaposition of possibly high-level skills and knowledge acquired before and recovered after the injury with substantial deficits caused by the injury
- A burst of progress, based on recovery of preinjury knowledge and skill, that may lead professionals to be overly optimistic about new learning
- Profound emotional struggles, based on loss of ability, friends, social status, and sense of self
- A need to shed possibly effective preinjury intellectual, academic, and social habits in order to learn new serviceable strategies

- A degree of confusion, disorientation, disinhibition, unawareness of deficits, and lack of self-control for which professionals may be unprepared, particularly in the early months after the injury

Clearly, these broadband domains suggest a wide array of problems for this patient population. At the same time, this array of concerns also highlights the need for treatment professionals to be aware of these possible problems and strategies for addressing them. In tandem with these general outcomes, more specific outcomes from a TBI have been described. A thorough review of these outcomes is beyond the scope of this chapter; however, the interested reader is referred to recent literature reviews of this topic (e.g., Cattelani, Lombardi, Brianti, & Mazzucchi, 1998; Snow & Hooper, 1994; Taylor & Alden, 1997).

Empirically Supported Interventions

For many disorders, relatively few empirically supported interventions exist (Lonigan, Elbert, & Johnson, 1998). This holds true for the treatment literature in the area of traumatic brain injury. For example, given the psychosocial and social-behavioral deficits evidenced in this population, one would imagine the psychotherapy literature would contain numerous efforts at validating specific treatments, but this simply is not the case. Nonetheless, there have been a number of efforts to provide treatment guidelines for children and adolescents with TBI, and some of these efforts have provided empirical evidence for their clinical efficacy.

In this regard, three major domains of intervention are discussed, with available validating support being presented: early rehabilitation efforts, cognitive rehabilitation, and school/educational interventions. In three other domains, behavioral therapies, family interventions, and medical treatments (e.g., hypothermia, pharmacology), literature is building that addresses children and adolescents with TBI (Kinsella, Ong, Murtagh, Prior, & Sawyer, 1999; Max et al., 1998; Slifer et al., 1996), but it is beyond the scope of this chapter to review these intervention domains. Suffice it to say that behavior analysis strategies and family interventions have been used with much success within the context of neurological rehabilitation (Kinsella et al., 1999; Pace & Colbert, 1996), and pharmacological interventions have received some support in their efforts to facilitate behavioral control and affective modulation following a TBI (Mahalick et al., 1998).

Early Rehabilitation Efforts

For more severe cases of TBI, a large number of children and adolescents require acute care (i.e., neurosurgery, acute rehabilitation) directly following the brain injury. Of patients hospitalized following a severe TBI, typical rehabilitation rates while in the hospital have ranged from 19% (Emanuelson & Wendt, 1998) to 84% (Mackay, Bernstein, Chapman, Morgan, & Milazzo, 1992). It appears that the strongest predictors of obtaining rehabilitation in a hospital setting were length of unconsciousness and length of acute-stage care. Typical methods for acute rehabilitation include physiotherapy, occupational therapy, and speech therapy.

Benefits from early rehabilitation following a TBI have been demonstrated by improvements in the areas of motor, sensory/perceptual, cognition, and language skills (Cope & Hall, 1982). Such improvements have been noted even for infants and toddlers (Bagnato & Mayes, 1986). Mackay et al. (1992) have proposed and demonstrated effectiveness of the following programmatic components of treatment during acute hospitalization: (1) trauma rehabilitation, (2) informing the patient's family about the head injury, (3) family involvement in therapy, (4) ongoing social service support, (5) information sharing between professionals through biweekly trauma and rehabilitation rounds, (6) ongoing support between trauma and rehabilitation, (7) formal family meetings, (8) use of a team approach in overall treatment, and (9) discharge planning by team members and family. With this program Mackay et al. (1992) were able to demonstrate significant reduction in length of coma, reduced total length of stay, and significant improvements in physical/motor, sensory/perceptual, and cognitive/language abilities following acute rehabilitation when compared with children and adolescents who received more typical care. The potential benefits of follow-up rehabilitation also should not be underestimated (Massagli, Michaud, & Rivara, 1996).

Cognitive Rehabilitation

Although the term "cognitive rehabilitation" has been used very broadly over the years, these treatments can be grouped into two different approaches: (1) those that attempt to repair damaged cognitive processes and (2) those that utilize compensatory strategies (Prigatano, Glisky, & Klonoff, 1996).

The goal of repairing damaged cognitive processes is to return the individual to preinjury levels of functioning. Therapy usually consists of multiple trials of stimuli designed (1) to facilitate further development of neuronal connections or (2) to make a functional portion of the brain assume new responsibilities. There is minimal support for this approach, particularly as the age of the individual increases (Schacter & Glisky, 1986). Recent work has reported neuronal branching in a damaged region following an injury (Mitchison, 1991); however, the problem is that it is not clear what the functional significance of this branching might be. Further, the studies that incorporate multiple trials to teach stimuli, such as words, indicate that although the recall of the word list may increase, the ability to generalize these skills to new or novel learning situations is very limited. This lack of generalizability does not support a hypothesis regarding the "repair" of underlying neurological structures and function (Ylvisaker & Szekeres, 1996).

An alternative approach assumes that damaged cognitive or neural mechanisms cannot be restored and instead focuses on utilizing compensatory strategies to obtain functional outcomes via related functional systems (Luria, 1980). This can be done through strategies for addressing specific areas of deficit (e.g., trying to improve memory via mnemonic strategies), compensatory devices (e.g., pad of paper), and/ or changes within the environment to facilitate learning in a structured setting. For example, although use of internal strategies (e.g., mnemonic strategies, verbal rehearsal) have been promising for individuals with milder impairments, little evidence indicates that even these individuals spontaneously use such strategies

(Beardmore, Tate, & Liddle, 1999). Because of the lack of long-term benefits seen with internal strategies, many professionals have turned more to external aids in their cognitive rehabilitation efforts (Harris, 1984). Prigatano et al. (1996) have noted that these aids range from environmental restructuring (e.g., labels on cupboards) to microcomputers (Suzman, Morris, Morris, & Milan, 1997). Kirsch, Levine, Lajiness, and Schnyder (1992) demonstrated that even some patients with severe memory impairments were able to use a microcomputer as an "interactive task guidance system" to cue their performance of real-world tasks (e.g., baking or cleaning).

Using case study methodology, Feeney and Ylvisaker (1995) were able to demonstrate reductions in maladaptive behaviors (e.g., aggression) and increases in work performance in three individuals who sustained TBIs during their adolescence through better establishing choice and routine. During the cognitive rehabilitation, the following three key aspects were incorporated: (1) analysis and restructuring of the individual's daily routine wherein the sequencing of the routine was negotiated between the individual and rehabilitation/instructional staff; (2) visual cues, in the form of photographs of activities, to help the individual stay organized and follow the routine; and (3) rehearsal prior to each component of the routine, along with review of performance after completion of each component. In addition to decreasing problem behaviors and increasing adaptive skills, these strategies would appear useful in facilitating independent functioning.

Ylvisaker and colleagues (Ylvisaker & Feeney, 1994; Ylvisaker & Szekeres, 1996) have suggested that this program, through planning and organization, promotes predictability and orderliness, which are important for children who may not be well oriented to routines and upcoming events. They also noted that it gives children a sense of control that they might otherwise gain through oppositional and manipulative behavior. This program also promotes goal setting, control of impulsivity, decision making, and development of the thought processes that are needed for thoughtful decision making. Similar to structuring an individual's daily routine, individual tasks can be broken down and restructured so as to minimize the organizational difficulties frequently seen in children and adolescents with TBI (Ylvisaker & Szekeres, 1996). It is important to note that these and other cognitive-behavioral strategies can be used to teach new skills, not just to remedy lost or impaired ones (Bergquist et al., 1994).

One of the primary needs related to cognitive rehabilitation is educating the family and individual about the child's limitations. Prigatano et al. (1996) propose that all individuals, in addition to receiving cognitive rehabilitation, should be helped to become more aware of residual deficits, as well as strengths, and recognize how these deficits affect everyday activities such as school, work, and relationships with others. This profile of abilities may shift over time, particularly during the first year or two following the injury, and it may be quantitatively, as well as qualitatively, different from preinjury status.

In general, the primary goals of cognitive rehabilitation are to promote recovery and to help individuals overcome barriers posed by their cognitive impediments (Ylvisaker et al., 1995). The specific strategy chosen for intervention and the extent of its deployment will depend on the severity of the injury, the resulting spared and impaired abilities, the surrounding milieu and general psychosocial supports, and the skills of the therapist. These variables notwithstanding, Prigatano, O'Brien, and Klonoff (1993) have provided several pragmatic guidelines for considering any type of cognitive retraining:

- Never underestimate the severity of the cognitive deficits
- Assume initially that an individual does not fully recognize the severity or impact of a cognitive and/or personality deficit
- Approach any cognitive retraining task with a collaborative-learning and problem-solving attitude
- Allow the individual to record and observe his or her own behaviors, and then encourage the individual to examine the intervenor in the same fashion
- Do not lecture the individual as to the deficits or the need for change
- Carefully record training activities and measure behavioral outcome on a regular basis
- Do not limit cognitive retraining activities to one-on-one sessions — in vivo situations are likely to prove more ecologically valid
- Watch the individual for an emotional reaction during the retraining activities
- Provide ample opportunities for practice in and out of the therapy setting
- Focus on cognitive retraining, as well as social-behavioral considerations

School/Educational Interventions

Along with acute rehabilitation, cognitive rehabilitation, and other types of intervention (e.g., behavioral therapies, pharmacology), care must be taken to prepare the child or adolescent for school or work reentry. Telzrow (1991) asserted that the process of educational consultation and programming should begin prior to the return of the student to the formal educational setting. Because hospital and rehabilitation facilities and schools are the two major service providers for children and adolescents with a TBI (Savage, 1997), it is imperative that these two systems overlap to provide continuity of care as the transition back to school takes place. In the "real world," however, these two systems have not been geared up to communicate with one another in a smooth or efficient fashion.

Initial transition of a child back into the school environment should evolve from an interdisciplinary school-based team, devoted exclusively to TBI and related medical problems, that works together to acquire additional information about the child and family's needs. The team members should try to ensure that educational efforts come from a common philosophical approach and plan, to offer alternative options for learning, to prepare the student for multiple transitions, to adapt the curriculum to meet the student's needs, and to establish a comprehensive individualized education plan (IEP; Blosser & Pearson, 1997). With these components in mind, a natural approach to educating children and adolescents following a TBI would be to (1) assess the student to identify abilities and needs, (2) develop a plan to meet these needs, and (3) identify the setting best suited to carrying out the individualized plan.

Aside from the necessary task of identifying strengths and weaknesses, the focus of a comprehensive assessment should be on the generation of practical recommendations. In the case of educational planning, particular attention should be paid to domains typically addressed within the school environment. Blosser and Pearson

(1997) pointed out the following six developmental domains for consideration when developing a curriculum for a student with a TBI:

- Adaptive domain: the area of the curriculum that addresses self-help, independent functioning, and personal and social responsibility
- Aesthetic domain: the area of the curriculum that addresses opportunities for creativity through such activities as art, music, and movement
- Cognitive domain: the area of the curriculum that addresses the understanding of time, area, volume, number, and classes (reading, math, written expression, problem solving, reasoning)
- Communication domain: the area of the curriculum that addresses the form, content, and use of language
- Sensorimotor domain: the area of the curriculum that addresses sensory awareness, exploration, differentiation based on sensory input, and small and large muscle development
- Social-emotional domain: the area of the curriculum that addresses management of self, as well as relationships with peers and adults

With the diverse consequences associated with TBI, it is common to see uneven profiles across the areas listed, especially during a period of recovery, and sensitivity to these types of profiles is critical from a treatment perspective. These profiles also are likely to change over time, with some areas being more amenable to interventions than others. Issues pertinent to skill deficits (i.e., inability to perform a task because of skill needs) versus performance deficits (i.e., inability to perform a task in selected situations despite having the requisite skills) should be addressed. To accommodate these changes over time, it has been recommended that individual plans be evaluated and adjusted more frequently than is typically done in the school system (Savage, 1997; Ylvisaker et al., 1995). Further, Ylvisaker, Hartwick, and Stevens (1991) recommend that planning and programming should be extended through the summer months in order to address the issues of maintenance and generalization of information. Finally, adolescents who have sustained a TBI may need an individual transition plan to identify goals and objectives for community reentry, (pre)vocational planning, and general adult functioning (West, Wehman, & Sherron, 1992).

Although a number of areas need to be addressed within an individualized program (e.g., IEP), cognitive and social-emotional difficulties typically become priorities for interventions within the school system because they tend to produce the most troubling questions for educational decision makers (Ylvisaker et al., 1995). The goal in both areas is to assist the student in reaching his or her highest potential. Increased behavioral benefits have occurred for general problem behaviors associated with a TBI and for social difficulty through the use of operant principles of behavior management (Feeney &Ylvisaker, 1995) and by utilizing peer involvement (Glang, Todis, Cooley, Wells, & Voss, 1997). Although providing consistent programming across settings facilitates generalization of behavioral control, maintenance of social benefits through peer involvement appears more problematic (Glang et al., 1997).

Although it is beyond the scope of this chapter to review the literature on behavior intervention strategies, as many of these types of interventions are reviewed elsewhere (e.g., Warzak, Mayfield, & McAllister, 1998), two key domains are imperative to successful school reintegration and academic adjustment: structure and motivation. It has been noted that children and adolescents following a TBI often demonstrate difficulties related to organizational functioning (Ylvisaker & Szekeres, 1996). By providing clear and structured tasks, students can focus on the academic task and not become overly distracted by instructional patterns. When presenting educational work to students following a TBI, it helps to ensure that the students can answer the following questions: What do I have to do? How much do I have to do? When am I finished? What do I do next? By providing the answers to these questions through a predetermined work system or strategy, independent work skills can be (re)established. It should be only at this point that new or more difficult academic tasks are presented. In order to teach any individual, the teacher must ensure that the child or adolescent is invested in the work being presented. The field of developmental disabilities provides us with some well-established techniques to increase and maintain motivation in children presenting with an uneven pattern of skills and weaknesses (Koegel et al., 1989). These include incorporation of a child's interests and strengths and interspersing difficult or new tasks with previously learned ones. High levels of motivation also lead to lower levels of frustration. Additional adjustments which may be important include more direct instruction techniques, repetition and practice, cueing, modeling, instructional pacing, decreased use of time limits, and providing immediate feedback regarding the individual's performance (Cohen, 1991).

Once a plan has been developed around the child or adolescent's needs and strengths, the academic setting best suited to reach the educational goals needs to be identified. Snow and Hooper (1994) suggest that placement decisions should consider the full range of services available in a school system in order to address the student's pending educational needs. One of the primary goals of the educational program is to increase the amount of time the student is served within the normal academic environment (Ylvisaker et al., 1995), although this process should be conducted in a systematic fashion and gauged carefully, given the potential unevenness in a child's postinjury functioning. A student may start in a more restrictive school setting in order to (re)learn academic strategies which, in turn, could later be applied to less restrictive settings.

Finally, once all of these concerns have been addressed, a remaining major issue relates to how information should be taught to the child so as to facilitate attainment of the predetermined goals and objectives. Glang, Singer, Cooley, and Tish (1992) describe what they call direct instruction techniques with students with TBI. These investigators described the features of direct instruction, including the assumption that all students can learn if instruction is presented in a logical and unambiguous manner. This technique is behavioral in nature and utilizes task analysis, shaping, modeling, and reinforcement. Unique features of the direct instruction model include the following: (1) skills are pretaught, (2) problem-solving strategies are developed, (3) wording of instructions is consistent, (4) corrections are built into the instructions to provide immediate practice with more difficult tasks, (5) mastery is ensured at each step of the learning process, and (6) a cumulative review of all skills ensures integration with previously learned materials. These investigators presented data for three case studies wherein a variety of techniques were illustrated across different subject materials. Systematic observations suggested positive increases beyond baseline data; however, the generalization of these findings was not examined. Although promising, Glang et al. (1992) noted that the direct instruction technique requires considerable training; nonetheless, this treatment effort represents one of the few research efforts to examine the effects of various teaching strategies for improving academic performance in children with TBI.

Integrating and Adapting Interventions in Real-World Settings

Attempting to integrate any kind of treatment into a "real world" setting is always the key to its clinical utility and ultimate success with a target population. With children and adolescents who have sustained a TBI, it is clear that any intervention will be put to the real-world test rapidly, and its ultimate utility will be determined by a highly critical audience of consumers (i.e., parents/families, teachers). In this regard, the application of many interventions into real-world settings likely has been met with a wide range of responses from consumers detailing what worked and, in particular, what did not work for their particular situation. Working with children and adolescents has "forced" the issues of intervention for students with TBI, largely because schools needed to have strategies to manage behavior, deal with affect, and ultimately continue to educate children who have been injured.

Consequently, professionals working with children and adolescents who have sustained a TBI have had to move out of their laboratories and into more ecological settings rapidly. For example, cognitive rehabilitation and cognitive retraining efforts have been conducted by a wide range of professionals in hospitals, rehabilitation settings, outpatient clinics, and schools. Although some professionals might argue "turf issues," it would seem that more children can be served by training many various professionals to execute such treatment strategies. Further, some efforts have even been made to take these strategies and techniques directly into the communities and high schools, with positive success being reported (Brett & Laatsch, 1998).

Similarly, educators working with students who have sustained a TBI clearly have had an advantage by having the large repertoire of special education strategies available to them. Although these strategies for teaching and managing behavior were not designed exclusively for children and adolescents with TBI, their potential application to this population of students is obvious. Further, these educational efforts have been advanced to an even greater degree by the inclusion of TBI as a special education classification under special education law. Schools must now identify and provide special education services to children and adolescents who have sustained a TBI.

Summary

This chapter is an attempt to alert the reader to key issues that could have an impact on treatment with this population. In addition to an overview of various issues related to TBI, such as definitional issues, risk factors, and outcomes, three major domains of treatment are described. Perhaps unlike some of the other disorders discussed in this book, the implementation of TBI treatment strategies into real-world settings likely has been swift, with consumers providing equally swift and critical feedback regarding the utility of specific treatment strategies. Professionals providing treatment services to this population also had the decided advantage of having a deep reservoir of empirically validated behavioral strategies, teaching techniques, and medical interventions that, although not piloted or specifically designed for a TBI population, clearly had immediate application to these children. Despite these apparent advantages, professionals providing treatment to this population of children continue to struggle with issues regarding treatment, and these issues will need to be addressed with respect to future treatment of students with TBI.

One key problem relates to education of the general public with respect to the nature of TBI. It is clear that many professionals working in schools, hospitals, and outpatient clinics, including some physicians, do not understand the nuances of TBI. Such education becomes critical to securing appropriate services for children, to tracking their progress across all domains in an effective manner, and to increasing the communication between families, hospitals, schools, and other community-based intervention sites. For example, despite the apparent availability of a wide array of special education treatment strategies, the lack of knowledge of the needs of TBI survivors likely has hindered the employment of these techniques for children with TBI in the school setting.

In the state of North Carolina we have embarked on several initiatives in this vein. One initiative has been directed toward the training of school psychologists in the area of TBI. This training initiative has included 42 hours of didactic instruction on TBI (introduction to the condition, advanced assessment, and treatment) and, for those who wish to work with such students, 30 hours of case supervision by a clinical neuropsychologist also is required. The ultimate impact of this training remains to be seen, but it is clear that the school psychologists needed this training to work more appropriately with these students. Another initiative, Project A.C.C.E.S.S. (Assuring Coordinated Care, Education, and Support for Survivors), is a federally funded, state-managed demonstration project in the state of North Carolina that was designed to address some of the education issues through timely screening and interventions, care coordination, family education, and follow-up support. A key part of this project was the development of the community transition coordinator positions that are located at three large hospitals in North Carolina. These individuals review patient charts to identify pediatric emergency room patients and inpatients who may have sustained a head injury. Information regarding TBI is then provided to the child's caregivers, and follow-up appointments are arranged as needed. Follow-up calls are made to the family during the first year at 1, 4, and 10 months postinjury, and any family concerns are addressed through referral to appropriate resources. This process clearly involves the family and community immediately following the TBI and, it is hoped, provides better education and improved care coordination for children.

Another associated problem relates to the development of multidisciplinary teams to address the needs of children and adolescents with TBI. Although many rehabilitation hospitals operate from a team model and generally are equipped to meet the needs of TBI survivors, schools are less equipped to deal with the needs of many children with TBI and other medical problems. Although a multidisciplinary team is mandated by special education law, the assessment, developmental needs, and ultimate educational placement of many students with TBI does not take into account the specific issues that can accompany these students. Understanding issues related to recovery, instructional planning and strategies, and the general dynamic nature of a TBI, particularly in the acute phase of recovery, are critical to working with these children in an appropriate fashion. The structuring of the multidisciplinary teams to make individuals more aware of the wide array of needs of these students would be critical. Also, the communication between medical and educational settings could be improved and, it is hoped, facilitate the smooth transition of students from hospitals and rehabilitation settings back to their schools. Too many cases continue to occur in which children are discharged from the hospital on Friday and begin school on Monday, with little or no planning having been done.

Another key area that requires continued vigilance is the area of prevention. One of the best ways to avoid the preceding problems is to avoid the occurrence of traumatic brain injury. Obviously, accidents happen, but prevention efforts have gone a long way toward lessening the chance of head injuries in many different situations. For example, although not specifically intended to prevent head injuries, statutes requiring the use of seat belts and car seats and the work of organizations such as Mothers Against Drunk Driving (M.A.D.D.) likely have saved lives and lessened the number of head injuries. More specific statutes that have explicitly addressed the issue of TBI, such as the use of bicycle helmets, also have contributed positively in this regard. Prevention efforts also have begun to focus on sports-related injuries, particularly as participation in selected sports (e.g., soccer, football) may contribute to the occurrence of TBI, but these efforts clearly will require more vigilance and work.

Finally, the field clearly would benefit from more systematic studies addressing specific assessment-treatment linkages for individuals with TBI. Although the field has been able to take advantage of existent techniques and strategies, their application to children and adolescents with different kinds of TBI will require further study.

REFERENCES

Annegers, J., Grabow, J., Kurland, L., & Laws, E. (1980). The incidence, causes, and secular trends of head trauma in Olmsted County, Minnesota, 1935–1974. *Neurology, 30,* 910–919.

Bagnato, S., & Mayes, S. D. (1986). Patterns of developmental and behavioral progress for young brain-injured children during interdisciplinary intervention. *Developmental Neuropsychology, 2,* 213–240.

Beardmore, S., Tate, R., & Liddle, B. (1999). Does information and feedback improve children's knowledge and awareness of deficits after traumatic brain injury? *Neuropsychology and Rehabilitation, 9,* 45–62.

Bergquist, T., Boll, T., Corrigan, J., Harley, J., Malec, J., Millis, S., & Schmidt, M. (1994). Neuropsychological rehabilitation: Proceedings of a consensus conference. *Journal of Head Trauma Rehabilitation, 9,* 50–61.

Bigler, E. (1990). Neuropathology of traumatic brain injury. In E. D. Bigler (Ed.), *Traumatic brain injury: Mechanisms of damage, assessment, intervention and outcome* (pp. 13–49). Austin, TX: Pro-Ed.

Blosser, J., & Pearson, S. (1997). Transition coordination for students with brain injury: A challenge schools can meet. *Journal of Head Trauma Rehabilitation, 12,* 21–31.

Brett, A. W., & Laatsch, L. (1998). Cognitive rehabilitation therapy of brain-injured students in a public high school setting. *Pediatric Rehabilitation, 2,* 27–31.

Brown, G., Chadwick, O., Shaffer, D., Rutter, M., & Traub, M. (1981). A prospective study of children with head injuries: III. Psychiatric sequelae. *Psychological Medicine, 11,* 63–78.

Cattelani, R., Lombardi, F., Brianti, R., & Mazzucchi, A. (1998). Traumatic brain injury in childhood: Intellectual, behavioural and social outcome into adulthood. *Brain Injury, 12,* 283–296.

Chadwick, O., Rutter, M., Brown, G., Shaffer, D., & Traub, M. (1981). A prospective study of children with head injuries: II. Cognitive sequelae. *Psychological Medicine, 11,* 49–61.

Christoffel, K. (1990). Violent death and injury in U. S. children and adolescents. *American Journal of Diseases of Children, 144,* 697–706.

Cohen, S. (1991). Adapting educational programs for students with head injuries. *Journal of Head Trauma Rehabilitation, 6,* 56–63.

Cooper, K., Tabaddor, K., Hauser, W., Schulman, K., Feiner, C., & Factor, P. (1983). The epidemiology of head injury in the Bronx. *Neuroepidemiology, 2,* 70–88.

Cope, D., & Hall, K. (1982). Head injury rehabilitation: Benefit of early intervention. *Archives of Physical Medicine and Rehabilitation, 63,* 433–437.

Craft, W., Shaw, D., & Cartlidge, N. (1972). Head injuries in children. *British Medical Journal, 4,* 200–203.

Eiben, C., Anderson, T., Lockman, L., Matthews, D., Dryja, R., Martin, J., Gottesman, N., O'Brian, P., & Witte, L. (1984). Functional outcome of closed head injury in children and young adults. *Archives of Physical Medicine and Rehabilitation, 65,* 168–170.

Emanuelson, I., & Wendt, L. (1998). Medical management in south-west Sweden of children and adolescents with serious traumatic brain injury. *Injury, 29,* 193–198.

Engberg, A. (1995). Severe traumatic brain injury: Epidemiology, external causes, prevention, and rehabilitation of mental and physical sequelae. *Acta Neurologica Scandinavica, 92,* (Suppl.), 70–71, 114–118.

Ewing-Cobbs, L., Fletcher, J. M., Levin, H. S., Francis, D. J., Davidson, K., & Miner, M. E. (1997). Longitudinal neuropsychological outcome in infants and preschoolers with traumatic brain injury. *Journal of the International Neuropsychological Society, 3,* 581–591.

Feeney, T., & Ylvisaker, M. (1995). Choice and routine: Antecedent behavioral interventions for adolescents with severe traumatic brain injury. *Journal of Head Trauma Rehabilitation, 10,* 67–86.

Fennell, E., & Mickle, J. (1992). Behavioral effects of head trauma in children and adolescents. In M. G. Tramontana & S. R. Hooper (Eds.), *Advances in child neuropsychology* (Vol. 1, pp. 24–49). New York: Springer.

Frankowski, R. (1985). Head injury mortality in urban populations and its relation to the injured child. In B. F. Brooks

(Ed.), *The injured child* (pp. 20–29). Austin, TX: University of Texas Press.

Glang, A., Singer, G., Cooley, E., & Tish, N. (1992). Tailoring direct instruction techniques for use with elementary students with brain injury. *Journal of Head Trauma Rehabilitation, 7*, 93–108.

Glang, A., Todis, B., Cooley, E., Wells, J., & Voss, J. (1997). Building social networks for children and adolescents with traumatic brain injury: A school-based intervention. *Journal of Head Trauma Rehabilitation, 12*, 32–47.

Goldstein, F., & Levin, H. (1987). Epidemiology of pediatric closed head injury: Incidence, clinical characteristics, and risk factors. *Journal of Learning Disabilities, 20*, 518–525.

Guyer, B., & Ellers, B. (1990). Childhood injuries in the United States. *American Journal of Diseases of Children, 144*, 649–652.

Harris, J. (1984). Methods of improving memory. In W. B. Moffat (Ed.), *Clinical management of memory problems* (pp. 46–62). London: Aspen.

Hooper, S. (1998). Individuals with traumatic brain injury. In A. S. Bellack & M. Hersen (Eds.), *Comprehensive clinical psychology* (pp. 137–153). New York: Pergamon Press.

Jaffe, K., Polissar, N., Fay, G., & Liao, S. (1995). Recovery trends over three years following pediatric traumatic brain injury. *Archives of Physical Medicine and Rehabilitation, 76*, 17–26.

Kampen, D., & Grafman, J. (1989). Neuropsychological evaluation of penetrating head injury. In M. D. Lezak (Ed.), *Assessment of the behavioral consequences of head trauma* (pp. 49–60). New York: Liss.

Kinsella, G., Ong, B., Murtagh, D., Prior, M., & Sawyer, M. (1999). The role of the family for behavioral outcome in children and adolescents following traumatic brain injury. *Journal of Consulting and Clinical Psychology, 67*, 116–123.

Kirsch, N. L., Levine, S. P., Lajiness-

O'Neill, R., & Schnyder, M. (1992). Computer-assisted interactive task guidance: Facilitating the performance of a simulated vocational task. *Journal of Head Trauma Rehabilitation, 7*, 13–25.

Klonoff, H., & Paris, R. (1974). Immediate, short-term and residual effects of acute head injuries in children: Neuropsychological and neurological correlates. In R. M. Reitan & L. A. Davison (Eds.), *Clinical neuropsychology: Current status and applications* (pp. 179–219). New York: Wiley.

Koegel, R., Schreibman, L., Good, A., Cerniglia, L., Murphy, C., & Koegel, L. (1989). *How to teach pivotal behaviors to children with autism: A training manual.* Santa Barbara: University of California.

Kraus, J. (1987). Epidemiology of head injury. In P. R. Cooper (Ed.), *Head injury* (2nd ed., pp. 1–19). Baltimore: Williams & Wilkins.

Kraus, J., Rock, A., & Hemyari, P. (1990). Brain injuries among infants, children, adolescents, and young adults. *American Journal of Diseases of Children, 144*, 684–691.

Lonigan, C. J., Elbert, J. C., & Johnson, S. B. (1998). Empirically supported psychosocial interventions for children: An overview. *Journal of Clinical Child Psychology, 27*, 138–145.

Luria, A. R. (1980). *The working brain.* New York: Basic Books.

Mackay, L., Bernstein, B., Chapman, P., Morgan, A., & Milazzo, L. (1992). Early intervention in severe head injury: Long-term benefits of formalized program. *Archives of Physical Medicine and Rehabilitation, 73*, 635–641.

Mahalick, D. M., Carmel, P. W., Greenberg, J. P., Molofsky, W., Brown, J. A., Heary, R. F., Marks, D., Zampella, E., Hodosh, R., & von der Schmidt, E. (1998). Psychopharmacologic treatment of acquired attention disorders in children with brain injury. *Pediatric Neurosurgery, 29*, 121–126.

Mahoney, W., D'Souza, B., Haller, A.,

Rogers, M., Epstein, M., & Freeman, J. (1983). Long-term outcome of children with severe head trauma and prolonged coma. *Pediatrics, 71,* 756–762.

Massagli, T., Michaud, L., & Rivara, F. (1996). Association between injury indices and outcome after severe traumatic brain injury in children. *Archives of Physical Medicine and Rehabilitation, 77,* 125–132.

Max, J. E., Arndt, S., Castillo, C. S., Bokura, H., Robin, D. A., Lindgren, S. D., Smith, W. L., Sato, Y., & Mattheis, P. J. (1998). Attention-deficit hyperactivity symptomatology after traumatic brain injury: A prospective study. *Journal of the American Academy of Child and Adolescent Psychiatry, 37,* 841–847.

Menkes, J. (1990). *Textbook of child neurology* (4th ed.). Philadelphia: Lea & Febiger.

Mitchison, G. (1991). Neuronal branching patterns and the economy of cortical wiring. *Proceedings of the Royal Society of London, Series B: Biological Sciences, 245,* 151–158.

National Head Injury Foundation (1985). *An educator's manual: What educators need to know about students with traumatic brain injury.* Framingham, MA: Author.

Pace, G., & Colbert, B. (1996). Role of behavior analysis in home and community-based neurological rehabilitation. *Journal of Head Trauma Rehabilitation, 11,* 18–26.

Prigatano, G., Glisky, E., & Klonoff, P. (1996). Cognitive rehabilitation after traumatic brain injury. In P. W. Corrigan & S. C. Yudofsky (Eds.), *Cognitive rehabilitation for neuropsychiatric disorders* (pp. 223–242). Washington, DC: American Psychiatric Press.

Prigatano, G., O'Brien, K., & Klonoff, P. (1993). Neuropsychological rehabilitation of young adults who suffer brain injury in childhood: Clinical observations. *Neuropsychological Rehabilitation, 3,* 411–421.

Rivara, F. (1984). Childhood injuries: III. Epidemiology of non-motor vehicle head trauma. *Developmental Medicine and Child Neurology, 26,* 81–87.

Rivara, F., & Mueller, B. (1986). The epidemiology and prevention of pediatric head injury. *Journal of Head Trauma Rehabilitation, 1,* 7–15.

Rutter, M., Chadwick, O., Shaffer, D., & Brown, G. (1980). A prospective study of children with head injuries: I. Design and methods. *Psychological Medicine, 10,* 633–645.

Savage, R. (1997). Integrating rehabilitation and education services for school-age children with brain injuries. *Journal of Head Trauma Rehabilitation, 12,* 11–20.

Schacter, D., & Glisky, E. L. (1986). Memory remediation: Restoration, alleviation, and the acquisition of domain-specific knowledge. In B. Uzzell (Ed.), *Clinical neuropsychology of intervention* (pp. 257–282). Boston: Martinus Nijhoff.

Slifer, K., Tucker, C., Gerson, A., Cataldo, M., Sevier, R., Suter, A., & Kane, A. (1996). Operant conditioning for behavior management during posttraumatic amnesia in children and adolescents with brain injury. *Journal of Head Trauma Rehabilitation, 11,* 39–50.

Snow, J., & Hooper, S. (1994). *Pediatric traumatic brain injury.* Thousand Oaks, CA: Sage.

Suzman, K. B., Morris, R. D., Morris, M. K., & Milan, M. A. (1997). Cognitive-behavioral remediation of problem solving deficits in children with acquired brain injury. *Journal of Behavior Therapy and Experimental Psychiatry, 28,* 203–212.

Taylor, H. G., & Alden J. (1997). Age-related differences in outcomes following childhood brain insults: An introduction and overview. *Journal of the International Neuropsychological Society, 3,* 555–567.

Telzrow, C. (1991). The school psychologist's perspective on testing students with traumatic brain injury. *Journal of Head Trauma Rehabilitation, 6,* 23–34.

Thompson, N., Francis, D., Stuebing, K.,

Fletcher, J., Ewing-Cobbs, L., Miner, M., Levin, H., & Eisenberg, H. (1994). Motor, visual-spatial, and somatosensory skills after closed head injury in children and adolescents: A study of change. *Neuropsychology*, 8, 333–342.

Warzak, W. J., Mayfield, J., & McAllister, J. (1998). Central nervous system dysfunction: Brain injury, postconcussive syndrome, and seizure disorder. In T. S. Watson & F. M. Gresham (Eds.), *Handbook of child behavior therapy: Issues in clinical child psychology* (pp. 287–309). New York: Plenum Press.

West, M., Wehman, P., & Sherron, P. (1992). Applications for use with traumatic brain injury. In P. Wehman (Ed.), *Life beyond the classroom: Transition strategies for young people with disabilities* (pp. 395–421). Baltimore: Brookes.

Ylvisaker, M., & Feeney, T. (1994). Communication and behavior: Collaboration between speech-language, pathologists and behavioral psychologists. *Topics on Language Disorders, 15,* 37–54.

Ylvisaker, M., Hartwick, P., & Stevens, M. (1991). School reentry following head injury: Managing the transition from hospital to school. *Journal of Head Trauma Rehabilitation, 6,* 10–22.

Ylvisaker, M., & Szekeres, S. (1996). Cognitive rehabilitation for children with traumatic brain injury. In P. W. Corrigan & S. C. Yudofsky (Eds.), *Cognitive rehabilitation for neuropsychiatric disorders* (pp. 263–296). Washington, DC: American Psychiatric Press.

Ylvisaker, M., Feeney, T., Maher-Maxwell, N., Meserve, N., Geary, P., & DeLorenzo, J. (1995). School reentry following severe traumatic brain injury: Guidelines for educational planning. *Journal of Head Trauma Rehabilitation, 10,* 25–41.

14

PETER G. SPRENGELMEYER
PATRICIA CHAMBERLAIN

Treating Antisocial and Delinquent Youth in Out-of-Home Settings

Estimates of the prevalence of delinquent and antisocial behavior in adolescent populations are difficult to derive because youths with these behaviors may present in either the mental health or juvenile justice systems. In the mental health system, a conservative population estimate of the prevalence of conduct disorder (6%; Institute of Medicine, 1989; Offord et al., 1987) would suggest that at any given time there are approximately 4 million youth in the United States who exhibit serious antisocial behavior (Kazdin, 1994). In 1995, the juvenile courts processed 1,714,300 youths (Office of Juvenile Justice and Delinquency Prevention [OJJDP], 1998), and this figure does not include the numerous youths already in the juvenile justice system prior to 1995. Of course, there is no clear way to know how many of these adolescents were reported to both the mental health and juvenile justice systems, and there is likely overlap between these estimates.

Increasing numbers of these youths have been deemed by the juvenile courts or the mental health system as being unable to be returned to their families. The American Public Welfare Association estimated that in 1990 there were 65,000 children and adolescents in residential care (U.S. Department of Health and Human Services, 1995), and the United States Department of Justice reported that 159,900 youths were ordered to out-of-home placements by juvenile courts in 1995 (OJJDP, 1998). Although point-prevalence figures for antisocial and delinquent behavior are difficult to determine, estimates can be made for youth in residential care who meet particular criteria. For example, the Office of Juvenile Justice and Delinquency Prevention (1999) conducted a census on October 29, 1997, of court-adjudicated youth under 21 years of age who were assigned to a residential bed because of a delinquent offense. With 94% of questioned facilities responding, 105,790 youth were found to be in residential care beds on this particular date.

An impressive body of research on the development of antisocial behavior from birth to adulthood has been accumulated during the past three decades (see Farrington, 1997, for a critical review). Although naturalistic prospective longitudinal studies have been extremely useful in identifying key developmental and behavioral precursors of delinquent and antisocial behavior, there remains an issue of how to draw conclusions about interventions from knowledge gained in these studies. For the most part, the models for treating youth with antisocial and delinquent behavior in out-of-home settings do not appear to have been influenced by findings from the research but rather to have been developed from within juvenile justice and mental health settings with virtually no reliance on this accumulated knowledge. In this chapter, a developmental model of antisocial behavior is examined, some alternative models of out-of-home care for adolescents with severe delinquency are reviewed, and an example of a theory-driven treatment that attempts to integrate research on developmental risk factors and predictors of delinquency is described.

Developmental Precursors of Delinquent and Antisocial Behavior

If theories about the development of delinquent behavior are to be useful to intervenors, they should concern themselves with a number of aspects, such as the timing of onset of problems, predictors of increases in severity of problems over time, and an examination of factors that are potentially influential at multiple levels (e.g., individual, interactional, and community).

Coercion theory (Patterson, Reid, & Dishion, 1992) is a developmental model of delinquent and antisocial behavior that attempts to include many of these aspects and that has received a great deal of empirical validation. This model strongly supports the view that despite the presence of other known risk factors (e.g., poverty, single-parent households), the development of delinquent behavior is mediated by parenting factors such as discipline consistency and fairness, adult supervision of youth behavior, and positive youth-adult relationships. Patterson et al. (1992) hypothesized that the development of antisocial behavior occurs in four primary stages. Behaviors within and between each stage are driven by interactions between the individual and the people that compose his or her social world, and therefore the context in which the behaviors occur is as important as the behaviors themselves in predicting future behaviors.

In the first stage, the parent is challenged by the youngster's difficult or noncompliant behaviors and does not deal constructively with child misbehavior in a way that works to effectively socialize the child. The parent(s) may resort to generally ineffective motivational tactics (e.g., yelling) to encourage compliance. This type of parent-child interaction pattern (child doesn't comply, parent yells) initiates a chain of coercive behaviors between parent and child. The parent tends to use inconsistent discipline with the child, at times giving in, at other times reacting with harsh punishment, and the child reacts with more noncompliance and aggressiveness. Across time, such patterns increase in intensity, duration, and predictive power. Eventually the pattern coalesces into a process characterized by parental requests, child refusals, and escalation by both parties. Clearly this is a gross oversimplification of the actual events and associated variables; however, these interactional sequences and their variants have been studied in homes of several hundred families and described by the Oregon group and others (Shaw & Winslow, 1997; Tremblay et al., 1992). A more complete account of all of the associated variables in problematic early childhood parent-child interchanges (e.g., socioeconomic status, child temperament, parenting skill, stress) is beyond the scope of this chapter. What is important here is that parents whose children display delinquent and antisocial behavior will often have interactional patterns with their children that are very firmly entrenched by the time their children reach adolescence.

The second stage of the coercion model is entered into when a child takes these reinforced, interactional patterns into other social environments, particularly the worlds of school and peers. Children who display high rates of noncompliant, oppositional, and aversive behavior have been consistently found to be rejected quickly by prosocial peers (Dishion, 1988; Patterson & Bank, 1989; Shinn, Ramsey, Walker, Stieber, & O'Neill, 1987) and to have difficulty completing academic work (Achenbach & Edelbrock, 1981). Both involved adults (e.g., teachers) and peers label the child as a "problem," and these now-labeled children tend to be excluded from a variety of activities that teach children to effectively relate to other people (e.g., sports, school activities). Simultaneously, such a problem child becomes increasingly proficient at using coercive strategies in social relationships, and interacting with him or her becomes an extremely aversive experience for everyone involved (Patterson et al., 1992). At home, parents tend to avoid interaction with the child, and parental knowledge about where the child is and what he or she is doing decreases. Thus children who show delinquent and antisocial behaviors will likely have long-standing difficulties at school and with peers, in addition to difficulties with parents.

The third stage of the coercion model begins when the rejected and undersupervised child links up with children who are living under similar circumstances and who have acquired similar behavioral repertoires. This link is facilitated through a continued lack of parental monitoring (or parental rejection) and is accelerated when siblings, neighborhood peers, or both are already involved in delinquent behaviors (Patterson et al., 1992). Through interactions within a deviant peer group, the child learns a whole new set of antisocial skills (e.g., stealing) and high-risk behaviors (e.g., substance use, unprotected sexual behavior). By mid- to late adolescence, youth who are heavily involved in such behaviors have developed a variety of skills that in the short run may benefit them in aversive environments, but they have not developed skills that will allow them to function well in conventional society. At this stage, youth are given the labels "delinquent" or "antisocial," and parents of these children become increasingly unaware of what their child is doing, where, or with whom. Thus, although the parents may serve as good sources of information about the history of these children, they may be too estranged from their children to serve as effective treatment agents.

The final stage of the coercion model begins as a youth becomes more completely independent of parents and family and enters the world of young adulthood. Once out on his or her own, a new set of issues arises, such as obtaining and maintaining employment; establishing an independent living arrangement; and negotiating the contexts, processes, and outcomes of romantic relationships, including extended family and children. Such life changes often come early in the lives of youths who are distant from their parents, drop out of school, and are heavily involved in deviant behavior. Individuals with long histories of poor social adjustment have difficulty meeting the intensive demands of these situations. Further, the existence and consequences of individual adjustment problems, such as substance abuse, depression, mental health problems, and antisocial behavior, interfere and create a dismal set of circumstances for the individual and those around him or her. Thus these youth often present for treatment with high expectations and low levels of life achievement.

The preceding developmental model traces the course of a typical trajectory between early parent-child conflict and later adolescent delinquent behavior. Such a trajectory is supported by the extant research, which clearly documents that those youth who engage in their first delinquent behaviors during early adolescence are at greatest risk for becoming chronic offenders (Farrington, 1983; Loeber, 1982). However, data across numerous studies conducted at the Oregon Social Learning Center and elsewhere suggest that one third to one half of all delinquent acts are committed by youth who are not part of this escalation process (Patterson, DeBaryshe, & Ramsey, 1989). This group of youth tend to have more normative social development (therefore greater social skills), and they tend to start their delinquent careers later in adolescence (Patterson et al., 1992). This group of youths does not show the same pattern of early parent-child problems, and antisocial behavior for these youths appears to be of shorter duration and lower intensity. Therefore, youths who are in this "late-starter" group would appear to be less likely to be targets for out-of-home care.

Models of Out-of-Home Treatment

As noted, a case can be made that many essential elements in the development and maintenance of antisocial and delinquent behaviors (especially in males) have been determined in the extant research. Surprisingly, however, large numbers of out-of-home treatment approaches for these behaviors virtually ignore this body of knowledge and in some cases employ program methods and practices that run counter to what research findings indicate would be helpful. A case in point is the reliance of most residentially based models on placing youth in group settings.

In their review of the role peers play in the development of delinquency and drug use, Thornberry and Krohn (1997) point out that as far back as the 1920s research has demonstrated a strong correlation between delinquency and peer associations and behaviors. More recently, the influence of negative peers on the development and escalation of delinquent behavior has been elevated to causal status in a number of studies (Dishion, McCord, & Poulin, 1999; Eddy & Chamberlain, 1999; Elliott & Menard, 1992). Yet during the past several years the popularity of group-based models, such as "boot camp" interventions, has been growing. Despite information about negative peer modeling and the positive influence of family or other mentoring adults, the boot camps typically include little or no family interaction and include extended incarceration with other delinquent youths. In these settings, delinquent youth are subjected to a variety of worklike and military-like experiences intended to provide constructive intervention and early support to a population of juvenile offenders (OJJDP, 1997). Yet there has been little or no research supporting the idea that lack of such rigor leads to the commission of delinquent offenses. Indeed, OJJDP (1997) reported that youth were equally likely to commit a subsequent offense whether or not they had participated in the boot camp program when controlled conditions were used (OJJDP, 1997). Such programs do serve to protect the public for the duration of the youth's incarceration but do little to deter further antisocial behavior.

Four Models

Four treatment models provide the basis for the majority of out-of-home programs for youth with delinquent and antisocial behaviors that are described in the literature.

1. *Positive Peer Culture.* Positive peer culture–based treatment approaches are founded on the idea that "the peer group has the strongest influence over the values, attitudes, and behavior of most youth" (Vorrath & Brendtro, 1985, p. 2). Within this paradigm, staff in a residential institution attempt to hold a group of adolescents responsible for their individual behavior and the impact of that behavior on other adolescents in the same group. Staff at an institution with a positive peer culture model work to create an atmosphere of caring and mutual concern among the youth and to use the group's social norms to promote growth. For example, when physical fights occur in a facility using a positive peer culture model, staff members are ultimately responsible for youths' safety, but group members are expected to protect one another from being hurt (Gold & Osgood, 1992). The positive peer culture model appears to be an inexpensive intervention approach because these programs are delivered to groups of adolescents, a practice embraced by many managed care and third-party payment structures. However, as noted previously, this idea runs counter to research on treatments for antisocial and delinquent youth, and giving the group a powerful and influential role in the treatment process could have iatrogenic effects (Chamberlain & Reid, 1998; Dishion & Andrews, 1995; McCord, 1997). Indeed, reviewers have suggested that the literature concerning treatment of delinquent and antisocial behaviors strongly points toward the need to remove antisocial youth from association with negative peers and that "ultimately, a successful prevention program will see children in the context of the family" (Coie & Jacobs, 1993).

2. *Reality Therapy.* Reality therapy (Glasser, 1965) has also formed the theoretical basis for many out-of-home treatment programs for delinquent and antisocial behavior problem youth. This model is based on the idea that individuals with behavioral problems need assistance in finding a more realistic manner of meeting their basic needs. Glasser (1965) states that the individual must accept responsibility for personal behavior and happiness and that this acceptance of responsibility requires active involvement with a key person. Treatment programs that use a reality therapy model take a variety of forms but typically include a group treatment delivery model. For example, Bratter (1973) reported on the use of a "drop-in" reality

therapy treatment group for adolescents who had concerns related to substance use. In a review of the literature regarding the effectiveness of reality therapy programs with adolescent substance abuse, Davidage and Forman (1998) concluded that serious methodological flaws limited the conclusions that could be drawn from the published research.

3. *Teaching Family Model.* Outcome studies of programs based on the teaching family model (TFM) have demonstrated promising outcomes for youth with delinquent and antisocial behavioral problems. The teaching family model uses a family-style group home setting to deliver treatment (e.g., Boys' Town). Treatment is based on social learning theory and includes the use of a token economy which emphasizes positive parent and peer relations (Braukmann & Wolf, 1987). Numerous studies have demonstrated a variety of positive changes during the program using the teaching family model (TFM). These include improvements in specific skill areas in the home and in school. Friman et al. (1996) found positive changes in follow-up on various psychological variables (e.g., sense of control) and in school performance for TFM youth compared with those who participated in other types of residential care. Other evaluations of the TFM model have failed to find evidence of sustained positive effects after youth leave their TFM placements (Kirigin, Braukmann, Atwater, & Wolf, 1982). TFM programs have been shown to operate at a substantially lower cost than traditional institutional placements for youth (Slot, Jagers, & Dangel, 1992).

4. *Treatment Foster Care.* Treatment foster care (TFC) is an out-of-home treatment model that has also shown positive effectiveness in addressing delinquent and antisocial behavior. TFC, like the teaching family model, is based on social learning theory, places youths with behavior problems in family-like settings, and addresses problem behaviors as they appear in a natural setting. Unlike teaching family homes, typically one and a maximum of two youths are placed in each TFC family home. The remainder of this chapter focuses on the theoretical underpinnings, practice methods, and empirical validation of the TFC model.

Theoretical Basis of TFC

TFC is a rapidly growing form of residential care that is being used with children and adolescents in a variety of situations. For example, TFC is frequently used as a step-down placement for children leaving residential care. TFC has also been used as an alternative to placement in more restrictive inpatient settings (Meadowcroft, Thomlison, & Chamberlain, 1994). Although the various implementations of the TFC model differ in terms of their theoretical underpinnings, most programs emphasize behavioral–social learning approaches, with systems and family therapy paradigms being second in popularity (Hudson, Nutter, Galaway, & Thomlison, 1991).

The Oregon TFC program was first developed to provide services and placement for severely delinquent youth (Chamberlain, 1990). This model uses social learning and, more specifically, coercion theory to inform program practices. Specifically, it is assumed that by the time a youth is presenting with delinquent behaviors, there has been a long history of problematic parent-child interactions. This history

TABLE 14.1 Adaptations of the Oregon TFC Model

Populations of youth served in TFC	Age	Funding source
Preschoolers with severe abuse/neglect and multiple disrupted foster placements (Fisher, Ellis, & Chamberlain, 1999)	3–7	Child welfare, mental health
Youth leaving the state mental hospital (Chamberlain & Reid, 1991)	9–18	Children's Bureau
Developmentally delayed youth with sexual acting out (Moore, Sprengelmeyer, & Chamberlain, in press)	8–18	Child welfare, mental health
Males from juvenile justice (Chamberlain & Reid, 1998)	12–18	Corrections, NIMH
Females from juvenile justice (Chamberlain, 1997)	12–18	Corrections, NIMH

is typically the result of chains of negative and escalating behavior that have been reinforced over time. During placement, the aim is to consistently reinforce the youths' adaptive behaviors and dissuade them from negative behaviors. This type of systematic intervention plan can be accomplished in a controlled setting such as TFC. Positive reinforcement for adaptive youth behavior and consistent sanctions for rule breaking can be carefully implemented through the interventions delivered daily by TFC parents in collaboration with trained program staff. Social learning theory suggests that interventions most likely to generalize to the youth's aftercare placement living setting are those that incorporate treatment characteristics that closely resemble the aftercare placement setting (e.g., the youth's home). The TFC treatment is delivered in a family home, which is a naturalistic setting that has the potential to maximize generalizability. A key feature of the Oregon TFC model involves working with the youth's parents or other aftercare placement resource while the youth is in the program to prepare them (and their youngster) for reunification. In this chapter, we focus on the application of TFC for youths referred from juvenile justice. In Table 14.1, adaptations of the Oregon TFC model for other populations of youngsters are shown.

The Oregon TFC model can be distinguished from the previously mentioned residential care options by a set of central program characteristics that emphasize consistent close supervision under which program youth are not permitted to associate with peers who have similar histories of criminal activity (Chamberlain, Ray, & Moore, 1996). Although both positive peer culture (PPC) and TFC program models attempt to hold youth accountable for problem behaviors and reinforce positive adjustment, the TFC model is guided by adults who are the youths' learning models rather than using peer models, as in PPC. In fact, time spent with peers versus adults has been used to measure the fidelity of the TFC treatment model (Eddy & Chamberlain, in press). TFC programs use adult-controlled discipline, and in a study comparing the daily practices in TFC and PPC programs, TFC foster parents reported greater adult control over when discipline was needed than adults in PPC. In TFC, adults determined what the discipline would be and who would administer it more often than they did in PPC (Chamberlain, Ray, & Moore, 1996). TFC programs also differ from many other out-of-home program models in that youth remain in the community interacting with school, peers, and a family rather than living in a milieu-based setting.

A number of practices are common in out-of-home placements for youths with delinquent and antisocial behaviors that are not part of the Oregon TFC intervention approach. For example, the TFC model does not rely on insight-based change processes. There is no empirical support for the notion that insight produces meaningful changes in adolescents with high rates of antisocial behavior, yet insight-oriented approaches are a common commodity in out-of-home treatment programs for these youth. Insight-based change is based on the assumption that once adolescents realize why they are behaving badly or making poor choices, they will change. Our clinical impression is that some adolescents with severe antisocial behavior problems have good insight into the causes and triggers of their problem behavior, but they are not skilled enough to change it. They also may have goals that are different from those of the adults around them, so they are not motivated to change. In other instances, their problem behaviors may be learned responses that have been functional (e.g., school truancy or disruptive behavior in class helps avoid revealing that one cannot read). Even though we are dealing with youth who are aggressive and violent, in the Oregon TFC program the use of holding or restraint-based behavioral controls is avoided. Not only do such practices have the capacity to retraumatize youths who might have previously been physically abused, but there is also no clear empirical support for their use. In addition, growing evidence shows that such practices encourage abuse by staff and may contribute to injuries or death to the children involved (Weiss, 1998).

Description of the Oregon TFC Model

The TFC model developed at the Oregon Social Learning Center has evolved from intervention work that began in the 1960s (Patterson & Brodsky, 1966). The Oregon Social Learning Center's TFC model was originally designed to provide an alternative to group residential care for severely delinquent male adolescents who were being diverted from commitment to the state training schools. The TFC intervention is designed to last approximately six months, with the youth starting in the TFC home and spending increasing amounts of time with the aftercare resource (e.g., biological parents). In TFC, community families are recruited, screened, and trained to provide treatment to the adolescent placed with them in conjunction with case management and therapy and are supervised throughout the program (see Chamberlain, 1994; Moore & Chamberlain, 1994, for detailed descriptions). Each of these aspects of the model is described briefly in the following sections.

Foster Parent Recruitment and Training

Both one- and two-parent families from diverse social, ethnic, and economic backgrounds have served as successful TFC parents. Efforts are made to select cohesive and nurturing families who are willing to work actively, consistently, and cooperatively toward specific behavioral goals with the youth who is placed with them. Recruitment occurs through word of mouth, newspaper ads, and direct referrals from current TFC parents. In addition to meeting the standard certification requirements for providing foster care, TFC parents agree to work with the youth placed in their home as active agents in the treatment program. In exchange for the extra effort and level of involvement and commitment that TFC parents make, they receive numerous support services and ongoing training.

Preservice Training and Ongoing Support

Foster parent training consists of direct teaching of basic behavior management skills (e.g., close supervision, fair and consistent discipline), methods for encouraging youth skill development and discouraging contact with delinquent peers (e.g., through involvement with prosocial activities and contact with the parents of peers), and techniques for dealing with problem situations through teaching and being nonreactive. The training takes the form of didactic instruction, role playing, and discussion. TFC parents are also taught to use a generic point/level system that will be individually tailored for the specific youth placed in their home.

Daily management of the child in the home, school, and community and supervision and monitoring of the youth is systematized through the use of the point/level program. School attendance, homework completion, and classroom behavior are tracked using a daily school card. This program outlines clear rules for unsupervised time. TFC parents respond daily with positive and negative consequences based on behaviors the youth is presenting. Serious rule violations or persistent difficulties are addressed with repetitive activities (e.g., sentence writing or work chores). TFC parents speak with a program person daily to discuss problem behaviors and points earned or lost, to collect data on the youth's behavior, and to examine emerging patterns. Weekly foster parent meetings give foster parents an opportunity for regular contact with the youth's case manager and allow discussion of changes to behavioral targets and treatment plans.

Case Management and Liaison Services

A case manager supervises the TFC parents' implementation of the point system. Prior to the youth's involvement in the program, he or she meets with the parents to explain how the point/level system operates. The case manager, who has a maximum caseload of 10 youths, conducts the weekly foster parent group meetings, coordinates the youth's TFC home with individual and family therapies, and is on call 24 hours a day for crisis intervention and consultation. Case managers also schedule home visits with biological parents (or other aftercare placement resource) that are coordinated with the assignments given to the biological parents or relatives in the family therapy sessions. Because of the extensive familiarity with social learning and developmental theories and system coordination issues necessary for this role, case managers must have broad experiences through formal education and applied work.

Individual Therapy

The youth's individual treatment occurs at least weekly and emphasizes building skills necessary for (1) negotiation and problem solving, (2) living successfully in a family setting, (3) modulation of anger expression, including techniques for expressing dissatisfaction and distress directly without violent retaliation, (4) development of an educational and occupational plan that incorporates the youth's interests and all identified academic strengths, and (5) prosocial peer involvement. In individual sessions, role playing, homework, and small rewards are used to motivate the youth and encourage the practice of appropriate behaviors. Specific targets of the interventions are defined by the individual therapist in conjunction with the case manager and by observing the youth in a variety of social settings. Individual therapists are typically master's-level individuals with training in the provision of. adolescent treatment.

Family Therapy

The youth's aftercare resource (typically a biological parent) is identified as early as possible in the treatment process, and the family therapist (typically also a master's-level individual) works with these individuals to implement supervision and discipline procedures that have been found to be effective in the TFC home. As the parent's skills develop, home visits become progressively longer. The case manager works during these visits to support the parents in the same manner in which the TFC parents are supported (e.g., phone consultations, crisis on-call). Aftercare parent groups are offered weekly for 12 months following the youth's return home.

Within a TFC program, the adolescent and family interact with a variety of individuals (case manager, individual therapist, and family therapist). Given the specific nature of each professional's relationship with the family, it is often possible for the treatment team to observe and intervene with problem behaviors in a manner that demonstrates respect for both the parents' and adolescent's positions. Importantly, the entire treatment team meets on a formal basis to coordinate treatment, and at these meetings a program director is responsible for supervision of team members and for maintaining treatment integrity.

Evidence for the Efficacy of TFC Programs

In examining the efficacy of the TFC programs, it is important to define the criteria for success. Although there have been a wide variety of different markers for success with the treatment of delinquent and antisocial behaviors, looking back to the developmental model described herein, it would appear to make sense that criteria be based on those factors that appear to contribute to the initiation or maintenance of the problem behaviors. For example, it is known that association with delinquent peers correlates with the initiation and maintenance of delinquent behavior, so a decrease in delinquent behavior that is to be sustained should be associated with changes in such patterns of association. To be truly effective, not only should such changes be seen across behavioral domains at the conclusion of the intervention, but these changes should also be sustained across time and should be associated with treatment success.

Chamberlain (1990) looked at the comparative effectiveness of TFC and group care models with delinquent adolescents matched for age, gender, and date of commitment to the state training school. Rates of incarceration for TFC youths were found to be lower than for group care youths at one- and two-year follow-up intervals. However, the small sample size (N = 32) and lack of random assignment limited the generalizability of these findings.

Improving on some of these limitations, Chamberlain and Reid (1991) examined the effectiveness of TFC in addressing the concerns of youth placed in the community following psychiatric hospitalization. Participants were 20 youth who were referred to the study at time of release and then randomly assigned either to the TFC group or to a services-as-usual control group. Of these participants, all but five had a diagnosis of conduct disorder, oppositional defiant disorder, or substance abuse/dependence when released from the hospital. Although the participants in the two groups were found not to significantly differ from each other in terms of diagnosis, family makeup, socioeconomic status, or rate of specific behavioral problems at intake, by the seven-month follow-up TFC youth were less likely than control youth to be re-hospitalized, to move to a more restrictive level of care, or to behave disruptively in their placements. Overall, TFC youth spent more time in community settings than did children in control groups.

The third and largest Oregon study on the effectiveness of TFC began in 1990 and involved the random assignment of 79 boys referred due to chronic and serious delinquency to TFC or group care programs. In addition to examining outcome variables, investigators studied four key variables thought to mediate the effectiveness of treatment. These included patterns of association with delinquent peers, type and amount of supervision and discipline, and quality of relationship with adult caretakers. Key outcomes examined included official and self-reported delinquency rates, drug use, school attendance and performance, and mental health status.

In this study, the TFC treatment provided was as previously described. The group care (GC) programs involved boys living with 6 to 15 other boys in a variety of congregate care settings, including family-style group homes, stand-alone group homes, or cottages within larger institutions. Participating boys were an average of 14 years old and had been arrested more than 13 times prior to entering the study. They averaged 1.4 previous out-of-home placements, excluding detention stays, and had spent an average of 80 days in detention during the previous year.

Data on outcomes are reported in Chamberlain and Reid (1998) and are briefly reviewed here. Official arrest rates at one year postdischarge showed that boys in TFC had statistically significantly fewer arrests (TFC mean = 2.6 arrests; GC mean = 5.4 arrests). Postdischarge self-reports of delinquent activities showed that TFC boys reported engaging in statistically significantly fewer delinquent activities, including serious and person crimes (self-reported criminal activities: TFC mean = 12.8; GC mean = 28.9). TFC boys also spent fewer days incarcerated that did boys in group care (means = 53 and 129 days, respectively).

Analyses of the factors that were thought to be mediators of treatment effects were also conducted. As reported in Eddy and Chamberlain (1999), association with delinquent peers during placement was a strong predictor of subsequent delinquency at one-year follow-up. Regardless of group assignment (TFC or GC), how well a boy was supervised, whether he received fair and consistent discipline, and the quality of his relationship with an adult caretaker all predicted rates of subsequent offending as measured by both official arrests and self-reports of criminal activity.

Summary

A central concern with any program that attempts to implement interventions across a variety of social contexts is the quality of the partnerships among the agencies and participants involved. There are a number of central participants whose cooperation is necessary for implementation of a successful TFC program. The agency administering the TFC program must have close and positive relationships with the funding source(s), local schools, juvenile probation and parole staff, area juvenile court judges, local court directors, foster parents, and foster care agencies. The most carefully constructed TFC program cannot succeed without support of these other individuals and agencies, and therefore careful strategies should be developed to initiate and maintain these relationships.

For example, it is essential that the TFC program have strong working relationships with its foster parents. Typically, local foster care or child welfare agencies can be joined in partnerships for initial screening and credentialing of foster parents. However, such agencies may not be adept at ongoing training and adherence across time to a particular treatment protocol. Therefore, the TFC agency may need to have an initial relationship with a child welfare agency and then work over time to maintain a more intense relationship with the individual foster parents. Relationships with parents are essential if the goal of reunification is to be realized. By the time their child is removed from the home, parents are often demoralized and hopeless and feel blamed by "the system." The treatment program needs to strike a balance between being supportive and sympathetic to the parents' struggle and being clear about their own rules and expectations for the youth. Parent involvement should be actively encouraged but not allowed to give the youth opportunities to escape from or undermine program rules. For example, it is important that parents enforce the same supervision rules during home visits that the youth has in the TFC home.

Despite its proven efficacy, there remain a large number of areas in which the TFC model needs to be investigated. For example, the effectiveness of the approach for dealing with the unique needs of females in the juvenile justice system is not known. The Oregon Social Learning Center has recently initiated such a study that will examine treatment process and outcomes for this understudied population. The long-term efficacy of the TFC approach is also unknown. Do youths who have initially positive outcomes in TFC have significantly better lives as adults than youths who remain embroiled in the delinquency process? Other issues, such as how TFC fits into a continuum or system of care, need to be studied. Preliminary evidence suggests that the TFC approach is a promising form of out-of-home care that is an effective alternative to more restrictive congregate-care approaches. Future studies are needed to examine the potential and limitations of this approach.

ACKNOWLEDGMENTS   Support for this project was provided by Grant No. R01 MH 54257 from the Center for Studies of Violent Behavior and Traumatic Stress, National Institute of Mental Health, U.S. Public Health Services, and Grant No. P50 MH 46690 from the Prevention Research Branch, National Institute of Mental Health, U.S. Public Health Services.

REFERENCES

Achenbach, T. M., & Edelbrock, C. S. (1981). Behavioral problems and competencies reported by parents of normal and disturbed children aged four through sixteen. *Monographs of the Society for Research in Child Development, 46* (1, Serial No. 188).

Bratter, T. (1973). Treating alienated, unmotivated drug-abusing adolescents. *American Journal of Psychotherapy, 27,* 585–598.

Braukmann, C. J., & Wolf, M. M. (1987). Behaviorally based group homes for juvenile offenders. In E. K. Morris & C. J. Braukmann (Eds.), *Behavioral approaches to crime and delinquency* (pp. 135–155). New York: Plenum Press.

Chamberlain, P. (1990). Comparative evaluation of specialized foster care for seriously delinquent youths: A first step. *Community Alternatives: International Journal of Family Care, 2,* 21–36.

Chamberlain, P. (1994). *Family connections: Treatment foster care for adolescents with delinquency.* Eugene, OR: Northwest Media.

Chamberlain, P. (1997). *Female delinquency: Treatment processes and outcomes* (Grant No. R01 MH 54257). Washington, DC: National Institutes of Mental Health, United States Public Health Service. Violence and Traumatic Stress Research Branch.

Chamberlain, P., & Moore, K. (1998). Models of community treatment for serious juvenile offenders. In J. Crane (Ed.), *Social programs that really work* (pp. 258–276). New York: Sage.

Chamberlain, P., Ray, J., & Moore, K. J. (1996). Characteristics of residential care for adolescent offenders: A comparison of assumptions and practices in two models. *Journal of Child and Family Studies, 5,* 285–297.

Chamberlain, P., & Reid, J. B. (1998). Comparison of two community alternatives to incarceration for chronic juvenile offenders. *Journal of Consulting and Clinical Psychology, 66,* 624–633.

Chamberlain, P. C., & Reid, J. B. (1991). Using a specialized foster care community treatment model for children and adolescents leaving the state hospital. *Journal of Community Psychology, 19,* 266–276.

Coie, J. D., & Jacobs, M. R. (1993). The role of social context in the prevention of conduct disorder. *Development and Psychopathology, 5,* 263–275.

Davidage, A. M., & Forman, S. G. (1998). Psychological treatment of adolescent substance abusers: A review. *Children and Youth Services Review, 10,* 43–55.

Dishion, T. J. (1988). A development model for peer relations: Middle childhood correlates and one-year sequelae.

Unpublished doctoral dissertation, University of Oregon, Eugene.

Dishion, T. J., & Andrews, D. W. (1995). Preventing escalation in problem behaviors with high risk young adolescents: Immediate and 1-year outcomes. *Journal of Consulting and Clinical Psychology, 63,* 538–548.

Dishion, T. J., McCord, J., & Poulin, F. (1999). When interventions harm: Peer groups and problem behavior. *Journal of Adolescent Research, 14,* 175–206.

Eddy, J. M., & Chamberlain, P. (in press). *Family management and deviant peer associations as mediators of the impact of treatment condition on youth antisocial behavior. Journal of Consulting and Clinical Psychology.*

Elliott, D. S., & Menard, S. (1992). *Delinquent friends and delinquent behavior: Temporal and developmental patterns.* Unpublished manuscript.

Farrington, D. P. (1983). Offending from 10–25 years of age. In K. T. Van Dusen & S. A. Mednick (Eds.), *Prospective studies of crime and delinquency* (pp. 17–37). Boston, MA: Kluwer-Nijhoff.

Farrington, D. P. (1997). A critical analysis of research on the development of antisocial behavior from birth to adulthood. In D. M. Stoff, J. Breiling, & J. D. Maser (Eds.), *Handbook of antisocial behavior* (pp. 234–240). New York: Wiley.

Fisher, P. A., Ellis, B. H., & Chamberlain, P. (1999). Early Intervention Foster Care: A model for preventing risk in young children who have been maltreated. *Children's Services: Social Policy, Research, and Practice, 2*(8), 159–182.

Friman, P. C., Osgood, D. W., Shanahan, D., Thompson, R. W., Larzelere, R., & Daly, D. L. (1996). A longitudinal evaluation of prevalent negative beliefs about residential placement for troubled adolescents. *Journal of Abnormal Child Psychology, 24,* 299–324.

Glasser, W. (1965). *Reality therapy: A new approach to psychiatry.* New York: Harper & Row.

Gold, M., & Osgood, D. W. (1992). *Personality and Peer influence in juvenile corrections.* Westport, CT: Greenwood Press.

Hudson, J., Nutter, R., Galaway, B., & Thomlison, B. (1991). *An annotated and cross referenced bibliography of treatment foster family-based programming.* Unpublished manuscript, University of Calgary, Calgary, Alberta, Canada.

Institute of Medicine (1989). *Research on children and adolescents with mental, behavioral and developmental disorders: Mobilizing a national initiative.* Washington, DC: National Academy Press.

Kazdin, A. E. (1994). Interventions for aggressive and antisocial children. In L. D. Eron, J. H. Gentry, & P. Schlegel (Eds.), *Reason to hope: A psychological perspective on violence and youth* (pp. 341–382). Washington, DC: American Psychological Association.

Kirigin, K. A., Braukmann, C. J., Atwater, J., & Wolf, M. M. (1982). An evaluation of achievement place (teaching-family) group homes for juvenile offenders. *Journal of Applied Behavior Analysis, 15,* 1–16.

Loeber, R. (1982). The stability of antisocial and delinquent child behavior: A review. *Child Development, 53,* 1431–1446.

McCord, J. (1997, April). *Some unanticipated consequences of summer camps.* Paper presented at the meeting of the Society for Research on Child Development, Washington, DC.

Meadowcroft, P., Thomlison, B., & Chamberlain, P. (1994). Treatment foster care services: A research agenda for child welfare. *Child Welfare, 33*(33), 565–581.

Moore, K. J., & Chamberlain, P. (1994). Treatment foster care: Toward development of community-based models for adolescents with severe emotional and behavioral disorders. *Journal of Emotional and Behavioral Disorders, 2*(1), 22–30.

Moore, K. J., Sprengelmeyer, P. G., &

Chamberlain, P. (in press). Community-based treatment for adjudicated delinquents: The Oregon Social Learning Center's "Monitor" multidimensional treatment foster care program. In S. I. Pfeiffer & L. A. Reddy, *Innovative mental health prevention programs for children.*

Office of Juvenile Justice and Delinquency Prevention (1997). *Boot camps for juvenile offenders.* Washington, DC: U.S. Department of Justice.

Office of Juvenile Justice and Delinquency Prevention (1998). *Juvenile Court statistics 1995.* Pittsburgh, PA: National Center for Juvenile Justice.

Office of Juvenile Justice and Delinquency Prevention (1999, March). *Juvenile offenders in residential placement, 1997.* (OJJDP Fact Sheet #96). Washington, DC: U.S. Department of Justice.

Offord, D. R., Boyle, M. H., Szatmari, P., Rae-Grant, N. I., Links, P. S., Cadman, D. T., Byles, J. A., Crawford, J. W., Munroe Blum, H., Byrne, C., & Woodward, C. A. (1987). Ontario Child Health Study: Six-month prevalence of disorder and rates of service utilization. *Archives of General Psychiatry, 44,* 832–836.

Patterson, G. R., & Bank, L. (1989). Some amplifying mechanisms for pathological processes in families. In M. R. Gunnar & E. Thelen (Eds.), *Systems and development: The Minnesota Symposia on Child Psychology* (Vol. 22, pp. 167–209). Hillsdale, NJ: Erlbaum.

Patterson, G. R., & Brodsky, G. (1966). A behaviour modification programme for a child with multiple problem behaviors. *Jouranl of Child Psychology and Psychiatry 1,* 277–295.

Patterson, G. R., DeBaryshe, B. D., & Ramsey, E. A. (1989). A developmental perspective on antisocial behavior. *American Psychologist, 44,* 329–335.

Patterson, G. R., Reid, J. B., & Dishion, T. J., (1992) *Antisocial boys.* Eugene, OR: Castalia.

Shaw, D. S., & Winslow, E. B. (1997). Precursors and correlates of antisocial behavior from infancy to preschool. In D. M. Stoff, J. Breiling, & J. D. Maser (Eds.), *Handbook of antisocial behavior* (pp. 148–158). New York: Wiley.

Shinn, M. R., Ramsey, E., Walker, H. M., Stieber, H., & O'Neill, R. E. (1987). Antisocial behavior in school settings: Initial differences in an at-risk and normal population. *Journal of Special Education, 21*(2), 69–84.

Slot, N. W., Jagers, H. D., & Dangel, R. F. (1992). Cross-cultural replication and evaluation of the Teaching Family Therapy Model for community-based residential treatment. *Behavioral Residential Treatment, 7,* 341–354.

Thornberry, T. P., & Krohn, M. D. (1997). Peers, drug use, and delinquency. In D. M. Stoff, J. Breiling, & J. D. Maser (Eds.), *Handbook of antisocial behavior* (pp. 218–233). New York: Wiley.

Tremblay, R. E., Masse, B., Perron, D., Le Blanc, M., Schwartzman, A. E., & Ledingham, J. E. (1992). Early disruptive behavior, poor school achievement, delinquent behavior, and delinquent personality: Longitudinal analyses. *Journal of Consulting and Clinical Psychology, 60,* 64–72.

U.S. Department of Health and Human Services. (1995). *Evaluating children's mental health systems* (Guidance for Applicants No. SM 95–02). Rockville, MD: Author.

Vorrath, H., & Brendtro, L. K. (1985). *Positive peer culture.* Chicago: Aldene.

Weiss, E. M. (1998, October 10–15). Deadly restraint. *The Hartford Courant* [Special reprint edition], pp. 1–16.

15

STANLEY J. HUEY JR.
SCOTT W. HENGGELER

Effective Community-Based Interventions for Antisocial and Delinquent Adolescents

Adolescents engage in higher rates of antisocial behavior and criminal activity than any other age group (Loeber, Farrington, & Waschbusch, 1998; Office of Technology Assessment, 1991). Although youth between the ages of 15 and 17 years comprised only 4% of the U.S. population in 1996, they accounted for 21% of arrests for burglary, 23% for robbery, 14% for rape, 10% for aggravated assault, 13% for murder, and 12% of total arrests (U.S. Bureau of the Census, 1997). When defined broadly to include minor delinquent acts (e.g., truancy, disobedience, vandalism), antisocial behavior is a common, if transient, occurrence over the normal course of childhood (Elliott, Ageton, Huizinga, Knowles, & Canter, 1983; Elliott, Huizinga, & Morse, 1986). Yet a large proportion of serious crimes is committed by a relatively small group of chronic and violent offenders (Loeber et al., 1998; Office of Technology Assessment, 1991), a substantial minority of whom go on to become adult offenders (Elliott, 1994; Farrington et al., 1990; Moffitt, 1993).

The societal costs of adolescent and adult antisocial behavior are considerable. Victims of violent crime often suffer immediate and long-term physical injury and psychological trauma (Hanson, Kilpatrick, Falsetti, & Resnick, 1995; Kilpatrick, Saunders, Veronen, Best, & Von, 1987; Resnick, Acierno, & Kilpatrick, 1997). The medical and mental health costs to these victims are estimated to exceed $10 billion annually (Miller, Cohen, & Rossman, 1993). When these costs are combined with estimates of lost productivity and property loss and with intangibles such as pain, suffering, and risk of death, the costs of criminal victimization may exceed $100 billion annually (Cohen, 1990; Miller, Cohen, & Wiersema, 1996). In addition, substantial costs are associated with the court processing, incarceration, and monitoring of adolescent offenders during probationary periods. For example, expenditures for operating public and private juvenile correctional facilities is estimated to exceed $2 billion annually (Office of Technology Assessment, 1991). Thus effective interventions for antisocial youth could yield substantial economic and health benefits to society.

Unfortunately, evidence for the effective treatment of antisocial behavior is ambiguous, with outcomes varying based on the treatment setting, sample characteristics, type of treatment, length of follow-up, and criteria for treatment success (Andrews et al., 1990; Antonowicz & Ross, 1994; Garrett, 1985; Gensheimer, Mayer, Gottschalk, & Davidson, 1986; Gottshalk, Davidson, Mayer, & Gensheimer, 1987; Lipsey, 1992; Mayer, Gensheimer, Davidson, & Gottschalk, 1986; Whitehead & Lab, 1989). Efforts to alter the short- and long-term trajectory of antisocial behavior have, generally, been minimally successful, with the typical treatment yielding only a 10% reduction in adolescent rearrests compared with control conditions (Lipsey, 1992; Lipsey, 1995). Recently, however, several intervention models have provided unambiguous evidence of effectiveness in treating serious antisocial behavior in youth (Elliott, 1998). These approaches appear to share at least two features deemed critical to achieving substantial, long-term reductions in arrest and incarceration rates. First, the treatments address the multiple factors that contribute to and maintain antisocial behavior. Second, they are truly community-based in that antisocial behavior is treated in the real-world contexts in which it occurs.

This chapter discusses these community-based delinquency interventions, as well as evidence for their long-term effectiveness. In addition, the empirical and theoretical underpinnings of these approaches are reviewed, as well as key treatment factors hypothesized as outcome mediators. Particular attention is given to two exemplary interventions, multisystemic therapy (MST; Henggeler, Schoenwald, Borduin, Rowland, & Cunningham, 1998) and functional family therapy (FFT; Alexander & Parsons, 1982), which have been described as "model" programs for violence prevention (Elliott, 1998) and which are considered among the most cost-effective approaches to crime reduction (Washington State Institute for Public Policy, 1998). First, however, the literature on the determinants of antisocial behavior is briefly reviewed to provide background on the complex array of factors that effective treatments must address.

Determinants of Antisocial and Delinquent Behavior

Antisocial behavior in adolescence is multidetermined by the reciprocal interplay among individual child characteristics and various features of the social ecology in which the youth is embedded (Dodge, 1993; Henggeler, 1991). The most prominent individual risk factors for antisocial behavior include early aggressive behavior, poor impulse control, antisocial attitudes, and deficient social perspective-taking (Hawkins et al., 1998; Lipsey & Derzon, 1998). Larger contextual predictors of antisocial behavior include early school difficulties, affiliation with deviant peers, and family management and interaction difficulties (Hawkins et al., 1998; Lipsey & Derzon, 1998). When these factors are considered in the context of "causal" modeling studies of antisocial behavior (Dishion, Patterson, & Kavanagh, 1992; Elliott, 1994; Elliott, Huizinga, & Ageton, 1985; LaGrange & White, 1985; Patterson, Capaldi, & Bank, 1991; Patterson & Dishion, 1985; Simcha-Fagan & Schwartz, 1986), several key patterns emerge. First, affiliation with deviant peers is nearly always a substantial, direct predictor of antisocial behavior. Second, family and parenting factors are linked directly to antisocial behavior, but also indirectly through their contribution to delinquent peer affiliation. Finally, school, neighborhood, and other community factors appear to exert their influence on delinquent behavior indirectly through their influences on family and peer factors.

Adding to this complexity are important developmental components that may exacerbate or attenuate the effects of these etiological factors. For example, age and developmental level may moderate the impact of certain contextual risks such as deviant peer affiliation (LaGrange & White, 1985; Patterson et al., 1991). Furthermore, differential patterns of prediction appear to exist for subclasses of delinquent behavior, including early versus late starters (Patterson et al., 1991) and aggressive versus nonaggressive versus substance-abusing offenders (Loeber, 1990).

Overall, findings from the extensive correlational and longitudinal literature strongly suggest that interventions that narrowly target only one or a few of the known risk factors for antisocial behavior will likely show limited effectiveness. Conversely, the findings suggest that complex, multifaceted interventions that are individualized and that address the multiple systems in which the delinquent youth is embedded should prove effective. Indeed, the model programs outlined next share such noteworthy characteristics.

Model Program Descriptions and Evidence for Effectiveness

Multisystemic Therapy (MST)

MST is a family-centered, home-based intervention that targets the multiple systems in which the antisocial youth is embedded. MST adopts Bronfenbrenner's social-ecological model of human development (Bronfenbrenner, 1979), which suggests that behavior problems are linked with the reciprocal interplay among individual child characteristics and various aspects of the youth's social ecology (Henggeler, Mihalic, Rone, Thomas, & Timmons-Mitchell, 1998; Henggeler, Schoenwald, et al., 1998). The social-ecological perspective is consistent with findings regarding the determinants of antisocial behavior, as well as with family systems conceptualizations of behavior (Minuchin, 1974). Thus MST therapists intervene primarily at the family level by (1) empowering caregivers with the skills they need to communicate with, monitor, and discipline the target youth effectively, (2) assisting caregivers in engaging the youth in prosocial activities while disengaging the youth from deviant peers, and (3) addressing existing individual and systemic barriers to effective parenting. To achieve these ends, MST is delivered within the family's natural environment (e.g., home, school, community) by therapists trained in the use of a variety of empirically supported techniques (Henggeler, Schoenwald, et al., 1998). In addition, MST therapists are guided by a set of nine principles which offer general guidelines that direct case conceptualization, treatment specification, and prioritization of specific interventions (Henggeler, Schoenwald, et al., 1998). MST is intensive (contact is daily when necessary) yet time-limited (services range from three to six months), requiring that therapist caseloads be fairly low compared with traditional services (caseloads range from four to six families).

To date, results from several randomized clinical trials demonstrate the long-term effectiveness of MST in reducing arrest rates, offense severity, and days incarcerated relative to control conditions. Three trials were conducted with violent and chronic juvenile offenders (Borduin et al., 1995; Henggeler, Melton, Brondino, Scherer, & Hanley, 1997; Henggeler, Melton, & Smith, 1992; Henggeler, Melton, Smith, Schoenwald, & Hanley, 1993), one with substance-abusing offenders (Henggeler, Pickrel, & Brondino, 1999), and one with a small sample of adolescent sexual offenders (Borduin, Henggeler, Blaske, & Stein, 1990). Compared with usual services or individual therapy, MST has reduced long-term arrests by as much as 63% and has reduced days incarcerated by as much as 64%. In addition, the effects of MST do not appear to be moderated by demographic characteristics (i.e., age, ethnicity, social class, arrest and incarceration history) or by preexisting problems in family, peer, or individual functioning (Borduin et al., 1995; Henggeler et al., 1992), indicating that MST is equally effective with youth and families from diverse backgrounds (Brondino et al., 1997).

Functional Family Therapy

FFT is a relatively brief, family-focused intervention representing an integration of family systems perspectives and behavioral strategies (Alexander et al., 1998). FFT proceeds through five sequential phases that involve (1) engaging families, (2) motivating families, (3) reducing risk factors while promoting protective factors, (4) developing concrete plans of action and implementing the plans while constantly monitoring process and outcome, and finally (5) "enhance[ing] the family's ability to impact multiple systems in which the family is embedded . . . , mobiliz[ing] community support systems (e.g., recovery services, nurse visitation) and modify [ing] deteriorated family-system relationships (e.g., with school, probation officers)" (Alexander et al., 1998, p. 13).

Initial validation trials demonstrated that FFT could reduce reoffending by as much as 60%, relative to control groups (Alexander, Barton, Schiavo, & Parsons, 1976; Alexander & Parsons, 1973; Klein, Alexander, & Parsons, 1977). However, these early trials possessed several characteristics that limited the potential generalizability of FFT. For example, this early version of FFT was very time-limited (10–12 sessions) and was conducted in university-based clinics. Furthermore, target youth were typically from White, middle-class, Mormon families and had committed "soft" delinquency offenses.

Subsequent replications of FFT, however, have been conducted by several teams of investigators with samples diverse in terms of cultural background, socioeconomic status, severity of offense, and locus of treatment delivery. For example, Barton and colleagues (Barton, Alexander, Waldron, Turner, & Warburton, 1985) provided home-based FFT to serious offenders, supplemented with job training and placement and school placement. At a 15-month follow-up, this intervention resulted in significantly lower rates of rearrest when compared with a matched control condition. Similarly, Gordon and colleagues (Gordon, Arbuthnot, Gustafson, & McGreen, 1988) conducted a quasi-experimental trial with lower-income, rural, court-referred delinquents with a range of previous status offenses, misdemeanors, and felonies. After an average of 25 contact hours, FFT resulted in reduced recidivism for delinquent males and females. In addition, they found FFT to be effective in reducing recidivism 2½ years posttreatment (Gordon et al., 1988), as well as 5 years later when the youth reached adulthood (Gordon, Graves, & Arbuthnot, 1995). Alexander et al. (1998) summarized the results of 11 published and unpublished clinical trials and found overall that FFT has produced nearly a 35% reduction in rearrest and other out-of-home placements compared with matched or randomly assigned comparison groups. Unfortunately, none of the published outcome studies of FFT conducted with serious offenders have involved random assignment to treatment conditions; thus claims about the effectiveness of FFT with this population should be considered quite promising, but tentative.

Mechanisms of Change

MST and FFT are also effective in improving functioning in those systems hypothesized to mediate the link between treatment and reductions in antisocial behavior. MST is effective at decreasing peer aggression (Henggeler et al., 1992) and improving school attendance (Brown, Henggeler, Schoenwald, Brondino, & Pickrel, 1999) among delinquent youth. At the family level, both MST and FFT have proven successful at improving several domains of family functioning, including intrafamilial communication and family interaction patterns (Alexander & Barton, 1976; Alexander & Parsons, 1973; Borduin et al., 1995; Henggeler et al., 1986; Parsons & Alexander, 1973), problematic parent-child relations (Brunk, Henggeler, & Whelan, 1987), family adaptability and cohesion (Borduin et al., 1995; Henggeler et al., 1992), and psychiatric symptomatology among caregivers (Borduin et al., 1995). Changes at the family level then appear to be directly linked to changes in youth antisocial behavior (Mann, Borduin, Henggeler, & Blaske, 1990). Furthermore, recent work (Huey, Henggeler, Brondino, & Pickrel, in press) suggests that therapist adherence to the MST protocol contributes indirectly to changes in delinquent behavior by improving family relations (i.e., family functioning, family cohesion, and parent monitoring) and decreasing the youth's affiliation with deviant peers. These findings conform with the "theory of change" advanced by both approaches (Alexander et al., 1998; Henggeler, Mihalic, et al., 1998).

Key Treatment Features

Successful interventions for antisocial youth share a number of overlapping key features related to treatment focus, breadth, and technique that appear to account for improved outcomes. Designation as a key treatment feature was determined using two primary criteria: (1) the extent to which the component represented a core aspect of the model programs presented, and (2) empirical support for the significance of the component as an outcome determinant. These features are neither novel nor arcane, as their relevance for the effective treatment of antisocial behavior has been argued by prominent reviewers for nearly two decades (Gendreau, 1996; Gendreau & Ross, 1979; Gendreau & Ross, 1987; Henggeler, 1994; Lipsey, 1992; Lipsey, 1995; McGuire & Priestley, 1995). Neither are these features unique to MST and FFT, although both approaches have been more successful than most at integrating these features within their respective treatment paradigms. With MST, nearly all of these features are encompassed by the nine treatment principles that guide MST interventions (Henggeler, Schoenwald, et al., 1998), whereas with FFT, they are more or less emphasized during distinct phases of treatment (Alexander et al., 1998).

Treatment Engagement

Engagement refers to the process whereby the therapist is perceived as supportive and helpful so that family members actively participate in the treatment process. The practice of actively engaging families in treatment collaboration and building a therapeutic alliance is central to both MST and FFT (Alexander et al., 1998; Henggeler, Schoenwald, et al., 1998) and indeed is an essential element to child and adult psychotherapy more broadly (Horvath & Luborsky, 1993; Shirk & Russell, 1996). Engagement is facilitated by several practices on the part of the therapist and treatment team, including: demonstrating respect for and sensitivity toward family beliefs and practices, acting as an advocate for the family, avoiding blaming the family, avoiding the impulse to impose change on the family rather than collaborating to attain family-defined goals, maintaining a strength focus, and reducing barriers to treatment accessibility (Alexander et al., 1998; Henggeler, Schoenwald, et al., 1998).

In theory, families who are engaged in treatment should be less inclined to terminate prematurely. Recent studies provide evidence that both MST and FFT are more successful than comparison conditions in retaining families. For example, in two recent clinical trials, MST demonstrated treatment completion rates of 98% (Henggeler, Pickrel, Brondino, & Crouch, 1996; Schoenwald, Ward, Henggeler, & Rowland, 2000), whereas 85% of families were retained in the most recent FFT trial (Gordon et al., 1988; Gordon et al., 1995). These rates compare quite favorably with standard levels of attrition found in traditional child mental health settings (Armbruster & Kazdin, 1994; Wierzbicki & Pekarik, 1993).

The links between treatment engagement efforts and caregiver responses to treatment have received some empirical support. For example, Patterson and Forgatch (1985) found that therapist efforts to teach or confront met with resistance by caregivers, whereas efforts to support and facilitate met with increased treatment compliance. Subsequently, families considered to be more resistant had higher rates of dropout and were perceived by therapists as being less successful cases (Chamberlain, Patterson, Reid, Kavanagh, & Forgatch, 1984). Similarly, Alexander and colleagues (Alexander et al., 1976) found that the ratio of supportive to defensive speech acts by clients in family treatment was associated with less frequent premature termination (Alexander et al., 1976). At a more global level, Szapocznik and colleagues (Santisteban et al., 1996; Szapocznik, Kurtines, Santisteban, & Rio, 1990;

Szapocznik et al., 1988) found that Hispanic families assigned to an engagement-enhanced family intervention were more likely to complete treatment than those receiving standard family treatment; however, they found that participation in the engagement-enhanced family intervention was not associated with improved clinical outcomes (Szapocznik et al., 1988). Together, these findings suggest that certain engagement strategies help retain families in treatment, but other methods may be needed to ensure effective treatment outcomes.

Focus on Strength

Social-ecological theories suggest that interventions that require families to make changes that are too discrepant from current family practices are unlikely to be sustainable in the long term (Gallimore, Goldenberg, & Weisner, 1993). Thus interventions should be strength-focused — reinforcing incremental progress toward treatment goals, building on competencies that family members already possess, and utilizing resources indigenous to the family and community. At the most basic level, maintaining a strength focus might involve providing verbal reinforcement for the client's efforts, homework completion, or treatment improvement. More complicated strength-focused interventions might involve enlisting the assistance of other natural agents to act as supports to family members.

With MST, one of the nine treatment principles highlights the importance of emphasizing positives throughout the course of treatment and of utilizing strengths as levers for change (Henggeler, Schoenwald, et al., 1998). Similarly, with FFT, there is a significant focus on the use of child, intrafamilial, and extrafamilial protective factors (e.g., supportive extended family, community resources) to mitigate the effects of risk factors that cannot readily be changed during the course of treatment (e.g., poverty, neighborhood violence; Alexander et al., 1998).

Taking a strength-focused approach is intuitively appealing, and empirical evidence supports its clinical utility. In particular, research suggests that therapy effects can be enhanced with the concurrent involvement of support figures in treatment (e.g., Wadden et al., 1990). For example, Higgins and colleagues (Higgins et al., 1993) found that adult cocaine users were 20 times more likely to achieve nine or more weeks of abstinence when a significant other was recruited to participate in treatment.

Intensiveness

Both MST and FFT are time-limited but intensive interventions. Generally, MST interventions last between three and six months and often occur several times per week. However, daily contact is sometimes required for families with the greatest need, particularly during the initial stages of treatment (Henggeler, Schoenwald, et al., 1998). The importance of MST "dosage" is supported by findings that MST "completers" demonstrate superior outcomes relative to MST "dropouts" (Borduin et al., 1995), a finding that contrasts with the effects of traditional child mental health services (Weisz, Weiss, & Langmeyer, 1987; Weisz, Weiss, & Langmeyer, 1989). Although early FFT clinical trials achieved impressive results treating families of "soft" delinquents with one session per week for a total of eight to twelve weeks (Alexander et al., 1976; Klein et al., 1977; Parsons & Alexander, 1973), recent work indicates that serious offenders require more intensive, home-based contact (Gordon et al., 1988).

This emphasis on intensity is consistent with results from several meta-analyses indicating that treatment intensity and duration have a moderate but significant influence on rates of rearrest (Gensheimer et al., 1986; Lipsey, 1992). However, it is important to note that the mere presence of intensive, family-focused services does not guarantee that the intervention will necessarily be of high quality or effective (Fraser, Nelson, & Rivard, 1997; Heneghan, Horwitz, & Levanthal, 1996).

Skills-Orientation, Using Behavioral Techniques

Meta-analytic findings clearly support the clinical efficacy of delinquency interventions that use behavioral or cognitive-behavioral strategies and are skill-oriented (Lipsey, 1992). This finding corresponds with evidence from several broad-based meta-analyses that demonstrate the superiority of behavioral and social learning interventions relative to more insight-oriented approaches for children (Weiss & Weisz, 1995; Weisz & Weiss, 1987; Weisz, Weiss, Han, Granger, & Morton, 1995).[1] MST and FFT succeed, in part, because they adopt intervention strategies that are pragmatic and action-oriented, with the goal of building concrete, generalizable skills in the youth and caregivers. Thus the therapeutic repertoire of MST and FFT therapists often includes a wide range of behavioral strategies, including contingency contracting; the use of reframing, diverting, and interrupting; communication training; and behavioral parent training. In addition, MST therapists must occasionally learn and integrate other empirically supported techniques to address such issues as caregiver depression (cognitive therapy) or drug dependence (community reinforcement approach). Guidelines for implementing these strategies are further specified in treatment manuals for both MST (Henggeler, Schoenwald, et al., 1998) and FFT (Alexander & Parsons, 1982).

Individualization and Flexibility

Interventions for antisocial youth should avoid a uniform "one-size-fits-all" approach by individualizing treatment to match the unique context of the target youth and family. Highly specified but rigidly manualized interventions that treat all antisocial youth as a homogenous group and fail to account for the family's needs and competencies are likely to prove less effective than more flexible approaches. To properly individualize treatment, both MST and FFT eschew formal assessment (e.g., achievement tests, personality inventories) but emphasize the importance of evaluating the particular factors that contribute directly and indirectly to the target youth's antisocial behavior (Alexander et al., 1998; Henggeler, Schoenwald, et al., 1998). Thus therapists obtain data from multiple sources within and across the systems in which the youth is embedded (e.g., family members, school personnel, caseworkers, court personnel) to evaluate the "fit" of the problem to the systemic context (Henggeler, Schoenwald, et al., 1998). The specifics of the intervention will then depend on the therapist's evaluation of the needs and strengths within and between relevant systems. Evidence from the adult psychotherapy literature suggests that "individualized" approaches are at least as effective as highly structured, standardized interventions, but only when the choices of "individualized" therapists are constrained to empirically supported strategies (Emmelkamp, Bouman, & Blaaw, 1994; Schulte, Kunzel, Pepping, & Schulte-Bahrenberg, 1992; Jacobson, Schmaling, Holtzworth-Monroe, Katt, Wood, & Follette, 1989).

Comprehensiveness

Given the pivotal role of primary caregivers and peers in the initiation and maintenance of antisocial behavior (see the preceding discussion), intervention at the family and peer level is of central importance. However, ample evidence suggests that for parents of disruptive and antisocial youth, compliance with therapy is often hampered by a host of factors "secondary" to the target problem, including economic distress, substance use, parent psychopathology, marital discord, and inadequate social support (Dumas & Wahler, 1983; Patterson & Chamberlain, 1988; Wahler, 1980; Wahler, Leske, & Rogers, 1979). If these barriers to treatment are left unaddressed, outcomes may suffer considerably (Patterson & Chamberlain, 1988).

Such barriers often require that therapists provide practical assistance to the family (e.g., transportation, arranging medical appointments, conflict mediation) or work with family members to develop assertion and planning skills to acquire needed resources on their own. In addition, circumstances may require the integration of MST with other empirically supported approaches for treating marital discord, substance dependence, and other potential barriers to caregiver functioning. For example, MST currently utilizes Higgins' community reinforcement approach (Budney & Higgins, 1998) when substance abuse or dependence interferes with the caregiver's ability to parent (Henggeler, Schoenwald, et al., 1998). However, both MST and FFT also target those systems outside the family unit (e.g., school, police) and the family's interactions with those systems (Alexander et al., 1998; Henggeler, Schoenwald, et al., 1998).

Promotion of Generalization

Treatment generalization is addressed by MST and FFT at two levels. First, clinicians focus on helping the family develop skills that extend to all family members and that persist after treatment ends. Second, therapists emphasize the reduction of delinquent behavior and related problems across multiple settings (e.g., home, school, neighborhood). Therapist intervention in extrafamilial systems may be direct, but the ultimate goal is to empower family members to interact effectively with these systems on their own. Generalization is thus facilitated when the therapist collaborates with caregivers in setting treatment goals and in devising and implementing treatment strategies. In addition, the home-based model of service delivery facilitates the generalization and maintenance of treatment gains by (1) encouraging a more valid assessment of the contingencies that contribute to and maintain antisocial behavior, (2) permitting the therapist to teach and monitor skills in the contexts in which they will actually be used, and (3) facilitating the use of natural reinforcers in the youth's ecology that are likely to be sustained beyond therapy (Gordon et al., 1988; Henggeler, Schoenwald, & Pickrel, 1995).

The long-term outcomes generated by MST (Borduin et al., 1995; Henggeler et al., 1997; Henggeler et al., 1992; Henggeler et al., 1993; Henggeler et al., 1996) and FFT (Barton et al., 1985; Gordon et al., 1988; Gordon et al., 1995; Klein et al., 1977) attest to the temporal generalizability of both treatments. Furthermore, in clinical trials that focused primarily on reducing antisocial behavior and rearrests, MST also had a secondary influence on drug use and abuse, drug-related arrests (Henggeler et al., 1991; Henggeler, Pickrel, et al., 1999), sexual offending (Borduin et al., 1990), and out-of-home placements (Henggeler et al., 1997; Henggeler et al., 1992; Henggeler, Rowland, et al., 1999; Henggeler, Pickrel, et al., 1999). Finally, compared with a control condition, FFT resulted in significantly lower rates of juvenile court involvement for the siblings of target youth (Klein et al., 1977), suggesting a generalizing effect beyond that of the intervention target.

Monitoring and Maintaining Treatment Fidelity

Meta-analytic and narrative reviews indicate that researcher involvement in the design and implementation of treatment, appropriate training of therapists, and monitoring of therapist fidelity are linked with favorable treatment outcomes for delinquent youth (Gendreau, 1996; Gensheimer et al., 1986; Lipsey, 1996). Yet treatment fidelity is often ignored as a relevant factor in the psychotherapy literature, representing one of the greatest threats to the internal validity of a treatment outcome study (Moncher & Prinz, 1991). In a broad meta-analysis of child and adolescent psychotherapy research, Kazdin, Bass, Ayers, and Rodgers (1990) found that only 19% of published studies monitored or evaluated treatment integrity. Similarly, Gensheimer et al. (1986) showed that over 40% of diversion programs for juvenile youth measured program implementation in some fashion, but that only 25% provided any evidence of deviations from the protocol or unplanned treatment variation. Both findings suggest that "weak" treatments with poor integrity may predominate in the child and family treatment literature, thereby compromising the practical utility of promising treatment approaches (Yeaton & Sechrest, 1981).

MST and FFT both include explicit protocols for monitoring and maintaining implementation fidelity (Alexander et al., 1998; Henggeler, Mihalic, et al., 1998). For both, therapist sessions are frequently audiorecorded and the tapes used to provide feedback and recommendations during supervision. Not surprisingly, Henggeler and colleagues found that therapist fidelity to the MST treatment principles was both a direct and indirect contributor to reduced rates of delinquent behavior, rearrests, and incarceration among juvenile offenders (Henggeler et al., 1997; Henggeler, Pickrel, et al., 1999; Huey et al., in press). Similarly, Alexander et al. (1976) found that treatment effectiveness was influenced by the structuring and relationship skills of therapists.

Other Promising Approaches

Other Comprehensive Approaches

Several additional interventions have demonstrated their effectiveness by addressing the multiple determinants of antisocial behavior. For example, Davidson's Community-Based Diversion Project (Davidson et al., 1977; Davidson, Redner, Blakely, Mitchell, & Emshoff, 1987) appears to possess many of the hallmarks of the exemplary approaches presented previously (e.g., being intensive, treatment in the youth's ecology, being strength-focused, using behavioral strategies) and has achieved substantial reductions in rearrests at follow-up relative to court-referred controls. However, several findings lead to some questions about its general application in the field. First, in the most recent clinical trial, an insight-oriented relationship therapy performed as well as community-based diversion (Davidson et al., 1987). Second, the only published replication to date by an independent investigator yielded no effects on recidivism (Emshoff & Blakely, 1983). Finally, no trials have been conducted under "real-world" conditions (e.g., using professional therapists).

The Youth Services Program (Collingwood & Genthner, 1980) and vocationally oriented psychotherapy (Shore & Massimo, 1966; Shore & Massimo, 1979) also targeted multiple risk factors and demonstrated substantial reductions in recidivism relative to controls. However, the effects of neither model have been replicated, and the published evaluations of both approaches have serious methodological problems (e.g., quasi-experimental design, small sample).

Vocational Interventions

Lipsey's meta-analysis revealed a seemingly paradoxical finding regarding the effectiveness of vocational interventions: whereas "employment-related" approaches are among the most effective interventions for delinquent youth, "vocational programs" are among the least effective (Lipsey, 1992; Lipsey, 1995; Lipsey & Wilson, 1998). This discrepancy is clarified when the key terms are defined — "vocational programs" usually provided training only, whereas "employment-related" programs provided work to the youth, often in addition to other relevant services. This finding complements an argument made by Shore (1972) that effective vocational interventions for youth need to be meaningful and challenging, while providing them with concrete opportunities. Indeed, when implemented in a comprehensive manner (e.g., education, training, placement in desirable or well-paying jobs), vocational interventions appear to be quite effective in reducing delinquent behavior (Odell, 1974; Shore & Massimo, 1966; Shore & Massimo, 1979; Walter & Mills, 1980). By providing quality training and access to a good job, a vocational intervention might significantly alter the youth's social ecology by exposing him or her to prosocial peers and by providing skills and resources necessary to enter the "opportunity structure" (Cloward & Ohlin, 1960). Conversely, vocational interventions that are loosely conceptualized or poorly implemented (e.g., group training with other delinquents, no job provision, undesirable or temporary jobs) appear to have a neutral or negative effect (Hackler, 1966; Johnson & Goldberg, 1983).

What Does Not Work?

Ample evidence shows that several broad categories of intervention do not reduce recidivism and in some cases may intensify the breadth and frequency of delinquent behavior.

Treating Antisocial Youth in Aggregate

Although peer group interventions for the prevention and treatment of antisocial behavior have proven quite popular, group approaches may have the unintended consequence of intensifying delinquent behavior in some youth (Dishion & Andrews, 1995; Fo & O'Donnell, 1975; Gottfredson, 1987; Hackler & Hagan, 1975; O'Donnell, Lydgate, & Fo, 1979). Although the mechanism for this iatrogenic effect is unclear, several authors have speculated that participation in such groups may facilitate and extend the antisocial youth's deviant social network (Dishion & Andrews, 1995; O'Donnell, 1992). Thus, although group approaches do not necessarily exacerbate antisocial behavior (see e.g., Chandler, 1973) and may be effective in treating less serious disruptive disorders (Hoag & Burlingame, 1997), extant evidence suggests that group interventions with antisocial youth, if implemented, should occur in settings in which prosocial peers predominate (e.g., Feldman, 1992).

Programs with Strong Punitive Elements

Recently, Lipsey (1992, 1995) demonstrated that deterrence-based programs with predominant punitive elements (e.g., shock incarceration, intense surveillance) resulted in roughly a 25% increase in reoffenses relative to control conditions. Similarly, a recent cost analysis of 16 prominent violence prevention approaches (Washington State Institute for Public Policy, 1998) indicated that boot camps — a favorite among "law and order" politicians — resulted in net financial losses compared with alternative approaches. As McGuire and Priestly (1995) explain, punitive programs often fail, in part because they fulfill few of the criteria necessary for punishment to be an effective mechanism of behavior change (e.g., immediacy, consistency, availability and reinforcement of alternative behaviors).

Traditional Counseling

Lipsey's meta-analysis found very low effect sizes for diffuse psychological interventions such as traditional counseling and casework (Lipsey, 1992, 1995),[2] suggesting that unstructured or eclectic approaches to treating delinquent youth are generally ineffective. When individual counseling does work, it usually incorporates skills-oriented, behaviorally based strategies (Gendreau, 1996; Reid & Hanrahan, 1981; Sheldon, 1994), although few of these efforts have been successfully replicated.

Integrating and Adapting Interventions in Real-World Settings

Currently, the vast majority of fiscal resources for addressing the problem of juvenile delinquency are devoted to highly restrictive settings (e.g., incarceration, hospitalization) with limited or no evidence supporting their effectiveness over less restrictive settings (Kutash & Rivera, 1994; Lyman & Campbell, 1996). Unfortunately, the effectiveness of traditional outpatient mental health services is also not supported in treating conduct-related or other problems of childhood (Weisz, 1991; Weisz, Bahr, & Donenberg, 1992; Weisz, Donenberg, Han, & Kauneckis, 1995; Weisz, Donenberg, Han, & Weiss, 1995).

In addition to their demonstrated long-term effectiveness in controlled clinical trials, MST and FFT both possess features that make them ideal alternatives to the usual community services. MST and FFT are both cost-effective and ecologically valid and have explicit mechanisms for maintaining treatment fidelity. MST has the strongest record in each of these areas. First, the cost-effectiveness of MST has been verified across several randomized trials by independent reporters (Henggeler et al., 1992; Schoenwald, Ward, Henggeler, Pickrel, & Patel, 1996; Washington State Institute for Public Policy, 1998). Second, ecological validity has been demonstrated in two randomized trials by the application of MST using professional therapists hired by community mental health centers (Henggeler et al., 1997; Henggeler et al., 1992). Finally, because the quality of therapist performance tends to deteriorate in "the field" (see, e.g., Fleischman, 1982; Henggeler et al., 1997), MST has explicit mechanisms for facilitating continued adherence to the MST protocol. To this end, MST is supported by a treatment manual, supervisory manual, and consultation manual which help ensure quality adherence to MST in community settings (Henggeler & Schoenwald, 1998; Henggeler, Schoenwald, et al., 1998; Schoenwald, 1998).

Unfortunately, several important barriers to the dissemination of these effective treatments remain. First, therapists, supervisors, and administrators are rarely held accountable to consumers or payers for outcomes. Reimbursement is based primarily on the provision of services rather than on therapeutic effectiveness, thus offering no assurances that consumers are receiving quality services. These funding mechanisms often support the use of more restrictive services over community-based services (Meyers, 1994). Second, in community settings, therapists are generally free to use whatever strategies they wish, with little attention to treatment integrity and minimal clinical oversight. As noted earlier, therapies that are diffuse and nonbehavioral with minimal fidelity to a prescribed treatment protocol are unlikely to make a difference with delinquent youth. Third, political expediency and public concerns about community safety contribute to the drive for punitive strategies and restrictive mental health services.

Future efforts to reduce such system barriers to the development of effective treatment programs might include providing (1) extensive training of therapists and supervisors in therapies with proven effectiveness in treating antisocial youth, and (2) strong financial and occupational incentives for the provider organization and therapists to provide empirically supported treatments. For example, in a recent MST clinical trial of youth with serious psychiatric problems (Henggeler, Rowland, et al., 1999), therapist pay and job security were tied to maintaining treatment fidelity. In the search to disseminate effective interventions to community settings, MST and FFT stand as models for effectively bridging the gap between research and real-world clinical practice with antisocial youth.

NOTES

1. See Casey & Berman (1985) for an exception.

2. Lipsey's most recent version of this meta-analysis (Lipsey & Wilson, 1998) shows individual counseling to yield a fairly respectable effect size of .46 — much higher than in previous analyses (Lipsey, 1992, 1995). However, further investigation suggests that this discrepancy may result, in part, from Lipsey's unique coding convention. For example, one of the eight treatments (Borduin et al., 1990) coded as individual counseling by Lipsey was actually multisystemic therapy!

REFERENCES

Alexander, J., Barton, C., Gordon, D., Grotpeter, J., Hansson, K., Harrison, R., Mears, S., Mihalic, S., Parsons, B., Pugh, C., Schulman, S., Waldron, H., & Sexton, T. (1998). *Blueprints for violence prevention: Functional family therapy*. Boulder, CO: Venture.

Alexander, J., & Parsons, B. V. (1982). *Functional family therapy*. Monterey, CA: Brooks/Cole.

Alexander, J. F., & Barton, C. (1976). Behavioral systems therapy for families. In D. H. L. Olson (Ed.), *Treating relationships* (pp. 167–188). Lake Mills, IA: Graphic.

Alexander, J. F., Barton, C., Schiavo, R. S., & Parsons, B. V. (1976). Systems-behavioral intervention with families of delinquents: Therapist characteristics, family behavior, and outcome. *Journal of Consulting and Clinical Psychology, 44*(4), 656–664.

Alexander, J. F., & Parsons, B. V. (1973). Short-term behavioral intervention with delinquent families: Impact on family process and recidivism. *Journal of Abnormal Psychology, 81*(3), 219–225.

Andrews, D. A., Zinger, I., Hoge, R. D., Bonta, J., Gendreau, P., & Cullen, F. T. (1990). Does correctional treatment work? A clinically relevant and psychologically informed meta-analysis. *Criminology, 28*(3), 369–404.

Antonowicz, D. H., & Ross, R. R. (1994). Essential components of successful rehabilitation programs for offenders. *International Journal of Offender Therapy and Comparative Criminology, 38*(2), 97–104.

Armbruster, P., & Kazdin, A. E. (1994). Attrition in child psychotherapy. In T. H. Ollendick & R. J. Prinz (Eds.), *Advances in clinical child psychology* (Vol. 16, pp. 81–108). New York: Plenum Press.

Barton, C., Alexander, J. F., Waldron, H., Turner, C. W., & Warburton, J. (1985). Generalizing treatment effects of functional family therapy: Three replications. *American Journal of Family Therapy, 13*(3), 16–26.

Borduin, C. M., Henggeler, S. W., Blaske, D. M., & Stein, R. J. (1990). Multisystemic treatment of adolescent sexual offenders. *International Journal of Offender Therapy and Comparative Criminology, 34*, 105–113.

Borduin, C. M., Mann, B. J., Cone, L. T., Henggeler, S. M., Fucci, B. R., Blaske, D. M., & Williams, R. A. (1995). Multisystemic treatment of serious juvenile offenders: Long-term prevention of criminality and violence. *Journal of Consulting and Clinical Psychology, 63*(4), 569–578.

Brondino, M. J., Henggeler, S. W., Rowland, M. D., Pickrel, S. G., Cunningham, P. B., & Schoenwald, S. K. (1997). Multisystemic therapy and the ethnic minority client: Culturally responsive and clinically effective. In D. K. Wilson, J. R. Rodrigue, & W. C. Taylor (Eds.), *Adolescent health promotion in minority populations* (pp. 229–250). Washington, DC: American Psychological Association.

Bronfenbrenner, U. (1979). *The ecology of human development: Experiments by nature and design.* Cambridge, MA: Harvard University Press.

Brown, T. L., Henggeler, S. W., Schoenwald, S. K., Brondino, M. J., & Pickrel, S. G. (1999). Multisystemic treatment of substance abusing and dependent juvenile delinquents: Effects on school attendance at posttreatment and 6-month follow-up. *Children's Services: Social Policy, Research, and Practice, 2,* 81–93.

Brunk, M., Henggeler, S. W., & Whelan, J. P. (1987). Comparison of multisystemic therapy and parent training in the brief treatment of child abuse and neglect. *Journal of Consulting and Clinical Psychology, 55*(2), 171–178.

Budney, A. J., & Higgins, S. T. (Eds.). (1998). *A community reinforcement plus vouchers approach: Treating cocaine addiction* (NIH Publication No. 98-4309). Rockville, MD: National Institute on Drug Abuse.

Chamberlain, P., Patterson, G., Reid, J., Kavanagh, K., & Forgatch, M. (1984). Observation of client resistance. *Behavior Therapy, 15,* 144–155.

Chandler, M. J. (1973). Egocentrism and antisocial behavior: The assessment and training of social perspective-taking skills. *Developmental Psychology, 9*(3), 326–332.

Cloward, R. A., & Ohlin, L. E. (1960). *Delinquency and opportunity: A theory of delinquent gangs.* New York: The Free Press.

Cohen, M. A. (1990). A note on the cost of crime to victims. *Urban Studies, 27*(1), 139–146.

Collingwood, T. R., & Genthner, R. W. (1980). Skills training as treatment for juvenile delinquents. *Professional Psychology, 11*(4), 591–598.

Davidson, W. S., II, Redner, R., Blakely, C. H., Mitchell, C. M., & Emshoff, J. G. (1987). Diversion of juvenile offenders: An experimental comparison. *Journal of Consulting and Clinical Psychology, 55*(1), 68–75.

Davidson, W. S., II, Seidman, E., Rappaport, J., Berck, P. L., Rapp, N. A., Rhodes, W., & Herring, J. (1977). Diversion program for juvenile offenders. *Social Work Research and Abstracts, 13,* 40–49.

Dishion, T. J., & Andrews, D. W. (1995). Preventing escalation in problem behaviors with high-risk young adolescents: Immediate and 1-year outcomes. *Journal of Consulting and Clinical Psychology, 63*(4), 538–548.

Dishion, T. J., Patterson, G. R., & Kavanagh, K. A. (1992). An experimental test of the coercion model: Linking theory, measurement, and intervention. In J. McCord & R. E. Tremblay (Eds.), *Preventing antisocial behavior: Interventions from birth through adolescence* (pp. 253–282). New York: Guilford Press.

Dodge, K. (1993). The future of research on the treatment of conduct disorder. *Development and Psychopathology, 5,* 311–319.

Dumas, J. E., & Wahler, R. G. (1983). Predictors of treatment outcome in parent training: Mother insularity and socioeconomic disadvantage. *Behavioral Assessment, 5*(4), 301–313.

Elliott, D. S. (1994). Serious violent offenders: Onset, developmental course, and termination—the American Society of Criminology 1993 Presidential Address. *Criminology, 32*(1), 1–21.

Elliott, D. S. (1998). *Blueprints for violence prevention.* Boulder, CO: Center for the Study and Prevention of Violence.

Elliott, D. S., Ageton, S. S., Huizinga, D., Knowles, B. A., & Canter, R. J. (1983). *The prevalence and incidence of delin-*

quent behavior: 1976–1980. Boulder, CO: Behavioral Research Institute.

Elliott, D. S., Huizinga, D., & Ageton, S. S. (1985). *Explaining delinquency and drug use.* Beverly Hills, CA: Sage.

Elliott, D. S., Huizinga, D., & Morse, B. (1986). Self-reported violent offending: A descriptive analysis of juvenile violent offenders and their offending careers. *Journal of Interpersonal Violence, 1*(4), 472–514.

Emmelkamp, P. M., Bouman, T. K., & Blaaw, E. (1994). Individualized versus standardized therapy: A comparative evaluation with obsessive-compulsive patients. *Clinical Psychology and Psychotherapy, 1,* 95–100.

Emshoff, J. G., & Blakely, C. H. (1983). The diversion of delinquent youth: Family-focused intervention. *Children and Youth Services Review, 5,* 343–356.

Farrington, D. P., Loeber, R., Elliott, D. S., Hawkins, J. D., Kandel, D. B., Klein, M. W., McCord, J., Rowe, D. C., & Tremblay, R. E. (1990). Advancing knowledge about the onset of delinquency and crime. In B. B. Lahey & A. E. Kazdin (Eds.), *Advances in Clinical Child Psychology* (Vol. 13, pp. 283–342). New York: Plenum Press.

Feldman, R. A. (1992). The St. Louis Experiment: Effective treatment of antisocial youths in prosocial peer groups. In J. McCord & R. E. Tremblay (Eds.), *Preventing antisocial behavior: Interventions from birth through adolescence* (pp. 233–252). New York: Guilford Press.

Fleischman, M. J. (1982). Social learning interventions for aggressive children: From the laboratory to the real world. *Behavior Therapist, 5,* 55–58.

Fo, W. S. O., & O'Donnell, C. R. (1975). The buddy system: Effect of community intervention on delinquent offenses. *Behavior Therapy, 6,* 522–524.

Fraser, M. W., Nelson, K. E., & Rivard, J. C. (1997). The effectiveness of family preservation services. *Social Work Research, 21,* 138–153.

Gallimore, R., Goldenberg, C. N., & Weisner, T. S. (1993). The social construction and subjective reality of activity settings: Implications for community psychology. *American Journal of Community Psychology, 21*(4), 537–559.

Garrett, C. J. (1985). Effects of residential treatment on adjudicated delinquents: A meta-analysis. *Journal of Research in Crime and Delinquency, 22*(4), 287–308.

Gendreau, P. (1996). Offender rehabilitation: What we know and what needs to be done. *Criminal Justice and Behavior, 23*(1), 144–161.

Gendreau, P., & Ross, B. (1979). Effective correctional treatment: Bibliotherapy for cynics. *Crime and Delinquency, 25,* 463–489.

Gendreau, P., & Ross, R. R. (1987). Revivification of rehabilitation: Evidence from the 1980s. *Justice Quarterly, 4*(3), 349–407.

Gensheimer, L. K., Mayer, J. P., Gottschalk, R., & Davidson, W. S. (1986). Diverting youth from the juvenile justice system: A meta-analysis of intervention efficacy. In S. J. Apter & A. P. Goldstein (Eds.), *Youth violence: Programs and prospects* (pp. 39–57). New York: Pergamon Press.

Gordon, D. A., Arbuthnot, J., Gustafson, K. E., & McGreen, P. (1988). Home-based behavioral-systems family therapy with disadvantaged juvenile delinquents. *American Journal of Family Therapy, 16*(3), 243–255.

Gordon, D. A., Graves, K., & Arbuthnot, J. (1995). The effect of functional family therapy for delinquents on adult criminal behavior. *Criminal Justice and Behavior, 22*(1), 60–73.

Gottfredson, G. D. (1987). Peer group intervention to reduce the risk of delinquent behavior: A selective review and a new evaluation. *Criminology, 25*(3), 671–714.

Gottshalk, R., Davidson, W. S., II, Mayer, J., & Gensheimer, L. K. (1987). Behavioral approaches with juvenile offenders: A meta-analysis of long-term treatment efficacy. In E. K. Morris & C. J. Braukmann (Eds.), *Behavioral approaches to crime and delinquency: A handbook of application, research, and concepts* (pp. 399–422). New York: Plenum Press.

Hackler, J. C. (1966). Boys, blisters, and behavior: The impact of a work program in an urban central area. *Journal of Research in Crime and Delinquency, 2,* 155–164.

Hackler, J. C., & Hagan, J. L. (1975). Work and teaching machines as delinquency prevention tools: A four-year follow-up. *Social Service Review, 49*(1), 92–106.

Hanson, R. F., Kilpatrick, D. G., Falsetti, S. A., & Resnick, H. S. (1995). Violent crime and mental health. In J. R. Freedy & S. E. Hobfoll (Eds.), *Traumatic stress: From theory to practice* (pp. 129–161). New York: Plenum Press.

Hawkins, J. D., Herrenkohl, T., Farrington, D. P., Brewer, D., Catalano, R. F., & Harachi, T. W. (1998). A review of predictors of youth violence. In R. Loeber & D. P. Farrington (Eds.), *Serious and violent juvenile offenders: Risk factors and successful interventions* (pp. 106–146). Thousand Oaks, CA: Sage.

Heneghan, A. M., Horwitz, S. M., & Levanthal, J. M. (1996). Evaluating intensive family preservation programs: A methological review. *Pediatrics, 97*(4), 535–542.

Henggeler, S. W. (1991). Multidimensional causal models of delinquent behavior and their implications for treatment. In R. Cohen (Ed.), *Context and development* (pp. 211–231). Hillsdale, NJ: Erlbaum.

Henggeler, S. W. (1994). A consensus: Conclusions of the APA Task Force Report on innovative models of mental health services for children, adolescents, and their families. *Journal of Clinical Child Psychology, 23,* 3–6.

Henggeler, S. W., Borduin, C. M., Melton, G. B., Mann, B. J., Smith, L. A.,

Hall, J. A., Cone, L., & Fucci, B. R. (1991). Effects of multisystemic therapy on drug use and abuse in serious juvenile offenders: A progress report from two outcome studies. *Family Dynamics and Addictions Quarterly, 1*(3), 40–51.

Henggeler, S. W., Melton, G. B., Brondino, M. J., Scherer, D. G., & Hanley, J. H. (1997). Multisystemic therapy with violent and chronic juvenile offenders and their families: The role of treatment fidelity in successful dissemination. *Journal of Consulting and Clinical Psychology, 65*(5), 821–833.

Henggeler, S. W., Melton, G. B., & Smith, L. A. (1992). Family preservation using multisystemic therapy: An effective alternative to incarcerating serious juvenile offenders. *Journal of Consulting and Clinical Psychology, 60*(6), 953–961.

Henggeler, S. W., Melton, G. B., Smith, L. A., Schoenwald, S. K., & Hanley, J. H. (1993). Family preservation using multisystemic treatment: Long-term follow-up to a clinical trial with serious juvenile offenders. *Journal of Child and Family Studies, 2*(4), 283–293.

Henggeler, S. W., Mihalic, S. F., Rone, L., Thomas, C., & Timmons-Mitchell, J. (1998). *Blueprints for violence prevention: Multisystemic Therapy.* Boulder, CO: Blueprints.

Henggeler, S. W., Pickrel, S. G., & Brondino, M. J. (1999). Multisystemic treatment of substance abusing and dependent delinquents: Outcomes, treatment fidelity, and transportability. *Mental Health Services Research, 1,* 171–184.

Henggeler, S. W., Pickrel, S. G., Brondino, M. J., & Crouch, J. L. (1996). Eliminating (almost) treatment dropout of substance abusing or dependent delinquents through home-based multisystemic therapy. *American Journal of Psychiatry, 153*(3), 427–428.

Henggeler, S. W., Rodick, J. D., Borduin, C. M., Hanson, C. L., Watson, S. M., & Urey, J. R. (1986). Multisystemic treatment of juvenile offenders: Effects on adolescent behavior and family interaction. *Developmental Psychology, 22*(1), 132–141.

Henggeler, S. W., Rowland, M. D., Randall, J., Ward, D. M., Pickrel, S. G., Cunningham, P. B., Miller, S. L., Zealberg, J. J., Hand, L. D., & Santos, A. B. (1999). *Home-based multisystemic therapy as an alternative to the hospitalization of youths in psychiatric crisis: Clinical outcomes, Journal of the American Academy of Child and Adolescent Psychiatry, 38,* 1331–1339.

Henggeler, S. W., & Schoenwald, S. K. (1998). *Multisystemic therapy supervisory manual: Promoting quality assurance at the clinical level.* Charleston, SC: MST Institute.

Henggeler, S. W., Schoenwald, S. K., Borduin, C. M., Rowland, M. D., & Cunningham, P. B. (1998). *Multisystemic treatment of antisocial behavior in children and adolescents.* New York: Guilford Press.

Henggeler, S. W., Schoenwald, S. K., & Pickrel, S. G. (1995). Multisystemic therapy: Bridging the gap between university- and community-based treatment. *Journal of Consulting and Clinical Psychology, 63*(5), 709–717.

Higgins, S. T., Budney, A. J., Bickel, W. K., Hughes, J. R., Foerg, F., & Badger, G. (1993). Achieving cocaine abstinence with a behavioral approach. *American Journal of Psychiatry, 150*(5), 763–769.

Hoag, M. J., & Burlingame, G. M. (1997). Evaluating the effectiveness of child and adolescent group treatment: A meta-analytic review. *Journal of Clinical Child Psychology, 26*(3), 234–246.

Horvath, A. O., & Luborsky, L. (1993). The role of the therapeutic alliance in psychotherapy. *Journal of Consulting and Clinical Psychology, 61*(4), 561–573.

Huey, S. J., Jr., Henggeler, S. W., & Brondino, M. J. (in press). *Mechanisms of change in multisystemic therapy: Reducing delinquent behavior through improved family and peer functioning. Journal of Consulting and Clinical Psychology.*

Jacobson, N. S., Schmaling, K. B., Holtzworth-Munroe, A., Katt, J. L., Wood, L. F., & Follette, V. M. (1989). Research-structured vs. clinically flexible versions of social learning–based marital therapy. *Behaviour Research and Therapy, 27*(2), 173–180.

Johnson, B. D., & Goldberg, R. T. (1983). Vocational and social rehabilitation of delinquents: A study of experimentals and controls. *Journal of Offender Counseling, Services, and Rehabilitation, 6*(3), 43–60.

Kazdin, A. E., Bass, D., Ayers, W. A., & Rodgers, A. (1990). Empirical and clinical focus of child and adolescent psychotherapy research. *Journal of Consulting and Clinical Psychology, 58*(6), 729–740.

Kilpatrick, D. G., Saunders, B. E., Veronen, L. J., Best, C. L., & Von, J. M. (1987). Criminal victimization: Lifetime prevalence, reporting to police, and psychological impact. *Crime and Delinquency, 33*(4), 479–489.

Klein, N. C., Alexander, J. F., & Parsons, B. V. (1977). Impact of family systems intervention on recidivism and sibling delinquency: A model of primary prevention and program evaluation. *Journal of Consulting and Clinical Psychology, 45*(3), 469–474.

Kutash, K., & Rivera, V. R. (1994). Residential services: Psychiatric hospitals and residential treatment centers. In K. Kutash & V. R. Rivera (Eds.), *Components of a system of care: What does the research say?* (pp. 7–24). Tampa, FL: University of South Florida Mental Health Institute, Research and Training Center for Children's Mental Health.

LaGrange, R. L., & White, H. R. (1985). Age differences in delinquency: A test of theory. *Criminology, 23,* 12–45.

Lipsey, M. W. (1992). The effect of treatment on juvenile delinquents: Results from meta-analysis. In F. Losel, D.

Bender, & J. Bliesener (Eds.), *Psychology and law: International perspectives* (pp. 131–143). Berlin, Germany: de Gruyter.

Lipsey, M. W. (1995). What do we learn from 400 research studies on the effectiveness of treatment with juvenile delinquents? In J. McGuire (Ed.), *What works: Reducing reoffending: Guidelines from research and practice* (pp. 63–78). Chichester, England: Wiley.

Lipsey, M. W., & Derzon, J. H. (1998). Predictors of violent or serious delinquency in adolescence and early adulthood. In R. Loeber & D. P. Farrington (Eds.), *Serious and violent juvenile offenders: Risk factors and successful interventions* (pp. 86–105). Thousand Oaks, CA: Sage.

Lipsey, M. W., & Wilson, D. B. (1998). Effective intervention for serious juvenile offenders: A synthesis of research. In R. Loeber & D. P. Farrington (Eds.), *Serious and violent juvenile offenders: Risk factors and successful interventions* (pp. 313–345). Thousand Oaks, CA: Sage.

Loeber, R. (1990). Development and risk factors of juvenile antisocial behavior and delinquency. *Clinical Psychology Review, 10*, 1–41.

Loeber, R., Farrington, D. P., & Waschbusch, D. A. (1998). Serious and violent juvenile offenders. In R. Loeber & D. P. Farrington (Eds.), *Serious and violent juvenile offenders: Risk factors and successful interventions* (pp. 13–29). Thousand Oaks, CA: Sage.

Lyman, R. D., & Campbell, N. R. (1996). Evaluating the effectiveness of residential and inpatient treatment. In R. D. Lyman & N. R. Campbell (Eds.), *Treating children and adolescents in residential and inpatient settings* (pp. 71–88). Thousand Oaks, CA: Sage.

Mann, B. J., Borduin, C. M., Henggeler, S. W., & Blaske, D. M. (1990). An investigation of systemic conceptualizations of parent-child coalitions and symptom change. *Journal of Consulting and Clinical Psychology, 58*(3), 336–344.

Mayer, J. P., Gensheimer, L. K., Davidson, W. S., & Gottschalk, R. (1986). Social learning treatment within juvenile justice: A meta-analysis of impact in the natural environment. In S. J. Apter & A. P. Goldstein (Eds.), *Youth violence: Programs and prospects* (pp. 24–38). New York: Pergamon Press.

McGuire, J., & Priestley, P. (1995). Reviewing "what works": Past, present and future. In J. McGuire (Ed.), *What works: Reducing reoffending: Guidelines from research and practice* (pp. 3–34). Chichester, England: Wiley.

Meyers, J. C. (1994). Financing strategies to support innovations in service delivery to children. *Journal of Clinical Child Psychology, 23*, 7–12.

Miller, T. R., Cohen, M. A., & Rossman, S. B. (1993). Victim costs of violent crime and resulting injuries. *Health Affairs, 12*, 186–197.

Miller, T. R., Cohen, M. A., & Wiersema, B. (1996, January). The extent and costs of crime victimization: A new look. *National Institute of Justice Research Preview*, 1–2.

Minuchin, S. (1974). *Families and family therapy*. Cambridge, MA: Harvard University Press.

Moffitt, T. E. (1993). Adolescence-limited and life-course-persistent antisocial behavior: A developmental taxonomy. *Psychological Review, 100*(4), 674–701.

Moncher, F. J., & Prinz, R. J. (1991). Treatment fidelity in outcome studies. *Clinical Psychology Review, 11*, 247–266.

Odell, B. N. (1974). Accelerating entry into the opportunity structure: A sociologically based treatment for delinquent youth. *Sociology and Social Research, 58*(3), 312–317.

O'Donnell, C. R. (1992). The interplay of theory and practice in delinquency prevention: From behavior modification to activity settings. In J. McCord & R. E. Tremblay (Eds.), *Preventing antisocial behavior: Interventions from birth through adolescence* (pp. 209–232). New York: Guilford Press.

O'Donnell, C. R., Lydgate, T., & Fo, W. S. O. (1979). The buddy system: Review and follow-up. *Child Behavior Therapy, 1*(2), 161–169.

Office of Technology Assessment. (1991). *Adolescent health: Background and the effectiveness of selected prevention and treatment services* (Vol. 2, OTA Publication No. OTA-H-468). Washington, DC: U.S. Government Printing Office.

Parsons, B. V., & Alexander, J. F. (1973). Short-term family intervention: A therapy outcome study. *Journal of Consulting and Clinical Psychology, 41*(2), 195–201.

Patterson, G. R., Capaldi, D., & Bank, L. (1991). An early starter model for predicting delinquency. In D. J. Pepler & K. H. Rubin (Eds.), *The development and treatment of childhood aggression* (pp. 139–168). Hillsdale, NJ: Erlbaum.

Patterson, G. R., & Chamberlain, P. (1988). Treatment process: A problem at three levels. In L. Wynne (Ed.), *State of the art in family therapy research: Controversies and recommendations* (pp. 189–223). New York: Family Process Press.

Patterson, G. R., & Dishion, T. J. (1985). Contributions of families and peers to delinquency. *Criminology, 23*(1), 63–79.

Patterson, G. R., & Forgatch, M. S. (1985). Therapist behavior as a determinant for client noncompliance: A paradox for the behavior modifier. *Journal of Consulting and Clinical Psychology, 53*(6), 846–851.

Reid, W. J., & Hanrahan, P. (1981). The effectiveness of social work: Recent evidence. In E. M. Goldberg & N. Connelly (Eds.), *Evaluative research in social care* (pp. 9–20). London: Heinemann Educational Books.

Resnick, H. S., Acierno, R., & Kilpatrick, D. G. (1997). Health impact of interpersonal violence: 2. Medical and mental health outcomes. *Behavioral Medicine, 23*(2), 65–78.

Santisteban, D. A., Szapocznik, J., Perez-Vidal, A., Kurtines, W. M., Murray, E. J., & LaPerriere, A. (1996). Efficacy of intervention for engaging youth and families into treatment and some variables that may contribute to differential effectiveness. *Journal of Family Psychology, 10*(1), 35–44.

Schoenwald, S. K. (1998). *Multisystemic therapy consultation manual.* Charleston, SC: MST Institute.

Schoenwald, S. K., Ward, D. M., Henggeler, S. W., Pickrel, S. G., & Patel, M. (1996). Multisystemic therapy treatment of substance abusing or dependent adolescent offenders: Costs of reducing incarceration, inpatient, and residential placement. *Journal of Child and Family Studies, 5*(4), 431–444.

Schoenwald, S. K., Ward, D. M., Henggeler, S. W., & Rowland, M. D. (2000). MST vs. hospitalization for crisis stabilization of youth: Placement outcomes 4 months post-referral. *Mental Health Services Research, 2,* 3–12.

Schulte, D., Kunzel, R., Pepping, G., & Schulte-Bahrenberg, T. (1992). Tailormade versus standardized therapy of phobic patients. *Advances in Behaviour Research and Therapy, 14,* 67–92.

Sheldon, B. (1994). Social work effectiveness research: Implications for probation and juvenile justice services. *Howard Journal, 33*(3), 218–235.

Shirk, S. R., & Russell, R. L. (1996). *Change processes in child psychotherapy: Revitalizing treatment and research.* New York: Guilford Press.

Shore, M. F. (1972). Youth and jobs: Educational, vocational, and mental health aspects. *Journal of Youth and Adolescence, 1*(4), 315–323.

Shore, M. F., & Massimo, J. L. (1966). Comprehensive vocationally oriented psychotherapy for adolescent delinquent boys: A follow-up study. *Ameri-*

can *Journal of Orthopsychiatry, 36,* 609–615.

Shore, M. F., & Massimo, J. L. (1979). Fifteen years after treatment: A follow-up study of comprehensive vocationally-oriented psychotherapy. *American Journal of Orthopsychiatry, 49*(2), 240–245.

Simcha-Fagan, O., & Schwartz, J. E. (1986). Neighborhood and delinquency: An assessment of contextual effects. *Criminology, 24*(4), 667–703.

Szapocznik, J., Kurtines, W., Santisteban, D. A., & Rio, A. T. (1990). Interplay of advances between theory, research, and application in treatment interventions aimed at behavior problem children and adolescents. *Journal of Consulting and Clinical Psychology, 58*(6), 696–703.

Szapocznik, J., Perez-Vidal, A., Brickman, A. L., Foote, F. H., Santisteban, D., Hervis, O., & Kurtines, W. M. (1988). Engaging adolescent drug abusers and their families in treatment: A strategic structural systems approach. *Journal of Consulting and Clinical Psychology, 56*(4), 552–557.

U.S. Bureau of the Census. (1997). *Statistical abstract of the United States.* Washington, DC: U.S. Government Printing Office.

Wadden, T. A., Stunkard, A. J., Rich, L., Rubin, C. J., Sweidel, G., & McKinney, S. (1990). Obesity in Black adolescent girls: A controlled clinical trial of treatment by diet, behavior modification, and parental support. *Pediatrics, 85*(3), 345–352.

Wahler, R. G. (1980). The insular mother: Her problems in parent-child treatment. *Journal of Applied Behavior Analysis, 13,* 207–219.

Wahler, R. G., Leske, G., & Rogers, E. S. (1979). The insular family: A deviance support system for oppositional children. In L. A. Hamerlynck (Ed.), *Behavioral systems for the developmentally disabled: I. School and family environments* (pp. 102–127). New York: Brunner/Mazel.

Walter, T. L., & Mills, C. M. (1980). A behavioral-employment intervention program for reducing juvenile delinquency. In R. R. Ross & P. Gendreau (Eds.), *Effective correctional treatment* (pp. 187–200). Toronto: Butterworth.

Washington State Institute for Public Policy. (1998). *Watching the bottom line: Cost-effective interventions for reducing crime in Washington.* Olympia, WA: Evergreen State College.

Weiss, B., & Weisz, J. R. (1995). Relative effectiveness of behavioral versus nonbehavioral child psychotherapy. *Journal of Consulting and Clinical Psychology, 63*(2), 317–320.

Weisz, J. (1991). Effectiveness of psychotherapy with children and adolescents: Controlled studies versus clinic data. In A. Algarin & R. M. Friedman (Eds.), *A system of care for children's mental health: Building a research base* (pp. 21–39). Tampa: Florida Mental Health Institute.

Weisz, J. R., Bahr, W., & Donenberg, G. R. (1992). The lab versus the clinic: Effects of child and adolescent psychotherapy. *American Psychologist, 47*(12), 1578–1585.

Weisz, J. R., Donenberg, G. R., Han, S. S., & Kauneckis, D. (1995). Child and adolescent psychotherapy outcomes in experiments versus clinics: Why the disparity? *Journal of Abnormal Child Psychology, 23*(1), 83–106.

Weisz, J. R., Donenberg, G. R., Han, S. S., & Weiss, B. (1995). Bridging the gap between laboratory and clinic in child and adolescent psychotherapy. *Journal of Consulting and Clinical Psychology, 63*(5), 688–701.

Weisz, J. R., & Weiss, B. (1987). Effectiveness of psychotherapy with children and adolescents: A meta-analysis for clinicians. *Journal of Consulting and Clinical Psychology, 55,* 542–549.

Weisz, J. R., Weiss, B., Han, S. S., Granger, D. A., & Morton, T. (1995). Effects of psychotherapy with children and adolescents revisited: A meta-analysis of treatment outcome studies. *Psychological Bulletin, 117*(3), 450–468.

Weisz, J. R., Weiss, B., & Langmeyer, D. B. (1987). Giving up on child psychotherapy: Who drops out? *Journal of Consulting and Clinical Psychology, 55*(6), 916–918.

Weisz, J. R., Weiss, B., & Langmeyer, D. B. (1989). On dropouts and refusers in child psychotherapy: Reply to Garfield. *Journal of Consulting and Clinical Psychology, 57*(1), 170–171.

Whitehead, J. T., & Lab, S. P. (1989). A meta-analysis of juvenile correctional treatment. *Journal of Research in Crime and Delinquency, 26*(3), 276–295.

Wierzbicki, M., & Pekarik, G. (1993). A meta-analysis of psychotherapy dropout. *Professional Psychology: Research and Practice, 24*(2), 190–195.

Yeaton, W. H., & Sechrest, L. (1981). Critical dimensions in the choice and maintenance of successful treatments: Strength, integrity, and effectiveness. *Journal of Consulting and Clinical Psychology, 49*(2), 156–167.

16

PAMELA J. BACHANAS
NADINE J. KASLOW

Depressive Disorders

Historically, much controversy has surrounded the topic of child and adolescent depression, particularly with regard to the existence and nature of the disorder (Kaslow, Morris, & Rehm, 1998). More recently, a consensus has emerged in the field that depressive disorders exist in children and that depression in youth represents a form of psychopathology that merits attention and intervention. Multiple views on the etiology, conceptualization, diagnosis, and treatment of the disorder can be found in the current literature. In this chapter, we begin by presenting a psychiatric perspective on the clinical characteristics of the disorder, as this perspective is the dominant one in the field. However, we believe that it is essential that this psychiatric perspective be integrated with a developmental psychopathology viewpoint. Next, we turn our attention to the epidemiology of depressive disorders in youth. Unfortunately, there is much less information on the prevalence and incidence of depressive disorders in youth than there is on other childhood disorders or on adult disorders. Following this is a brief summary of the developmental precursors and consequences of the disorder from a psychosocial perspective. A discussion of empirically supported psychosocial intervention and prevention programs for depressed children and adolescents follows. We conclude with some comments regarding the challenges associated with transferring these empirically supported intervention models into a broad array of community settings with diverse populations.

Clinical Characteristics

Several studies have shown that, when proper assessment and standardized diagnostic criteria are applied, the symptoms of clinical depression in children and adolescents are similar but not identical to those manifested by depressed adults (Birmaher, Ryan, & Williamson, 1996; Ryan et al., 1987). Thus we begin our discussion of the clinical characteristics of the primary depressive disorder diagnoses according to the *Diagnostic and Statistical Manual of Mental Disorders* (*DSM-IV*; American Psychiatric Association, 1994). This is followed by a review of the symptoms and conditions that commonly co-occur with depression in youth.

Major Depressive Disorder

According to the *DSM-IV*, major depressive disorder (MDD) in children and adolescents is characterized by the presence of five or more of the following symptoms for a two-week period: depressed or irritable mood; anhedonia; significant weight loss or gain; sleep disturbance; psychomotor retardation or agitation; fatigue or loss of energy; feelings of worthlessness or inappropriate guilt; concentration difficulties or indecisiveness; and thoughts of death or suicide. At least one of the symptoms must be either depressed mood, irritability, or anhedonia, and these symptoms must represent a change from previous functioning and cause distress or impairment. According to the *DSM-IV*, there are some characteristic symptoms of MDD that change with age — most notably, irritability, somatic complaints, and social withdrawal are particularly common in children, whereas psychomotor retardation, hypersomnia, and delusions are less common in prepuberty than in adolescence or adulthood.

Dysthymic Disorder

Dysthymic disorder (DD) in children and adolescents is characterized by chronically depressed or irritable mood, plus two or more of the following symptoms: appetite disturbance; sleep disturbance; decreased energy; low self-esteem; concentration problems; and feelings of helplessness. The duration of these symptoms need only be one year (rather than two years, as in adults) to make the diagnosis of DD in children and adolescents.

Adjustment Disorder with Depressed Mood

Adjustment disorder with depressed mood (ADDM), characterized by depressive symptoms that reflect a maladaptive reaction to an identifiable psychosocial stressor, must occur within three months of the onset of the stressor and may not last for more than six months following the resolution of the stressor. ADDM is diagnosed when a child's symptoms do not meet criteria for MDD or DD but are of significant concern to warrant treatment.

Comorbidity

Epidemiological studies have shown high rates of comorbidity in children and adolescents with MDD, with rates of comorbidity for anxiety disorders between 20% and 70%, for disruptive disorders (conduct, oppositional defiant, and attention deficit) between 10% and 50%, and for substance use approximately 25% (Angold & Costello, 1993; Birmaher, Ryan, & Williamson, 1996; Kashani et al., 1987). In addition, MDD often co-occurs with eating disorders, particularly in adolescents (Rhode, Lewinsohn, & Seeley, 1991). Data reveal that approximately 70% of youngsters with early-onset DD have a superimposed MDD and that 50% have other preexisting psychiatric disorders, including anxiety disorders (40%), conduct disorders (30%), attention-deficit/hyperactivity disorder (24%), and elimination disorders (15%; Kovacs & Gatsonis, 1994). In general, comorbid diagnoses appear to influence the duration of the depressive episode, suicide attempts or behaviors, functional outcome, response to treatment, and utilization of mental health services (Birmaher, Ryan, Williamson, Brent, Kaufman, et al., 1996; Kovacs, Goldston, & Gatsonis, 1993).

Epidemiology

Prevalence Rates

The prevalence of depression varies depending on the age, gender, and sociocultural background of the child; the specific diagnostic category; the nature of the population (e.g., clinical versus community); the informant (e.g., child, parent, teacher, clinician); the method of data collection (e.g., reports by child, parent, teacher, peer, clinician); and inconsistencies in sampling and measurement (Fleming & Offord, 1990; Mufson & Moreau, 1997). Prevalence rates for mood disorders in community samples range from 0.4% to 2.5% in children and between 0.4% and 8.3% in adolescents (Birmaher, Ryan, Williamson, Brent, Kaufman, et al., 1996). Prevalence rates range from 13% to 59% in clinical samples (Birmaher, Ryan, & Williamson, 1996). The lifetime prevalence rates of MDD in adolescents range from 15% to 20%, rates that are consistent with those reported among adults (Birmaher, Ryan, Williamson, Brent, Kaufman, et al., 1996). Epidemiological data on dysthymic disorders in youth is sparse; however, the extant data reveals a point prevalence rate from 0.6% to 1.7% in children and 1.6 to 8.0% in adolescents (Kashani et al., 1987; Lewinsohn, Clarke, Seeley, & Rhode, 1994).

Age

Rates of depressive disorders increase with age (Fleming & Offord, 1990). Depressive disorders in infants and preschoolers are rare or impossible to diagnose with the current criteria (Trad, 1987). Depressive conditions are more likely to begin to emerge in prepubertal youth, and prepubertal depression is associated with a strong genetic loading for depression (Weissman, Warner, Wickramaratne, & Prusoff, 1988). There is a threefold increase in the prevalence of depressive disorders between ages 6 and 11 and 12 and 16 (Fleming & Offord, 1990). An interplay of factors explains the age trends in depressive conditions, including measurement artifacts, attainment of puberty, decrease in protective factors and/or increase in risk factors, and an age-by-gender interaction (Harrington, 1993).

Gender

There are no consistent sex differences in rates of depression in prepubertal youth (Angold, 1988). However, by age 15, females are twice as likely as males to receive a depressive diagnosis, and this sex difference persists into adulthood (Nolen-Hoeksema & Girgus, 1994). Females are more likely than males to carry risk factors for depression even prior to early adolescence, but these risk factors lead to depression only in the light of the challenges that increase in frequency during early adolescence (Nolen-Hoeksema & Girgus, 1994). Risk factors include sex-role socialization patterns, cognitive styles and coping patterns, number and nature of stresses encountered in early adolescence, and differential maladaptive behavioral expressions of distress (Petersen et al., 1993). Although some argue that differential hormonal changes associated with puberty contribute to the emergence of sex differences (Brooks-Gunn & Warren, 1989), others refute this assertion (Angold & Rutter, 1992).

Clinical Course

Depressive episodes in children and adolescents tend to be of relatively long duration, with protracted time to recovery (Hanna, 1992). Specifically, only 50% of youth recover from a depressive episode within one year. Further, depressive disorders tend to recur, and the greater number of prior episodes, the greater the likelihood of future episodes of mood disorders in childhood, adolescence, and adulthood (Hanna, 1992; Harrington, 1992). In a longitudinal nosologic study of the natural history of depressive conditions, Kovacs (1989) found that the age of onset for MDD was 8–14, whereas DD and ADDM showed average age of onset to be 6–13 and 8–12 years of age, respectively. Average length of episode for ADDM, MDD, and DD are six months, eight months, and three years, respectively. Although children with ADDM appear to have a reasonably good short-term prognosis, those with MDD and DD are at significant risk in later childhood, adolescence, and adulthood for future psychiatric difficulties (e.g., mood disorders, disruptive behavior disorders, suicidal behavior), psychosocial impairments (low self-esteem, interpersonal difficulties) and physical health problems (Birmaher, Ryan, Williamson, Brent, Kaufman, et al., 1996; Fleming, Boyle, & Offord, 1993; Harrington, 1992; Kandel & Davies, 1986; Kovacs, Aksikal, Gastonis, & Parrone, 1994; McCauley & Myers, 1992; Rao et al., 1995). Factors that influence the course of depressive disorders include parental mood disorders (Warner, Weissman, Fendrich, Wickramaratne, & Moreau, 1992), family environment, comorbid psychiatric disorders, age, and sex (Harrington, 1992; McCauley et al., 1993). It is important to note, however, that not all individuals with a history of depressive episodes during childhood or adolescence experience recurrent bouts of depression, and a sizable number have good social adjustment (Rao et al., 1995).

Developmental Precursors and Consequences

A biopsychosocial model can be used to classify the major developmental precursors and consequences of depression in youth. Biological variables include sleep and neuroendocrine abnormalities. Psychological factors include cognitive styles and affective functioning. Social factors include family functioning, peer relations, and the sociocultural context. Because this chapter focuses on psychosocial interventions, we will review only the psychological and social precursors and consequences of youth depression. However, the reader is referred to the work of Emslie, Weinberg, Kennard, and Kowatch (1994) for a discussion of the neurobiological aspects of depression in children and adolescents.

Psychological Factors

AFFECTIVE FUNCTIONING. In the affective domain, depressed youth verbalize a pattern of emotional experiences similar to those reported by depressed adults. Specifically, depressed children and adolescents report high levels of sadness, anger, self-directed hostility, and shame (Blumberg & Izard, 1985). In nonverbal domains, depressed youth, particularly those in an inpatient psychiatric service, show slow activity (latency, gestures, self-movements), flat affect (intonation, facial expressiveness), and outward signs of sadness (e.g., tearfulness; Kazdin, Sherick, Esveldt-Dawson, & Racurello, 1985). Research also reveals that depressed youth exhibit affect regulation difficulties; they utilize fewer and more maladaptive emotion regulation strategies (e.g., withdrawal and aggression) than their nondepressed peers (Garber, Braafladt, & Zeman, 1991).

COGNITIVE STYLE. Depression has also been associated with a negative cognitive style. Similar to their adult counterparts, depressed youth often have low self-esteem, high self-criticism, significant cognitive distortions (e.g., negative view of self, world, and future), impairments in information processing (e.g., using dysfunctional schemas to negatively interpret their experiences and evaluate their behavior), a feeling of lack of control over negative events (helplessness), and a sense of hopelessness about their future (Garber & Hilsman, 1992; Kaslow, Brown, & Mee, 1994). Youth who are exposed to stressful life events and who have negative styles of interpreting and coping with stress are at particularly high risk for developing depressive symptoms (Garber & Hilsman, 1992).

Social Factors

FAMILY FUNCTIONING. Having a depressed parent places children at increased risk for the development of depression and other psychiatric disorders. Children of depressed parents are three times more likely to have an episode of MDD during their lifetime and are at high risk for other behavioral disturbances (e.g., school problems, suicidal behavior; Birmaher, Ryan, & Williamson, 1996; Weissman et al., 1987). Parental loss through death is another well-documented family risk factor for depression in adolescence, particularly for girls (Wells, Deykin, & Klerman, 1985).

The quality of familial relationships has been associated with depression in youth (Puig-Antich et al., 1993). Specifically, family relational patterns associated with depressive symptoms in youth include: insecure parent-child attachment, low levels of family cohesion and support, inappropriate levels of family control, high levels of conflict and poor conflict resolution skills, difficulties with affect regulation, dysfunctional communication patterns, and a poor fit between child temperament and family interaction style (Kaslow, Deering, & Ash, 1996; Kaslow et al., 1998).

PEER RELATIONS.   Depressed children and adolescents often experience impairments in their social relationships and school functioning. For example, depressed children have fewer "best" friendships and a lower ability to make and maintain positive peer relationships, are more often teased, and are rated by their peers as having more negative social behaviors than their nondepressed counterparts (Puig-Antich et al., 1985a; Rudolph, Hammen, & Burge, 1994). These interpersonal difficulties often persist even after remission of a depressive episode (Puig-Antich et al., 1985b). Depressed youth also report experiencing more stressful life events than their nondepressed peers and are exposed to high levels of stress prior to becoming depressed (Birmaher, Ryan, & Williamson, 1996; Williamson et al., 1998).

SOCIOCULTURAL CONTEXT.   Data regarding the impact of sociocultural variables on the epidemiology of depressive disorders is relatively sparse. Although some studies reveal an inverse relation between depressive symptoms and social class, other research does not confirm such an association (Angold, 1988; Harrington, 1993). However, some data suggest that low socioeconomic status predicts recurrence of major depressive episodes in adolescence and adulthood (Rao et al., 1995). Similarly, no consistent picture has emerged that links ethnicity and the epidemiology of depressive conditions in childhood. For example, some studies report higher rates of depressive disorders in young African American males as opposed to their Caucasian counterparts, whereas others indicate no effect of race (Harrington, 1993).

Empirically Supported Treatments

Intervention research literature on child and adolescent mood disorders has lagged behind the treatment literature both of other childhood disorders and of adult depression. Historically, the intervention literature has been characterized by theoretical writings, case reports, and small-scale single-participant designs. Interventions for depressed youth have included psychodynamic, cognitive-behavioral, interpersonal, group, and family approaches. Only recently have empirically based outcome studies been conducted that have met some of the criteria for well-established or probably efficacious interventions (Chambless et al., 1996). For an intervention to be deemed well established, at least two good between-group design experiments must demonstrate efficacy in one of the following ways: (1) superiority to pill or psychological placebo or to another treatment; or (2) equivalency with an already established treatment in experiments with adequate statistical power ($n \geq 30$/group). The experiments must be conducted in accordance with a treatment manual, sample characteristics must be detailed, and at least two different investigators or investigatory teams must demonstrate intervention effects. For an intervention to be classified as probably efficacious, either two experiments must demonstrate that the intervention is more effective than a wait-list condition or one or more experiments must meet all criteria for a well-established treatment except for the requirement that treatment effects be shown by two different research teams.

This section reviews intervention studies conducted with depressed children and adolescents that are group designs, that incorporate treatment manuals or clearly defined intervention techniques, and that provide pre- and postintervention data. Few of the published studies to date meet the criteria for well-established or probably efficacious interventions (Kaslow & Thompson, 1998). We include both psychosocial treatment outcome studies and prevention studies that target "at-risk" children based on elevated self-reported levels of depressive symptoms. We conclude this section with a brief description of pharmacological interventions.

Cognitive-Behavioral Interventions

Given the widespread support for cognitive-behavioral interventions with depressed adults, child clinicians and researchers have turned their attention to examining cognitive-behavioral strategies for depressed youth from a developmentally informed perspective. Although these studies employ relatively small samples, the findings are quite promising. When adapting adult cognitive-behavioral interventions to children, several developmental modifications must be incorporated into the intervention programs. First, given that children's memory and attentional capacities are limited, they may benefit from short and repetitive treatment sessions. Second, because of children's limited verbal capacities, they may be engaged most effectively when games, activities, and stories are incorporated into the treatment protocols. Third, because children are dependent on and influenced by their families, family involvement in treatment may be beneficial and even necessary (Kaslow & Racusin, 1994).

There are many similarities among the cognitive-behavioral intervention programs for depressed youth, and many utilize similar intervention strategies. A description of the cognitive-behavioral techniques frequently used in these interventions is provided in Table 16.1. In the following section, we briefly review empirically supported cognitive-behavioral interventions for depressed children and depressed adolescents, conclude with our perspective on which interventions are most likely to be effective, and offer strategies that can be implemented in many clinical settings.

INTERVENTIONS WITH CHILDREN. The first empirical investigation of treatment for depressed children compared the efficacy of 10-session role-play, cognitive-restructuring, attention-placebo, and waiting-list conditions for fifth- and sixth-graders with elevated self-reported depression scores and teacher referrals (Butler, Miezitis, Friedman, & Cole, 1980). This study was undertaken in an elementary school; the interventions were conducted by graduate students in applied psychology. The role-play intervention, devised for this study, targeted social problem-solving training and rehearsal of social skills. In the cognitive-restructuring condition, influ-

TABLE 16.1   Descriptions of commonly used cognitive-behavioral techniques for treating child and adolescent depression (adapted from Stark, Swearer, Kurowski, Sommer, & Bowen, 1996).

Technique	Description
Activity scheduling	Purposeful scheduling of enjoyable and goal-directed activities.
Anger management strategies	Coaching on leaving the situation; going to do something enjoyable; using words rather than actions to express anger; doing something physical and demanding, such as exercise; using relaxation techniques to reduce physical tension.
Problem-solving strategies	Identifying and defining the problem; using positive self-talk to counter pessimism and foster motivation; generating alternative solutions; using consequential thinking (e.g., predicting the likely outcomes for each possible solution); reviewing possible solutions, choosing one, and enacting the plan; evaluating progress toward solving the problem.
Altering faulty information processing	Redirecting attention from negative thoughts and feelings to more pleasant emotions and positive thoughts; using self-monitoring of positive events and pleasant emotions.
Altering automatic thoughts	Drawing awareness to the tendency to think negatively; therapist modeling more adaptive thoughts to replace child's negative thoughts and rehearsing them with the child.
Changing dysfunctional schema	Using cognitive restructuring techniques such as evaluating the evidence for the maladaptive thought, considering alternative interpretations, thinking about what really would happen if the undesirable event occurred (e.g., decatastrophizing).
Changing negative self-evaluations	Using cognitive restructuring techniques to help children more realistically and reasonably evaluate their performances, possessions, and personal qualities.
Behavioral strategies	Role-playing examples and therapist modeling of these techniques.

enced by the work of Beck, Rush, Shaw, and Emery (1979) and of Ellis (1962), depressive cognitive patterns were identified, and the children were taught to develop more adaptive cognitions. Although both experimental conditions were effective, children in the role-play group showed comparatively fewer self-reported depressive symptoms and better functioning in the classroom. No follow-up was conducted.

Stark, Reynolds, and Kaslow (1987) compared 12-session group interventions of self-control therapy (based on the work of Rehm, 1977), behavioral problem-solving therapy (based on the work of Lewinsohn, 1974), and a waiting-list control condition for fourth- through sixth-graders with elevated self-reported depression scores.

This study was implemented in a school setting; interventions were led by graduate students and postdoctoral fellows in clinical and school psychology. The self-control groups were taught adaptive self-monitoring, self-evaluating, self-consequating, and appropriate causal attributions. The behavioral problem-solving group consisted of education, self-monitoring of pleasant events, and group problem-solving directed toward improving social behavior. Postintervention and eight-week follow-up assessments found that children in both active interventions reported a reduction of depressive symptoms; participants on the waiting list reported minimal change.

In a subsequent study in which the primary treatment intervention was based on a combination of Rehm's (1997) self-control model and Lewinsohn's (1974) behavioral model, Stark, Rouse, and Livingston (1991) evaluated self-control therapy for fourth-through seventh-graders with high levels of depressive symptoms. This cognitive-behavioral treatment, consisting of 24 to 26 sessions and conducted in a school setting by graduate students in school psychology, included self-control and social skills training, cognitive restructuring, and problem-solving techniques. This experimental intervention was compared with a traditional counseling condition designed to control for nonspecific elements of therapy. Both conditions incorporated monthly family contacts. At postintervention and seven-month follow-up, both groups revealed decreased self-reported depression on a paper-and-pencil measure. Interestingly, however, at postintervention, graduate students who were blind to treatment condition rated children in the cognitive-behavioral group as more improved on a semistructured interview than youth in the counseling condition. Children in the cognitive-behavioral intervention also reported fewer depressive cognitions at postintervention than their peers in the counseling condition. These data suggest that interventions that target cognitions may enhance adaptive cognitive processing more than interventions not designed to address directly dysfunctional cognitions.

Rehm and Sharp (1996) examined a psychoeducational intervention based on self-control theory in a large, urban multicultural school setting. The sample consisted of fourth- and fifth-graders who were nominated by school personnel based on descriptions of depressed behavior and who had elevated depressive symptom scores. The intervention was conducted by school psychology interns and graduate students in clinical and counseling psychology. At postintervention, there were significant decreases in self-reported depressive symptoms, marked improvements in social skills, and more adaptive attributional styles. No follow-up data are reported.

Liddle and Spence (1990) randomly assigned 7- to 11-year-olds with elevated depressive symptoms on self-report measures and a diagnostic interview to one of three groups for eight weeks: a social-competence training group, an attention-placebo control group, and a no-treatment control group. This study was conducted in private Catholic schools by postdoctoral fellows in clinical psychology. The social-competence training condition, based on a combination of cognitive and behavioral models, included social skills training, interpersonal problem-solving techniques, and cognitive restructuring regarding social situations. Although all groups reported fewer depressive symptoms at postintervention and three-month follow-up, no differential treatment effects were found and no changes in social competence were revealed.

Kahn, Kehle, Jenson, and Clark (1990) compared three psychoeducational group interventions (cognitive-behavioral, relaxation training, self-modeling) and a wait-list control group for 10–14-year-olds selected on the basis of self- and parent reports and clinical interviews. These psychoeducational groups met in a large suburban middle school and were led by a school psychologist or school counselor. The cognitive-behavioral intervention incorporated the Coping with Depression course of Lewinsohn, Antonuccio, Steinmetz, and Teri (1984), a relaxation training program similar to that used by Reynolds and Coats (1986), and a self-modeling approach in which individuals repeatedly view videotapes of themselves exhibiting only positive behaviors (Dowrick, 1983). Decreases in depressive symptoms and improved self-esteem were noted in children in all three experimental conditions relative to the wait-list control group. Improvements were maintained at one-month follow-up. There were no significant differences between the experimental conditions.

Weisz, Thurber, Sweeney, Proffitt, and LeGagnoux (1997) conducted an eight-session cognitive-behavioral program, entitled the Primary and Secondary Control Enhancement Training Program, with third- to sixth-grade elementary school students with elevated depression scores. The treatment program focused on (1) primary control (changing objective conditions to fit one's wishes; e.g., through activity selection and goal attainment) and (2) secondary control (changing oneself to buffer the impact of objective conditions; e.g., altering depressogenic thinking, practicing mood-enhancing cognitions). The treatment program took place at the children's school and was conducted by graduate students in clinical psychology. The experimental group showed greater reductions in depressive symptoms than the control group, and the treatment effects were maintained at nine-month follow-up.

Taken together, these studies show that cognitive-behavioral intervention approaches are efficacious in ameliorating depressive symptoms in children. In addition, the strategies employed by Stark and colleagues appear to have the strongest empirical support, as they meet criteria for "probably efficacious treatments" given the multiple treatment outcome studies demonstrating effectiveness (Kaslow & Thompson, 1998). Further, Stark and coworkers (1996) have described their intervention techniques in detail, making them available to clinicians to modify and adapt to clinic populations and settings as needed. It is also possible to incorporate their intervention strategies into an individual or family therapy format; however, the effectiveness of this has not yet been empirically tested. Although there appears to be strong evidence for the efficacy of cognitive-behavioral interventions for depressed children, there are several limitations to these studies that should be noted. All of the studies reviewed herein were conducted with nonreferred children in nonclinical settings, which may affect their generalizability to clinic populations in community settings. In addition, there are no data regarding which specific component(s) of these multifaceted interventions may be most beneficial for which problems. Despite these limitations, these treatment programs offer promising results and provide effective strategies for intervening with depressed children.

INTERVENTIONS WITH ADOLESCENTS.   Similar to the treatment literature for depressed children, intervention studies with depressed adolescents have primarily investigated the effectiveness of cognitive-behavioral strategies. It is important to note, however, that developmental transitions occur in adolescence which must be taken into account when implementing intervention programs. Specifically, adolescence is characterized by the transition from concrete to formal operational thought and the capacity for metacognition. In addition, biological, psychological, and social developmental changes occur during puberty. Consequently, treatment approaches must consider the adolescent's cognitive and internal psychological processes, as well as his or her psychosocial environment and relationships (e.g., peers, family, social activities). A review of the empirically supported cognitive-behavioral treatment outcome studies with adolescents follows.

Reynolds and Coats (1986) conducted the first treatment outcome study of adolescent depression. Nonreferred high school students who self-reported high levels of depressive symptoms were assigned randomly to 10 sessions of self-control therapy akin to the treatment delineated by Rehm (1997), to 10 sessions of relaxation training in accord with the strategies articulated by Lewinsohn (1974), or to a wait-list control condition. All sessions were conducted in the high school and were led by graduate students in school psychology. Posttreatment and five-week follow-up results revealed that both experimental conditions were more effective than the control condition in reducing depression and anxiety and enhancing academic self-concept. No differences were found between the active treatment conditions.

Fine, Forth, Gilbert, and Haley (1991) compared a 12-week social skills training group with a therapeutic support group for psychiatric outpatient adolescents who met diagnostic criteria for major depressive disorder or dysthymic disorder. Both groups were conducted by a male-female cotherapy dyad that included one experienced and one less experienced mental health professional (psychiatrist, psychologist, social worker, psychiatric nurse). The social skills groups, based on Lewinsohn's social skills model, taught specific skills, including recognizing feelings, assertiveness, communication skills, and social problem solving. In the therapeutic support groups, discussions of common concerns were facilitated and adaptive ways to address difficult situations were addressed. At posttreatment, youth in the support groups had less clinical depression and higher self-concepts than those in the social skills groups. At nine-month follow-up, between-group differences were no longer evident; adolescents in the support groups maintained their gains and those youth who had participated in the social skills group continued to improve.

The most sophisticated cognitive-behavioral treatment outcome study has been conducted by Lewinsohn, Clarke, Hops, and Andrews (1990) with depressed adolescents in schools. These interventions were led by graduate students in clinical, counseling, or educational psychology or social work. Lewinsohn and colleagues (1990) assigned high school students aged 14–18 with *DSM-IV* depressive disorders to one of three groups: a 14-session cognitive-behavioral group treatment for the adolescent only; a group in which concurrent cognitive-behavioral treatment was given to the depressed adolescent and his or her parents for 7 sessions, and a wait-list control group. The cognitive-behavioral intervention, based on the Coping with Depression course for adults, was adapted to address the concerns and competencies of adolescents and focused on experiential learning and skills training (increasing pleasant activities, relaxing, controlling depressive thoughts, improving social interaction and communication, and practicing negotiation and conflict resolution skills). The seven-session complementary parent intervention was aimed at enhancing parents' capacity to reinforce and promote their adolescent's adaptive changes to increase the likelihood that treatment effects would be maintained and generalized. Posttherapy, fewer adolescents in the active treatment groups met criteria for depression, and they showed greater reductions in self-reported depressive and anxious symptoms and maladaptive cognitions and more involvement in positive events compared with youth in the wait-list condition. Gains were maintained at two-year follow-up. Although a trend indicated that the adolescent-and-parent condition was more effective than the adolescent-only condition, only a few between-group differences reached statistical significance.

Lewinsohn, Clarke, Rhode, Hops, and Seeley (1996) replicated the Lewinsohn et al. (1990) study using the Coping with Depression course with two modifications: skills training was presented throughout the course and a follow-up condition was added. Specifically, one third of adolescents received booster sessions every four months for two years; one third were assessed every four months but received no booster sessions; and one third were assessed annually with no booster sessions. Recovery rates posttreatment were superior in both treatment groups compared with the wait-list control; however, again the two treatment groups did not significantly differ. With regard to the impact of the maintenance booster program on depression recurrence rates following treatment-mediated recovery, the booster sessions did not significantly prevent recurrence of MDD. However, they were associated with significantly faster depression recovery among participants who had not fully recovered from their index depressive episode by the end of the acute treatment phase (Clarke, Rhode, Lewinsohn, Hops, & Seeley, 1999). These findings emphasize the importance of following some individuals for ongoing treatment beyond the time limits specified by the research study.

Brent and colleagues (1997) compared cognitive-behavioral therapy, systematic-behavioral family therapy, and nondirective supportive treatment with teens (aged 13–18) who met diagnostic criteria for MDD. Participants received 12 to 16 sessions of therapy over three to four months provided by therapists with master's degrees in a clinic setting. All groups showed equivalent improvement on depressive diagnoses; however, participants in the cognitive-behavioral therapy condition showed a lower rate of MDD at the end of treatment and a higher rate of remission compared with those in the systematic-behavioral family therapy and nondirective supportive therapy conditions. In addition, decreases in suicidality were greatest for the cognitive-behavioral therapy and family therapy groups. Youth who did not evidence significant improvements in response to the interventions were those with a clinical referral source, comorbid anxiety disorder, high level of cognitive distortion, and hopelessness (Brent et al., 1998). Conversely, rapid responders to these interventions, compared with intermediate responders and initial nonresponders, had had less severe MDD at the outset of treatment. No between-group differences were noted with regard to comorbid conditions, severity of cognitive distortion, suicidal ideation, or social class (Renaud et al., 1998). In a subsequent follow-up study, Brent, Kolka, Birmaher, Baugher, and Bridge (1999) found that more than half of the adolescents in the study required additional treatment beyond that provided in the clinical trial. Severity of depressive symptomatology and comorbid disorders were predictors of need for additional treatment.

The previously cited studies offer promising evidence that cognitive-behavioral intervention programs are effective in reducing depressive symptomatology in adolescents. Several of the studies reviewed have the advantage of having been conducted with clinic-referred teens in mental health settings, thereby more closely resembling the population and setting most clinicians will encounter. Further, several of the treatment programs (e.g., Clarke et al., 1999, and Brent et al., 1999) produced long-term follow-up data, which has provided critical information on the importance of going beyond prepackaged treatment programs with a limited number of sessions for fully treating the depression. This has been shown to be particularly important for teens who present with severe depressive symptomatology and comorbid diagnoses, which is how many teens in clinic and community settings will present. The intervention programs of Clarke and colleagues (1999) have obtained the most empirical support to date and appear to meet criteria as a "probably efficacious treatment" given the multiple treatment outcome studies reporting positive findings (Kaslow & Thompson, 1998). These clinician-researchers have also provided fairly detailed descriptions of their programs so that clinicians can modify and adapt their strategies as indicated (cf. Clarke & Lewinsohn, 1986). Similar to the literature on depressed children, the adolescent intervention studies do not offer data on which specific components or techniques are most effective in treating specific problems. However, overall, these treatment programs offer promising results of cognitive-behavioral strategies that address depressed teens' psychological and psychosocial issues.

Interpersonal/Family Interventions

As noted previously, some of the cognitive-behavioral intervention programs have incorporated a parent program (Lewinsohn et al., 1990, 1996; Stark et al., 1991), but there are limited data to support the enhanced efficacy of cognitive-behavioral interventions when parent involvement is included. Other studies have evaluated treatments that emphasize the role of interpersonal and family factors in depression, including: (1) interpersonal psychotherapy for depression and (2) family psychoeducational programs.

INTERPERSONAL THERAPY. Interpersonal therapy for adolescents (IPT-A; Mufson, Moreau, Weissman, & Klerman, 1993) was modified from interpersonal therapy for adults. This intervention is a brief, time-limited psychotherapy aimed at decreasing depressive symptomatology and improving interpersonal functioning by enhancing communication skills in significant relationships (Klerman, Weissman, Rounsaville, & Chevron, 1984). IPT was developed on the premise that regardless of what the underlying cause of the depression is, the depression is inextricably intertwined with the individual's interpersonal relationships.

IPT-A is a psychoeducational treatment approach designed for use with adolescents aged 12–18 with an acute-onset MDD. It uses a developmental perspective to address common interpersonal issues of adolescence, including age-appropriate independence from family of origin, authority and peer conflicts, and romantic relationships with peers. The therapeutic strategies include education, clarification of feelings and expectations, development of communication skills, and role playing.

After a 12-week open trial of individual interpersonal psychotherapy for clinically depressed adolescents in an outpatient psychiatric clinic, adolescents who were treated by a clinical child psychologist reported decreases in depressive symptoms, no longer met criteria for a depressive disorder, and evidenced improvements in other psychological symptoms and in physical distress (Mufson et al., 1994). IPT-A also appeared to improve overall social functioning. In a recent study of IPT-A with 32 clinic-referred adolescents who met criteria for MDD, Mufson, Weissman, Moreau, and Garfinkel (1999) found that teens who received IPT-A reported a greater decrease in depressive symptoms and greater improvement in overall social functioning, in functioning with friends, and in specific problem-solving skills compared with teens in the control group who received clinical monitoring.

FAMILY PSYCHOEDUCATION. Brent, Poling, McKain, and Baugher (1993) examined a two-hour psychoeducational program for parents of suicidal adolescents with mood disorders who were followed in an outpatient clinic. This psychoeducational program was led jointly by a psychiatrist and a social worker and emphasized knowledge and coping strategies (Poling, 1989). For some parents, attendance at this program was associated with a small increase in knowledge about mood disorders and a slight modification of dysfunctional beliefs about the etiology, course, and treatment of adolescent depression. No follow-up data are reported.

In sum, the limited data regarding interpersonal psychotherapy for depression in youth are promising. Given the dearth of empirical studies that focus on family interventions for depressed youth, despite data suggesting that family variables play a critical role in the development and maintenance of depression in youth, and given the fact that a number of investigators currently are undertaking systematic evaluation of family-oriented prevention programs (Brent et al., 1997; Brent et al., 1993; Diamond & Siqueland, 1995; Kaslow, Mintzer, Meadows, & Grabill, in press; Schwartz, Kaslow, Racusin, & Carton, 1998), it is premature to draw conclusions about the efficacy of this treatment approach. However, we feel these intervention strategies are worthy of attention by clinicians, as many therapists will address interpersonal and relationship issues with teens in individual therapy in clinic settings. Similarly, many parents of teens present to clinicians requesting family intervention. These strategies, although not extensively evaluated empirically, offer theoretically grounded and clinically relevant treatment techniques for intervening with depressed teens and their families. Further, they follow a specific treatment program that again offers intervention strategies clinicians can modify and adapt for use in their setting (cf. Mufson et al., 1993).

Prevention Programs

When devising and implementing intervention programs for depressed children and adolescents, we encourage consideration of the relatively new prevention literature. A number of the approaches used to treat depression in youth have been used in a preventative context. For the most part, these prevention efforts have been psychoeducational in nature, and most incorporate cognitive-behavioral interventions (Rehm & Sharp, 1996). Although many of these prevention programs have been conducted in school settings, some efforts that have targeted at-risk youth (e.g., children of depressed parents) have been undertaken in clinical settings. Some of the prevention efforts conducted to date have incorporated universal interventions delivered to all members of a population, whereas others have used targeted interventions delivered to a subgroup of high-risk youth (e.g., individuals with early signs of a mood disorder; children of depressed parents). Prevention trials for depression are recent, although a number of programs designed for youth following stressful events (e.g., divorce, bereavement) have implications for preventing depression (Asarnow, 1990). These programs have targeted children from first grade through high school. The major empirical prevention studies are discussed next.

PREVENTION PROGRAMS FOR YOUTH WITH ELEVATED DEPRESSIVE SYMPTOMS. Jaycox, Reivich, Gillham, and Seligman (1994) explored the efficacy of a group cognitive and social problem-solving program for 10- to 13-year-olds with elevated depressive symptoms and parental conflict. The cognitive component of the program was based on the work of Ellis (1962) and Beck et al. (1979). This study was conducted in suburban schools, and the preventive intervention was led by doctoral students in clinical psychology. Results revealed greater diminution of symptoms for youth in the experimental than control condition at postintervention and six-month follow-up. In a subsequent study, Gillham, Reivich, Jaycox, and Seligman (1995) assessed the same group of children over a two-year follow-up period. The investigators found that children in the prevention group reported fewer depressive symptoms through the two-year follow-up and that moderate to severe symptoms were reduced by half compared with children in the control group (Gillham et al., 1995).

Rice, Herman, and Petersen (1993) used a psychoeducational approach to teach adaptive cognitive and behavioral skills to seventh-graders in both rural (working class) and suburban (middle to upper middle class) school settings. The 16-session preventive intervention was based primarily on Clarke and Lewinsohn's (1986) Coping with Depression manual and the work of Goldstein, Sprafkin, Gershaw, and Klein (1980) on teaching prosocial skills. Participants in the preventive intervention reported increases in perceived coping ability and perceived control over challenging events, improved peer relationships, and enhanced family relationships, whereas no significant improvements were noted in those youth who did not receive the intervention. Additionally, whereas the preadolescents in the preventive intervention condition noted a decrease in negative life events, control participants revealed a notable increase in negative life events. No follow-up data were reported.

Clarke and colleagues (1995) compared a 15-session after-school preventive intervention program (a modification of the Coping with Depression: Adolescent version course) with a treatment-as-usual control condition for ninth- and tenth-graders with self-reported depressive symptoms who did not meet diagnostic criteria for a mood disorder. The groups were held in suburban high schools and were led by master's-level school psychologists and school counselors with considerable experience and training. A survival analysis indicated that at a 12-month follow-up, adolescents in the experimental group were less likely than controls to meet diagnostic criteria for a mood disorder. These findings support the utility of prevention programs in reducing the risk for mood disorders in vulnerable youth.

PREVENTION PROGRAMS FOR CHILDREN OF DEPRESSED PARENTS.   Related prevention efforts focus on children at high risk for depression (e.g., children of affectively ill parents). In an outpatient clinic, Beardslee and colleagues (1993) compared clinician-based and lecture-based cognitive psychoeducational prevention programs for addressing family members' behaviors and attitudes toward depression. Families in the clinician-based group were more positive about the program and developed more adaptive attitudes and behaviors for coping with stress than did families in the lecture-based program. These changes may be associated with improved parental management of high-risk children and more adaptive child coping, both of which may decrease the child's risk for depression (Beardslee et al., 1993). A three-year follow-up study conducted with the families who participated in the project revealed that although both preventive interventions produced long-term changes in behaviors and attitudes, parents in the clinician-facilitated intervention reported more benefit (Beardslee, Wright, Rothberg, Salt, & Versage, 1996). In addition, children in the clinician-facilitated group reported greater understanding of parental affective disorder and evidenced better adaptive functioning following the completion of the intervention (Beardslee et al., 1997).

Taken together, these prevention efforts, which are in their infancy, yield promising results. Many of these programs utilize the same intervention strategies as those reviewed for depressed children and adolescents; however, they target children at risk for mood disorders rather than children who meet diagnostic criteria for mood disturbance. In general, these techniques appear to be effective for both depressed and at risk youth. Given the increased interest of national funding agencies in early intervention in primary care settings to prevent onset and development of mental illness in children and adolescents, these prevention programs offer important and timely intervention strategies for reducing the risk of childhood mood disorders. These programs are especially relevant for children who are known to be at risk for mood disorders given their family history (e.g., children of depressed parents) or current life circumstances (e.g., death of a parent). In addition, given that depressive disorders recur and interfere with a child's development and functioning throughout childhood and adolescence, additional attention should be devoted to developing and evaluating relapse prevention programs.

Pharmacological Interventions

For adults, the effectiveness of antidepressant medication is well established, but there have been relatively few studies of the usefulness of antidepressant medications in youth, and they have yielded mixed results. A review of placebo-controlled studies of tricyclic antidepressants (e.g., imipramine, nortriptyline, amitriptyline) in young people between ages 6 and 18 years found that the difference between treatment with medication and placebo was too small to be clinically significant (Hazell, O'Connell, Heathcote, Robertson, & Henry, 1995). Also, tricyclic antidepressants are often associated with significant side effects in youth, especially cardiac changes, and an overdose is potentially lethal (Ryan, 1992). However, over the past two decades, these medications have been used frequently in clinical practice with depressed children and adolescents.

The reports that selective serotonin reuptake inhibitors (SSRIs) are efficacious in the treatment of adults with major depression have led to the use of these medications in children. SSRIs include fluoxetine (Prozac), sertraline (Zoloft), paroxetine (Paxil), and fluvoxamine (Luvox). These medications have a relatively benign side-effect profile and low lethality after an overdose and are easily administered, with once-per-day dosing. From 1989 to 1994, SSRI prescriptions for children and adolescents increased fourfold (Birmaher, Ryan, Williamson, Brent, & Kaufman, 1996). Early open studies demonstrated the effectiveness of treating depressed adolescents with fluoxetine (Boulos, Kutcher, Gardner, & Young, 1992; Colle, Belair, DiFeo, Weiss, & LaRoche, 1994). However, a placebo-controlled double-blind study of a small sample of adolescents did not find significant differences between treatment with fluoxetine and placebo (Simeon, Dinicola, & Ferguson, 1990). More recently, Emslie and colleagues (1997) conducted a more methodologically sound eight-week double-blind study with a large sample of children and adolescents and found fluoxetine to be superior to placebo in treating acute depression. These children had severe, persistent depressive symptoms. Despite the lack of a great number of methodologically sophisticated studies that document the usefulness of medication in treating depressed children, many child psychiatrists advocate their use. More controlled studies with large samples are needed before definitive statements can be made about the efficacy of SSRIs for treating childhood depression.

Although empirical support for pharmacological interventions for child and adolescent depression is equivocal, clinical practice reveals that medication in conjunction with psychological interventions may be helpful for certain youth. Specifically, children and adolescents who exhibit neurovegetative symptoms (e.g., sleep disturbance, appetite disturbance, concentration difficulties, psychomotor agitation or retardation) may not be able to benefit from psychotherapy until some symptom relief is achieved. For these youth, early pharmacologic intervention may be indicated. For other young people, minimal response to psychological interventions or deterioration in functioning may signal the need for a medication trial. The practice parameters of the American Academy of Child and Adolescent Psychiatry (1998) also suggest that children and adolescents with nonrapid cycling bipolar depression and psychotic depression should be considered for antidepressant medication, in addition to youth with severe depressive symptoms that prevent effective psychotherapy and depression that fails to respond to an adequate trial of psychotherapy.

Integrating and Adapting Interventions in Real-World Settings

Issues in Adopting and Implementing Research-Based Interventions

Despite the growing number of empirically supported and effective interventions for depressed youth, these interventions are rarely being adopted in "real-world" settings such as primary care clinics, community mental health centers, hospitals, schools, and clinician's offices. A number of reasons have been hypothesized to explain the disparity between clinical research findings and actual clinical practice. These issues must be considered when attempting to apply research findings on child and adolescent depression to the real world.

First, most treatment studies have used restricted samples. Specifically, many of these studies use only youth at risk for depression (e.g., elevated depressive symptoms rather than a depressive disorder) or youth with depressive disorders that either are not severe (e.g., no significant suicidal ideation or behavior) or that do not co-occur with other psychological (e.g., substance abuse, attention-deficit/hyperactivity disorder) or medical disorders (e.g., cancer, HIV). Many depressed youth who present for care in the community evidence more severe psychopathology and comorbid psychological and medical disorders. Thus, when adapting these interventions to real-world settings, practitioners may need to extend the length of the interventions (e.g., increase the number of sessions, add booster sessions), add commonly used strategies for comorbid problems, and increase family involvement to more fully address the complexity of issues presented by the child (Jellinek, 1999).

Second, the empirically tested and supported treatments for depression in youth are based on treatment manuals. Most clinicians in the field have concerns about using treatment manuals for a variety reasons. Most notably, mental health practitioners often report that the use of manuals makes it more difficult to establish a therapeutic alliance with a child and limits their ability to tailor treatment to the unique needs of each child (Collins et al., 1997). Because issues of forming a secure attachment with the child and empathically addressing the child's affective distress and interpersonal dynamics are central when working with depressed youth, clinicians may need to view treatment manuals as guides rather than directives on the conduct of sessions, to adapt the manual flexibly to each individual case, and to integrate the material in the manual with other treatment strategies as appropriate (Addis, 1997).

Third, many, although not all, of the interventions tested have used a group format. Many clinicians predominantly work individually with children and may not have the training, resources (e.g., space, funding for supplies), or a large enough caseload size to conduct structured group interventions. Given that there is strong empirical support for the use of group interventions, more practitioners could benefit from training in group therapy for children. Further, they may need to be creative in finding ways to partner with other clinicians or agencies in order to obtain the necessary space, resources, and caseload to conduct groups.

Fourth, many of these studies do not include the child's family actively in the intervention. Given that "depression runs in families" and that many depressed youth reside in families characterized by dysfunctional interactional patterns (Kaslow et al., 1996), many health and mental health care professionals prefer intervention approaches that are family-sensitive and that include the child's family. Therefore, clinicians may want to consider adding a family component to current child-based interventions and can be guided by the interpersonal family therapy model developed by Kaslow and colleagues (Kaslow et al., in press; Schwartz et al., 1998).

Fifth, many of the interventions have been developed with children from specific cultural and economic groups and thus may not be generalizable to the broad array of children commonly seen by mental health professionals (Collins et al., 1997). As such, when adopting empirically supported intervention programs, it behooves the clinician to make culturally competent modifications that may include: selecting a treatment modality that is congruent with the cultural values of the community in which the child is embedded, introducing the child and family's cultural values directly into the intervention, using techniques to bridge cultural differences, developing networks in the minority community to enhance family's access to and involvement in care, and increasing the accessibility and acceptability of the interventions for non–English-speaking participants by recruiting bilingual and bicultural staff (Mufson & Moreau, 1997).

Sixth, given the gender differences in the rates and expression of depression in youth, as well as the interaction of age and gender in rates of youth depression, the failure of most of the interventions developed by researchers to attend to gender-specific issues in a developmentally sensitive fashion is of concern to many therapists who may be interested in utilizing empirically supported interventions. When using empirically supported interventions with depressed youth, therapists should make modifications based on the child's gender and age. These modifications may relate to the topics covered and the emphasis placed on certain symptoms and issues. For example, for adolescent females, interventions must address body image concerns, sexuality, teenage pregnancy, and the differential socialization practices that result in higher levels of helplessness and lower self-esteem in females. In contrast, interventions for younger males should target appropriate expression of sadness and anger, effective strategies for managing angry impulses (e.g., alternatives to bullying), and appropriate impulse control and behavior management strategies for those depressed males with comorbid externalizing problems.

Seventh, many have asserted that the bulk of empirically supported interventions fail to consider the ecological models of influence that maintain a child's depression (Ammerman & Hersen, 1997; Mufson & Moreau, 1997). The multiple ecological community influences on depressed youth, which may include poverty, family and community violence, inadequate education, parental psychopathology, and substance abuse, often serve to impede the child's and family's psychosocial development and functioning and negatively affect the efficacy of potential interventions (Ammerman & Hersen, 1997). Interventions with depressed youth, when conducted in the community, must address these broader influences to be effective in reducing children's depressive symptoms and enhancing affective, cognitive, and interpersonal functioning.

Eighth and finally, the majority of the research-based interventions for youth depression are steeped in cognitive-behavioral psychology. However, many practitioners do not primarily espouse a cognitive-behavioral approach to care but rather practice psychotherapy integration. Thus many practitioners are likely to incorporate cognitive-behavioral strategies into a more broad-based treatment model. Therefore, it behooves clinical researchers and practitioners to work collaboratively to develop intervention programs that are compatible with the integrative approach to psychotherapy.

Impediments to Care and Obstacles to Improvement

Often, there are many factors that impede depressed youth's access to care or that interfere with a depressed child's capacity to benefit from the available services. For empirically supported interventions to be implemented and effective in community settings, these impediments to care and obstacles to improvement must be addressed. Commonly cited barriers include: the fact that depressed youth often are ignored or neglected because they are less troublesome to most adults than are youth with externalizing disorders; the limited availability of services that specifically target depressed youth; poverty and associated limitations in resources such as transportation, insurance, money to pay for services, and caretaker availability to attend sessions; and the unwillingness of caregivers to participate in the child's treatment due to parental psychopathology and substance use and/or the stigma associated with mental health services (Mufson & Moreau, 1997). In addition, researchers may have an easier time recruiting and retaining participants because they may reimburse the children for attending sessions, whereas interventions occurring in the real world typically require payment from the recipients of care. Further, the highly selective method of obtaining participants in most intervention studies is in stark contrast to the broad array of youth who require services for their depression and related problems. To overcome the aforementioned barriers to care, practitioners need to develop culturally competent, developmentally informed, and gender-sensitive interventions; to actively engage the child's social support network and develop a partnership with significant people in the child's life; to serve as resource persons, not just as therapists in the traditional sense, for the child and his or her family, to develop alliances with a broad range of community-based agencies; and to work in active collaboration with an interdisciplinary team (Mufson & Moreau, 1997).

Examples: Interventions with Depressed Youth in Real-World Settings

The following are three brief examples of attempts to apply empirically grounded interventions for depressed youth in community settings.

COMMUNITY INTERVENTION FOR ABUSED AND DEPRESSED AFRICAN AMERICAN ADOLESCENT FEMALES AND THEIR FAMILIES. First, Kaslow and colleagues have modified their brand of interpersonal family therapy (Kaslow et al., in press; Schwartz et al., 1998) for working with depressed adolescent, African American females from low-income families who have a history of childhood maltreatment. Specifically, they have partnered with the Turner Foundation, the Georgia Campaign for Adolescent Pregnancy Prevention (G-CAPP) under the leadership of Jane Fonda, African American church groups, child protective services in Georgia, Boys' and Girls' Clubs, YMCA youth groups, and an inner-city hospital to provide a community-based family intervention for these depressed adolescent females.

This theory-driven model incorporates interventions derived from cognitive-behavioral psychology, family systems approaches, and attachment theory. The treatment model is described in a culturally informed intervention manual that addresses topics particularly relevant to these young people and their families (e.g., racial identity, prevention of teen pregnancy, poverty). The manual uses examples specific to the population being targeted, and the handouts and audiovisual aids used are culturally appropriate. The interventions, which are conducted in a 10-session multiple-family group format, are conducted by African American therapists who engage in active outreach to the families. This includes a flexible definition of "family" members with regard to participation in the intervention, provision of resources to enhance participation (e.g., bus and subway tokens), reminder phone calls, flexibility in scheduling, and an emphasis on helping the family to secure a variety of resources that will enable them to enhance the quality of their lives. The program is conducted in community organizations, such as local churches, as these are places in which the families feel more comfortable in participating.

WORKING IN PRIVATE PEDIATRICIANS' OFFICES. A second effort in the early stages of development relates to a national movement toward screening children and adolescents for depression in pediatricians' offices and then offering identified youth targeted mental health services based on previously developed empirically supported interventions. This approach builds on currently existing models of care in pediatric psychology based in primary care settings (Schroeder, 1996). These interventions plan to target such groups of youth as those with elevated levels of depressive symptoms with or without other internalizing or externalizing problems, youth at risk for depression (e.g., children of divorce, youth with depressed parents), and youth who frequently visit pediatricians' offices and/or who present with physical complaints (e.g., stomach aches, headaches) with no known organic etiology. Once such a child is identified, the child and his or her family are offered a family and psychoeducationally oriented skill-building intervention that focuses on enhancing competencies and building resilience in order to reduce depressive symptoms and decrease one's risk for depression. The strategies used are borrowed from already existing empirically supported intervention programs, but only those techniques needed to address a particular child's difficulties are implemented. These interventions, which are conducted in a developmentally and culturally informed manner, are implemented by mental health professionals working closely with pediatricians.

MULTIDISCIPLINARY APPROACH TO WORKING IN AN ADOLESCENT PRIMARY CARE CLINIC. One final example highlights the importance of providing care for depressed youth and youth at risk for depression using a multidisciplinary approach. Based on the findings that many young people who need mental health treatment do not receive it and that contact with medical providers enhances chances of obtaining professional help for emotional problems such as depression (Saunders, Resnick, Hoberman, & Blum, 1994), Bachanas, Morris, Lewis, Sirl, and Sawyer (1999) have developed an interdisciplinary approach to treating high-risk inner-city youth. This program is based in an outpatient clinic of an inner-city children's hospital and provides comprehensive care to teens at risk for pregnancy, sexually transmitted diseases, HIV, and substance abuse. Many of these teens present with or endorse depressive symptoms (Bachanas et al., 1999).

Medical providers screen for depression and other psychological and behavioral problems, and mental health providers assess and intervene with teens during their medical visits. In addition, mental health providers are available for ongoing mental health follow-up in the clinic, which includes individual, family, and group psychotherapy, as well as pharmacological treatments. Attempts are made to modify empirically supported psychosocial treatments to an individual or family model of intervention in a manner consistent with the underlying theory of the intervention protocol on which the treatment is based. This interdisciplinary approach to treatment engages depressed youth in mental health care who may otherwise not have been identified as needing services and provides these youth with access to a more comprehensive array of services, such as medical care, health education, family planning, educational resources, and social services (e.g., housing, transportation, Medicaid, shelters).

Summary

Depressive disorders, either in isolation or comorbid with other conditions, occur in a significant percentage of children and adolescents in the general population and in a high percentage of clinical samples. Although there are many similarities in the clinical pictures of depressed children and adolescents and depressed adults, the unique developmental characteristics of youth result in varying manifestations of the disorder over the life span. When diagnosing a depressive disorder in a child or adolescent, it is essential to incorporate information obtained from a multitrait, multimethod, and multiinformant assessment. This enables the clinician to develop a comprehensive picture of the depressed child's functioning across neurobiological, cognitive, affective, familial, and interpersonal domains. In addition, the child's age, gender, and ethnic and economic backgrounds need to be taken into account in understanding the youth's symptom picture.

Depression in childhood and adolescence can be a serious condition that interferes with the child's development and functioning, even on remission from a depressive episode. Depressions in youth tend to persist over time and to recur and thus necessitate treatment. The limited data on empirically supported primary, secondary, and tertiary prevention efforts reveal that some form of psychosocial treatment is better than no treatment at all in ameliorating depressive symptoms and disorders and improving the course of the disorder. However, insufficient data exist to support the superiority of any given treatment.

Unfortunately, there have been limited attempts to apply the empirically supported interventions for depressed youth to real-world settings. Some of the lessons learned thus far with regard to taking research findings into the community are as follows. First, the interventions and materials need to be tailored to address the specific concerns of the developmental, gender, and cultural group being targeted. Second, the interventions need to be broad based and able to accommodate a broad range of symptoms, psychological problems, family issues, and social concerns. Third, it is essential to work with personnel from various agencies who already have connections with young people and their families to engage depressed youth in intervention programs. Fourth, depressed youth often do not present to mental health professionals but rather to other health care providers. Thus they may be particularly likely to access services provided in primary care settings. Given the current health care climate, interventions in these primary care settings need to be brief and targeted. Fifth, providing interdisciplinary and comprehensive services in community settings, such as primary care clinics, schools, and community mental health centers, allows youth access to more community resources that address the socioecological context within which the youth is embedded. This increased access to resources enhances the likelihood that children and adolescents will be able to benefit from the interventions targeting their depression. Sixth, in addition to developing programs that target depressed youth, prevention interventions that target youth at risk for depression are necessary.

In order to develop interventions for depressed youth that are empirically supported and applicable to and utilized in real-world settings, it will be necessary for clinical researchers and practitioners to work collaboratively. This will enable us to gather empirical support for community-based approaches to care for depressed youth. Such collaborations also will increase the likelihood that interventions that are empirically supported in clinical research settings are appropriate for use by mental health professionals in a broad array of contexts.

REFERENCES

Addis, M. E. (1997). Evaluating the treatment manual as a means of disseminating empirically validated psychotherapies. *Clinical Psychology: Science and Practice, 4*, 1–11.

American Academy of Child and Adolescent Psychiatry. (1998). Practice parameters for the assessment and treatment of children and adolescents with depressive disorders. *Journal of the American Academy of Child and Adolescent Psychiatry, 37*, 63S–83S.

American Psychiatric Association. (1994). *Diagnostic and statistical manual of mental disorders* (4th ed.). Washington, DC: American Psychiatric Association.

Ammerman, R. T., & Hersen, M. (1997). Prevention and treatment with children and adolescents in the real world context. In R. T. Ammerman & M. Hersen (Eds.), *Handbook of prevention and treatment with children and adolescents* (pp. 3–12). New York: Wiley.

Angold, A. (1988). Childhood and adolescent depression: I. Epidemiological and aetiological aspects. *British Journal of Psychiatry, 152*, 601–617.

Angold, A., & Costello, E. (1993). Depressive comorbidity in children and adolescents: Empirical, theoretical, and methodological issues. *American Journal of Psychiatry, 150*, 1779–1791.

Angold, A., & Rutter, M. (1992). Effects of age and pubertal status in a large clinical sample. *Development and Psychopathology, 4*, 5–28.

Asarnow, J. (1990). Psychosocial intervention strategies for the depressed child: Approaches to treatment and prevention. *Child and Adolescent Psychiatric Clinics of North America, 1*, 257–283.

Bachanas, P. J., Morris, M. K., Lewis, J. K., Sirl, K., & Sawyer, M. (1999, August). Predictors of sexual self-efficacy in African American adolescents: Implications for HIV prevention. Paper presented at the meeting of the American Psychological Association, Boston, MA.

Bachanas, P. J., Sirl, K. S., Morris, M. K., Lewis, J. K., & Sawyer, M. K. (1999,

August). Predictors of risky sexual behavior for African-American female adolescents: Developmental implications for HIV prevention. Paper presented at the CDC/NIMH National HIV Prevention Conference, Atlanta, GA.

Beardslee, W., Salt, P., Porterfield, K., Rothberg, P., Van de Velde, P., Swatling, S., Hoke, L., Moilanen, D., & Wheelock, I. (1993). Comparison of preventive interventions for families with parental affective disorder. *Journal of the American Academy of Child and Adolescent Psychiatry, 32,* 254–263.

Beardslee, W. R., Wright, E., Rothberg, P. C., Salt, P., & Versage, E. (1996). Response of families to two preventive intervention strategies: Long-term differences in behavior and attitude change. *Journal of the American Academy of Child and Adolescent Psychiatry, 35,* 774–782.

Beardslee, W. R., Wright, E. J., Salt, P., Drezner, K., Gladston, T. R., Versage, E. M., & Rothberg, P. C. (1997). Examination of children's responses to two preventive intervention strategies over time. *Journal of the American Academy of Child and Adolescent Psychiatry, 36,* 196–204.

Beck, A. T., Rush, A. J., Shaw, B. F., & Emery, G. (1979). *Cognitive therapy of depression.* New York: Guilford Press.

Birmaher, B., Ryan, N. D., & Williamson, D. E. (1996). Depression in children and adolescents: Clinical features and pathogenesis. In K. I. Shulman, M. Tohen, & S. P. Kutcher (Eds.), *Mood disorders across the life span* (pp. 51–81). New York: Wiley.

Birmaher, B., Ryan, N. D., Williamson, D. E., Brent, D. A., & Kaufman, J. (1996). Childhood and adolescent depression: A review of the past 10 years (part 2). *Journal of the American Academy of Child and Adolescent Psychiatry, 35,* 1575–1583.

Birmaher, B., Ryan, N. D., Williamson, D. E., Brent, D. A., Kaufman, J., Dahl, R. E., Perel, J., & Nelson, B. (1996).

Childhood and adolescent depression: A review of the past 10 years (part 1). *Journal of the American Academy of Child and Adolescent Psychiatry, 35,* 1427–1439.

Blumberg, S. H., & Izard, C. E. (1985). Affective and cognitive characteristics of depression in 10- and 11-year old children. *Journal of Personality and Social Psychology, 49,* 194–202.

Boulos, C., Kutcher, S., Gardner, D., & Young, E. (1992). An open naturalistic trial of fluoxetine in adolescents and young adults with treatment-resistant major depression. *Journal of Child and Adolescent Psychopharmacology, 2,* 103–111.

Brent, D., Holder, D., Kolko, D., Birmaher, B., Baugher, M., Roth, C., Iyengar, S., & Johnson, B. (1997). A clinical psychotherapy trial for adolescent depression comparing cognitive, family, and supportive therapy. *Archives of General Psychiatry, 54,* 877–885.

Brent, D. A., Kolko, D. J., Birmaher, B., Baugher, M., & Bridge, J. (1999). A clinical trial for adolescent depression: Predictors of additional treatment in the acute and follow-up phases of the trial. *Journal of the American Academy of Child and Adolescent Psychiatry, 38,* 263–271.

Brent, D., Poling, K., McKain, B., & Baugher, M. (1993). A psychoeducational program for families of affectively ill children and adolescents. *Journal of the American Academy of Child and Adolescent Psychiatry, 32,* 770–774.

Brent, D. A., Kolko, D. J., Birmaher, B., Baugher, M., Bridge, J., Roth, C., & Holder, D. (1998). Predictors of treatment efficacy in a clinical trial of three psychosocial treatments for adolescent depression. *Journal of the American Academy of Child and Adolescent Psychiatry, 37,* 906–914.

Brooks-Gunn, J., & Warren, M. P. (1989). Biological and social contributions to negative affect in young adolescent girls. *Child Development, 60,* 40–55.

Butler, L., Miezitis, S., Friedman, R., & Cole, E. (1980). The effect of two school-based intervention programs on depressive symptoms in preadolescents. *American Education Research Journal,* 17, 111–119.

Chambless, D., Sanderson, W., Shoham, V., Johnson, S., Pope, K., Crits-Cristoph, P., Baker, M., Johnson, B., Woody, S., Sue, S., Beutler, L., Williams, D., & McCurry, S. (1996). An update on empirically validated therapies. *Clinical Psychologist,* 49, 5–18.

Clarke, G., Hawkins, W., Murphy, M., Sheeber, L., Lewinsohn, P., & Seeley, J. (1995). Targeted prevention of unipolar depressive disorder in an at-risk sample of high school adolescents: A randomized trial of a group cognitive intervention. *American Academy of Child and Adolescent Psychiatry,* 34, 312–321.

Clarke, G., & Lewinsohn, P. (1986). *The Coping with Depression course: Adolescent version.* Eugene, OR: Oregon Research Institute.

Clarke, G., Rhode, P., Lewinsohn, P., Hops, H., & Seeley, J. (1999). Cognitive-behavioral treatment of adolescent depression: Efficacy of acute group treatment and booster sessions. *Journal of the American Academy of Child and Adolescent Psychiatry,* 38, 272–279.

Colle, L. M., Belair, J. F., DiFeo, M., Weiss, J., & LaRoche, C. (1994). Extended open-label fluoxetine treatment of adolescents with major depression. *Journal of Child and Adolescent Pharmacology,* 4, 225–232.

Collins, M. H., Loundy, M. R., Brown, F. L., Hollins, L. D., Eckman, J., & Kaslow, N. J. (1997). Applicability of criteria for empirically validated treatments to family interventions for pediatric sickle cell disease (SCD). *Journal of Developmental and Physical Disabilities,* 9, 293–309.

Diamond, G., & Siqueland, L. (1995). Family therapy for the treatment of depressed adolescents. *Psychotherapy: The ory, Research, Practice, Training,* 32, 77–90.

Dowrick, D. (1983). Self-modeling. In P. Dowrick & S. Biggs (Eds.), *Using video: Psychological and social applications* (pp. 105–124). New York: Wiley.

Ellis, A. (1962). *Reason and emotion in psychotherapy.* New York: Stuart.

Emslie, G. J., Rush, A. J., Weinberg, W. A., Kowatch, R. A., Hughes, C. W., Carmody, T., & Rintelmann, J. (1997). A double-blind, randomized, placebo-controlled trial of fluoxetine in children and adolescents with depression. *Archives of General Psychiatry,* 54, 1031–1037.

Emslie, G. J., Weinberg, W. A., Kennard, B. D., & Kowatch, R. A. (1994). Neurobiological aspects of depression in children and adolescents. In W. M. Reynolds & H. F. Johnston (Eds.), *Handbook of depression in children and adolescents* (pp. 143–165). New York: Plenum Press.

Fine, S., Forth, A., Gilbert, M., & Haley, G. (1991). Group therapy for adolescent depressive disorder: A comparison of social skills and therapeutic support. *Journal of the American Academy of Child and Adolescent Psychiatry,* 30, 79–85.

Fleming, J., Boyle, M., & Offord, D. (1993). The outcome of adolescent depression in the Ontario Child Health Study follow-up. *Journal of the American Academy of Child and Adolescent Psychiatry,* 32, 28–33.

Fleming, J. E., & Offord, D. R. (1990). Epidemiology of childhood depressive disorders: A critical review. *Journal of the American Academy of Child and Adolescent Psychiatry,* 29, 571–581.

Garber, J., Braafladt, N., & Zeman, J. (1991). The regulation of sad affect: An information-processing perspective. In J. Garber & K. A. Dodge (Eds.), *The development of emotion regulation and dysregulation* (pp. 208–240). New York: Cambridge University Press.

Garber, J., & Hilsman, R. (1992). Cognitions, stress, and depression in children and adolescents. *Child and Adolescent Psychiatric Clinics of North America, 1,* 129–167.

Gillham, J., Reivich, K., Jaycox, L., & Seligman, M. E. P. (1995). Prevention of depressive symptoms in school children: Two year follow-up. *Psychological Science, 6,* 343–351.

Goldstein, A., Sprafkin, R., Gershaw, N., & Klein, P. (1980). *Skill-streaming the adolescent.* Champaign, IL: Research Press.

Hanna, G. L. (1992). Natural history of mood disorders. *Child and Adolescent Psychiatric Clinics of North American, 1,* 169–181.

Harrington, R. (1992). Annotation: The natural history and treatment of child and adolescent affective disorders. *Journal of Child Psychology and Psychiatry, 33,* 1287–1302.

Harrington, R. (1993). *Depressive disorder in childhood and adolescence.* New York: Wiley.

Hazell, P., O'Connell, D., Heathcote, D., Robertson, J., & Henry, D. (1995). Efficacy of tricyclic drugs in treating child and adolescent depression: A meta-analysis. *British Medical Journal, 310,* 897–901.

Jaycox, L., Reivich, K., Gillham, J., & Seligman, M. E. P. (1994). Prevention of depressive symptoms in school children. *Behavioral Research and Therapy, 32,* 801–816.

Jellinek, M. S. (1999). Commentary on "A clinical trial for adolescent depression: Predictors of additional treatment in the acute and follow-up phases of the trial by Brent and colleagues." *Journal of the American Academy of Child and Adolescent Psychiatry, 38,* 270–271.

Kahn, J., Kehle, T., Jenson, W., & Clark, E. (1990). Comparison of cognitive behavioral, relaxation, and self-modeling interventions for depression among middle-school students. *School Psychology Review, 19,* 196–211.

Kandel, D. B., & Davies, M. (1986). Adult

sequelae of adolescent depressive symptoms. *Archives of General Psychiatry, 43,* 255–262.

Kashani, J. H., Beck, N. C., Hoeper, E. W., Fallahi, C., Corcoran, C. M., McAllister, J. A., Rosenberg, T. K., & Reid, J. C. (1987). Psychiatric disorders in a community sample of adolescents. *American Journal of Psychiatry, 144,* 584–589.

Kaslow, N. J., Brown, R. T., & Mee, L. (1994). Cognitive and behavioral correlates of childhood depression: A developmental perspective. In W. M. Reynolds & H. F. Johnston (Eds.), *Handbook of depression in children and adolescents* (pp. 97–121). New York: Plenum Press.

Kaslow, N. J., Deering, C. G., & Ash, P. (1996). Relational diagnosis of child and adolescent depression. In F. W. Kaslow (Ed.), *Handbook of relational diagnosis and dysfunctional family patterns* (pp. 171–185). New York: Wiley.

Kaslow, N. J., Mintzer, M. B., Meadows, L. A., & Grabill, C. M. (in press). A family perspective on assessing and treating childhood depression. In E. Bailey (Ed.), *Working with children: Using the family as a resource in children's therapy.* New York: Norton.

Kaslow, N. J., Morris, M. K., & Rehm, L. P. (1998). Childhood depression. In R. J. Morris & T. R. Kratochwill (Eds.), *The practice of child therapy* (3rd ed., pp. 48–90). Boston: Allyn & Bacon.

Kaslow, N. J., & Racusin, G. R. (1994). Family therapy for depression in young people. In W. M. Reynolds & H. F. Johnston (Eds.), *Handbook of depression in children and adolescents* (pp. 345–363). New York: Plenum Press.

Kaslow, N. J., & Thompson, M. P. (1998). Applying the criteria for empirically supported treatments to studies of psychosocial interventions for child and adolescent depression. *Journal of Clinical Child Psychology, 27,* 146–155.

Kazdin, A. E., Sherick, R. B., Esveldt-Dawson, K., & Racurello, M. D. (1985).

Nonverbal behavior and childhood depression. *Journal of the American Academy of Child and Adolescent Psychiatry, 24,* 303–309.

Klerman, G., Weissman, M., Rounsaville, B., & Chevron, E. (1984). *Interpersonal psychotherapy for depression.* New York: Basic Books.

Kovacs, M. (1989). Affective disorder in children and adolescents. *American Psychologist, 44,* 209–215.

Kovacs, M., Aksikal, S., Gastonis, C., & Parrone, P. L. (1994). Childhood-onset dysthymic disorder. *Archives of General Psychiatry, 51,* 365–374.

Kovacs, M., & Gatsonis, C. (1994). Secular trends in age at onset of MDD in a clinical sample of children. *Journal of Psychiatric Research, 28,* 319–329.

Kovacs, M., Goldston, D., & Gatsonis, C. (1993). Suicidal behaviors and childhood-onset depressive disorders: A longitudinal investigation. *Journal of the American Academy of Child and Adolescent Psychiatry, 32,* 8–20.

Lewinsohn, P. (1974). A behavioral approach to depression. In R. M. Friedman & M. M. Katz (Eds.), *Psychology of depression: Contemporary theory and research* (pp. 157–185). New York: Wiley.

Lewinsohn, P., Antonuccio, D., Steinmetz, J., & Teri, L. (1984). *The coping with depression course: A psychoeducational intervention for unipolar depression.* Eugene, OR: Castalia Press.

Lewinsohn, P., & Clarke, G. (1999). Psychosocial treatments for adolescent depression. *Clinical Psychology Review, 19,* 329–342.

Lewinsohn, P., Clarke, G., Hops, H., & Andrews, J. (1990). Cognitive-behavioral treatment for depressed adolescents. *Behavior Therapy, 21,* 385–401.

Lewinsohn, P., Clarke, G., Rhode, P., Hops, H., & Seeley, J. (1996). A course in coping: A cognitive-behavioral approach to the treatment of adolescent depression. In E. D. Hibbs & P. S. Jensen (Eds.), *Psychosocial treatments for child and adolescent disorders: Empirically based strategies for clinical practice* (pp. 109–135). Washington, DC: American Psychological Association.

Lewinsohn, P. M., Clarke, G. N., Seeley, J. R., & Rhode, P. (1994). Major depression in community adolescents: Age at onset, episode duration, and time to recurrence. *Journal of the American Academy of Child and Adolescent Psychiatry, 33,* 809–818.

Liddle, B., & Spence, S. (1990). Cognitive behavior therapy with depressed primary school children: A cautionary note. *Behavioural Psychotherapy, 18,* 85–102.

McCauley, E., & Myers, K. (1992). Family interactions in mood disordered youth. *Child and Adolescent Psychiatric Clinics of North America, 1,* 111–127.

McCauley, E., Myers, K., Mitchel, J., Calderon, R., Schloredt, K., & Treder, R. (1993). Depression in young people: Initial presentation and clinical course. *Journal of the American Academy of Child and Adolescent Psychiatry, 32,* 714–722.

Mufson, L., & Moreau, D. (1997). Depressive disorders. In R. T. Ammerman & M. Hersen (Eds.), *Handbook of prevention and treatment with children and adolescents* (pp. 403–430). New York: Wiley.

Mufson, L., Moreau, D., Weissman, M., & Klerman, G. (1993). *Interpersonal psychotherapy for depressed adolescents.* New York: Guilford Press.

Mufson, L., Moreau, D., Weissman, M., Wickramaratne, P., Martin, J., & Samoilov, A. (1994). Modification of interpersonal psychotherapy with depressed adolescents (IPT-A): Phase I and II studies. *Journal of the American Academy of Child and Adolescent Psychiatry, 33,* 695–705.

Mufson, L., Weissman, M. M., Moreau, D., & Garfinkel, R. (1999). Efficacy of interpersonal therapy for depressed adolescents. *Archives of General Psychiatry, 56,* 573–579.

Nolen-Hoeksema, S., & Girgus, J. S. (1994). The emergence of gender differences in depression during adolescence. *Psychological Bulletin, 115,* 424–443.

Petersen, A. C., Compas, B. E., Brooks-Gunn, J., Stemmler, M., Ey, S., & Grant, K. E. (1993). Depression in adolescence. *American Psychologist, 48,* 155–168.

Poling, K. (1989). *Living with depression: A survivor manual for families.* Pittsburgh, PA: University of Pittsburgh, Western Psychiatric Institute and Clinic.

Puig-Antich, J., Kaufman, J., Ryan, N., Williamson, D., Dahl, R., Lukens, E., Todak, G., Ambrosini, P., Rabinovich, H., & Nelson, B. (1993). The psychosocial functioning and family environment of depressed adolescents. *Journal of the American Academy of Child and Adolescent Psychiatry, 32,* 244–253.

Puig-Antich, J., Lukens, E., Davies, M., Goetz, D., Brennan-Quattrock, J., & Todak, G. (1985a). Psychosocial functioning in prepubertal major depressive disorder: I. Interpersonal relationships during the depressive episode. *Archives of General Psychiatry, 42,* 500–507.

Puig-Antich, J., Lukens, E., Davies, M., Goetz, D., Brennan-Quattrock, J., & Todak, G. (1985b). Psychosocial functioning in prepubertal major depressive disorder: II. Interpersonal relationships after sustained recovery from affective episode. *Archives of General Psychiatry, 42,* 511–517.

Rao, U., Ryan, N. D., Birmaher, B., Dahl, R. E., Williamson, D. E., Kaufman, J., Rao, R., & Nelson, B. (1995). Unipolar depression in adolescents: Clinical outcome in adulthood. *Journal of the American Academy of Child and Adolescent Psychiatry, 34,* 566–578.

Rehm, L. P. (1977). A self-control model of depression. *Behavior Therapy, 8,* 787–804.

Rehm, L. P., & Sharp, R. (1996). Strategies for childhood depression. In M. A. Reinecke, F. M. Dattilio, & A. Freeman (Eds.), *Cognitive therapy with children and adolescents: A casebook for clinical practice* (pp. 103–123). New York: Guilford Press.

Renaud, J., Brent, D., Baugher, M., Birmaher, D., Kolko, D., & Bridge, J. (1998). Rapid response to psychosocial treatment for adolescent depression: A two year follow-up. *Journal of the American Academy of Child and Adolescent Psychiatry, 37,* 1184–1190.

Reynolds, W., & Coats, K. (1986). A comparison of cognitive-behavioral therapy and relaxation training for the treatment of depression in adolescents. *Journal of Consulting and Clinical Psychology, 54,* 653–660.

Rhode, P., Lewinsohn, P. M., & Seeley, J. R. (1991). Comorbidity of unipolar depression: II. Comorbidity with other mental disorders in adolescents and adults. *Journal of Abnormal Psychology, 100,* 214–222.

Rice, K., Herman, M., & Petersen, A. (1993). Coping with challenge in adolescence: A conceptual and psycho-educational intervention. *Journal of Adolescence, 16,* 235–251.

Rudolph, K., Hammen, C., & Burge, D. (1994). Interpersonal functioning and depressive symptoms in childhood: Addressing the issues of specificity and comorbidity. *Journal of Abnormal Child Psychology, 22,* 355–371.

Ryan, N. D. (1992). The pharmacologic treatment of child and adolescent depression. *Psychiatric Clinics of North America, 15,* 29–40.

Ryan, N. D., Puig-Antich, J., Ambrosini, P., Rabinovitch, H., Robinson, D., Nelson, B., Iyengar, S., & Twomey, J. (1987). The clinical picture of major depression in children and adolescents. *Archives of General Psychiatry, 44,* 854–861.

Saunders, S., Resnick, M., Hoberman, H., & Blum, R. (1994). Formal help-seeking behavior of adolescents identifying themselves as having mental health problems. *Journal of the American Academy of Child and Adolescent Psychiatry, 33,* 718–728.

Schroeder, C. (1996). Psychologists and pediatricians in collaborative practice. In R. J. Resnick & R. H. Rozensky (Eds.), *Health psychology through the life-span: Practice and research opportunities* (pp. 109–131). Washington, DC: American Psychological Association.

Schwartz, J. A., Kaslow, N. J., Racusin, G. R., & Carton, E. R. (1998). Interpersonal family therapy for childhood depression. In V. B. V. Hasselt & M. Hersen (Eds.), *Handbook of psychological treatment protocols for children and adolescents* (pp. 109–151). Mahwah, NJ: Erlbaum.

Simeon, J., Dinicola, V., & Ferguson, H. (1990). Adolescent depression: A placebo-controlled fluoxetine treatment study and follow-up. *Progress in Neuropsychopharmacology and Biological Psychiatry, 14,* 791–795.

Stark, K. D., Reynolds, W. M., & Kaslow, N. J. (1987). A comparison of the relative efficacy of self-control therapy and behavior problem-solving therapy for depression in children. *Journal of Abnormal Child Psychology, 15,* 91–113.

Stark, K. D., Rouse, L., & Livingston, R. (1991). Treatment of depression during childhood and adolescence: Cognitive behavioral procedures for the individual and family. In P. Kendall (Ed.), *Child and adolescent therapy* (pp. 165–206). New York: Guilford Press.

Stark, K. D., Swearer, S., Kurowski, C., Sommer, D., & Bowen, B. (1996). Targeting the child and the family: A holistic approach to treating child and adolescent depressive disorders. In E. D. Hibbs & P. S. Jensen (Eds.), *Psychosocial treatments for child and adolescent disorders: Empirically based strategies for clini-*

cal practice (pp. 207–238). Washington, DC: American Psychological Association.

Trad, P. V. (1987). *Infant and childhood depression: Developmental factors.* New York: Wiley.

Warner, V., Weissman, M., Fendrich, M., Wickramaratne, P., & Moreau, D. (1992). The course of major depression in the offspring of depressed parents. *Archives of General Psychiatry, 49,* 795–801.

Weissman, M. M., Gammon, G. D., John, K., Merikangas, K. R., Prusoff, B., & Sholomskas, D. (1987). Children of depressed parents: Increased psychopathology and early onset of depression. *Archives of General Psychiatry, 44,* 847–853.

Weissman, M. M., Warner, V., Wickramaratne, P., & Prusoff, B. (1988). Early onset major depression in parents and their children. *Journal of Affective Disorders, 15,* 269–277.

Weisz, J., Thurber, C., Sweeney, L., Proffitt, V., & LeGagnoux, G. (1997). Brief treatment of mild to moderate child depression using primary and secondary control enhancement training. *Journal of Consulting and Clinical Psychology, 65,* 703–707.

Wells, V., Deykin, E., & Klerman, G. (1985). Risk factors for depression in adolescents. *Psychiatric Development, 3,* 83–108.

Williamson, D. E., Birmaher, B., Frank, E., Anderson, B. P., Matty, M. K., & Kupfer, D. J. (1998). Nature of life events and difficulties in depressed adolescents. *Journal of the American Academy of Child and Adolescent Psychiatry, 37,* 1049–1057.

17

RONALD T. BROWN
MICHELLE MACIAS

Chronically Ill Children and Adolescents

Chronic disease refers to disease states that have symptoms with a protracted course and involvement of one or more organ system (e.g., heart, lung, blood, brain). The percentage of children with severe long-term disease has more than doubled in the past two decades, partly because of technological advances in medical and surgical care. Approximately 10% to 20% of children and adolescents experience one or more chronic health conditions by the age of 18 years; about 2% to 4% of children have a disease of such severity that it regularly interferes with usual daily activities (Behrman & Vaughan, 1996).

Many chronic pediatric disorders are associated with marked medical and psychological morbidity (i.e., disruption of normal developmental processes and adaptive competencies; Roberts, 1995; Routh, 1988; Russo & Varni, 1982). Behavioral factors (e.g., diet, treatment nonadherence, and substance abuse) are important in predicting the onset, course, and prognosis of many disorders and injuries and therefore contribute to disease and injury onset and maintenance (Brannon & Feist, 1997). Table 17.1 presents a summary of disorders from major pediatric subspecialties, the incidence of the disorders, and examples of relevant psychological aspects.

Developmental Precursors and Consequences

Children and adolescents with chronic illness are predicted to have optimal adaptation to their disease state when protective or resistance factors outweigh risk factors (Wallander & Thompson, 1995). Protective or resistance factors include intrapersonal variables (e.g., temperament, problem-solving skills), social-ecological factors

TABLE 17.1 Disorders for Major Pediatric Subspecialties

Subspecialty	Condition	Incidence	Representative Psychological Aspects
Trauma (surgery)	Orthopedic trauma	20,000,000/year that require treatment	Coping with intense postinjury pain, adjustment to disfigurement
	Burns	100,000 with permanent disability	
Cardiology	Congenital heart defects	6–8/1,000 live births	Impaired cognitive function secondary to hypoxia, parental guilt about responsibility for anomaly, restriction of activity secondary to blood thinner used in valve replacement
			Acquired heart defects
Endocrinology	Diabetes mellitus	1.9/1,000	Nonadherence with complex self-care regimen, damaged self-concept and peer relations
	Short stature	1.9/1,000	
Gastroenterology	Encopresis	1.5/100	Coercive parent-child interactions, impaired child self-esteem, reinforcement of sick behaviors, familial dysfunction
	Abdominal pain	10/100	
Hematology	Sickle cell disease	.36/1,000 (1/500 African American)	Recurrent pain, cognitive changes, chronic arthritic pain
	Hemophilia	1.13/1,000 (.25/1,000 males)	
Infectious disease	AIDS	5–10/100,000	Cognitive deterioration, depression, alterations in mental status
	Menigitis		
Neonatology	Brochopulmonary displasia	7.1/100	Feeding disorders, developmental delays, defects in sleep regulation
	Apnea	7.1/100	
Nephrology	Renal failure	2/1,000	Treatment nonadherence, cognitive symptoms, muscle weakness, body composition changes
	Cushing's syndrome		
Neurology	Migraine headaches	5/100	Stress, medication-induced changes in cognitive functioning
	Seizures	5.2–8/1,000	
Oncology	Leukemia		Coping with aversive medical diagnostic and treatment procedures, pain, treatment-related cognitive changes, death and dying issues
	Solid tumors		
Pulmonology	Asthma	10–15/100	Activity restrictions, repeated hospitalizations, decreased life expectancy
	Cystic fibrosis	.5/1,000	

(e.g., stable family environment, adequate social support systems, adequate financial resources), and stress processing (e.g., adaptive coping strategies). Risk factors include disease and disability parameters (e.g., disease type, severity of symptoms, central nervous system [CNS] involvement), inadequate adaptive competencies, and a high frequency of psychosocial stressors.

Risk Factors

Psychological risk factors are multidimensional and influenced by many elements that can complicate disease presentation or management (Wallander & Thompson, 1995). These elements include severity of disease, biological and genetic risk factors, environmental influences, decreased competency in daily living activities, and psychosocial stressors.

DISEASE AND DISABILITY PARAMETERS   Disease and disability parameters are biological dimensions that combine to cause disease, exacerbate severity of disease, and influence children's overall adjustment to disease. Biological risk factors include genetically based disorders (e.g., cystic fibrosis, Down syndrome), teratogenic agents (e.g., alcohol, tobacco, cocaine), and medically based disorders (e.g., congenital heart disease, intrauterine growth retardation, prematurity).

Genetic disorders.   Many chronic diseases are genetically based. In many conditions a genetic component exists that reflects either a chromosomal abnormality or more subtle genetic defects that may influence key biological processes (Thompson & Gustafson, 1996). Most common are autosomal recessive patterns in which an affected child inherits a disease-causing gene from each parent. Examples are cystic fibrosis and sickle cell disease (SCD). Sex-linked ("X-linked") disorders are passed on the X chromosome from an asymptomatic carrier mother to affected sons (e.g., hemophilia, muscular dystrophy).

Intrauterine growth retardation, prematurity, and low birth weight.   Low birth weight frequently results from intrauterine growth retardation, prematurity, or both; these children are at particular risk for multiple health problems (McCormick, 1985). Variables related to low birth weight include poor nutrition and low maternal weight gain during pregnancy, specific obstetrical complications (e.g., high blood pressure, preeclampsia, and infections), smoking, abuse of drug substances, and poor access to and use of prenatal care programs (Institute of Medicine, 1988). An inverse linear relationship exists between the frequency of risk factors and the level of mental abilities among children who are classified as low-birth-weight neonates (Liaw & Brooks-Gunn, 1994).

Teratogens.   Teratogenic agents are substances transferred from the mother to the developing fetus that can cause systemic malformations and other structural defects. Alcohol, opiates (e.g., heroin, methadone), cocaine, anticonvulsant medications (e.g., phenobarbital, phenytoin, valproic acid), and lead are extensively studied teratogens that affect CNS development. Alcohol is unequivocally associated with systemic structural defects (CNS, somatic growth, facial dysmorphology; Streis-sguth, Barr, Sampson, Darby, & Martin, 1989), as well as with cognitive and behavioral differences. Other drug substances such as cocaine, heroin, and phency-clidine may also affect CNS functioning (Chasnoff, Burns, Schnoll, & Burns, 1985; Chasnoff, Griffith, Freier, & Murray, 1992).

Disease severity.   Much of the literature in pediatric psychology indicates little association between severity of a disease and psychological adaptation (Thompson & Gustafson, 1996). In support of this notion, no differences were found in self-reported anxiety of children with severe asthma versus children with mild or moderate asthma (Wamboldt, Fritz, Mansell, McQuaid, & Klein, 1998), although children with complex heart disease were rated by parents as being more withdrawn and having more social problems compared with peers diagnosed with innocent murmurs (Casey, Sykes, Craig, Power, & Mulholland, 1996). Few research diagnostic criteria exist for quantifying severity of disease among various chronic illness groups.

FUNCTIONAL INDEPENDENCE   Functional independence is determined by competencies in activities of daily living. Few studies have focused on functional independence or adaptive behaviors of children with chronic illness. Age, sex, and mental abilities have been found to be efficient predictors of adaptive competencies across a variety of domain categories, with higher adaptive functioning associated with younger children, girls, and higher intellectual functioning (Brown, Eckman, Baldwin, Buchanan, & Dingle, 1995), although family and demographic variables may mediate this association (Carlson-Green, Morris, & Krawiecki, 1995; Devine, Brown, Lambert, Donegan, & Eckman, 1998). School absenteeism has been used as a variable to assess functional limitation and has been found to be associated with children's self-reports of psychosocial problems, activity limitations, and specific health conditions (i.e., SCD; Fowler, Johnson, & Atkinson, 1985; Weitzman, 1986).

PSYCHOSOCIAL STRESSORS   Psychosocial stressors are illness-related difficulties, major life events, and daily stressors. Illness-related difficulties refer to the sequelae of the disease or trauma, including stress resulting from school absenteeism or limitations on activities that require physical exertion. A child's illness and treatment regimen may be stressors that deplete the child's environmental or interpersonal resources, resulting in impaired psychosocial functioning. Major life events consist of major external changes, either positive or negative. Daily stressors are minor annoyances that occur during the normal course of the day. Over the past decade, studies have generally found that the stress associated with daily hassles and the use of avoidance coping account for much of the variance in children's adaptation to the disease process (Thompson & Gustafson, 1996). Investigators have found that severity of disease is associated with life stressors and may be mediated by serious noncompliance with medical regimens (Goldston, Kovacs, Obrosky, & Ivengar, 1995), and more adverse life events have been associated with higher mortality rates (Moss, Bose, Wolters, & Brouwers, 1998).

Resistance Factors

INTRAPERSONAL FACTORS Intrapersonal factors include the child's temperament, social competence, motivation, self-esteem, and problem-solving abilities. These characteristics may influence a child's adaptation to a chronic illness in combination with disease and disability factors and family variables and are associated with psychosocial adjustment. A chronic illness is a risk factor that may predispose some children to diminished self-concept and self-esteem, although it is not necessarily a sufficient condition (Nassau & Drotar, 1995). Social competencies and self-esteem are likely mediated by a number of variables, including severity of disease, functional limitations imposed by the disease, and degree of social support available from peers (Pendley, Dahlquist, & Dreyer, 1997).

SOCIAL-ECOLOGICAL FACTORS

Family functioning. Social-ecological factors include the family environment and family members' adaptation, social support systems, and family utilitarian resources (e.g., intact, divorced, presence of siblings, family income and health care financing, parental responsibilities and leisure time, parental education level). The family environment appears to be an important predictor of adaptation to the disease by the children who are ill and their caregivers (Kazak, Segal-Andrews, & Johnson, 1995; Thompson, Gustafson, Hamlett, & Spock, 1992). In addition, compelling support has been provided for the interrelation of family structure, child adjustment, and management of disease (Overstreet et al., 1995; Silver, Stein, & Dadds, 1996). Greater levels of cohesive and adaptive family functioning have been found to buffer the potential detrimental effects of caring for hard-to-manage, chronically ill children (Ievers, Brown, Lambert, Hsu, & Eckman, 1998). More adaptive family relationships and parental psychological adjustment are positively associated with better psychological adaptation for children with chronic disease (Drotar, 1997).

Financial resources. Clearly, children's health problems are strongly associated with poverty (for a review, see Tarnowski, Brown, & Simonian, 1998). Many of these health conditions have their origins in the poor education of their caregivers and a childhood experience of inadequate care (Tarnowski, Brown, & Simonian, 1998). Consequently, poverty also is a significant risk factor for poor management of chronic illness in children, which has been attributed to a lack of resources, decreased ability to obtain existing services, and the lack of appropriate adherence necessary to manage complicated disease regimens.

STRESS PROCESSING Stress processing consists of coping strategy variables and cognitive appraisal. Coping strategies typically have been conceptualized as adaptive, active, or engagement types of coping, but also include avoidance or disengagement coping. In addition, children who experience control over their illness are better adjusted than those who do not (Weithorn & McCabe, 1988). A self-perceived lack of a predictable association between one's behavior and the outcome of events may lead to feelings of helplessness in the child and may also be a risk factor for depression (Abramson, Seligman, & Teasdale, 1978).

Coping has been studied extensively in the pediatric literature, particularly as it affects disease management and adaptation (Balfour, White, Schiffrin, Dougherty, & Dufresne, 1993; Reid, Dubow, Carey, & Dura, 1998; Tyc, Mulhern, & Bieberich, 1997). The association between styles of coping and children's adjustment in negotiating the stressors of a chronic illness or disability has been the topic of numerous studies (Frank, Blount, & Brown, 1997; Lewis & Kliewer, 1996; Phipps, Fairclough, & Mulhern, 1995; Phipps & Srivastava, 1997), and research affirms the importance of coping in predicting adjustment in children with chronic illness.

Adaptation

Adaptation refers to the psychological functioning and personal adjustment of children who suffer from chronic disease. The vast number of studies pertaining to adaptation have been categorized as either epidemiologic, clinical, or meta-analytic (for a review, see Thompson & Gustafson, 1996). Conclusions from these epidemiological studies were that children with chronic illness are at significant risk for difficulties in psychological adjustment, including behavioral and emotional problems, problems with self-esteem, social adjustment, peer relationships, and difficulties with academic performance (for a review, see Thompson & Gustafson, 1996).

Two comprehensive meta-analytic reviews examined studies of emotional and behavioral adjustment of chronically ill children (Bennett, 1994; Lavigne & Faier-Routman, 1992). Conclusions reveal that children with chronic physical illnesses had higher levels of adjustment problems, but they were not found to differ from their typically developing peers, as determined by test norms (Lavigne & Faier-Routman, 1992). Similarly, ratings of depressive symptoms in children with chronic physical illnesses have been found to be above the mean of comparison control groups (Bennett, 1994). However, no direct association has been found between illness type and psychological adjustment (Wallander & Thompson, 1995).

Empirically Supported Interventions

The field of pediatric psychology recently entered a tertiary stage of evolution with the development of empirically validated treatment research. In fact, it has been recommended that this research be conducted to test theoretical models that were previously primarily correlational in design (Thompson & Gustafson, 1996). Programs of intervention research in pediatric psychology have been conceptualized within the domains of school performance and peer relations, parenting and family systems research, adherence research, and pain management (Thompson & Gustafson, 1996).

Integrating and Adapting Interventions to Real-World Settings

Mental health providers are most frequently consulted when problems such as adherence, parenting issues, and pain management are interfering with medical care. Unfortunately, these difficulties are not usually addressed in a proactive manner. Intervention typically is sought when problems have escalated and the child and family are frustrated and less amenable to appropriate therapeutic services. In inpatient settings, consultation is sometimes initiated by staff who are encountering behavioral difficulties with either the child or the family that are impeding the smooth operation of the hospital ward. The mental health provider must advocate for the child and be a skilled negotiator between the medical staff and the patient. Working through these difficulties requires diplomacy and sensitivity to the issues of the patient, the family, and the other health care providers.

Ideally, children with chronic illnesses are managed by a multidisciplinary team on an inpatient and outpatient basis (Gillman & Mullins, 1991). The optimal team profile includes an individual skilled in biopsychosocial issues and proficient in various medical services. Issues of cost containment, time constraints, and multiple providers make coordinating such a service a challenging task. Multidisciplinary teams are likely to work most successfully when roles are clearly delineated, relationships are well established, and a realistic expectation exists of what services can be appropriately provided. Frequently, mental health providers can be effective leaders and mediators when they possess the sensitivity and social skills necessary to navigate the complex structure within a busy medical service. To accomplish this mission, staff liaison must educate all levels of health care providers. Direct communication and sustaining productive working relationships with key team members are essential ingredients in this process. The mental health provider can help by assessing the various opinions of staff and by building a consensus so that a treatment plan can be successfully implemented.

Gillman and Mullins (1991) suggested that parents, medical staff, and mental health professionals participate in an initial care conference. In this meeting, participants discuss and describe roles and responsibilities for each team member. To encourage compliance with this program, regular conferences that assess progress and determine needed modifications are scheduled. When consensus is achieved, the program plan is outlined, distributed to team members, and placed in the patient's chart.

Successful outcomes are contingent on parental knowledge, understanding, and acceptance and support for the care plan. This aspect is particularly important because parents are sometimes deferential to medical personnel, especially at large medical centers, and may be reluctant to voice their opinions. Parental freedom of expression and support are key factors in managing adherence, pain, and behavioral issues. Family participation in the various psychosocial intervention components is crucial to success of the program. This is especially true in medical conditions (e.g., abdominal pain, headaches, asthma) that result from familial dysfunction (e.g., marital discord, alcohol and substance abuse, physical and other abuse) or are exacerbated by familial stressors.

School Performance and Peer Relations

Few studies in pediatric psychology have evaluated programs designed to enhance peer relationships and to reintegrate children to school (Sexson & Madan-Swain,

1993). The theoretical rationale underlying these programs is to assure normalization of developmental processes by assuring a smooth transition to the classroom.
In one study, the efficacy of a school reintegration program for children with cancer
was investigated (Katz, Varni, Rubenstein, Blew, & Hubert, 1992). The program
included preliminary intervention activities that involved both parents and children, conferences with school personnel about essential issues of the illness and its
management, classroom presentations to peers explaining the illness and associated
treatments, and follow-up contact with school personnel as needed. Children
receiving the intervention program, relative to comparison controls, exhibited better
adjustment when returning to school, fewer internalizing behavioral problems as
reported by both parents and children, and greater physical and social competencies
reported by parents and the children. More important, teachers rated the children
who participated in the program as evidencing better school adjustment relative
to the control group.

Social-skills training has been helpful for reintegrating child cancer survivors to
school (Varni, Katz, Colegrove, & Dolgin, 1993). Such programs are based on
the theoretical tenets that peer social support enhances adaptation to illness and
psychosocial adjustment. The children who received the social problem-solving
training evidenced fewer adjustment difficulties and greater teacher and peer support as compared with children who received only routine school reintegration
services. More important, higher perceived support from classmates was associated
with fewer symptoms of depression and anxiety and fewer externalizing behavioral
difficulties.

In short, intervention studies designed to facilitate reintegration to school and
socialization with peers have demonstrated efficacy in enhancing adjustment. Successful integration into school and socialization with peers are important developmental tasks of childhood, and assistance with these efforts is an important ingredient in successful adjustment.

Family Systems and Parenting

As noted previously, the family is a mediator of children's successful adaptation to
disease and serves as a moderator of adjustment difficulties. Despite the compelling
body of pediatric psychology literature attesting to the importance of the family, few
studies have actually tested family-system–focused interventions. In one promising
exception, however, adolescents with diabetes and their families participated in a
multifamily group designed to promote independent problem-solving skills and
effective communication. These adolescents evidenced improvements in metabolic functioning relative to controls at the three- and six-month follow-up periods
(Satin, La Greca, Zigo, & Skyler, 1989), although no differences were found in
adolescents' or their parents' perceptions of family functioning.

As another example, the efficacy of a "culturally and developmentally sensitive"
intervention program for children with SCD and their families, who were of low
socioeconomic status, was evaluated (Kaslow et al., 1997, p. 213). The children
participating in the experimental intervention group were described as being more

improved and having increased knowledge of SCD in comparison with controls. However, there were few differences between the groups.

Kazac and colleagues (1996) completed a randomized controlled prospective outcome study of a combined psychological and pharmacological intervention relative to pharmacotherapy alone for procedurally related distress associated with the medical management of children with leukemia. The psychological intervention involved parents assuming the primary role in providing distraction, guided imagery, and externally oriented play for younger children. Child and parent psychological distress in both conditions was compared using mothers' and nurses' ratings. Their ratings of child distress revealed less distress in the group that received a combined pharmacologic and psychological intervention relative to the group that received pharmacotherapy alone. The findings emphasize the importance of teaching children to cope successfully during stressful procedures. The investigation underscores the primary role of parents as change agents in promoting children's successful adaptation to those stressful procedures.

In summary, few studies have examined family interventions as a means to enhance both disease adaptation and psychological adjustment for children with various chronic illnesses. Clearly, additional research is needed in this area, particularly studies designed to improve family communication and adaptation patterns as children and adolescents negotiate the stressors of a chronic illness. Programs based on this research will need to be evaluated for their success in mediating parents' and children's adaptation to the disease process, their psychological adjustment, and their overall quality of life.

Adherence

Adherence refers to the extent to which an individual's behavior agrees with advice given by health care providers. Much of the literature concerning adherence in pediatrics has come from the research on antibiotic therapies for the treatment of otitis media and the use of inhalers for the management of asthma (Dunbar-Jacob, Dunning, & Dwyer, 1993). The research on adherence has been limited to a few diagnostic categories examined within a few developmental periods; most studies have been conducted either with school-age children or toddlers. Researchers have generally focused on medication administration, although a few investigators have examined such factors as appointment keeping and dietary studies (Thompson & Gustafson, 1996). Thompson and Gustafson (1996) have observed that the "majority of research on pediatric adherence has been atheoretical" (p. 253).

Three distinct models have been elucidated in the adherence literature: the health-belief model, the self-regulation model, and the systems-theory model (Thompson & Gustafson, 1996). The health-belief model focuses on the role of perceived benefits versus perceived costs in adhering to health care recommendations. Implementing the health-belief model, Slimmer and Brown (1985) used group decision-making counseling and a balance-sheet procedure with parents of children diagnosed with attention-deficit/hyperactivity disorder (ADHD) to enhance adherence to the drug regimen. Parents discussed alternative ways to handle their child with ADHD and subsequently rank-ordered their decision alternatives.

Parents were encouraged to discuss their experiences and seek clarification when they did not comprehend a specific point. The decision-making counseling increased parental awareness of the importance of deliberating about their decisions and also increased adherence. The discussion focused on behavioral actions, as well as psychological mechanisms.

The children's health-belief model similarly describes the role of specific cognitive processes underlying adherence behavior. These cognitive processes include memory, causal thinking, and personal control (Iannoti & Bush, 1993). Parents modeling the home administration of factor replacement therapy for children with hemophilia (Sergis-Deavenport & Varni, 1983) and teaching children with diabetes to self-inject insulin (Gilbert et al., 1982) are examples of training specific cognitive processes that underlie adherence behaviors.

The efficacy of behavioral parent training for children with cystic fibrosis and their parents was examined in another study (Stark, Powers, Jelalian, Rape, & Miller, 1994). The program was designed to target maladaptive mealtime behavior and included the use of differential attention, contingent privileges, setting realistic expectations of behavior at mealtime, and the introduction of new or nonpreferred foods. Parents' attention to disruptive behavior decreased, attention to appropriate eating increased, and parental control at meals increased. The children demonstrated an increase in appropriate behavior, a decrease in disruptive behavior, and an increase in caloric intake and weight. The researchers demonstrated that regulation of the external environment is an efficacious method to improve adherence and health outcome.

Several investigators have demonstrated the efficacy of medical supervision in enhancing adherence to medical regimens, including administration of anticonvulsant medication for children with seizure disorders (Dawson & Jamieson, 1971) and administration of insulin for children with insulin dependent diabetes mellitus (IDDM) (Delamater et al., 1990). External regulation of the environment with telephone calls or visual cues such as appointment cards is also useful (Casey, Rosen, Glowasky, & Ludwig, 1985). Families who received telephone calls demonstrated the highest adherence to appointments compared with groups receiving either patient education or no interventions. Telephone calls also were efficacious for monitoring adolescents' smoking behavior (McConnell, Biglan, & Severson, 1984). Visual cues (e.g., a clock printed on the prescription label) were useful for children and adolescents with various acute illnesses (Lima, Nazarian, Charney, & Lahti, 1976).

Reinforcement procedures are also efficacious in enhancing adherence regimens in children and adolescents. For example, the use of a reinforcement strategy (i.e., a coupon earned for each kept appointment that later could be traded for a prize) for adherence to appointments at an allergy and asthma clinic was evaluated (Finney, Lemanek, Brophy, & Cataldo, 1990). Although the intervention was effective for some of the children participating in the study, the improvement dissipated following termination of the reinforcement program. Clearly, a major problem with reinforcement programs is their failure to be generalized and maintained once the treatment program has been discontinued (La Greca & Schuman, 1995).

The efficacy for internal regulation of behavior is less compelling than the demonstrated success of external regulation of behavior. For example, blood glucose monitoring in adolescents was examined, comparing a self-monitoring condition with a combined condition of self-monitoring and reinforcement (Wysocki, Green, & Huxtable, 1989). The outcome was that for the group participating in the combined condition, blood glucose testing remained at baseline; the adolescents participating in the self-monitoring condition evidenced significant decline in the frequency of blood glucose monitoring. La Greca and Schuman (1995) concluded that self-monitoring likely has little utility in fostering adherence to complex medical regimens. In part, they attribute this to the daily record keeping necessary for self-monitoring and the limited benefits of the procedure for the adolescents participating in treatment.

Family relations and family knowledge about disease are key components for adherence. However, few researchers tested the family system as a means of enhancing adherence (La Greca & Schuman, 1995). A six-week multifamily intervention program for adolescents with diabetes was examined in one study (Satin, La Greca, Zigo, & Skyler, 1989). Treatment conditions included multifamily sessions that emphasized communication skills, problem solving, and family support for the adolescents' self-care. This multifamily condition also was studied in combination with a condition in which parents simulated having diabetes for a week and obtained their own daily glucose levels, maintained a dietary program, and sustained an exercise regimen. Relative to a wait-list control condition, self-care with the diabetes regimen and metabolic control were enhanced by the multifamily intervention program even six months following the treatment program. These results underscore the importance of the family in enhancing adherence behaviors.

Some intervention research examined the combinations of several intervention programs that involved parents and children with the goal of enhancing adherence. Baum and Creer (1986) studied the efficacy of self-monitoring compared with the combination of self-management, self-monitoring, and parental involvement in the therapeutic program. The children in the self-management condition were more likely to manage an asthma attack themselves without seeking adult attention, although no differences were revealed in medication adherence between the two groups. Consistent with these findings, another study provided evidence that suggested that parent and child involvement in the self-monitoring of the diabetes regimen enhanced metabolic control one and two years following the initial diagnosis relative to a conventional treatment and supportive counseling condition (Delamater et al., 1990). Finally, a multimodal intervention that emphasized peer and parent support, education, self-monitoring, and medical supervision was associated with increased self-care and prevention of a decreased metabolic control relative to a standard care condition (Anderson, Wolf, Burkhart, Cornell, & Bacon, 1989).

Intervention approaches have been divided into educational and behavioral strategies (Haynes, 1976). Improvement rates for adherence generally range from 64% for educational interventions to 85% for behavioral interventions and 88% for the combination of educational and behavioral interventions. Despite such improvements, adherence studies have limitations that include small sample sizes, brief treatment durations (with most being less than six months), failure to identify the efficacy of specific components in combined intervention programs, and failure to match specific intervention programs to the specific adherence barriers of patients and their families (La Greca & Schuman, 1995).

Pain Management

Current theory supports the notion that children's and parents' behaviors interact to influence coping with painful procedures and with chronic and recurrent pain (Thompson & Gustafson, 1996). Children of mothers who used more active coping strategies (i.e., problem solving and seeking social support) for chronic pain have been found to manage their pain more effectively than children of mothers who used more passive and palliative techniques (i.e., avoidance and wishful thinking; Sharpe, Brown, Thompson, & Eckman, 1994). The developmental stage of the child also influences tolerance and expression of pain. For example, older children possess a more complex and precise understanding of pain relative to their younger peers. Preschool children possess preoperational thought patterns and may develop causal explanations that are egocentric in interpreting the origins of their pain. Most children and adolescents adequately negotiate the pain associated with their chronic illness (Thompson & Gustafson, 1996). However, a small subset of children become preoccupied with pain, which disrupts developmental tasks associated with childhood and adolescence such as attending school and participation in social activities (McGrath et al., 1986).

Researchers have concentrated on therapeutic interventions for pain. Interventions focus on improving children's ability to cope with painful medical procedures and assisting children in managing stressors from pain associated with chronic illness. Underlying these therapies is the reinforcement of coping behaviors rather than pain- or stress-related behaviors (Jay, 1988). Thus, in the management of painful procedures and chronic pain that may be associated with a long-term illness, parents and caregivers are taught to support their children's active coping efforts by coaching them in the use of behavior and cognitive techniques. These techniques include distraction, avoiding the use of assurance and explanation, and supporting children's active coping strategies. The rationale for these techniques is that the experience of pain involves the interaction of psychological and organic factors. Thus recent conceptualizations of pain have emphasized the interplay among sensory, affective, neurochemical, and motivational factors (Brown, Tanaka, & Donegan, 1998).

Environment may serve to elicit, sustain, or diminish the expression of pain and coping behaviors (Thompson & Gustafson, 1996). For this reason, it is necessary to determine the child's history and experience with pain from multiple sources (e.g., home, clinic, school; Tarnowski, Brown, Dingle, & Dreelin, 1998). As Thompson and Gustafson (1996) observed, "thoughts and feelings serve as the volume (control) for the pain signals and can be used for self-regulation" (p. 287). In addition, psychological factors such as attention, anxiety, history of learning, cultural experiences of pain, attributional meaning of pain, and the developmental status of the child influence the expression of pain in children and adolescents. Consequently, younger children incorporate specific familial and cultural issues in coping with pain, whereas adolescents are likely to assimilate peer social supports into their management of pain (Holden, 1995).

Transforming these assumptions into clinical practice requires that the clinician "establish the context and meaning of pain" (Thompson & Gustafson, 1996, p. 287) for the child so that thinking patterns can be altered to assist children in coping effectively with pain. Therapeutic efforts focus on keeping children from viewing pain as punishment for their behavior or illness. Efforts are also made to assist children in coping with pain rather than curing pain and in minimizing the impact of pain on daily activities so that they can resume typical developmental tasks of childhood.

Numerous behavioral and cognitive methods exist to help children manage painful medical procedures and chronic pain. Brown et al. (1998) reviewed procedures for progressive muscle relaxation, biofeedback, and imagery that decrease sympathetic nervous system activity and result in decreased oxygen consumption and respiration, increased skin resistance, and production of alpha waves. For example, during biofeedback, a child is taught to recognize physiological activity and to differentiate between relaxation and tension. This technique is particularly appropriate for children who have attained concrete operational thought, because biofeedback provides a concrete recognition of various emotional states by means of auditory or visual signals (Tarnowski & Brown, 1995). The use of biofeedback is particularly effective for pain associated with headaches (McGrath, 1991).

Another technique used to manage pain is imagery. Through this process, the child produces a pleasant mental image that incorporates visual, auditory, or kinesthetic images and ultimately results in a relaxation response (Tarnowski & Brown, 1995). Pederson (1995) investigated the physiological, psychological, and behavioral effects of an imagery procedure conducted during a cardiac catheterization. Children in the imagery condition displayed fewer distress behaviors during catheterization than children in the control group. In further support of these findings, relaxation and imagery training were found to reduce cancer-treatment-related pain (Syrjala, Donaldson, Davis, Kippes, & Carr, 1995), although another study found that imagery did not result in diminution of sensory pain (Pederson, 1995).

With distraction, the child's attention is diverted from the painful stimuli and focused on another stimulus. Distraction is grounded in the theoretical tenet that the cognitive processes of attention and concentration may weaken neuronal impulses evoked by noxious stimuli (Tarnowski & Brown, 1995). Various distraction techniques are available, including video games, hand squeezing, counting backwards, and other activities that might refocus the child's attention from the original painful stimuli. Distraction has been demonstrated to be a viable strategy in ameliorating children's perceptions of pain during venipuncture (needle sticks; Vessey, Carlson, & McGill, 1994). The effects of distraction and parental reassurance on children's reactions to injections were compared in another study (Gonzalez, Routh, & Armstrong, 1993). Children in the distraction condition exhibited less behavioral distress than children in either the reassurance group or the control group.

Based on the theory that pain behaviors may be inadvertently reinforced by significant others (e.g., teachers, parents, health care providers), operant or contingency management techniques are frequently used in the management of children's pain. Consistent with the notion that pain behavior is influenced by environment, the contingencies that reinforce pain behaviors are first identified. These variables may include avoidance behaviors (e.g., missed days from school) and familial and emotional factors. The factors most likely to be affected by intervention are identified, and a system of reinforcement is established to reward incompatible behaviors. Contingency management programs are most productive when health care providers and the caregivers are involved in the program and when rewards are contingent on specific behavioral criteria (Tarnowski & Brown, 1995).

The stress-inoculation method, developed by Turk (1978), uses a combination of relaxation, imagery, and contingency management to decrease observed and self-reported stress (Dahlquist, Gil, Armstrong, Ginsberg, & Jones, 1985). Stress inoculation is especially appealing to pediatric patients and their families because there are no invasive physical procedures (Miller, Manne, & Palevsky, 1998). Stress inoculation is generalizable and improvement is sustained over time (Tarnowski & Brown, 1995; Tarnowski, Brown, Dingle, & Dreelin, 1998).

Stress inoculation may be useful within a family systems model. Family members help the child cope with painful medical procedures, and they work collaboratively with medical staff in managing the child's chronic pain. Soliciting family support in the pain management process is critical to the success of such a program for several reasons. For example, any pain management program is contingent on parents' compliance with the various components of the program. Also, family stress may exacerbate pain in children (Maron & Bush, 1991). Finally, children's strategies for managing pain are highly associated with their parents' strategies (Walker, Garber, & Greene, 1993).

In keeping with this model, in another study parents were taught to coach their children in the use of coping behaviors during painful injections (Powers, Blount, Bachanas, Cotter, & Swan, 1993). Whereas parents learned coping-promoting behaviors, children learned specific coping techniques and concomitantly displayed less behavioral distress. Similarly, children who received a family intervention incorporating cognitive-behavioral techniques were shown to have higher rates of pain remission, lower levels of relapse, and fewer activity restrictions compared with children who received standard pediatric care (Sanders, Shepherd, Cleghorn, & Woolford, 1994). Kazak et al. (1996) evaluated a combined pharmacological-psychological protocol, the Analgesia Protocol for Procedures in Oncology. The interventions were individualized and included various cognitive-behavioral approaches in which parents assumed primary responsibility for the interventions. Those children who received the combined intervention of pharmacotherapy and psychological intervention displayed less distress relative to a group that received pharmacotherapy alone. The findings underscore the importance of the family and the efficacy of a multitreatment approach in managing children's pain resulting from stressful procedures.

Summary

Over the past two decades, medical technological advances have resulted in significantly increased survival rates for many childhood chronic illnesses. As mortality has decreased, increased focus on psychosocial issues has become a part of standard care. These children and their families are faced with many challenges and stressors associated with the multiple demands of living with a chronic illness. Attention is focused on the psychological adaptation of children and their families to a chronic illness. The literature does not indicate any single or specific pattern of psychological adaptation to disease; rather, many factors predict adjustment. Because these factors influence developmental progression and outcome, identifying and understanding them is important. Guided by the risk-resistance adaptation model, our review of the literature indicates that risk factors that influence psychological adjustment include severity of disease, adaptive competencies (i.e., functional independence), psychosocial stressors, or some combination. In addition, socioecological factors (i.e., family functioning, social class), interpersonal factors (i.e., temperament, problem-solving skills), and stress processing abilities may either moderate or mediate the impact of these risk factors on adjustment.

Empirically validated interventions in the pediatric literature are still in their infancy. Generally, the few available studies include interventions that target school performance, peer relationships, family systems issues, adherence, and management of pain. Intervention studies that focus on pain management have been the most informative. This research validates previous correlational studies that suggested that psychosocial factors predict overall psychological adjustment and disease adaptation. Methodological design and empirical validation of these interventions may be improved by using the pain management studies as a referent for future research in this area. The foundation for such interventions should follow from existing correlation data. Multisite, collaborative studies will increase sample size and enhance power so that experimental error is avoided. Follow-up studies of these treatment programs will assure assessment of the durability and generalizability of these programs. Further, treatment fidelity is an important variable to consider. Finally, investigators must carefully choose the assessment battery so it reflects appropriate ecological and psychometric validity.

The clinical arena does not always parallel research, and research does not always guide clinical practice. Because of these inconsistencies, clinical practice is not always justifiable. It is hoped that the health care crisis in this country will encourage clinicians to use resources wisely and ultimately use empirically validated assessment and interventions as a standard of care. Undoubtedly, this will require increases in federal funding for clinical research and training. As a hoped-for result, psychosocial and physical morbidities will be reduced and quality of life will be enhanced for children with chronic illness and their families.

REFERENCES

Abramson, L. Y., Seligman, M. E. P., & Teasdale, J. D. (1978). Learned helplessness in humans: Critique and reformulation. *Journal of Abnormal Psychology, 87,* 29–74.

Anderson, B. J., Wolf, F. M., Burkhart, M. T., Cornell, R. G., & Bacon, G. E. (1989). Effects of peer group intervention on metabolic control of adolescents with IDDM: Randomized outpatient study. *Diabetes Care, 3,* 179–183.

Balfour, L., White, D. R., Schiffrin, A., Dougherty, G., & Dufresne, J. (1993). Dietary disinhibition, perceived stress, and glucose control in young, type 1 diabetic women. *Health Psychology, 12,* 33–38.

Baum, D., & Creer, T. (1986). Medication compliance in children with asthma. *Journal of Asthma, 23,* 49–59.

Behrman, R. E., & Vaughan, V. C. (1996). *Nelson textbook of pediatrics.* Philadelphia: Saunders.

Bennett, D. S. (1994). Depression among children with chronic medical problems: A meta-analysis. *Journal of Pediatric Psychology, 19,* 149–170.

Brannon, L., & Feist, J. (1997). *Health psychology* (3rd ed.). Pacific Grove, CA: Brooks/Cole.

Brown, R. T., Eckman, J., Baldwin, K., Buchanan, I., & Dingle, A. D. (1995). Protective aspects of adaptive behavior in children with sickle cell syndrome. *Children's Health Care, 24,* 205–222.

Brown, R. T., Tanaka, O., & Donegan, J. E. (1998). Pediatric pain management. In L. Phelps (Ed.), *A practitioner's handbook of health related disorders in children* (pp. 501–513). Washington, DC: American Psychological Association.

Carlson-Green, B., Morris, R. D., & Krawiecki, N. (1995). Family and illness predictors of outcome in pediatric brain tumors. *Journal of Pediatric Psychology, 20,* 769–784.

Casey, F. A., Sykes, D. H., Craig, B. G., Power, R., & Mulholland, H. C. (1996). Behavioral adjustment of children with surgically palliated complex congenital heart disease. *Journal of Pediatric Psychology, 21,* 335–352.

Casey, R., Rosen, B., Glowasky, A., & Ludwig, S. (1985). An intervention to improve follow-up of patients with otitis media. *Clinical Pediatrics, 24,* 149–152.

Chasnoff, I. J., Burns, W. J., Schnoll, S. H., & Burns, K. A. (1985). Cocaine use in pregnancy. *New England Journal of Medicine, 313,* 666–669.

Chasnoff, I. J., Griffith, D. R., Freier, C., & Murray, J. (1992). Cocaine/polydrug use in pregnancy: Two-year follow-up. *Pediatrics, 89,* 284–289.

Dahlquist, L. M., Gil, K., Armstrong, D. I., Ginsberg, A., & Jones, B. (1985). Behavior management of children's distress during chemotherapy. *Journal of Behavior Therapy and Experimental Psychiatry, 16,* 325–329.

Dawson, K. P., & Jamieson, A. (1971). Value of blood phenytoin estimation in management of childhood epilepsy. *Archives of Diseases of Childhood, 46,* 386–388.

Delamater, A. M., Bubb, J., Davis, S. G., Smith, J. A., Schmidt, L., White, N. H., & Santiago, J. V. (1990). Randomized prospective study of self-management training with newly diagnosed diabetic children. *Diabetes Care, 13,* 492–498.

Devine, D., Brown, R. T., Lambert, R., Donegan, J. E., & Eckman, J. (1998). Predictors of psychosocial and cognitive adaptation in children with sickle cell syndromes. *Journal of Clinical Psychology in Medical Settings, 5,* 295–313.

Drotar, D. (1997). Relating parent and family functioning to the psychological adjustment of children with chronic health conditions: What have we learned? What do we need to know? *Journal of Pediatric Psychology, 22,* 149–165.

Dunbar-Jacob, J., Dunning, E. J., & Dwyer, K. (1993). Compliance research in pediatric and adolescent populations: Two decades of research. In N. P. Krasneger, L. Epstein, S. B. Johnson, & S. J. Yaffe (Eds.), *Developmental aspects of health compliance behavior* (pp. 29–51). Hillside, NJ: Erlbaum.

Finney, J. W., Lemanek, K. L., Brophy, C. J., & Cataldo, M. F. (1990). Pediatric appointment keeping: Improving adherence in a primary care allergy clinic.

Journal of Pediatric Psychology, 15, 571–579.

Fowler, A. G., Johnson, M. P., & Atkinson, S. S. (1985). School achievement and absence in children with chronic health conditions. *Journal of Pediatrics, 106,* 683–687.

Frank, N. C., Blount, R. L., & Brown, R. T. (1997). Attributions, coping, and adjustment in children with cancer. *Journal of Pediatric Psychology, 22,* 563–576.

Gilbert, B. O., Johnson, S. B., Spillar, R., McCallum, M., Silverstein, J. H., & Rosenbloom, A. (1982). The effects of a peer-modeling film on children learning to self-inject insulin. *Behavior Therapy, 13,* 186–193.

Gillman, J. B., & Mullins, L. L. (1991). Pediatric pain management: Professional and pragmatic issues. In J. P. Bush & S. W. Harkins (Eds.), *Children in pain: Clinical and research issues from a developmental perspective* (pp. 117–148). New York: Springer-Verlag.

Goldston, D. B., Kovacs, M., Obrosky, D. S., & Ivengar, S. (1995). A longitudinal study of life events and metabolic control among youths with insulin-dependent diabetes mellitus. *Health Psychology, 14,* 409–414.

Gonzalez, J. C., Routh, D. K., & Armstrong, F. D. (1993). Effects of maternal distraction versus reassurances on children's reactions to injections. *Journal of Pediatric Psychology, 18,* 593–604.

Haynes, R. B. (1976). Strategies for improving compliance: A methodologic analysis and review. In D. L. Sackett & R. B. Haynes (Eds.), *Compliance with therapeutic regimens* (pp. 69–82). Baltimore: Johns Hopkins University Press.

Holden, P. (1995). Psychosocial factors affecting a child's capacity to cope with surgery and recovery. *Seminars in Preoperative Nursing, 4,* 75–79.

Iannoti, R. J., & Bush, P. J. (1993). Toward a developmental theory of compliance. In N. A. Kasneger, L. Epstein, S. B. Johnson, & S. J. Yaffe (Eds.), *Developmental aspects of health compliance behavior* (pp. 59–76). Hillsdale, NJ: Erlbaum.

Ievers, C. E., Brown, R. T., Lambert, R. G., Hsu, L., & Eckman, J. R. (1998). Family functioning and social support in the adaptation of caregivers of children with sickle cell syndromes. *Journal of Pediatric Psychology, 23,* 378–381.

Institute of Medicine (1988). *Prenatal care: Reaching mothers, reaching infants.* Washington, DC: National Academy Press.

Jay, S. M. (1988). Invasive medical procedures: Psychological intervention and assessment. In D. K. Routh (Ed.), *Handbook of pediatric psychology* (pp. 401–425). New York: Guilford Press.

Kaslow, K. J., Collins, M. H., Loundy, M. R., Brown, F., Hollins, L. D., & Eckman, J. (1997). Empirically validated family interventions for pediatric psychology: Sickle cell disease as an exemplar. *Journal of Pediatric Psychology, 22,* 213–227.

Katz, E. R., Varni, J. W., Rubenstein, C. L., Blew, A., & Hubert, N. (1992). Teacher, parent, and child evaluative ratings of school reintegration intervention for children with newly diagnosed cancer. *Children's Health Care, 21,* 69–75.

Kazak, A., Penati, B., Boyer, B., Himelstein, B., Brophy, P., Waibel, M. K., Blackall, G. F., Daller, R., & Johnson, K. (1996). A randomized controlled prospective outcome study of a psychological and pharmacological intervention protocol for procedural distress in pediatric leukemia. *Journal of Pediatric Psychology, 21,* 615–631.

Kazak, A. E., Segal-Andrews, A. M., & Johnson, K. (1995). Pediatric psychology research and practice: A family/systems approach. In M. C. Roberts (Ed.), *Handbook of pediatric psychology* (2nd ed., pp. 84–104). New York: Guilford Press.

La Greca, A. M., & Schuman, W. B. (1995). Adherence to prescribed medical regimens. In M. C. Roberts (Ed.), *Handbook of pediatric psychology* (2nd ed., pp. 55–83). New York: Guilford Press.

Lavigne, J., & Faier-Routman, J. (1992). Psychological adjustment to pediatric physical disorders: A meta-analytic review. *Journal of Pediatric Psychology, 17,* 133–157.

Lewis, H. A., & Kliewer, W. (1996). Hope, coping, and adjustment among children with sickle cell disease: Tests of mediator and moderator models. *Journal of Pediatric Psychology, 21,* 25–41.

Liaw, F., & Brooks-Gunn, J. (1994). Cumulative familial risks and low-birth-weight children's cognitive and behavioral development. *Journal of Clinical Child Psychology, 23,* 360–372.

Lima, J., Nazarian, L., Charney, E., & Lahti, C. (1976). Compliance with short-term antimicrobial therapy: Some techniques that help. *Pediatrics, 57,* 383–386.

Maron, M., & Bush, J. P. (1991). Burn injury and treatment pain. In J. P. Bush & S. W. Harkins (Eds.), *Children in pain: Clinical and research issues from a developmental perspective* (pp. 275–295). New York: Springer-Verlag.

McConnell, S., Biglan, A., & Severson, H. H. (1984). Adolescents' compliance with self-monitoring and physiological assessment of smoking in natural environments. *Journal of Behavioral Medicine, 7,* 115–122.

McCormick, M. C. (1985). The contribution of low birth weight to infant mortality and childhood morbidity. *New England Journal of Medicine, 312,* 82–90.

McGrath, P. J. (1991). Intervention and management. In J. P. Bush & S. W. Harkins (Eds.), *Children in pain: Clinical and research issues from a developmental perspective* (pp. 85–119). New York: Springer-Verlag.

McGrath, P. J., Dunn-Geier, J., Cunningham, S. J., Brunette, R., D'Astoris, J., Humphreys, P., Latter, J., & Keene, D. (1986). Psychological guidelines for helping children cope with chronic benign intractable pain. *Clinical Journal of Pain, 1,* 229–233.

Miller, D. L., Manne, S., & Palevsky, S. (1998). Brief report: Acceptance of behavioral interventions for children with cancer: Perceptions of parents, nurses, and community controls. *Journal of Pediatric Psychology, 23,* 267–271.

Moss, H., Bose, S., Wolters, P., & Brouwers, P. (1998). A preliminary study of factors associated with psychological adjustment and disease course in school-age children affected with the human immunodeficiency virus. *Journal of Developmental and Behavioral Pediatrics, 19,* 18–25.

Nassau, J. H., & Drotar, D. (1995). Social competence in children with IDDM and asthma: Child, teacher, and parent reports of children's social adjustment, social performance, and social skills. *Journal of Pediatric Psychology, 20,* 187–204.

Overstreet, S., Goins, J., Chen, R. S., Holmes, C. S., Greer, T., Dunlap, W. T., & Frentz, J. (1995). Family environment and the interrelation of family structure, child behavior, and metabolic control for children with diabetes. *Journal of Pediatric Psychology, 20,* 435–444.

Pederson, C. (1995). Effect of imagery on children's pain and anxiety during cardiac catheterization. *Journal of Pediatric Nursing, 10,* 365–374.

Pendley, J. S., Dahlquist, L. M., & Dreyer, Z. (1997). Body image and psychosocial adjustment in adolescent cancer survivors. *Journal of Pediatric Psychology, 22,* 29–43.

Phipps, S., Fairclough, D., & Mulhern, R. K. (1995). Avoidant coping in children with cancer. *Journal of Pediatric Psychology, 20,* 217–232.

Phipps, S., & Srivastava, D. K. (1997). Repressive adaptation in children with cancer. *Health Psychology, 15,* 521–528.

Powers, S. W., Blount, R. L., Bachanas, P. J., Cotter, M. W., & Swan, S. C.

(1993). Helping preschool leukemia patients and their parents cope during injections. *Journal of Pediatric Psychology, 18,* 681–695.

Reid, G. J., Dubow, E. F., Carey, T. C., & Dura, J. R. (1998). Contribution of coping to medical adjustment and treatment responsibility among children and adolescents with diabetes. *Journal of Developmental and Behavioral Pediatrics, 15,* 327–335.

Roberts, M. C. (Ed.). (1995). *Handbook of pediatric psychology* (2nd ed.). New York: Oxford University Press.

Routh, D. K. (Ed.). (1988). *Handbook of pediatric psychology.* New York: Guilford Press.

Russo, D. C., & Varni, J. W. (1982). *Behavioral pediatrics: Research and practice.* New York: Plenum Press.

Sanders, M. R., Shepherd, R. W., Cleghorn, G., & Woolford, H. (1994). The treatment of recurrent abdominal pain in children: A controlled comparison of cognitive-behavioral family intervention and standard pediatric care. *Journal of Consulting and Clinical Psychology, 62,* 306–314.

Satin, W., La Greca, A. M., Zigo, M. A., & Skyler, J. S. (1989). Diabetes in adolescence: Effects of multifamily group intervention and parent simulation of diabetes. *Journal of Pediatric Psychology, 14,* 259–275.

Sergis-Deavenport, E., & Varni, J. (1983). Behavioral assessment and management of adherence to factor replacement therapy in hemophilia. *Journal of Pediatric Psychology, 8,* 367–377.

Sexson, S. B., & Madan-Swain, A. (1993). School reentry for the child with chronic illness. *Journal of Learning Disabilities, 26,* 115–125.

Sharpe, J. N., Brown, R. T., Thompson, N. J., & Eckman, J. (1994). Predictors of coping with pain in mothers and their children with sickle cell syndrome. *Journal of the American Academy of Child and Adolescent Psychiatry, 39,* 1246–1255.

Silver, E. J., Stein, R. E. K., & Dadds, M. R. (1996). Moderating effects of family structure on the relationship between physical and mental health in urban children with chronic illness. *Journal of Pediatric Psychology, 21,* 43–56.

Slimmer, L. W., & Brown, R. T. (1985). Parents' decision-making process in medication administration for control of hyperactivity. *Journal of School Health, 55,* 221–225.

Stark, L. J., Powers, S. W., Jelalian, E., Rape, R. N., & Miller, D. L. (1994). Modifying problematic mealtime interactions of children with cystic fibrosis and their parents via behavioral parent training. *Journal of Pediatric Psychology, 19,* 751–768.

Streissguth, A. P., Barr, H. M., Sampson, P. D., Darby, B. L., & Martin, D. C. (1989). IQ at age 4 in relation to maternal alcohol use and smoking during pregnancy. *Developmental Psychology, 25,* 3–11.

Syrjala, K. L., Donaldson, G. W., Davis, M. W., Kippes, M. E., & Carr, J. E. (1995). Relaxation and imagery and cognitive-behavioral training reduce pain during cancer treatment: A controlled clinical trial. *Pain, 63,* 189–198.

Tarnowski, K. J., & Brown, R. T. (1995). Psychological aspects of pediatric disorders. In M. Hersen & R. T. Ammerman (Eds.), *Advanced abnormal child psychology* (pp. 393–410). Hillside, NJ: Erlbaum.

Tarnowski, K. J., Brown, R. T., Dingle, A. D., & Dreelin, E. (1998). Management of pediatric pain. In R. T. Ammerman & J. V. Campo (Eds.), *Handbook of pediatric psychology and psychiatry* (Vol. 2, pp. 1–15). Needham Heights, MA: Allyn & Bacon.

Tarnowski, K. J., Brown, R. T., & Simonian, S. (1998). Social class. In T. H. Ollendick & W. K. Silverman (Eds.), *Developmental issues in the clinical treatment of children and adolescents* (2nd ed.). New York: Plenum Press.

Thompson, R. J., Jr., & Gustafson, K. E.

(1996). *Adaptation to chronic childhood illness*. Washington, DC: American Psychological Association.

Thompson, R. J., Jr., Gustafson, K. E., Hamlett, K. W., & Spock, A. (1992). Stress, coping, and family functioning in the psychological adjustment of mothers of children with cystic fibrosis. *Journal of Pediatric Psychology, 17,* 573–585.

Turk, D. C. (1978). Cognitive behavioral techniques in the management of pain. In J. P. Foreyt & D. P. Rathjen (Eds.), *Cognitive behavior therapy* (pp. 199–232). New York: Plenum Press.

Tyc, V. L., Mulhern, R. K., & Bieberich, A. A. (1997). Anticipatory nausea and vomiting in pediatric cancer patients: An analysis of conditioning and coping variables. *Journal of Developmental and Behavioral Pediatrics, 18,* 27–33.

Varni, J. W., Katz, E. R., Colegrove, R., Jr., & Dolgin, M. (1993). The impact of social skills training on the adjustment of children with newly diagnosed cancer. *Journal of Pediatric Psychology, 18,* 751–767.

Vessey, J. A., Carlson, K. L., & McGill, J. (1994). Use of distraction with children during an acute pain experience. *Nursing Research, 43,* 369–372.

Walker, L., Garber, L., & Greene, J. (1993). Psychosocial correlates of recurrent childhood pain: A comparison of patients with recurrent abdominal pain, organic illness, and psychiatric disorders. *Journal of Abnormal Psychology, 102,* 248–258.

Wallander, J. L., & Thompson, R. J., Jr. (1995). Psychosocial adjustment of children with chronic physical conditions. In M. C. Roberts (Ed.), *Handbook of pediatric psychology* (2nd ed., pp. 124–141). New York: Guilford Press.

Wamboldt, M. Z., Fritz, G., Mansell, A., McQuaid, E. L., & Klein, R. B. (1998). Relationship of asthma severity and psychological problems in children. *Journal of the American Academy of Child and Adolescent Psychiatry, 37,* 943–950.

Weithorn, L. A., & McCabe, M. A. (1988). Emerging ethical and legal issues in pediatric psychology. In D. K. Routh (Ed.), *Handbook of pediatric psychology* (pp. 567–606). New York: Guilford Press.

Weitzman, M. (1986). School absence rates as outcome measures in studies of children with chronic illness. *Journal of Chronic Disease, 39,* 799–808.

Wysocki, T., Green, L., & Huxtable, K. (1989). Blood glucose monitoring by diabetic adolescents: Compliance and metabolic control. *Health Psychology, 8,* 267–284.

18

PATRICIA M. CRITTENDEN
ANDREA LANDINI
ANGELIKA H. CLAUSSEN

A Dynamic-Maturational Approach to Treatment of Maltreated Children

This chapter is intended to describe those specific treatments that are most suitable for maltreated children. The topic seems straightforward, but, in fact, it presents some serious difficulties. First, although it is clear that maltreated children can be helped by treatment (Stevenson, 1999), it is not clear which treatments are most helpful to which children (Kolko, 1998). Second, it is not clear that treatment of abused and neglected children differs in any substantial way from treatment of numerous other forms of emotional and behavioral dysfunction. It has been argued that one of the reasons for this lack of precision is that existing studies are poorly designed. Although that is certainly true, even if the studies were improved, there would remain a lack of clarity about exactly what is being treated and precisely what the outcomes should be. Put another way, a theory of treatment is needed. This chapter presents a "dynamic-maturational" perspective on treatment of emotional and behavioral disorder.

Most approaches to intervention are based on a set of assumptions regarding the relation of a set of causal conditions to a set of detrimental outcomes. For example, physical abuse plus the correlates of abuse (such as poverty, broken families, stress, etc.) are seen as causal to an assortment of symptoms (such as depression, anxiety, aggression, etc.). Primary prevention attempts to eliminate the causal conditions, whereas most psychiatric treatment attempts to control or eliminate the symptoms. In both cases, however, the question of why these conditions are associated with these symptoms often remains unaddressed, as does the process by which the connection between them can be modified. In this chapter we ask what the causal conditions have in common that might explain their detrimental effects and why these outcome symptoms might have developed. That is, we attempt to move beyond a description of the problem and its response to treatment to explain why the risk factors and symptoms require change and how that change might best be structured.

Further, rather than applying a medical model, in which treatment is an attempt to return the patient as nearly as possible to the predisease condition, we use an intervention model. The intent of intervention is to provide a catalytic interruption in a maladaptive interpersonal process that will change the process in a designated manner. Using Bowlby's notion of developmental pathways, intervention does not return the individual to some younger, more idyllic period. Intervention introduces experiences that expand future possibilities in ways that account for early experiences and what was learned in the past without limiting the individual's future to only the narrow range of environments that fit this early experience. Specifically, we ask whether different treatments or treatment techniques can modify an individual's developmental pathway in ways that make possible a wider array of adaptive solutions to life problems. We begin with a short review of what is known about the condition of maltreated children.

The Condition of Maltreated Children

Early work on child abuse and neglect tended to lump all forms and severities of maltreatment together. Increasingly, however, studies have tried to cluster children on the basis of similar sorts of experiences, for example, physical abuse, physical neglect, and sexual abuse. Use of these distinctions has led to greater clarity regarding the relation between causal conditions and effects on children. Nevertheless, the fact that many children are both abused and neglected has tended to reduce the utility of these distinctions. Furthermore, the tendency to dichotomize children's experience as either abusive or nonabusive has reduced our ability to identify variables that differentially affect development in all children. Finally, researchers have been slow to consider development as an important variable both in creating vulnerability to particular forms of parental behavior and also in affecting the sorts of symptoms that may result from maltreatment. For example, being hit by a parent may have very different meanings and effects when a child is 2 months old versus 18 months old versus 5 or 15 years old. Very few studies have considered maltreatment from such a fine-grained developmental perspective. One study that considered variables as dimensions and analyzed the data in terms of child age found that among school-aged children harsh discipline was related in a linear manner to later aggressive behavior and that this was associated with distorted processing of social information (Weiss, Dodge, Bates, & Pettit, 1992). There was no effect for infants and preschool-aged children. This finding suggests that (1) the issue is not abuse per se but rather that harsh discipline has predictable effects and (2) the effects differ by age even to the point of being absent when, possibly, the child is not mature enough to use or retain some of the information present in the experience. It should be remembered, however, that effects are defined by the assessments used; when these are age-specific, there can appear to be no effect even though unassessed effects exist. For example, when children are assessed with verbal measures, there is a particular risk of false negative findings for events that occurred very early in life.

Causal Conditions

One of the clearest and most frequently replicated findings is that physical abuse and neglect are associated with aspects of social disadvantage such as poverty, living in a single-parent family, low parental education, underemployment, residence in dangerous neighborhoods, and frequent changes of residence. All of these conditions either increase the probability of children's exposure to danger or reduce parents' ability to protect children. Moreover, when the variance associated with these conditions is partialed out first, they account for most of the evidence of psychological difficulty, particularly long-term difficulty, that is attributed to maltreatment (Stevenson, 1999). That is, the evidence does not support the notion that it is the abuse or neglect per se that cause the detrimental outcomes that are associated with maltreatment; these outcomes are better explained as degree of exposure to endangering conditions. A comprehensive study of 2,250 unselected women, some of whom had experienced physical or sexual abuse or neglect as children, found that maltreatment of all types raised the probability of psychopathology and that the symptoms were unrelated to the form of maltreatment (Mullen, Martin, Anderson, Romans, & Herbison, 1996). Stevenson concludes that it would be inappropriate and not in the child's best interest to provide treatment that was centered solely around the issue of maltreatment. Instead he recommends that a clear understanding of the network of influences that effect children is essential to focusing treatment properly (Stevenson, 1999). We propose that this network is defined by danger or the perception of being endangered, that is, anxiety.

Psychological and Behavioral Effects

The behavioral and psychological effects of physical abuse and neglect include anxiety, fearfulness, external locus of control, insecure attachment, low self-esteem, passivity, depression, lowered IQ, delay in acquiring vocabulary regarding internal states, delay in expressive language, distractibility, hypervigilance, hyperactivity, compulsive behavior, avoidance in social relationships, aggression, juvenile delinquency, deficits in processing of information about social relationships, substance abuse, and anxiety disorders (see reviews by Cicchetti & Olson, 1990; Crittenden, 1998; Erickson & Egeland, 1996; Youngblade & Belsky, 1990). For sexual abuse, the outcome symptoms are quite similar except for the inclusion of symptoms related to sexuality, for example, sexual dysfunction, age-inappropriate sexual behavior, sexual behavior problems, revictimization, and perpetration of sexual abuse (Browne & Finkelhor, 1986; Green, 1993; Kendall-Tackett, Williams, & Finkelhor, 1993; Malinosky-Rummell & Hanson, 1993). It should be noted, however, that researchers studying sexual abuse generally seek evidence of sexual outcomes, whereas researchers studying physical abuse and neglect generally do not. Consequently, the presence of sexual problems in about one third of sexually abused children can be asserted with some confidence, whereas the absence of such difficulties is less certain in cases of physical abuse and neglect. An important finding from studies in which maltreated children are compared with other disturbed children is that there is no systematic difference in the array or severity of symptomatology (Kendall-Tackett et al., 1993).

Although these lists of symptoms are quite comprehensive and overlap greatly with the symptoms of other forms of emotional and behavioral disorder, Rutter (1983) points out the need to find patterns both among the symptoms and between symptoms and risk factors in order to identify the processes underlying them. That is, Rutter suggests seeking evidence of the functional organization of behavior and using information about these functions to organize more precise and effective treatment strategies. In the almost 20 years since that recommendation was made, more detailed information has accumulated, but an understanding of the function of the symptoms that maltreated children display has not been achieved.

Protective Factors

Much less is known about protective factors in children's environment or experience than about risk factors. Nevertheless, a few conditions or experiences are mentioned repeatedly in the literature. These are the presence of (1) a caregiving member of the family who supports the child by offering protection, counsel, or even just listening empathically to the child; (2) a close sibling relationship; (3) an adult outside the family (such as a teacher or neighbor) who gives recognition and support to the child; and (4) aspects of the child's disposition that foster adaptation (e.g., intelligence, sociability, and academic competence; Garmezy & Masten, 1994; Jenkins & Smith, 1990; Kendall-Tackett et al., 1993; Quinton & Rutter, 1988; Werner & Smith, 1992). Three of these conditions refer to a protective and/or comforting attachment figure, or surrogate attachment figure, and all of them may be, in part, outcomes of the child's adaptation. That is, the abilities to attract and maintain protective and comforting relationships or to display competence may themselves be a function of how the child adapts to his or her experience. Possibly, good adaptation generates the potential for further adaptive functioning.

Treatments That Work

When considering the empirical data on the effectiveness of treatment of children who have experienced abuse or neglect in any of its various forms, three issues should be considered. First, are maltreated children different in some important way from other children in need of treatment and, if there is a difference, does it imply a need for unique forms of treatment? Second, how much impact is treatment likely to have on children's functioning? Third, which treatments are most effective at yielding the desired change? Possibly, however, the central question is, what should be treated and for what purpose? The studies reviewed here do not address the final question, and discussion of it is reserved for the next section.

Design Limitations

Before reviewing the existing studies on treatment of children, it should be noted that the quantity and quality of the studies limits very greatly both the breadth of our knowledge and our certainty regarding the findings. This is particularly true if only studies of maltreated children are considered. Furthermore, very few studies have been carried out that compare treatment strategies on samples of participants who were randomly assigned to treatment groups. In addition, sample sizes are often very small, and the range of outcome measures used quite limited.

The Findings

Are maltreated children different from other disturbed children in ways that have implications for treatment? According to Stevenson's (1999) review of the treatment literature, there is no basis at present for presuming that maltreatment is unique from other forms of behavioral or emotional disorder. Certainly the range of symptoms is essentially identical. However, the importance of the abuse or neglect as an independent contributing factor cannot be dismissed altogether. Based on the findings of Holmes (1995), adults who had a history of childhood abuse, as compared with those without such history, responded less fully to psychological treatment. If, however, abuse contributes something unique, it is not yet clear what that is, whether all forms of maltreatment have this effect, whether it affects treatment only in adulthood, or whether factors in childhood, for example, age at the time of abuse, family functioning after the abuse, and so forth, affect availability or readiness for treatment.

How much of an effect does treatment have on maltreated children? Studies that do not use a control group suggest that treatment of maltreated children may have a positive effect. Waiting-group comparison studies clarify this: four out of five studies cited by Stevenson (1999) demonstrated a positive effect for treatment. The one study with a randomized control group also found beneficial effects for treatment. The small number of studies and the lack of similarity in type of treatment and outcome variables precludes drawing conclusions regarding the efficacy of specific treatments. Reviews of studies of treatment of maltreating parents suggests that they, too, benefit from treatment, but the studies do not indicate whether treatment of parents has beneficial effects on maltreated children (Schellenbach, 1998; Stevenson, 1999). Thus treatment appears to have beneficial, but relatively unspecified, effects (Oates & Bross, 1995; Wolfe & Wekerle, 1993). More important, however, the majority of maltreating parents receive neither parent training nor psychotherapy, even though it is well known that essentially all of them are untreated victims of maltreatment during their own childhoods.

There is a somewhat larger body of studies of treatment for child sexual abuse. Studies without control groups (the majority of treatment studies) indicate a lessening of symptoms over time among sexually abused children but cannot attribute this to the provision of treatment (Finkelhor & Berliner, 1995). Alternative explanations include regression to the mean and spontaneous recovery. Indeed, when control groups were used, there is little evidence that treatment made a difference (Stevenson, 1999). When randomized assignment to treatment groups is employed in the research design, the consistent result is that treatment is more effective than no treatment. Because of the paucity and incomparability of the studies, no meaningful conclusions can be drawn at this time regarding the effectiveness of various types of treatment on different aspects of functioning. Further, studies address only short-term reduction of negative symptoms (12 months posttreatment or less) and do not indicate what effect treatment has overall on children's development.

If one considers the more basic issue of the effects of psychological treatment on disturbed children (thus not limiting the studies to maltreated children), there is strong evidence that treatment is effective and that it is generally about as effective as treatment of adults. One meta-analysis found an effect size of .93 (Shapiro & Shapiro, 1982). This estimate, however, may be inflated as compared with outcomes for normal clinic populations not involved in treatment research. Again, however, it is necessary to point out that long-term effects and diagnosis-specific or treatment-specific effects cannot be determined from the existing literature.

Which treatments are most effective at yielding the desired change? It is abundantly clear that there are insufficient data to answer this question. There are some limited data to indicate that cognitive-behavioral and behavioral treatment may alleviate some types of symptoms for some population of children and that psychoanalytic treatment lacks evidence of effectiveness (Cohen & Mannarino, 1996; Downing, Jenkins, & Fisher, 1988; Weisz, Weiss, Han, Granger, & Morton, 1995). Further, multicomponent programs work, but the contribution of specific components is unknown (Schellenbach, 1998). This lack of precision is a necessary consequence of the limited number of adequately designed studies that compare alternative treatment approaches with equivalent and randomly selected samples. However, even if there were adequately designed studies, it is unlikely that differences favoring one form of psychotherapy over another would be found. Indeed, if the literature on psychotherapy with adults is indicative of effects with children, no differences between treatment types will be found (Lambert & Bergin, 1994; Luborsky, Singer, & Luborsky, 1975; Smith & Glass, 1977).

It is possible, however, that randomized designs, as they have been used to date, may not be a sound approach to testing the efficacy of alternative treatment approaches. That is, if some treatments were more appropriate for some individuals and other treatments were best suited to a different set of individuals, then a randomized design would wipe out effects. Put another way, for a randomized design to yield a meaningful result, the sample must be uniform with regard to the variable(s) that are critical to treatment success. If symptoms are the critical variable, most of the existing research is probably sound. However, if symptoms can serve a variety of psychological functions, then it is possible that some treatments address specific functions better than others. This finding would be lost in studies that randomize patients who are similar with regard to symptom but heterogeneous with regard to the function of the symptom. This addresses the issue of whether a treatment that works in general (in a group design) works for each particular individual to which it is applied (the basic clinical question; Howard, Moras, Brill, Martinovitch, & Lutz, 1996). In addition, existing studies emphasize individual variables without tying these adequately to theory or to the measurement of outcomes. Indeed, there is little consensus on what constitutes successful treatment. Is it adaptive behavior, sense of well-being, or changed personality structure (Strupp, 1996)? Certainly, the last named cannot be measured by mere symptom reduction or self-reported improved feelings. Thus the question of the purpose of psychotherapy becomes critical to understanding which treatment approaches best accomplish that purpose. With regard to this and with an eye to the discussion of theory that follows, it is relevant to note that, in one study, 79% of queried children indicated that the single most important component of therapy was helping them to prevent further abuse (Hyde, Bentovim, & Monck, 1995).

Theories to Explain the Effects of Maltreatment on Children

Theory regarding the process by which maltreatment of children is transformed into maladaptive behavior has progressed from single-cause theories to multiple-cause additive theories to systemic theories. The factors involved range from the specific nature of the maltreatment itself to the individual, dyadic, and family environment to the larger social and cultural context. Few researchers or clinicians would now eliminate any of these influences from consideration. Nevertheless, the progression of the last 30 years from very simplistic theories to highly complex, inclusive, and systemic theories has its costs as well. The more comprehensive theories make it more difficult (1) conceptually to define the problem and (2) practically to design efficient and effective interventions. A means of aggregating relevant information without reducing either its generalizability or its sensitivity to individual differences is needed. The approach taken here emphasizes the function of symptoms and strategic patterning of symptoms with regard to the issues of self-protection and comfort.

To date the most useful approaches have been models that combine essential aspects of children's context with an understanding of how children's maturing mental capacity processes information about experience to generate responses (Cicchetti & Sroufe, 1978; Crittenden, 2000; Sroufe & Rutter, 1984). Crittenden and Ainsworth (1989) have emphasized the importance of caregiving adults (i.e., attachment figures) protecting or failing to protect children from threat. They considered the absence of such protection a "critical cause" of child maltreatment and its effects. More recent work by researchers in both attachment and other areas has focused on the mental processes by which exposure to danger is transformed into distorted attributions of meaning and maladaptive behavior (Crittenden, 1997; Dodge & Frame, 1982; Dodge & Steinberg, 1983; Rieder & Cicchetti, 1989; Weiss et al., 1992). Another recent development is the consideration of two aspects of parents' roles as attachment figures to children: protection of children when they are in danger and provision of comfort when children feel distressed (Crittenden, 1999). The influence of these ideas on the development of psychopathology is considered in the next section.

A Dynamic-Maturational Theory of Danger and Anxiety

Parents function to provide their children with a safe and secure base from which to learn how to live safely and comfortably both within their family and in the world outside the family. When children are not safe, they can be expected to respond in ways that would increase their safety, either by attempting to elicit adult protection or by reducing the probability of eliciting adult threats. When children feel unsafe, that is, when they are anxious or uncomfortable, they can be expected to act in ways that would increase parental attention and reassurance or, if that fails, that create the appearance of invulnerability. These simple statements about behavioral contingencies and regulation of feeling states may be central to the display of symptoms shown by unsafe and/or uncomfortable children and thus to the construction of treatment. That is, children may attempt to reduce the probability of danger to themselves by: (1) doing those behaviors associated with subsequent safety and not doing those behaviors associated with subsequent danger; and (2) using feelings of anxiety to focus their attention on possible sources of danger (and away from safe situations and activities) and to attract the attention and caregiving of potentially protective people. Framed this way, we could say that maltreating parents fail to protect their children adequately or to comfort them sufficiently under conditions of real or perceived danger, including conditions in which the parent is the source of danger.

One of the advantages of this formulation is that it creates a way to think about the relation of maltreatment (the dangerous event) to children's symptoms. Furthermore, because it is phrased in terms of universal conditions and processes, this formulation could explain the functioning of both maltreated children and nonmaltreated disturbed children. Because the data on characteristics of maltreated and disturbed children and on treatment efficacy suggest these two groups of children are drawn from a single population, a theory that encompasses both groups would be very helpful to constructing and selecting appropriate treatment strategies. In the following sections, an elaboration of this perspective is offered in which these two functions, using temporal contingencies to reduce the probability of dangerous events and using feelings of anxiety to focus both children's and caregivers' attention on children's safety, are considered. This elaboration ties symptoms to children's strategies for achieving safety and comfort. This, in turn, provides a basis for considering therapeutic interventions.

Strategies Based on Temporal Contingencies

Behavioral theory provides a very simple way to understand some of the symptoms that maltreated and other disturbed children show. Specifically, when a particular act has preceded an aversive (i.e., self-threatening) outcome, repetition of that act may be inhibited in the future. When a self-threatening event is expected and does not occur, protective properties may be attributed to the act that preceded the nonoccurrence of danger. In the future, this presumed protective act may be repeated whenever danger is expected. These two preconsciously learned attributions of meaning to the relation between self-behavior and dangerous events can lead to inhibitions and compulsions that function to protect the self. These are learned attributions that serve a self-protective function and that may be accurate or erroneous — that is, they may reflect superstitious learning.

Put in terms of information processing, inhibition and compulsion are indicators of self-reflexive, procedural, dispositional representational models that function to protect the self from danger. By procedural is meant that the representations are in procedural memory, a nonverbal, nonconscious memory system that contains information about what to do in specific circumstances. Because procedural memory is precortical, it operates very rapidly; thus in the event of imminent danger it can be more protective than more slowly processed conscious thought. When the outcome of procedural functioning is safety, the process rarely becomes conscious and, therefore, continues to operate in an unchanged manner. Such representations create a disposition to act in a particular manner. Acting with inhibition or compulsion in response to the expectation of danger (based on past experience with danger) constitutes a basic strategy for self-protection. This transformation of sensory information based on the temporal order of events, that is, "cognitive" information, tells *when* in the flow of one's own behavior danger can be expected (Crittenden, 1995, 1997).

Strategies Based on Anxious Arousal

Current neurological evidence indicates that in mammalian species certain kinds of stimuli, processed through the limbic system, lead to (1) physiological arousal (in preparation to fight or flee), (2) increased alertness, and (3) perceived feelings of anxiety. Initially, the signals that initiate this process are innate (i.e., genetically transmitted) and consist of extreme forms of sensory stimulation, for example, darkness/brilliant light, loud noises/intense silence, crowds/isolation, painful touch/light hair-raising touch. With experience, the sensory attributes that accompany experienced danger elicit arousal. In other words, anxiety is an affective state that functions to increase vigilance to possible danger and preparation for self-protection. "Affective" information is not tied to a specific known source of danger but rather signals a change in the probability of danger based on some aspect of the context. Thus this information is less specific, less focused, and more inclusive than cognitive information. Affect tells *where* there may be a higher probability of danger. Anxious arousal may occur when there is, in actuality, no danger.

In information-processing terms, processing of sensory information through the limbic system creates a self-reflexive, imaged dispositional representation. Like procedural representations, imaged representations are precortical, operate very rapidly, and are strengthened through a process of negative reinforcement each time the individual experiences anxiety, responds in an anxious manner, and remains unharmed. Behaviorally, this will appear as agitation, a bias toward rapid attentional shifts (i.e., scanning of the environment for signals of danger), anxiety, attention seeking, and dependence. The opposite condition is one of comfort. One of the most reliable means of achieving comfort, especially in infancy and childhood, is through contact with an attachment figure, especially one who provides rhythmic stroking or rocking, speaks in a low murmuring voice, and holds the child gently close. That is, the innate elicitors of feelings of comfort consist of the opposite sensory signals as feelings of anxiety (learned elicitors can include anything, including comfort itself). Children's display of anxiety tends to elicit precisely these comforting behaviors from caregivers. When children are comfortably near caregivers, they are, in fact, usually safer than when at a distance; even in cases of maltreatment, young children would almost certainly die without the care and protection of the very parents who also maltreat them. Put another way, displaying anxiety (or any of its symptomatic behaviors) functions as a self-protective strategy by eliciting adult caregiving and protection.

Cortical Integration

Both cognitive and affective information use transformations of sensory stimulation to generate predictions about danger and safety. Each creates a dispositional representation that contains the possibility of error. However, because these transformations are processed differently through the brain, the sources of error are different. Therefore, when the attributions in one memory system are erroneous, the representations will usually differ. Cortical processing creates the possibility for selecting and acting on one representation in preference to the other. Specifically, cortical processing permits more thorough analysis of the sensory input (through the sensory cortices) and comparison of a wider array of information (through the hippocampus and prefrontal cortex). All of this, however, takes time. If the threat of danger is perceived as immediate or extremely self-threatening, time cannot be wasted. The representation that motivates self-protection will regulate behavior. Although this often leads to unnecessary self-protective functioning, it maximizes safety. Thus the greater an individual's exposure to prior danger or anxiety, the more the individual is likely to respond self-protectively at a preconscious level, and the less likely he or she will be to engage in cortical processing that could correct erroneous information and fine-tune representational models. This is true for everyone, but it is especially important for children who are unable, for lack of mental and experiential maturity, to completely process information.

A Strategic Perspective on Behavioral and Emotional Disorder

The discussion of attribution of meaning to information and the behavioral correlates of various attributions is directly applicable to how children, especially threatened children, solve problems regarding danger and how those solutions can be construed as psychopathology. Three patterns that reflect the mental processes described previously can be identified, and these three parallel the attachment patterns identified by Ainsworth (1979, 1985) and expanded by Crittenden (1995).

TYPE B   Some children live in safe and comforting circumstances; this promotes mental integration. The more integration that occurs before action is taken, the better fitting the action taken will be. It will reflect the use of both cognition and affect to construct a balanced dispositional representation of the child's situation. In attachment terms, the child will be a Type B child who is safe and feels secure. In the terms of the dynamic-maturational model being proposed here, the child will be using a mental strategy of integrating and balancing cognitive and affective information and a behavioral strategy of communicating with others about needs and desires in the expectation that needs will be met and desires attended to. The Type B strategy is the most adaptive strategy when conditions are safe and caregivers are responsive to children's need for safety and comfort. Under conditions of safety, it is not associated with risk for emotional or behavioral disturbance.

TYPE A   Other children experience actual danger or the feeling of insecurity. Under these conditions, children may curtail cortical processing and act self-protectively. If previous experience with temporal contingencies tied to the presence of danger is the basis for the expectation of danger, children will inhibit danger-eliciting behavior or will exhibit a presumed protective behavior or both. In either case, children may implicitly attribute safety to their own behavior, and this is what they will modify. When this modified behavior effectively reduces the probability of danger, that is, when it actually functions self-protectively, children will both tend to use the rapid, precortical "cognitive" strategy and also come to believe that they control and are responsible for outcomes. What will be observed are overcontrolled, anxious children who are rarely angry or disruptive, who are solicitous of adults, aware of their feelings, perspectives, and intentions, who meet adults' expectations whether these be for caregiving of adults, obedience to adults, or independence from adults, and who may seem inhibited or show compulsive forms of behavior. Although children will understand very little about their own feelings and desires, use of the Type A strategy will lower the risk of angry, dangerous outbursts from powerful adults and increase the probability of protective attention from physically and psychologically withdrawn adults. The strategy will, in other words, increase the probability of safety. In attachment terms, these children will use a Type A "avoidant" (infancy term) or "inhibited" (preschool term) strategy.

TYPE C   Some children live in relatively safe circumstances, but, because of the unpredictability of their parents' attention and caregiving, the ineffectiveness of the parents' comforting behavior, or both, the children do not feel secure. To the contrary, their feelings are aroused, and they feel anxious. Unlike Type A children, they cannot find a predictable pattern of temporal contingencies tied to their behavior. Because the children cannot identify the source of danger, cognition is not an informative transformation of information. Instead, there is only the unfocused feeling of anxiety. This is displayed as physiological arousal, perceptual vigilance, agitation, and active bids to others for attention and protection. These, in turn, tend to elicit attention and comforting behavior from others. That is, anxiety tends to elicit positively reinforcing behavior. If the reinforcement is delivered on an unpredictable, intermittent schedule of positive reinforcement of negative affect (e.g., anxiety, anger, distress), these behaviors will be maintained at a high frequency and intensity in spite of (1) attempts to extinguish the behavior, (2) punishment of the behavior, or (3) positive reinforcement of incompatible behaviors.

If the child's anxious behavior results in parental attention and comforting, the child will relax. Such a mild Type C strategy carries little, if any, risk for psychopathology. If the parent is either (1) preoccupied and, therefore, unresponsive or (2) responsive but not comforting (for example, being angry or distressed), then the child may escalate the behavior to gain the desired attention and comfort. The child may become provocative. He or she will do the opposite of what the parent wants in order to gain attention. If the attention is angry, the child will become disarmingly sweet, with intensified signals of vulnerability and innocence. If the parent is placating, the child will continue to be demanding and provocative. In either case, the strategy is one of intensely exaggerated displays of negative affect that are used to regulate parental attention. This strategy of nonverbal communication of alternating affective states requires the parent's presence; in young children, we call this dependency. It also requires that children not permit their attention to be diverted to other things (i.e., with regard to other activities, such children display a deficit of attention). Further, their conduct becomes "uncontrolled," their moods appear to shift rapidly and intensively (i.e., "disregulated" affect), and, as their anxiety increases, they become actively agitated (e.g., "hyperactive"). Some parents habituate to this; they give up and let the anxious child run wild. In such cases, the child's behavior may escalate to risk-taking behavior; the issue of safety and comfort is put directly before the parent.

One effect of this strategy is to increase parental availability and predictability. However, as the child's efforts to achieve this become more extreme, there is also an increasing probability of parental anger. In some cases, anger is expressed abusively and in other cases as rejection. Thus the Type C strategy of affective communication both elicits parental attention and comfort and, in its extreme forms, may also elicit abuse or rejection.

SYMPTOMS AND STRATEGIES   A major contribution of dynamic-maturational theory is that it interprets the meaning of symptoms in terms of their predictable function with regard to the child's safety and comfort. It explains why and how the symptoms are associated with causal conditions. If the clusters of symptoms are strategies that serve a self-protective function, they may reflect an adaptive response, given the context in which the child lives. For example, under conditions of war, hypervigilance, anxiety, and intense wariness of strangers are both adaptive and self-protective but are associated with psychopathology during the peacetime that follows. When countries, neighborhoods, or families expose children to danger or fail to make them feel safe, self-protective strategies are to be expected. When the danger can be successfully reduced by parents or when parents adequately comfort children, the most adaptive strategy would be the Type B strategy. When a present danger is predictable and tied temporally to the child's behavior, the most adaptive strategy would be a Type A strategy of inhibition or compulsion or both. When there is no actual danger but the parent is unable for any reason to comfort the child, the most adaptive strategy is a Type C strategy of split, exaggerated, and alternated negative affect. When the danger is both unpredictable and uncomforted, an A/C combination of strategies is likely.

Based on the proposition that danger and threat of danger elicit strategies that employ "symptom" behaviors, it would be expected that children who experience more severe danger and at younger ages would most often display Type A strategies, including inhibition, compulsive behaviors, and perceptual vigilance. Children who experienced danger at later ages or with less severity, as well as children who experienced only the threat of danger or the uncertainty of safety, would more frequently use Type C strategies, including agitated, attention-getting, affectively intense, unpredictable patterns of behavior. Type C, in other words, would frequently be associated with emotional and behavioral disturbance, with or without maltreatment.

In all cases, the strategies would be associated with certain behavioral responses, that is, symptoms. From the perspective of dynamic-maturational theory, it is the condition of danger and distress that is undesirable, as opposed to the strategic and self-protective responses to these conditions. Maladaptation occurs when the self-protective strategies are applied to conditions with different characteristics. This includes applying (1) the A or C strategies to safe and comfortable contexts, (2) the A strategy to an unpredictable environment or the Type C strategy to a predictable one, or (3) the B strategy to an unsafe environment. In cases of mismatch, the strategies can become endangering or disruptive. Treatment can both reduce the disruptive symptoms and, more importantly, enable the child to construct more adaptive dispositional representational models to motivate behavior.

A Dynamic-Maturational Perspective on the Treatment of Behavioral and Emotional Disorder

Danger and Adaptation

The central notion behind the dynamic-maturational perspective is that previous experience with danger and feelings of being unsafe are two ways of predicting future safety. Thus they constitute a fundamental basis around which individuals organize thought and behavior. Use of this simple postulate enables well-adjusted, disturbed, and maltreated children to be conceptualized from a single perspective. When children have been exposed to danger or felt themselves unsafe, their mental strategies are expected to overestimate the probability of danger; this maximizes the probability of identifying danger. Similarly, their behavioral strategies function to prevent danger (for predictable, known danger) or to elicit attention and care-giving (for unpredictable, unidentified danger). In both cases, but especially in that of unpredictable and unknown danger, the strategies often employ behaviors that are considered psychopathological. The evaluation of the adaptiveness of the behavior, however, ultimately depends on its function for the child. This, in turn, is tied to the context in which the behavior is used. When behavior that was learned and used adaptively in one context, for example, the family, is applied in another, for example, school or other relationships, it may function maladaptively. The primary goal of treatment should be to enable children to represent accurately a range of contexts that differ in terms of safety and security, to organize a variety of self-protective and exploratory strategies, and to select and implement those specific strategies that function most adaptively with regard to immediate conditions in each context.

This goal cannot be met, however, while children or adults are living in dangerous or threatening circumstances. Consequently, for children living in dangerous circumstances, the first step in the process of providing ameliorative treatment is reducing the danger. Depending on the situation, this can be accomplished through acknowledgment of the problem and temporary restraints on family members' behavior, supervision of the household, relocation of the family, removal of dangerous adults, removal of the child,[1] and/or teaching the child self-protective strategies. Only when safety is relatively probable can treatment of psychological problems be undertaken constructively. Treatment can then focus on reducing feelings of being unsafe and strategies for self-protection.

From a dynamic-maturational perspective, symptoms are a measure of the lengths to which individuals feel they must go in order to be or feel safe. Under dangerous or threatening conditions, it is reasonable to limit other aspects of development in order to survive. Under safe conditions, overattribution of danger limits developmental progress and threatens personal safety and relationships. That is, highly inhibited, compulsive, anxious, or distrustful behavior limits greatly an individual's ability to participate in safe and secure relationships. Thus extreme forms of the self-protective A and C strategies are adaptive under conditions of danger or threat of danger but maladaptive under conditions of safety and security.

Treatment and Developmental Processes

Children's age (i.e., their developmental maturation) affects the risk conditions to which they are vulnerable, their mental and behavioral potential for constructing self-protective strategies, and the extent of family involvement necessary for treatment to be successful.

INFANCY AND EARLY CHILDHOOD   Particularly with infants and preschool-aged children, the primary dangers are in the home, and children's potential to protect themselves or regulate their environment is very limited. Treatment that does not emphasize parents cannot be successful (Crittenden, 1992b). Indeed, because infants and young children cannot think about their situation and instead can only "know" through experience, parents are essential. They determine the context to such an extent that treating the infant and placing him with unchanged parents is futile, whereas treating the parent without treating the infant can be entirely successful at changing the infant's functioning. Ironically, the effects of intervening "successfully" with infants and young children are sometimes devastating to their parents. When a parent sees her child being more cooperative, loving, or settled when in someone else's care, she feels destroyed and ashamed. Permitting such experiences reduces the probability that the parent will become a successful parent (Crittenden, 1983). For this reason, direct intervention with infants should probably be reserved for cases in which the infant is unlikely to return home. The same principle holds true for preschool-aged children, but less extremely so. Surely some nursery situations can be managed, but even so, if the mother feels that her role as mother has been usurped, harm will be done. On the other hand, involving the parent in parent-infant or parent-child psychotherapy or interactional guidance has been shown to be highly effective for both parent and child (Svanberg, 1998).

THE SCHOOL YEARS AND ADOLESCENCE   The school years constitute a transition from the family to the larger community. Parents need parenting guidance that is focused on the specific developmental competencies and problems of their children (Wolfe, Edwards, Manion, & Koverola, 1988). Children benefit from intervention that includes peers and their relationships with peers (Fantuzzo, Jurecic, Stovall, Hightower, Goins, & Schachtel, 1988).

By adolescence the situation is almost reversed: the extrafamilial environment is very important, mental and behavioral capacity are approaching adult levels, and life away from and independent of the parents' home becomes an increasingly viable possibility. Adolescents' emerging ability to reflect on their own behavior and on their behavior in different relationships provides both new means for conducting treatment and a new focus for the content of treatment. Nevertheless, it should be remembered that adolescents are not adults: they have little experience with abstract, self-reflective processes and are not yet fully able to live independent of protective parents. This struggle between desired independence and real aspects of dependency might explain why family therapists so often receive referrals with adolescents as designated patients. Although it is true that adolescents have maturational features that allow individual, self-motivated integrative work, family approaches that emphasize recognition of procedural interpersonal processes and interpersonal discussion of these often seem even more relevant than in school years. Indeed, given that adolescents are just on the cusp of full cortical functioning, treatment strategies that emphasize clarity with regard to procedural, imaged, semantic, and episodic knowledge may be particularly timely in preparing adolescents for the adult task of integration.

ADULTHOOD The central, ongoing task of adulthood is integration, that is, assimilation and accommodation in Piaget's terms, of past experience such that it can be applied productively to the present and future. For adults who have learned to use several strategies and to recognize that others have alternate perspectives, adulthood provides experiences that facilitate integration. Specifically, marriage and child rearing foster perspective taking, in the first case, with a same-aged partner and, in the second, with a child whose developmental status is different from the adult's. These experiences (or similar experiences that require similar integrative functioning) may be requisite for achievement of personal integrity.

This readiness for integration is the desired state for parents, but it is not achieved by all adults as they enter marriage and become parents. This is particularly true for parents of disturbed and maltreated children. The literature on maltreating parents refers to parents as perpetrators, offenders, or the nonoffending partners of abusers. This overlooks the well-known fact that most maltreating parents were the victims of maltreatment in their own childhoods. Moreover, almost none of them had the benefit of treatment. That is, they are being punished for doing what was done (without societal concern) to them by their parents in their childhood. They have carried into adulthood the very sorts of problems that are being treated or hopefully prevented in their children. If the parents were perceived as adult victims in addition to perpetrators, it would become clear that they have (1) decades of history of mistreatment, (2) little experience of an empathic adult caregiver who could understand their perspective, and (3) little experience with making implicit information explicit and integrating discrepant forms of information into regulation of their own behavior. Recognition of these conditions could promote the provision of developmentally relevant treatment to the parents of disturbed and maltreated children. Such an approach, as opposed to an accusatory approach, might promote successful treatment of both parents and their children.

The Therapeutic Relationship

CONSENT AND NONVERBAL NEGOTIATION OF RELATIONSHIPS   Unlike adults and, to some extent, adolescents, young children cannot consent to treatment or evaluate for themselves its beneficial or detrimental qualities. Nor can they participate in the process of therapy in a self-aware and reflective manner. This produces several differences in treatment of children as compared with that of adults. First, therapists who treat children bear a greater responsibility than therapists who treat adults to safeguard the child's interests. This includes not jeopardizing the child's relationship with his or her caregivers, for example, by tying the child preferentially to the therapist; not behaving so as to create doubt, worry, or suspicion on the parents' part; and not promoting the child's use with parents of strategies that might incur further risk. Second, because young children function primarily on the basis of procedural and imaged memory, these will necessarily be central to the treatment techniques selected. Although treatment may facilitate verbalization of what is known implicitly, the reflective processes used in adult treatment will not be the primary method used. Again, therapists who work with children need to be especially alert to their processes, because techniques based on procedural and imaged memory generally place relatively more control in the hands of the therapist than do explicitly verbal techniques. Third, possibly one of the most effective contributions of treatment is facilitation of the child's expression of his or her own perspective and the empathic acceptance of the validity of this perspective by the therapist. Especially when children live with parents who cannot perceive or tolerate the child's perspective, this may not only comfort the child but may also promote keeping the child's representations open to new input, including the child's own perspectives. This holds true even for infants. Fourth, therapists can assist children to predict and understand actions taken to reduce danger, especially those that children often perceive as more dangerous than the maltreatment itself—for example, the removal of a member of the family from the household. Again, it may be important that children both share their own perspective with an empathic person and have the opportunity to see that there can be different possible perspectives on the same action. Fifth, this openness may be the basis on which the therapist can assist the child to construct and implement new strategies. The risk here is that the new strategies may confuse or displease the parent. This danger is a reminder that children's safety, allegiance, and comfort lie with their parents. Forms of therapy that exclude the parents themselves and/or that do not include the parents' perspectives may do no good and may even do harm.

Effective treatment of children should facilitate children's adaptation both at home and in other contexts. Often this will mean augmenting children's repertoire of strategies (as opposed to replacing those learned with the child's parents). Better yet, parents will participate in the process of change, thus enabling their children to use less rigidly self-protective strategies at home.

DANGER Much of the literature on treatment describes therapists as sources of safety and comfort and indicates that establishing trust is preliminary to more in-depth psychological work. The dynamic-maturational perspective is somewhat different. Danger is seen as part and parcel of life; there are no people, places, or relationships that are completely and uniformly safe. Even therapists make mistakes, mistime their interventions, behave with insufficient knowledge, and occasionally behave out of self-interest in ways that are harmful to their clients and patients. In this way, therapists are human; learning to manage this aspect of human relationships is central to recovery from exposure to danger or fear of danger. That is, therapy is not simply about putting past danger in the past; it is also about learning from that danger what is important to self-protection in the future and carrying that information forward in the form of strategic patterns of thought and behavior that can be applied to important relationships outside therapy. Part of the process for accomplishing this requires that the client or patient use his or her self-protective strategies to cope with the failure of trust. Possibly, then, a more accurate preliminary condition to therapeutic work is to convey that using multiple models and perspectives is not only possible and acceptable, but an advantage. Thus the child's or adolescent's perspective is accepted and articulated explicitly, the symptoms are seen as serving a function, and the child's concern for safety is respected even if it leads to areas of dysfunction; but at the same time other perspectives are explored.

In part, then, therapy is about experiencing an examined relationship in which the child can identify current strategies, thus becoming better able to regulate when and how they will be used in the future. (This is the function of "transference.") It is also about becoming confident that one can withstand the threats inherent in even the best relationships and survive the occasional failures of trust. That is, therapy is similar to actual intimate relationships in that it addresses topics that are central to the self and the self in intimate relationships; of these, the safety of the self is crucial. Therapy is different from naturally occurring relationships in that (1) it is not itself one of these relationships and (2) threats to the self are regulated so as to be relatively few, executed with awareness and intention by the therapist to serve the patient or client's interests (as opposed to the therapist's), and gauged so as to require only small and almost certainly possible steps forward in strategic competence. One might say that therapy is a purposefully engineered relationship that functions to make other relationships safer. In this sense, the therapist's role is catalytic. The therapist's job is not to make the change but rather to help initiate change and to assist during its initial stages. Put another way, if the therapist were to be trusted, were to make the change, and were to provide comfort as a powerful and knowing person, then the changes made and the processes started could not be sustained after the end of therapy and, ultimately, would make no real sense.

In addition, therapy provides an opportunity to expand the child's repertoire of strategies in a protected environment, thus promoting adaptation in a wider range of circumstances. For maltreated and disturbed children, a particular challenge is learning to manage those relationships that are largely safe, protective, and comforting, that is, relationships that fit the Type B strategy. Trust, in both oneself and also others, is inherent in the Type B strategy of open and direct communication of thoughts and feelings, together with negotiation of others' perspectives. This necessarily exposes individuals to others' failure of empathy, to conflicting interests, and to treachery. Consequently, the Type B strategy can be a naively endangering strategy under dangerous circumstances. Under some dangerous circumstances and all deceptively dangerous circumstances, the Type B strategy is not adaptive. Because no relationship is perfectly safe and entirely comforting, use of the Type B strategy always incurs some vulnerability to pain and treachery. Trust reflects an informed willingness, born of strategic competence to protect the self, to tolerate this vulnerability.

Selecting Treatment Techniques

An important notion in the dynamic-maturational perspective is that the Type A and C strategies constitute opposite mental and behavioral strategies. A corollary of this is that some treatment techniques that promote correction of the distortions inherent in one strategy may augment the distortions of the other strategy. That is, selection of an inappropriate treatment strategy may increase the child's psychological problems or exacerbate the symptoms or both; see, for example, data offered by Heibert-Murphy, De Luca, and Runtz (1992) and Nelki and Watters (1989). Nevertheless, precisely focused techniques produce more easily measured results than global unspecified strategies or generalized support.

Unfortunately, there may be an inverse relation between the precision of measurement of outcomes and the overall importance of the outcome. Indeed, it may be that the process of treatment, by modeling and enacting means of managing interpersonal engagement, may itself be the most powerful and important aspect of treatment. This, of course, presumes that the process promotes both reflective integration and transfer of emerging competencies to actual life circumstances. This alternating process of standing back to view complexity and then engaging in real-life complexity is not well reflected in most forms of intervention or therapy. Family therapy constitutes an exception, albeit one that uses relatively imprecise assessment and treatment techniques.

Awareness of children's strategies could assist in the selection of appropriate treatment techniques. For example, many Type A children inhibit expression of negative feelings, especially anger, fear, and desire for comfort; treatment techniques that encourage them to focus on and express these feelings may be helpful, whereas techniques that encourage them to take other people's perspectives may augment the distortion of their existing strategy. Type C children, on the other hand, are strongly motivated by negative affect; they need to be encouraged to attend to others' feelings and to regulate their display of affect in ways that reduce its arousing function. In general, treatment techniques for children using a Type A strategy should help children to augment their awareness of their own feelings and perspectives and to accept imperfection in themselves. Treatment techniques for children using a Type C strategy should enable them to identify predictable patterns of consequences, to differentiate complex feeling states, and to regulate and communicate feelings at a moderate intensity. For all children, there is a need to learn to tolerate ambiguity, uncertainty, and complexity, to negotiate perspectives and shared control with others, and to use different strategies in different contexts. For some examples of how treatment techniques might be associated with the Type A and C self-protective strategies, see Table 18.1; this list is not definitive and there are no empirical data at present to confirm or disconfirm the proposed associations. Generating such data is an appropriate goal of future research.

Assessing Attachment

Pattern of attachment is a central construct in the approach offered here. At present, there is a wide range of assessments of pattern of attachment across the life span. It should be noted, however, that only some of these assess the full range of patterns described by the dynamic-maturational model and that none of these are simple self-report or checklist measures. A set of suitable assessments is described in Crittenden (1998, 1999).

People and Contexts

Children do not live in isolation. They are not maltreated in isolation and they do not develop emotional or behavioral disorder in isolation. There are always people whose interactions with children strongly affect children's functioning and contexts whose characteristics facilitate or limit children's development. For these reasons, almost no one recommends individual psychological treatment of children in the absence of attention to their family and context. The differences in perspectives have to do with (1) the breadth of involvement beyond the child (e.g., the school or peers), (2) the means of involvement (e.g., directly with the family, as in family therapy, or among professionals who deal with different people in the child's system), (3) management of differences in allegiance and needs (e.g., issues of confidentiality and legal responsibility, competing needs of family members, professionals' personal and discipline-based differences in priorities), and (4) the degree of integration of services (i.e., multidisciplinary teams, different therapists for each family member, or central coordination and control of services).

What is striking about this list is that it often threatens professionals who sometimes resist expanding their perspective to include people other than their designated client or patient, who frequently find the priorities of other professional disciplines to be skewed, and who generally fear yielding control to others. Families are less worried about these issues and instead seek coordinated services, desire participation in all parts of the service plan, and complain about confusing treatment plans. Typically, intervention with maltreated children uses multidisciplinary teams to combine multiple levels and types of service aimed at the array of problems affecting maltreating families. Nevertheless, the outcome has been less cohesive and integrated than may be required for effective treatment of the psychological and behavioral consequences of abuse and neglect. This can lead to fragmented, competing, and confusing service delivery (Crittenden, 1992a).

One reason for families' frequent failure to cooperate with treatment plans is that they feel a loss of control. Their inclusion in the decision-making process about their own lives is usually limited to signing service contracts and being mentioned in policy statements. Parental attendance at multidisciplinary decision-

TABLE 18.1 Examples of Intervention Techniques with Differential Effects on Memory Systems and Types A and C Children.

1. *Technique:* Reinforcement contingencies negotiation (behavioral contracting between parents and child).
   Memory systems affected: Procedural (contingencies), semantic (discussion of these).
   Effect on Type A children: Superficial change. Advantages: feelings, opinions, and needs of the child are acknowledged, expressed, and negotiated (but only for children for whom a degree of awareness already exists). Risk: increased belief by the child that his or her behavior is central to family outcomes (i.e., that the child bears more than personal responsibility).
   Effect on Type C children: Essential to change. Advantages: Expectation of predictability, leading to reduced anxiety. Augmentation of ability to tolerate frustration, to decenter from one's own perspective, to negotiate needs, and to share planning with the parent. Risks: Escalation of negative child behavior in response to changed contingencies, resulting in parents' inability to maintain the contingencies (hence a return to unpredictability but at a higher level of disruptiveness).

2. *Technique:* Progressive muscular relaxation (Jacobson, 1938) with focused imagery.
   Memory systems affected: Imaged.
   Effect on Type A children: Beneficial (especially in situations such as severe tonic-clonic stuttering or motor tics among compulsive children). Advantages: Reduction of internal distress, more adequate functioning. Risks: None.
   Effect on Type C children: Superficial. Advantages: Few; type C children usually resist the technique. Risks: It can slightly disorganize the management of affect by focusing attention away from arousing stimuli. It can also lead to symptom substitution if the function of agitated arousal is not addressed.

3. *Technique:* Self-Instructional Training (Meichenbaum, 1977).
   Memory systems affected: Procedural, semantic.
   Effect on Type A children: Not very effective. Advantages: Increased performance. Risks: Reduction in behavioral flexibility and emotional awareness because the ability to impose temporal order on information and to set aside feelings in favor of performance is already overdeveloped.
   Effect on Type C children: Beneficial. Advantages: More ability to control internal states and to tolerate frustration and less perception of being controlled by others (e.g., attention-deficit disorder with hyperactivity [ADHD] in which there is a deficit in the mediation between, and temporal ordering of, stimuli and enacted responses). Risks: Few, as long as the goal is selected by the child or adolescent. If it is not, the technique is either wasted or the potential source of a battle with therapist or family.

4. *Technique:* Classic cognitive techniques (A-B-C form where A = an event, B = thoughts during the event, and C = feelings during the reaction; Beck, 1976; Ellis, 1962).
   Memory systems affected: Semantic, episodic.
   Effect on Type A children: Very little efficacy. Advantages: Some effect if more emphasis is put on the "C" stage and on somatic images as opposed to the semantic connotations of emotions. Risks: Increased analytical distancing of self from experience.
   Effect on Type C children: Beneficial. Advantages: Improved ability to describe events semantically, order them temporally, and thus regulate internal affective states (e.g., anxiety disorders, "school" phobia). Risks: Because thoughts are treated as central to motivation, the power of feelings to motivate Type C children's behavior may be overlooked, thus leaving unchanged their dependence on affect to organize behavior.

5. *Technique:* Moviola (reviewing past life episodes both forward and backward and from a distance and close up on segments; Guidano, 1991).
   Memory systems affected: Imaged (zooming in), semantic (zooming out), episodic.
   Effect on Type A children: Beneficial. Advantages: Emphasis on zooming in to examine the body images tied to affect can increase children's awareness of their own feelings. Risks: Emphasis on temporal sequencing can augment the existing distortions in Type A children.
   Effect on Type C children: Beneficial. Advantages: Emphasis on viewing the episode in "slow motion" so as to identify the temporal sequencing, that is, zooming out, improves Type C children's understanding of causal relations. Risks: Emphasis on affective states can augment the existing distortions in Type C children.

TABLE 18.1   Continued

---

6. *Technique:* Family sculpting (Papp, 1976).

Memory systems affected: Imaged (somatic images), semantic (when discussed verbally).

Effect on Type A children: Beneficial. Advantages: Identification of child's affective state in cases of inhibition (including severe psychosomatic inhibition). Risks: Exposure of the child to parents' disapproval.

Effect on Type C children: Limited effectiveness, unless it is used to increase verbal differentiation of affective states and to recognize others' affective states. Risks: Very arousing, so the limited ability to regulate emotional state and the affect contagion can lead to affective and behavioral disorganization. In addition, the difficulty of Type Cs to accept directions can make the application of the technique a struggle, shifting the focus from the experience of the sculpture itself to a power struggle of the family with the therapist.

---

making meetings is rare, and, when it occurs, parents generally listen rather than have substantial input to decisions. Yet family acceptance of the plan is so essential for the success of the plan that any and all professionals could refuse to participate and the plan could go forward; but without the family, there is no plan.

Alternatives, although rare in Western countries, exist. Prior to the professionalization of mental health treatment early in this century, all "treatment" was managed in the family-community context. An example of this traditional process is approximated in New Zealand for Maori (aboriginal) child protection cases. When a child's welfare is jeopardized, a planning meeting is called. Family, neighbors, lay personnel (religious leaders, etc.), and professionals are invited. Although professionals manage the meeting, the extended family takes primary responsibility for its members and their problems. The ultimate solution must be accepted by the family, which then takes responsibility for its implementation. More so than the Western process, this procedure (1) gathers all components of the child's developmental context and (2) places responsibility in the hands of those who must implement change while (3) still accessing the full range of professional resources. Such an approach reflects the actual location of power, responsibility, and context-specific knowledge. Compared with usual professional practices, it is a radically traditional strengths approach.

Summary

Whom Should We Treat?

Maltreated children constitute one end of a spectrum of endangerment. The more advantaged end consists of well-functioning children who are generally safe and usually both comfortable and comforted. Between these is a range of children who are less confident of their safety and less safe; some of these children are identified as emotionally disturbed or behaviorally disordered. In addition, the parents of maltreated and disturbed children are the untreated adult victims of childhood endangerment and threat; through their parenting practices, they introduce their children to self-protective strategies that are suitable to self-threatening conditions. Finally, because children live in interpersonal environments and use their strategies to regulate these, treatment must attend to the needs and behavior of family members, relevant authority figures (for example, teachers), and acquaintances (for example, neighbors and peers). Successful treatment of interpersonal problems cannot be focused on a single individual in isolation from the contributions, needs, and perspectives of other people.

What Are We Treating?

Currently, most treatment is directed toward the reduction of behavioral symptoms, whereas, in the past, the goal was usually structural personality change. A dynamic-maturational perspective seeks an intermediary level of specificity. The goal of treatment is to enable children and their parents to organize their mental processes and behavior so as to live in reasonable safety and comfort in a varied range of environments while concurrently being able to attend to aspects of life other than safety and comfort. This implies that treatment must address the issue of physical and psychological safety. Because many risk factors associated with emotional and behavioral disorder are indicative of threat of danger or lack of resources to protect children from danger, reduction of these is relevant to children's treatment. Successful treatment also requires that symptoms be considered in terms of both what elicits them and their likely outcomes; symptoms, in other words, should be considered as evidence of underlying self-protective strategies. Awareness of these strategies and expansion of children's repertoire of strategies are considered more important than reduction of symptom display (indeed, this can often be accomplished most effectively using pharmacological therapies). In this regard, treatment techniques that impose on children or force them to accept what they fear, for example, "holding therapies," may reduce symptoms but increase psychological harm by substituting inhibition and compliance for strategic attempts by the child to create predictable effects. What are we treating? We are treating the effects of danger and the perception of being unsafe. The role of treatment is to reduce the impact of danger and increase the possibility of safety and comfort for both children and their parents.

How Do We Treat the Effects of Danger?

Treatment uses strategically guided therapeutic relationships to improve children's real-life relationships. Both specific treatment techniques and the process of organizing these techniques function to enable children and their parents to adapt their behavior to the variety of relationships and contexts that constitute their lives. This does not mean teaching children and parents to use the Type B strategy exclusively. To the contrary, because danger is a naturally occurring aspect of every life, good treatment facilitates the development of an array of strategies suitable for the range of human conditions. That is, effective treatment assists individuals to maintain representational models that are open to new information and that constantly undergo a process of concatenated integration and reintegration as new experiences and newly maturing psychological processes make new syntheses possible. This facilitates a lifelong process of generating an increasingly refined repertoire of interpersonal strategies. Furthermore, good treatment does not attend solely to the needs of any one family member in preference to those of others. Successful family life and interpersonal relationships of all types require balancing each individual's needs and desires with those of others. Treatment should both exemplify and teach this process. When it is successful, psychological treatment enables formerly threatened individuals to turn their attention to other aspects of life.

A good treatment model is not a set of approved or best techniques; to the contrary, good treatment is a process of selecting sets of techniques, each tied to the unique features of specific individuals and families, that function to (1) increase safety and comfort and (2) prepare individuals to maintain the process of adaptation for themselves. Such a model is based on the postulate that mental and behavioral processes are evolved to promote self-protection and that both prior experience and feelings of anxiety or comfort inform the process of adaptation. Thus the model postulates two basic strategies and the integration of these over the course of a lifetime to generate an array of strategies that promote safety and comfort under almost all possible conditions and in almost all possible contexts. The model itself favors no particular behavioral strategy. Instead, the strategy that best fits current circumstances is deemed most adaptive. On the other hand, the model places ultimate priority on a mental process of open and direct consideration of all information, awareness of distortions of information and behavior, and conscious implementation of all behavioral strategies when they are the most appropriate strategy. The model favors self-reflection as the means by which behavior can be freed from the constraints of unique developmental histories so as to be applied adaptively to the changing conditions of each life. The dynamic-maturational model promotes flexibility and variability of behavior, regulated by a conscious and reflective mind. Establishing this is a lifelong process. Successful treatment prepares children and their parents to engage fruitfully in this process.

ACKNOWLEDGMENTS   The authors appreciate the assistance of Furio Lambruschi on Table 18.1 and of P. O. Svanberg in the development of this chapter.

NOTE

1. Removal of the child is one of the most frequently used forms of intervention in cases of maltreatment. It is unclear, however, whether it is intended primarily to help the child or to punish the parent. Certainly, it is rarely accompanied by other forms of intervention with the child or the parent. To the contrary, placement often functions more like warehousing children while adults delay difficult decisions. However, removal of children from their attachment figures, including maltreating attachment figures, always involves the trauma of loss or separation, as well as the stress of having to adapt to new people and households. This often leads to further behavioral disorder that, in turn, jeopardizes placements. Multiple placements, accompanied by repeated assaults of children's security, are more common than single or permanent placements, and maltreatment in placement is more common than in the general population. The point is that removal of children from their parents is

a dangerous act that should be undertaken only when there is immediate threat of permanent injury to the child that cannot be prevented or substantially reduced by improved service to the family.

REFERENCES

Ainsworth, M. D. S. (1979). Infant-mother attachment. *American Psychologist, 34,* 932–937.

Ainsworth, M. D. S. (1985). Patterns of infant-mother attachment: Antecedents and effects on development. *Bulletin of the New York Academy of Medicine, 61,* 771–791.

Beck, A. T. (1976). *Cognitive therapy and emotional disorders.* New York: International Universities Press.

Browne, A., & Finkelhor, D. (1986). Impact of child sexual abuse: A review of the literature. *Psychological Bulletin, 99,* 66–77.

Cicchetti, D., & Olson, K. (1990). The developmental psychopathology of child maltreatment. In M. Lewis & S. M. Miller (Eds.), *Handbook of developmental psychopathology* (pp. 261–279). New York: Plenum Press.

Cicchetti, D., & Sroufe, L. A. (1978). An organizational view of affect: Illustration from the study of Down's Syndrome infants. In M. Lewis & L. Rosenblum (Eds.), *The development of affect* (pp. 309–350), New York: Plenum Press.

Cohen, J. A., & Mannarino, A. P. (1996). A treatment outcome study for sexually abused preschool children: Initial findings. *Journal of the Academy of Child and Adolescent Psychiatry, 35,* 42–50.

Crittenden, P. M. (1983). The effect of mandatory protective daycare on mutual attachment in maltreating mother-infant dyads. *International Journal of Child Abuse and Neglect, 3,* 297–300.

Crittenden, P. M. (1992a). The social ecology of treatment: A case study of a service system for maltreated children. *American Journal of Orthopsychiatry, 17,* 1–13.

Crittenden, P. M. (1992b). Treatment of anxious attachment in infancy and early childhood. *Development and Psychopathology, 4,* 575–602.

Crittenden, P. M. (1995). Attachment and psychopathology. In S. Goldberg, R. Muir, & J. Kerr (Eds.), *John Bowlby's attachment theory: Historical, clinical, and social significance* (pp. 367–406), New York: Analytic Press.

Crittenden, P. M. (1997). Toward an integrative theory of trauma: A dynamic-maturational approach. In D. Cicchetti & S. Toth (Eds.), *Rochester Symposium on Developmental Psychopathology: Vol. 10. Risk, trauma, and mental processes* (pp. 34–84). Rochester, NY: University of Rochester Press.

Crittenden, P. M. (1998). Dangerous behavior and dangerous contexts: A thirty-five-year perspective on research on the developmental effects of child physical abuse. In P. Trickett (Ed.), *Violence to children* (pp. 11–38). Washington, DC: American Psychological Association.

Crittenden, P. M. (1999). Danger and development: The organization of self-protective strategies. In J. I. Vondra & D. Barnett (Eds.), *Monographs of the Society for Research in Child Development: Vol. 64, No. 3 Atypical attachment in infancy and early childhood among children at developmental risk.* (pp. 145–171).

Crittenden, P. M. (2000). A dynamic-maturational model of the function, development, and organization of human relationships. In R. S. L. Mills & S. Duck (Eds.), *Developmental psychology of personal relationships* pp. 199–218. Chichester, England: Wiley.

Crittenden, P. M., & Ainsworth, M. D. S.

(1989). Child maltreatment and attachment theory. In D. Cicchetti & V. Carlson (Eds.), *Handbook of child maltreatment* (pp. 432–463). New York: Cambridge University Press.

Dodge, K. A., & Frame, C. L. (1982). Social cognitive biases and deficits in aggressive boys. *Child Development, 53,* 620–635.

Dodge, K. A., & Steinberg, M. S. (1983). Attributional bias in aggressive adolescent boys and girls. *Journal of Social and Clinical Psychiatry, 1,* 312–321.

Downing, J., Jenkins, S. J., & Fisher, G. L. (1988). A comparison of psychodynamic and reinforcement treatment with sexually abused children. *Elementary School Guidance Counseling, 22,* 291–298.

Ellis, A. (1962). *Reason and emotion in psychotherapy.* New York: Stuart.

Erickson, M. F., & Egeland, B. (1996). Child neglect. In J. Briere, L. Berliner, J. Bulkey, C. Jenny, & T. Reid (Eds.), *APSAC Handbook on Child Maltreatment* (pp. 158–174). Thousand Oaks, CA: Sage.

Fantuzzo, J. W., Jurecic, L., Stovall, A., Hightower, A. D., Goins, C., & Schachtel, D. (1988). Effects of adult and peer social initiations on the social behavior of withdrawn, maltreated preschool children. *Journal of Consulting and Clinical Psychology, 56,* 34–39.

Finkelhor, D., & Berliner, L. (1995). Research on treatment of sexually abused children: A review and recommendations. *Journal of the Academy of Child and Adolescent Psychiatry, 34,* 1408–1423.

Garmezy, N., & Masten, A. (1994). Chronic adversities. In M. Rutter, L. Hersov, & E. Taylor (Eds.), *Child and adolescent psychiatry* (pp. 191–208). Oxford, England: Blackwell Scientific Publications.

Green, A. H. (1993). Child sexual abuse: Intermediate and long-terms effects and intervention. *Journal of the American Academy of Child and Adolescent Psychiatry, 32,* 890–902.

Guidano, V. F. (1991). *The self in process.* New York: Guilford Press.

Heibert-Murphy, D., De Luca, R., & Runtz, M. (1992). Group treatment for sexually abused girls: Evaluation outcome. *Families in Society, 73,* 205–213.

Holmes, T. R. (1995). A history of childhood abuse as a predictor variable: Implications for outcome research. *Research on Social Work Practice, 5,* 297–308.

Howard, K. I., Moras, K., Brill, P. L., Martinovitch, Z., & Lutz, W. (1996). Evaluation of psychotherapy: Efficacy, effectiveness, and patient progress. *American Psychologist, 51,* 1059–1064.

Hyde, C., Bentovim, A., & Monck, E. (1995). Some clinical and methodological implications of a treatment outcome study of sexually abused children. *Child Abuse and Neglect, 19,* 1387–1399.

Jacobson, E. (1938). *Progressive relaxation.* Chicago: University of Chicago Press.

Jenkins, J. M., & Smith, M. A. (1990). Factors protecting children in disharmonious homes: Maternal reports. *Journal of the American Academy of Child and Adolescent Psychiatry, 29,* 60–69.

Kendall-Tackett, K. A., Williams, L. M., & Finkelhor, D. (1993). Impact of sexual abuse on children: A review and synthesis of recent empirical studies. *Psychological Bulletin, 113,* 164–180.

Kolko, D. (1998). Treatment and intervention: For child victims of violence. In P. Trickett (Ed.), *Violence to children* (pp. 213–249). Washington, DC: American Psychological Association.

Lambert, M. J., & Bergin, A. E. (1994). The effectiveness of psychotherapy. In J. C. Norcross & M. R. Goldstein (Eds.), *Handbook of psychotherapy integration* (4th ed., pp. 143–189). New York: Wiley.

Luborsky, L., Singer, B., & Luborsky, L. (1975). Comparative studies of psychotherapies: Is it true that "Everyone has won and all must have prizes"? *Archives of General Psychiatry, 32,* 995–1008.

Malinosky-Rummell, R., & Hanson, D. J. (1993). Long-term consequences of childhood physical abuse. *Psychological Bulletin, 114,* 68–79.

Meichenbaum, D. (1977). *Cognitive-behavior modification: An integrative approach.* New York: Plenum Press.

Mullen, P. E., Martin, J. L., Anderson, J. C., Romans, S. E., & Herbison, G. P. (1996). The long-term impact of the physical, emotional, and sexual abuse of children: A community study. *Child Abuse and Neglect, 20,* 7–21.

Nelki, J. S., & Watters, J. (1989). A group for sexually abused children: Unraveling the web. *Child Abuse and Neglect, 13,* 369–375.

Oates, R. K., & Bross, D. C. (1995). What have we learned about treating child physical abuse? A literature review of the past decade. *Child Abuse and Neglect, 19,* 463–473.

Papp, P. (1976). Family choreography. In P. J. Guerin (Ed.), *Family therapy: Theory and practice.* New York: Gardner Press.

Quinton, D., & Rutter, M. (1988). *Parenting breakdown: The making and breaking of intergenerational links.* Avebury, England: Gower.

Rieder, C., & Cicchetti, D. (1989). Organizational perspective on cognitive control functioning and cognitive-affective balance in maltreated children. *Developmental Psychology, 25,* 382–393.

Rutter, M. (1983). Stress, coping, and development: Some issues and some questions. In N. Garmezy & M. Rutter (Eds.), *Stress, coping and development in children* (pp. 1–41). New York: McGraw-Hill.

Schellenbach, C. J. (1998). Child maltreatment: A critical review of research on treatment for physically abusive adults. In P. Trickett (Ed.), *Violence to children* (pp. 251–268). Washington, DC: American Psychological Association.

Shapiro, D. A., & Shapiro, D. (1982). Meta-analysis of comparative therapy studies: A replication and refinement. *Psychological Bulletin, 92,* 581–604.

Smith, M. L., & Glass, G. V. (1977). Meta-analysis of psychotherapy outcome studies. *American Psychologist, 32,* 752–760.

Sroufe, L. A., & Rutter, M. (1984). The domain of developmental psychopathology. *Child Development, 55,* 17–29.

Stevenson, J. (1999). The treatment of the long-term sequelae of child abuse. *Journal of Child Psychology and Psychiatry, 40,* 89–111.

Strupp, H. (1996). The tripartite model and the *Consumer Reports* study. *American Psychologist, 51,* 1017–1024.

Svanberg, P. O. (1998). Attachment, resilience, and prevention. *Journal of Mental Health*-UK, 7(6), 543–578.

Weiss, B., Dodge, K. A., Bates, J. E., & Pettit, G. S. (1992). Some consequences of early harsh discipline: Child aggression and maladaptive social information processing style. *Child Development, 63,* 1312–1335.

Weisz, J. R., Weiss, B., Han, S. S., Granger, D. A., & Morton, T. (1995). Effects of psychotherapy with children and adolescents revisited: A meta-analysis of treatment outcome studies. *Psychological Bulletin, 117,* 450–468.

Werner, E. E., & Smith, R. S. (1992). *Overcoming the odds.* Ithaca, NY: Cornell University Press.

Wolfe, D., Edwards, B., Manion, I., & Koverola, C. (1988). Early interventions for parents at risk for child abuse and neglect: A preliminary investigation. *Journal of Consulting and Clinical Psychology, 56,* 40–47.

Wolfe, D. A., & Wekerle, C. (1993). Treatment strategies for child physical abuse and neglect: A critical progress report. *Clinical Psychology Review, 13,* 473–500.

Youngblade, L. M., & Belsky, J. (1990). The social and emotional consequences of child maltreatment. In R. Ammerman & M. Hersen (Eds.), *Children at risk: An evaluation of factors contributing to child abuse and neglect* (pp. 109–146). New York: Plenum Press.

19

DAVID M. GARNER
JULIE J. DESAI

Eating Disorders in Children and Adolescents

The increased recognition of eating disorders among adolescent and young adult women, as well as of the dangerous physical and psychological consequences of eating disorders, has resulted in a rapid increase in theoretical formulations and research involving pathogenesis and treatment. This research has led to a divergence in etiological viewpoints, as well as a convergence of opinion, with regard to the usefulness of practical intervention strategies. Although current knowledge has yet to lend support to any one theoretical viewpoint, one of the most enduring theoretical orientations for understanding eating disorders has been a risk factor model that accounts for the development and maintenance of symptoms through the interaction of cultural, biological, and psychological predisposing factors (Garner & Garfinkel, 1980). According to the risk factor model, these features are manifested differently within the context of a heterogeneous patient population (Garfinkel & Garner, 1982). This heterogeneity must be appreciated to fully understand and to competently treat this group of patients.

The aim of this chapter is to first provide background regarding diagnostic and prevalence of eating disorders and then to discuss the risk factor model, including major cultural, biological, and psychological factors that have been hypothesized to predispose individuals to eating disorders. This will be followed by an overview of the major perpetuating factors that need to be understood in treating eating disorders. Finally, empirically supported treatments, including family therapy and cognitive-behavioral, interpersonal, and pharmacological therapies will be discussed, along with a rationale for integrating and sequencing interventions.

Diagnosis

The current requirements for a diagnosis of anorexia nervosa, according to the *Diagnostic and Statistical Manual of Mental Disorders* (*DSM-IV*; American Psychiatric Association, 1994), are summarized as follows: (1) refusal to maintain a body weight over a minimally normal weight for age and height; (2) intense fear of gaining weight or becoming fat, even though underweight; (3) disturbance in the way that body weight, size, or shape is experienced; (4) amenorrhea in females (absence of at least three consecutive menstrual cycles). The *DSM-IV* suggests that weight loss leading to maintenance of a body weight 15% below norms or failure to achieve expected weight gain during a period of growth are characteristic of the disorder.

The *DSM-IV* (1994) divides anorexia nervosa into two diagnostic subtypes: (1) restricting type and (2) binge eating/purging type. The restricting type is defined by rigid restriction of food intake without bingeing or purging. The binge eating/purging type is defined by stringent attempts to limit intake, which is punctuated by episodes of binge eating and of self-induced vomiting and/or laxative abuse. This diverges from previous conventions in which anorexia nervosa was subdivided simply on the basis of the presence or absence of binge eating. The rationale for dividing anorexia nervosa patients on the basis of bingeing and purging rather than binge-eating alone rests on two observations. First, there are significant medical risks associated with compensatory behaviors such as self-induced vomiting and laxative abuse. Second, recent research has indicated that patients who purge, even if they do not engage in objective episodes of binge eating, display significantly more psychosocial disturbance than nonpurging patients (Garner, Garner, & Rosen, 1993). Patients who regularly engage in bulimic episodes report greater impulsivity, social and sexual dysfunction, substance abuse, general impulse control problems (e.g., lying and stealing), family dysfunction, and depression as part of a general picture of more conspicuous emotional disturbance when compared with patients with the restricting subtype of anorexia nervosa (Garner et al., 1993). In contrast, patients with restricting anorexia nervosa have been described as being overly compliant but at the same time obstinate, perfectionistic, obsessive-compulsive, shy, introverted, interpersonally sensitive, and stoical.

The criteria for diagnosis of bulimia nervosa according to the *DSM-IV* are summarized as follows: (1) recurrent episodes of binge eating (a sense of lack of control over eating; eating a larger amount of food in a certain period of time than would be considered normal for most people under similar circumstances); (2) recurrent inappropriate compensatory behavior(s) in order to prevent weight gain (e.g., vomiting, abuse of laxatives, diuretics, or other medications, fasting or excessive exercise); (3) a minimum average of two episodes of binge eating and inappropriate compensatory behaviors per week over the previous three months; (4) self-evaluation is unduly influenced by body shape and weight; (5) the disturbance does not occur exclusively during episodes of anorexia nervosa. Bulimia nervosa patients are further divided into purging and nonpurging subtypes based on the regular use of self-induced vomiting, laxatives, or diuretics (APA, 1994). Although binge eating is the key symptom identifying bulimia nervosa, agreement has not been achieved about the definition of this behavior in the disorder. For example, the requirement that binges must be "large" is inconsistent with research indicating that a significant proportion of "binges" reported by bulimia nervosa patients involve small amounts of food (cf. Garner, Shafer, & Rosen, 1992).

The *DSM-IV* (1994) delineates a large and heterogeneous diagnostic category, Eating Disorder, Not Otherwise Specified (EDNOS), for individuals with clinically significant eating disorders who fail to meet all of the diagnostic criteria for anorexia nervosa or bulimia nervosa. However, the specific terminology of this diagnostic category may result in misinterpretations regarding the clinical significance of such eating problems, as they may be mistakenly perceived as being of less importance. This view is inaccurate, as the clinical picture for individuals diagnosed with EDNOS can be as highly complex and serious as for those who meet the diagnostic criteria for anorexia nervosa and bulimia nervosa (Walsh & Garner, 1997).

Binge eating disorder (BED) is included in the *DSM-IV* as a category requiring further study. Although there is merit in adopting binge eating disorder into the diagnostic nomenclature, it is critical to remain aware of the fact that binge eating and associated psychological symptoms, particularly in the obese, may be attributed to standard weight loss treatments (cf. Garner & Wooley, 1991). BED has been proposed to apply to individuals who suffer from serious distress or impairment as a result of binge eating but who do not qualify for a diagnosis of bulimia nervosa because they do not regularly engage in inappropriate compensatory behaviors such as self-induced vomiting and the abuse of laxatives and/or medications. Despite those differences, individuals who fit into the separate *DSM-IV* categories also share many common features, especially pertaining to the degree of emphasis that is placed on body weight in self-assessment.

The *DSM-IV* criteria for the BED diagnosis include (1) eating a quantity of food that most people would consider large under similar circumstances within a specific period of time, and (2) an associated sense of loss of control with regard to eating behavior. Additionally, the behavior must occur within the context of three of the five subsequent items: (1) eating quickly, (2) eating beyond the point of satiety, (3) eating for reasons other than physical hunger, (4) eating in isolation due to self-consciousness regarding the quantity of food consumed, or (5) experiencing self-deprecating, depressive, or guilty feelings after overeating. Marked distress as a result of binge eating must be present, and the binge eating should occur for two days per week for a duration of six months (APA, 1994).

Incidence and Prevalence

Incidence rates are defined as the number of new cases in the population per year, whereas prevalence rates refer to the actual number of cases in the population at a certain point in time. Data on incidence and prevalence rates of eating disorders have been limited, as many estimates have been derived exclusively from self-report instruments and on samples which may not reflect demographic differences in base rates. Estimates of incidence based on detected cases in a primary care practice yielded rates of 8.1 per 100,000 persons per year for anorexia nervosa and 11.5 for bulimia nervosa (Hoek et al., 1995). The most sophisticated prevalence studies using strict diagnostic criteria report rates of about 0.3% for anorexia nervosa and about 1% for bulimia nervosa among young females in the community (Fairburn & Beglin, 1990; Hoek, 1993). These results contrast with questionnaire surveys that find that as many as 19% of female students report bulimic symptoms. Nonetheless, there is consensus that anorexia nervosa and bulimia nervosa occur in 1% to 4% of female high school and college students (cf. Fairburn & Beglin, 1990, Kreipe, 1995). Subclinical variants of eating disorders are represented in certain subgroups, in which there is increased pressure to diet or to maintain a thin shape. Research demonstrates a high incidence of suspected and actual cases among ballet dancers, professional dancers, wrestlers, swimmers, skaters, and gymnasts (cf. Garner, Rosen, & Barry, 1998). Case reports of anorexia nervosa in young children exist (Fosson, Knibbs, Bryant-Waugh, & Lask, 1987), but there is agreement that it is very rare in this age group (Jaffe & Singer, 1989). However, many children present with subclinical variants of eating disorders which fail to meet the strict *DSM-IV* criteria (Bryant-Waugh & Lask, 1995).

Predisposing Factors

A comprehensive understanding of anorexia and bulimia nervosa involves examining those factors which predispose individuals to each of the eating disorders, and theory should be able to depict the range of developmental experiences that interacts with those factors to initiate and maintain symptom expression in their various clinical presentations. Although the current models fail to stipulate these features in detail, the quality and quantity of research and clinical observations have augmented the understanding of eating disorders, resulting in more specific treatment recommendations.

In the past few decades, the conceptualization of eating disorders as "multidetermined" has taken the place of single-factor causal theories (Garner, 1993). Symptomatic patterns denote the final common pathways that result from the interchange of the three broad categories of predisposing factors depicted in Figure 19.1. This model stipulates that cultural, individual (psychological and biological), and familial causal factors interact with each other in various ways, leading to the

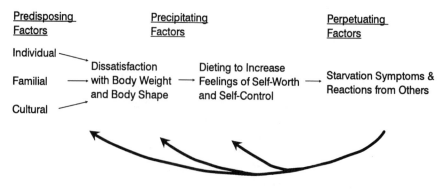

FIGURE 19.1   Eating disorders as multidetermined disorders.

development of eating disorders. Less is known about the precipitating factors, except that dieting is customarily an early element. The most useful advancements in treatment have been derived from a heightened appreciation of the perpetuating effects of starvation with its psychological, emotional, and physical consequences (Figure 19.1).

Cultural Factors

Eating disorders involve an intense preoccupation with fatness, leading to extreme attempts to control body weight. For several decades, the fashion, entertainment, and publishing industries have bombarded women with role models for physical attractiveness who are so gaunt as to represent virtually no women in the actual population; this has resulted in restrictive dieting and increased vulnerability to eating disorders (Garner, 1997). A strong concern about physical appearance appears to predate the appearance of eating disorders (Rastam, 1992). Research has shown that dieting to lose weight and fear of fatness are common in girls as young as 7 years old; these attitudes and behaviors escalate significantly during adolescence, particularly among those at the heavier end of the weight spectrum (Button, Loan, Davies, & Sonuga-Barke, 1997; Edlund, Halvarsson, & Sjödén, 1995). It has been shown that the risk of developing an eating disorder is eight times higher in dieting than in nondieting 15-year-old girls (Patton, Johnson-Sabine, Wood, Mann, & Wakeling, 1990). Those exposed to more pressure to diet, such as athletes participating in sports that emphasize leanness for performance or appearance, are at greater risk of eating disorders (Garner et al., 1998). In North America, disordered eating patterns appear to be equally common among Caucasian and Hispanic females, less common among Black and Asian females, and most common among Native Americans (Crago, Shisslak, & Estes, 1996). A thorough understanding of eating disorders demands a full appreciation of the cultural forces that have encroached on young girls and women over the past several decades. One of the most destructive has been the unyielding pressure to diet and engage in rigid weight controlling strategies to fulfill unrealistic standards for thinness (Garner, 1997). The strong impact of cultural factors on norms associated with dieting and other weight control measures has led to the conclusion that eating disorders may develop even in those individuals who lack underlying personality disturbances or family dysfunction, even though secondary disruption in both areas may exist when the individual presents for an initial assessment (Garner, 1997).

Individual Factors

During the last decade, there has been intense interest in the relationship between eating disorders and personality disorders. A number of recent reports have indicated that almost two thirds of eating-disordered patients receive a concurrent diagnosis of personality disorder diagnosis, with borderline personality disorder being reported as particularly common (Bulik, Sullivan, Joyce, & Carter, 1995; J. Cooper et al., 1988; Gillberg, Rastam, & Gillberg, 1995; Johnson, Tobin, & Dennis, 1990; Levin & Hyler, 1986). Levin and Hyler (1986) assessed 24 bulimia nervosa patients and found that 15 (63%) met diagnostic criteria for personality disorder, with 6 (25%) fulfilling the diagnosis for borderline personality disorder. Similarly, Bulik et al. (1995) found at least one personality disorder in 63% of a sample of 76 women with bulimia nervosa. Fifty-one percent of the personality disorders were in Cluster C (specifically, avoidant, obsessive-compulsive, or dependent personality disorders), 41% in Cluster B (particularly, borderline or histrionic), and 33% in Cluster A (paranoid, schizoid, or schizotypal). In an earlier evaluation of 35 patients with eating disorders, Gartner, Marcus, Halmi, and Loranger (1989) found that 57% met the DSM-III-R (APA, 1987) diagnostic criteria for at least one form of personality disorder, with borderline, self-defeating, and avoidant disorders being the most common. Two or more Axis II diagnostic criteria were met by 40% of the patients, and 17% fulfilled all of the criteria for five to seven personality disorder diagnoses. Wonderlich, Swift, Slotnick, and Goodman (1990) interviewed 46 eating-disordered patients and reported that 72% met criteria for at least one personality disorder. Obsessive-compulsive personality disorder was common among patients with restricting anorexia. Histrionic and borderline personality disorder diagnoses were common among bulimic groups. Johnson, Tobin, and Dennis (1990) followed patients one year after an initial assessment and found that those who initially scored above a threshold on the self-report Borderline Syndrome Index had a worse prognosis in terms of eating behavior and general psychiatric symptoms. Gillberg et al. (1995) found that obsessive-compulsive and avoidant personality disorders were particularly common in a study that compared 51 anorexia nervosa patients with an age-matched community sample.

Arguing that borderline assessment measures are confounded by certain eating symptoms, Pope and Hudson (1989) challenged the interpretation that borderline personality disorder is overrepresented among eating disorders. For example, bulimic eating patterns may be used to satisfy the DSM-III-R criterion of poor impulse control for borderline personality disorder, making the association between disorders tautological. Nevertheless, the tendency toward poor impulse regulation has been identified as a negative prognostic sign in eating disorders (e.g., Hatsukami, Mitchell, Eckert, & Pyle, 1986; Sohlberg, Norring, Holmgren, & Rosmark, 1989). Results from research on the incidence and prevalence of personality disorders in anorexia nervosa are inconsistent. Some studies indicate remarkably high rates, with avoidant personality disorder occurring in as many as 33% of anorexic restricters and borderline personality disorder occurring in almost 40% of anorexic bulimic patients (Piran, Lerner, Garfinkel, Kennedy, & Brouilette, 1988). Other studies suggest that personality disorders are relatively uncommon in anorexia nervosa (Herzog, Keller, Sacks, Yeh, & Lavori, 1992; Pope & Hudson, 1989). Impulse-control problems, such as self-mutilation, suicide attempts, and stealing, are reported in a subgroup of anorexia nervosa patients, particularly those with purging and/or bulimic symptoms (Garner, Garner, & Rosen, 1993). Although personality disturbances are not uniform in eating disorders, their presence suggests meaningful subtypes that may be relevant to treatment planning and prognosis.

There has been considerable interest and controversy in recent years regarding the role of sexual abuse as a risk factor for the development of eating disorders. Clinical accounts and the observation in some studies of a high incidence of sexual abuse in eating disorder patient samples (Oppenheimer, Howells, Palmer, & Chaloner, 1985; Sloan & Leichner, 1986) were followed by further clinical reports and numerous empirical studies that yielded conflicting findings (Fallon & Wonderlich, 1997). Fallon and Wonderlich summarized the literature and concluded that: (1) childhood sexual abuse appears to be positively associated with bulimia nervosa; (2) there is less evidence for this association in anorexia nervosa; (3) childhood sexual abuse does not appear to be a specific risk factor for eating disorders (i.e., it is no higher for eating-disordered patients than for psychiatric controls); (4) childhood sexual abuse does appear to be associated with greater levels of comorbidity among those with eating disorders, but there is not strong evidence that it predicts a more severe eating disorder; and (5) a more complex approach to the definition of sexual abuse has led to better prediction of later disturbances in eating. It is indisputable that a significant subgroup of women from some clinical eating-disorder samples have a history of sexual abuse and that careful assessment and treatment is important in the process of dealing with resulting feelings of shame, distrust, and anger (Fallon & Wonderlich, 1997).

Familial and Developmental Factors

The role of the family and its relative contribution to the development of eating disorders have been prominent in descriptions of the disorder (cf. Garfinkel & Garner, 1982). Regardless of their theoretical orientations, writers have examined the potential familial contribution to the development of both anorexia nervosa and bulimia nervosa (cf. Garner & Garfinkel, 1997). The structural approach, conceived by Minuchin and his colleagues (Minuchin, Rosman, & Baker, 1978), was considered a significant progression within the domain of family therapy. These theorists specified many characteristics representative of the interactions that occur within families of eating-disordered patients, including enmeshment, overprotectiveness, rigidity, and poor conflict resolution. In a controlled trial examining the efficacy of family therapy for anorexia nervosa, Russell, Szmukler, Dare, and Eisler (1987) found that family therapy was superior to individual therapy for younger patients. This study, as well as clinical experience, suggests that family therapy should be routinely employed as the treatment of choice for young eating-disordered patients.

There have been a number of psychodynamically oriented writers who have suggested that eating disorders evolve from particular developmental experiences. These accounts have been based primarily on clinical experience; however, they have been very popular in guiding clinical interventions with eating disorders. Early psychodynamically oriented writings on eating disorders accentuated the viewpoint that eating disorders represent a repudiation of adult femininity. Crisp (1965), who expanded and refined this theme, maintains that the fear of the psychological and biological experiences related to achieving adult weight pertains to the core psychopathology of anorexia nervosa and bulimia nervosa. Following this viewpoint, starvation is used as the main mechanism to prevent psychobiological maturity, because it results in a return to prepubertal appearance and hormonal status. Some developmental theorists have conceptualized eating disorders as resulting from differing types of parenting failures. Both Bruch (1973) and Selvini-

Palazzoli (1974) provided a developmental paradigm suggesting that the mother superimposes her own inaccurate perceptions of the child's needs onto the child, invalidating the child's experiences. Accordingly, this results in an arrest of cognitive development, which is manifested in debilitating feelings of ineffectiveness that appear later in adolescent struggles for autonomy and control of the body. Bruch (1973) theorized that these early parenting failures produce basic deficits in self-awareness, including the manner in which the body is perceived and experienced.

Goodsitt (1997) has used a self-psychology perspective to explain eating disorders as a reflection of developmental arrest in the separation-individuation process. In accordance with this conceptualization, the eating-disordered individual's lack of a cohesive sense of self is a consequence of the primary caregiver's failure to provide essential functions (mirroring, tension regulation, and integration) during development. The overconcern with eating and repeated episodes of bingeing and vomiting provide the individual with organizing and tension-regulating mechanisms to assist in managing essential deficits in "self-structures." The symptomatic behaviors displayed by the eating-disordered individual serve to organize events and provide extreme stimulation to help anesthetize the suffering and void which permeate the eating-disordered individual's life.

Strober (1997) has intertwined developmental theory, psychobiology, and personality genetics to provide a meaningful understanding of the adaptive mechanisms responsible for the spectrum of symptoms observed among eating-disordered patients. He synthesizes current psychoanalytic concepts of development with constructs denoting (1) that individual differences may be expected in the internal regulators of arousability or temperament that organize self-experiences and (2) that heritable personality traits and their presumed biological substrata set limits within which behavior patterns are expressed.

There is some evidence of genetic vulnerability to eating disorders, particularly for anorexia nervosa. In studies of approximately 100 twin pairs culled from selected twin case report summaries and from twin studies indicate concordance rates of more than 50% for monozygotic twin pairs compared with less than 10% for dizygotic twins (Garfinkel & Garner, 1982; Holland, Sicotte, & Treasure, 1988). These studies suggest that there may be a genetic component to the transmission of anorexia nervosa; however, it is not at all clear what is inherited. Is it the specific disorder, a particular personality trait associated with the disorder, or a general vulnerability to psychiatric disturbance? Moreover, the concordance data on twins reared together does not conclusively distinguish between genetic and environmental transmission (Holland et al., 1988).

Perpetuating Factors

It may not be apparent from an initial assessment whether depression, low self-esteem, psychological distress, personality features, and social maladjustment reported by eating-disordered patients signal fundamental emotional deficits or are secondary elaborations resulting from weight loss and chaotic dietary patterns. These and other symptoms identified in human semistarvation studies and in research on the consequences of dieting may perpetuate eating disorders (Garner,

Vitousek, & Pike, 1997). Findings from these studies indicate that striking changes in personality traits can occur with relatively small reductions in body weight and that these may perpetuate eating disorders by making coping more difficult or by aggravating preexisting psychopathology. Patients with bulimia nervosa report depression, general psychological distress, and personality disturbance, including traits that would indicate borderline personality disorder on initial assessment; however, the speed of the marked improvement in these psychological features once eating symptoms have been brought under control with treatment suggests that they may be secondary to the eating disorder rather than indicative of enduring emotional deficits (Garner et al., 1990).

Assessment

Assessment should be considered integral to the ongoing treatment process. Various approaches to information gathering have been developed for eating disorders, including standard clinical interviews, semistructured interviews, behavioral observation, standardized self-report measures, symptom checklists, clinical rating scales, self-monitoring procedures, and standardized test means. There are three broad areas of focus in the assessment process: (1) the assessment of specific symptom areas that allow the diagnosis of the eating disorder, (2) the measurement of other attitudes or behaviors characteristic of eating disorders, (3) the identification and measurement of associated psychological and personality features that are indicative of overall psychosocial functioning (Crowther & Sherwood, 1997).

Assessment should include careful questioning regarding the duration and frequency of binge eating, as well as extreme measures designed to control body weight, such as vomiting, laxative abuse, and excessive exercise. It should also cover weight-controlling behaviors such as use of other drugs or alcohol to control appetite, chewing and spitting food out before swallowing, prolonged fasting, and vigorous exercise for the purpose of controlling body weight. Diabetic patients may manipulate insulin levels to control weight, and patients taking thyroid replacement may alter their dosage to control their weight (Garfinkel & Garner, 1982).

Marked personality changes that mimic primary personality disorders may actually stem from prolonged undernutrition. The assessment should include a careful evaluation of premorbid personality features. Patients may recall being sociable and more confident prior to the onset of the disorder. As the disorder has progressed, they may have become more sullen and isolated from others. Other patients describe a passive, compliant, and reserved premorbid personality style. Formal personality testing may be useful in some cases; however, the confounding of primary and secondary symptoms is a concern (Crowther & Sherwood, 1997). When primary personality disturbance is identified, it usually means a longer duration of therapy with a more difficult course. Adaptations are required for patients whose disorder is complicated by substance, physical, or sexual abuse.

In many cases, standardized self-report measures can be efficient in gathering information regarding eating behavior and other symptoms common in those with eating disorders. The Eating Disorder Inventory-2 (EDI-2; Garner, 1991) is a standardized, multiscale measure that adds three subscales to the original EDI.

The EDI-2 is specifically aimed at assessing a range of psychological characteristics clinically relevant to eating disorders. It consists of three subscales for tapping attitudes and behaviors relating to eating, weight, and shape (Drive for Thinness, Bulimia, Body Dissatisfaction), in addition to eight subscales that assess more general organizing constructs or psychological traits clinically relevant to eating disorders (Ineffectiveness, Perfection, Interpersonal Distrust, Interoceptive Awareness, Maturity Fears, Asceticism, Impulse Regulation, and Social Insecurity). In clinical settings, the EDI-2 is designed to provide information helpful in understanding the patient, planning treatment, and assessing progress. In nonclinical settings, the EDI-2 is intended as an economical means of identifying individuals who have "subclinical" eating problems or those who may be at risk for developing eating disorders.

Empirically Supported Interventions

The quantity of psychotherapeutic options accessible to eating-disordered patients has proliferated in the past decade, and the principal approaches to psychotherapy have been explained well and have been accompanied by the development of alternate treatment choices (Garner & Garfinkel, 1997). The wisdom of considering integration of different psychotherapeutic procedures is increasingly evident with the demonstrated effectiveness of different forms of treatment (Garner & Needleman, 1997). There has been recent interest in "stepped-care," "decision-tree," or "integration" models which rely on standard rules for the delivery of the various treatment options (Garner & Needleman, 1997). Figure 19.2 illustrates a tentative decision-making paradigm for sequencing and integrating treatments for people with eating disorders. Various treatment options (i.e., hospitalization, family therapy, self-help, and individual therapy) are represented by the sharp-cornered boxes, and pertinent questions (i.e., those associated with symptoms, patient characteristics, responses to previous treatments) related to deciding the type of treatment are characterized by curved-cornered boxes. Not all existing treatment alternatives are incorporated in the figure, but it focuses on those which are supported both clinically and empirically.

Family Therapy

Family therapy is the initial treatment choice for patients who are young and/or living at home (see Figure 19.2). As mentioned earlier, Russell et al. (1987) found that family therapy was superior to individual therapy for younger patients. Family therapy is an essential component of treatment for patients who are young and/or living at home and should also be strongly considered as a therapeutic adjunct for older patients (living outside of the home) who experience family discord. The recommendation of family therapy for young patients is based on both a practical and a theoretical rationale. Practically, parents are responsible for the well-being of the patient and can serve as powerful agents of change by providing guidance and assistance to facilitate the implementation and achievement of treatment goals because they reside within the child's physical environment. Family members also

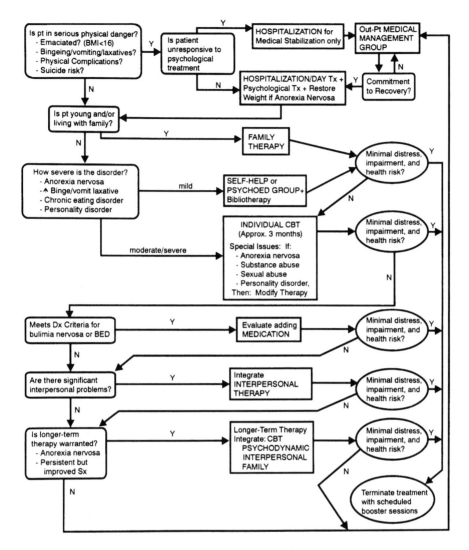

FIGURE 19.2 General guidelines for integration and sequencing major treatment options for eating-disordered patients. Begin in the upper left corner with the question "Is pt in serious physical danger?" Further criteria for decision making, including symptom areas, patient characteristics, and response to previous treatments, are indicated by boxes with rounded corners (mostly on the left side of the figure). The treatment options are represented by boxes with sharp corners (hospitalization, family therapy, self-help/education, individual therapy, etc.). The figure does not delineate all treatment alternatives or all considerations for decision making. However, it does include the main interventions for which there is good clinical and/or empirical support and key variables to consider in determining the most appropriate type and intensity of treatment. Abbreviations: pt, patient; BMI, body mass index; 5×/wk, five times a week; Dx, diagnostic; BED, binge-eating disorder; Tx, treatment; CBT, cognitive-behavioral therapy; Sx, symptoms.

need therapeutic direction in learning how to cope with the eating-disordered patient and to deal with their own feelings in an effective manner. Family therapists have persuasively maintained their stance that eating disorders may be indicative of discord, dysfunctional roles, or disturbed interactional patterns within the family context (Dare & Eisler, 1997; Minuchin et al., 1978; Selvini-Palazzoli, 1974). The following list depicts some of the most common problematical themes:

1. The parents and identified patient may display denial regarding the seriousness of the eating disorder and will require assistance in accurately labeling the eating disorder without minimizing or maximizing the importance of behavioral symptoms.
2. Parents of younger patients might need assistance in establishing an effective parenting style, as feelings of guilt and fear may have prevented them from maintaining firm and clear behavioral guidelines consistent with recovery. Unless unrealistic parental expectations are directly related to the problem, it is suggested that parents maintain their expectations in those areas which are unrelated to food and eating (i.e., bedtime, chores, language, treatment of siblings/parents). Treatment interventions should be developmentally appropriate for the child and should be within the boundaries of the family's value system.
3. Parents will need help in understanding and respecting the patient's need for autonomy and self-expression through traits, interests, and values which may differ from expectations set by the family.
4. Parental attitudes regarding weight, shape, thinness, or fitness may be inappropriate at times, and unsuitable eating patterns and beliefs about food, eating, or exercise should be identified and addressed using practical interventions to interrupt any possible problem developing areas.
5. An eating disorder can deflect members of the family away from potentially threatening developmental expectations that emerge in the transition to puberty. It can function as a maladaptive solution to the adolescent's struggle to achieve autonomy in a family in which any move toward independence is perceived as a threat to family unity. It can also become a powerful diversion, enabling the parents and the child to avoid major sources of conflict.
6. The identified patient's symptoms may be functional within a disturbed family context, and the meaning systems that underlie the resulting interactional patterns need to be identified and corrected. Problematic family interactional patterns which need to be addressed include enmeshment, overprotectiveness, inadequate mechanisms for resolving conflicts, and inappropriate parent-child allegiances which undermine the marital relationship (Minuchin et al., 1978).

Lask and Bryant-Waugh (1997) describe four critical factors to prevent the maintenance of the child's eating disorder: (1) cohesion, (2) consistency, (3) communication, and (4) conflict resolution. Parents must consider these factors when their child is being treated for an eating disorder, as they bear moral and legal responsibilities for the child's welfare. In addition to having basic education and information, the parents must maintain cohesiveness and present a unified team front to best help the child. Parents must also remain consistent in their interactions so the child knows what to expect. Finally, the integration of family therapy with long-term individual therapy may be strategic in addressing physical and sexual abuse within the family (Andersen, 1985; Garner, Garfinkel, & Bemis, 1982).

Cognitive-Behavioral Therapy

Cognitive-behavioral therapy (CBT) has become the standard treatment for bulimia nervosa and forms the theoretical base for much of the treatment of anorexia nervosa. As indicated in Figure 19.2, CBT should be considered the treatment of choice for patients whose age does not mandate family therapy and whose symptoms range from moderate to severe. The CBT for bulimia nervosa developed by Fairburn and colleagues (Fairburn, 1985; Fairburn, Marcus, & Wilson, 1993) emphasizes the following major points: (1) self-monitoring of food intake, bingeing, and purging episodes, as well as thoughts and feelings which trigger these episodes; (2) regular weighing; (3) specific recommendations, such as the introduction of avoided foods and meal planning designed to normalize eating behavior and curb restrictive dieting; (4) cognitive restructuring directed at habitual reasoning errors and underlying assumptions that are relevant to the development and the maintenance of the eating disorder; and (5) relapse prevention.

There have now been more than 25 controlled-treatment studies of bulimia nervosa, and they provide very encouraging findings (McKisack & Waller, 1997; Mitchell, Raymond, & Specker, 1993). In a long-term prospective follow-up of 91 eating-disordered patients from two randomized controlled trials involving CBT, behavior therapy (BT), and focal interpersonal therapy (FIT), Fairburn et al. (1995) found that those bulimia nervosa patients who received BT did poorly, whereas those who received CBT or FIT did markedly better. Compared with participants in the BT condition, those receiving FIT were twice as likely to be in remission (defined as no longer meeting a *DSM-IV* diagnosis for an eating disorder), and those in the CBT condition were more than three times as likely to be in remission. Similarly, about half of the patients who received CBT or FIT were completely abstinent from all key behavioral symptoms such as binge eating, vomiting, and laxative and diuretic abuse compared with 18% of those receiving BT.

In the case of anorexia nervosa, CBT has been recommended largely on clinical grounds (Garner, 1986; Garner & Bemis, 1982, 1985; Garner & Rosen, 1990; Garner, Vitousek, & Pike, 1997; Vitousek & Orimoto, 1993). Case studies and preliminary research provide some grounds for optimism (Channon, DeSilva, Hemsley, & Perkins, 1989; Cooper & Fairburn, 1984); however, current data are insufficient to warrant meaningful conclusions regarding effectiveness.

There are many areas of overlap between the versions of CBT offered for anorexia and bulimia nervosa; however, there are also important differences that have implications for clinical care (Garner et al., 1997). A major focus for both disorders is the patient's underlying assumption that "weight, shape, or thinness can serve as the sole or predominant referent for inferring personal value or self-worth" (Garner & Bemis, 1982, p. 142). Fear of body weight gain is a central theme for both anorexia and bulimia nervosa; however, most bulimia nervosa patients can be reassured that treatment will probably result in little weight gain. In contrast, in anorexia nervosa, therapeutic strategies must be aimed at actual weight gain in the face of the implacable wish to maintain a low weight. Establishing a sound and collaborative therapeutic relationship is particularly important in anorexia nervosa because it becomes a fulcrum for gradually helping the patient to relinquish the myriad of ego-syntonic symptoms. As indicated in Figure 19.2, CBT is modified for anorexia nervosa. It is typically longer in duration, and the targets for cognitive interventions are broad, encompassing a wider range of personal and interpersonal subject domains than typical for bulimia nervosa (Garner et al., 1997). These modifications address the marked deficits that impede normal psychosocial functioning in many of these patients. Thus cognitive interventions are aimed not only at beliefs that maintain extreme dieting and chronic weight suppression but also at fundamental assumptions associated with interpersonal conflicts, feelings of ineffectiveness, struggles with autonomy, and fears associated with psychosocial development (Garner & Bemis, 1982; Garner et al., 1997). Components of interpersonal therapy and family therapy are often integrated into longer term CBT for anorexia nervosa (see Figure 19.2). In the subset of anorexia nervosa patients who do not engage in binge eating and in those who show no obvious serious physical complications, there may be extraordinary resistance to complying with the therapeutic objectives of weight gain. As long as there is gradual improvement in symptoms (see Figure 19.2), outpatient therapy is recommended; however, if the patient's condition deteriorates, hospitalization must be considered. Outpatient medical management (group therapy) should be considered if there is a protracted therapeutic impasse. Such an impasse often takes the form of apparent psychological insights that invariably fail to translate into symptomatic change.

Interpersonal Therapy

For almost a decade, the prevailing view was that CBT's effectiveness with eating disorders was tied to cognitive and behavioral methods aimed specifically at overconcern about weight and shape that is responsible for restrictive dieting and extreme weight-controlling behaviors. Changing these attitudes presumably relaxed restrictive dieting and relieved the biological tension created by chronic attempts to suppress body weight. However, a series of studies using interpersonal psychotherapy (IPT) adapted to bulimia nervosa has prompted reexamination of earlier speculations regarding the specific mechanisms of action in the treatment of binge eating (Fairburn et al., 1995). This happened because IPT does not directly focus on eating problems. IPT was originally proposed by Klerman, Weissman, Rounsaville, and Chevron (1984) as a short-term treatment for depression. The IPT treatment process is divided into three stages (Fairburn, 1997). The first stage involves identifying of the interpersonal problems that led to the development and maintenance of the eating problems. The second stage consists of a therapeutic contract for working on these interpersonal problems. The final stage addresses issues related to termination. Fairburn et al. (1991) found IPT somewhat less effective than CBT at the end of treatment; however, patients who received IPT gradually improved during the follow-up period, so that after one year both treatments were equally effective (Fairburn, Jones, Peveler, Hope, & O'Connor, 1993). These findings are maintained over the longer term, with patients receiving CBT or interpersonal therapy doing significantly better than those receiving behavior therapy (Fairburn et al., 1995). This pattern of improvement during follow-up was not found in a study of another very different form of interpersonally oriented therapy, supportive-expressive therapy (Garner, Rockert, Garner, Davis, & Olmsted, 1993). These findings suggest that the interpersonal therapies offered in the Oxford trials by Fairburn and colleagues contain specific therapeutic ingredients that facilitate change. Further support for the effectiveness of IPT comes from Wilfley et al. (1993) in a study of nonpurging bulimic patients, many of whom presented with obesity. They found both CBT and IPT equally effective in reducing binge eating, assessed both at the end of treatment and at one-year follow-up.

The evidence that certain interpersonal therapies are as effective with binge eating as CBT has implications for the decision process illustrated in Figure 19.2. It could be argued that there should be no priority for either IPT or CBT as the initial treatment of choice for bulimia nervosa because both treatments are equally effective in the long term. Certainly a therapist well trained in one of the interpersonal therapies described by Fairburn (1997) should not be encouraged to abandon this form of treatment in favor of CBT. However, we are still inclined to recommend CBT as the preferred initial treatment at this time because it has been shown to have a more rapid effect on symptoms. Moreover, the efficacy of IPT for bulimia nervosa has been demonstrated in just one center, compared with many studies in support of CBT. If the findings from the Oxford trials are replicated in other centers, then IPT may become another "standard" initial treatment for bulimia nervosa. At this time, there is no empirical basis for suggesting that IPT should be differentially applied to patients on the basis of premorbid features such as interpersonal conflicts. However, integrating IPT into treatment should be considered for bulimia nervosa patients who fail to respond favorably to an initial course of CBT when interpersonal conflicts predominate, as indicated in Figure 19.2. The IPT orientation should also be a leading candidate for integration into longer term psychotherapy for anorexia nervosa patients or for others with persistent symptoms.

Pharmacotherapy

As depicted in Figure 19.2, medication is generally not indicated for anorexia nervosa, although it should be considered for those patients with bulimia nervosa or binge-eating disorder who fail an initial trial of cognitive-behavioral therapy. After reviewing the research in this area, Raymond, Mitchell, Fallon, and Katzman (1994) have suggested that medication should not be "the primary mode of therapy with patients with bulimia nervosa" (p. 241). This conclusion is based on the following observations: (1) psychological interventions have been shown to be very effective, (2) high dropout rates are reported in most medication studies, (3) there are risks of drug side effects, and (4) data suggest high relapse rates with drug discontinuation. In a meta-analysis using 9 double blind, placebo-controlled medication trials (870 participants) and 26 randomized psychosocial studies (460 participants), Whittal, Agras, and Gould (1999) reported that CBT produced significantly larger-weighted effect sizes for all indices of treatment outcome.

Tricyclic antidepressants may be considered as an alternative for some patients who fail a course of fluoxetine, but side effects, such as high dropout rates and greater lethality with overdose, may be a source of concern when treating some patients (Leitenberg et al., 1994). Similarly, MAOIs may be useful in a small minority of patients who fail using fluoxetine and tricyclics. There is some evidence that patients who fail on one tricyclic may benefit from changing to an alternative medication (see Mitchell et al., 1993). Importantly, the specific decision not to prescribe medication may be therapeutic (Raymond et al., 1994).

There is still little evidence for change to the early recommendations that pharmacotherapy has a very limited value with emaciated anorexia nervosa patients and should never be the sole treatment modality (Garfinkel & Garner, 1982). Occasionally patients may benefit from medication to deal with overwhelming anxiety, severe depression, or intolerable gastric discomfort after meals, but this only applies to a small minority of patients (Andersen, 1985; Garfinkel & Garner, 1982; Garfinkel & Walsh, 1997).

Thus, in the decision-tree approach for treating eating disorders, antidepressant medication should be considered as an adjunct or possibly an alternative for bulimia nervosa patients who fail to respond to psychosocial therapies or for those whose affective symptoms are clearly impeding progress in other forms of treatment. Drug treatments have generally not proven effective for anorexia nervosa.

Integrating and Adapting Interventions

A major premise in this chapter has been that eating disorders are multidetermined and heterogeneous syndromes that result from the interplay of biological, psychological, familial, and sociocultural predisposing factors. In this sense, they are probably best understood as final common pathways that appear to have different psychological points of entry. Within this overall context, this chapter has selectively reviewed diagnostic issues, major etiological formulations, and associated psychopathology applied to eating disorders. An important direction for future research will be the clearer specification of the relative contribution of particular biological, psychological, and interpersonal predisposing features considered relevant to eating disorders. It is hoped that the extraordinary clinical and research interest in personality disorders, depression, sexual abuse, and addictive behaviors as related to eating disorders will continue to lead to improved understanding. Further research is clearly needed to determine the precise nature and the significance of the observed associations. If past research to date is any indication of future findings, the within-diagnostic-group variability will continue to be as noteworthy as the between-group differences.

Managed Care Considerations with Eating Disorders

During the 1980s, there were a convergence of extraordinary economic incentives for inpatient care, surging demands for clinical services, and widespread misinformation regarding optimal treatment which led to the unnecessary hospitalization of many eating-disordered patients who could have been easily managed at a less intensive level of care. The earlier abuse of inpatient treatment led to an understandable backlash by insurers, resulting in denial of hospital coverage or extreme limitations of coverage for eating-disordered patients, putting many at unnecessary risk for chronic illness or death. This has created a major problem in the treatment of eating disorders, because it is well established in the treatment literature that even the most ambitious treatment for patients with severe eating disorders requires more time and expense than is routinely allowed in the benefits packages for many patients. If insufficient time is devoted to treatment, few patients recover, and this has very negative economic consequences for insurers as well as sufferers. Research has shown that discharging anorexia nervosa patients before they achieve a reasonable goal weight is associated with relapse (Baran, Weltzin, & Kaye, 1995). Even though treatment is a time-consuming and expensive process, it is an economical alternative if it leads to recovery, because a chronic eating disorder inflicts a heavy price both in monetary and emotional terms. There has been a growing trend to treat eating disorders in specialized treatment settings (as opposed to general hospital wards) because experienced staff may be able to manage more severely disturbed patients at a lower level of care than in traditional hospitalization (i.e., partial hospitalization or intensive day treatment). We have found intensive day treatment (seven hours a day, five days a week) to be preferable to inpatient care because the structure for meal times and the possibility for intensive therapy it provides is sufficient for most patients to make behavioral changes without requiring them to be totally disengaged from the supports and the therapeutic challenges outside of the hospital.

Summary

It is now evident that certain patients respond relatively quickly to brief interventions, in contrast to others who require more intensive and protracted treatments. Perhaps the most significant goal for future research will be the identification of traits, personality features, or background factors that predict differential response to treatment. Even better would be a taxonomy that yields an accurate match between patient characteristics and treatment type. Recent advances in research on psychopathology and treatment efficacy warrant genuine optimism with regard to bulimia nervosa. Less is known about personality and response to treatment for anorexia nervosa because of the relative absence of controlled treatment research into this eating disorder. It is hoped that controlled treatment research will assume a high priority and that the results will generate the same level of progress as is now evident with bulimia nervosa.

REFERENCES

American Psychiatric Association. (1987). *Diagnostic and statistical manual of mental disorders* (3rd ed., rev.). Washington, DC: American Psychiatric Association.

American Psychiatric Association. (1994). *Diagnostic and statistical manual of mental disorders* (4th ed.) Washington, DC: American Psychiatric Association.

Andersen, A. E. (1985). *Practical comprehensive treatment of anorexia nervosa and bulimia.* Baltimore, MD: Johns Hopkins University Press.

Baran, S. A., Weltzin, T. E., & Kaye,

W. H. (1995). Low discharge weight and outcome in anorexia nervosa. *American Journal of Psychiatry, 152,* 1070–1072.

Bruch, H. (1973). *Eating disorders: Obesity, anorexia nervosa and the person within.* New York: Basic Books.

Bryant-Waugh, R., & Lask, B. (1995). Annotation: Eating disorders in children. *Journal of Child Clinical Psychiatry, 36,* 191–202.

Bulik, C., Sullivan, P., Joyce, P., & Carter, F. (1995). Temperament, character, and personality disorder in bulimia nervosa. *Journal of Nervous and Mental Disease, 183,* 593–598.

Button, E. J., Loan, P., Davies, J., & Sonuga-Barke, E. J. S. (1997). Self-esteem, eating problems, and psychological well-being in a cohort of schoolgirls aged 15–16: A questionnaire and interview study. *International Journal of Eating Disorders, 21,* 39–47.

Channon, S., DeSilva, P., Hemsley, D., & Perkins, R. (1989). A controlled trial of cognitive behavioral and behavioral treatment of anorexia nervosa. *Behavioral Research and Therapy, 27,* 529–535.

Cooper, J. L., Morrison, T. L., Bigman, O. L., Abramowitz, S. I., Levin, S., & Krener, P. (1988). Mood changes and affective disorder in the bulimic binge-purge cycle. *International Journal of Eating Disorders, 7,* 469–474.

Cooper, P. J., & Fairburn, C. G. (1984). Cognitive behavioral treatment for anorexia nervosa: Some preliminary findings. *Journal of Psychosomatic Research, 28,* 493–499.

Crago, M., Shisslak, C. M., & Estes, L. S. (1996). Eating disturbances among American minority groups: A review. *International Journal of Eating Disorders, 19,* 239–248.

Crisp, A. H. (1965). Clinical and therapeutic aspects of anorexia nervosa: Study of 30 cases. *Journal of Psychosomatic Research, 9,* 67–78.

Crowther, J., & Sherwood, N. (1997). Assessment. In D. M. Garner & P. E. Garfinkel (Eds.), *Handbook of treatment for eating disorders* (pp. 34–49). New York: Guilford Press.

Dare, C., & Eisler, I. (1997). Family therapy for anorexia nervosa. In D. M. Garner & P. E. Garfinkel (Eds.), *Handbook of treatment for eating disorders* (pp. 307–326). New York: Guilford Press.

Edlund, B., Halvarsson, K., & Sjödén, P. (1995). Eating behaviours, and attitudes to eating, dieting, and body image in 7-year-old Swedish girls. *European Eating Disorders Review, 3,* 1–14.

Fairburn, C. G. (1985). Cognitive-behavioral treatment for bulimia. In D. M. Garner & P. E. Garfinkel (Eds.), *Handbook of psychotherapy for anorexia nervosa and bulimia* (pp. 160–192). New York: Guilford Press.

Fairburn, C. G. (1997). Interpersonal psychotherapy for bulimia nervosa. In D. M. Garner & P. E. Garfinkel (Eds.), *Handbook of treatment for eating disorders* (pp. 278–294), New York: Guilford Press.

Fairburn, C. G., & Beglin, S. J. (1990). Studies of the epidemiology of bulimia nervosa. *American Journal of Psychiatry, 147,* 401–408.

Fairburn, C. G., Jones, R., Peveler, R. C., Carr, S. J., Solomon, R. A., O'Connor, M. E., Burton, J., & Hope, R. A. (1991). Three psychological treatments for bulimia nervosa: A comparative trial. *Archives of General Psychiatry, 48,* 463–469.

Fairburn, C. G., Jones, R., Peveler, R. C., Hope, R. A., & O'Connor, M. (1993). Psychotherapy and bulimia nervosa: the longer-term effects of interpersonal psychotherapy, behavior therapy and cognitive behavior therapy. *Archives of General Psychiatry, 50,* 419–428.

Fairburn, C. G., Marcus, M. D., & Wilson, G. T. (1993). Cognitive-behavioral therapy for binge eating and bulimia nervosa. In C. G. Fairburn & G. T.

Wilson (Eds.), *Binge eating: Nature, assessment, and treatment* (pp. 361–404). New York: Guilford Press.

Fairburn, C. G., Norman, P. A., Welch, S. L., O'Connor, M. E., Doll, H. A., & Peveler, R. C. (1995). A prospective study of outcome in bulimia nervosa and the long-term effects of three psychological treatments. *Archives of General Psychiatry, 52,* 304–312.

Fallon, P., & Wonderlich, S. (1997). Sexual abuse and other forms of trauma. In D. M. Garner & P. E. Garfinkel (Eds.), *Handbook of treatment for eating disorders* (pp. 394–414). New York: Guilford Press.

Fosson, A., Knibbs, J., Bryant-Waugh, R., & Lask, B. (1987). Early onset anorexia nervosa. *Archives of Disease in Childhood, 62,* 114–118.

Garfinkel, P. E., & Garner, D. M. (1982). *Anorexia nervosa: A multidimensional perspective.* New York: Brunner/Mazel.

Garfinkel, P. E., & Walsh, B. (1997). Drug therapies. In D. M. Garner & P. E. Garfinkel (Eds.), *Handbook of treatment for eating disorders* (pp. 229–247). New York: Guilford Press.

Garner, D. M. (1986). Cognitive therapy for anorexia nervosa. In K. D. Brownell & J. P. Foreyt (Eds.), *Handbook of eating disorders* (pp. 301–327). New York: Basic Books.

Garner, D. M. (1991). *Eating Disorder Inventory-2: Professional Manual.* Odessa, FL. Psychological Assessment Resources.

Garner, D. M. (1993). Pathogenesis of anorexia nervosa. *Lancet, 341,* 1631–1635.

Garner, D. M. (1997). Psychoeducational principles in treatment. In D. M. Garner & P. E. Garfinkel (Eds.), *Handbook of treatment for eating disorders* (pp. 145–177). New York: Guilford Press.

Garner, D. M., & Bemis, K. M. (1982). A cognitive-behavioral approach to anorexia nervosa. *Cognitive Therapy and Research, 6,* 123–150.

Garner, D. M., & Bemis, K. M. (1985). Cognitive therapy for anorexia nervosa. In D. M. Garner & P. E. Garfinkel (Eds.), *Handbook of psychotherapy for anorexia nervosa and bulimia* (pp. 107–146). New York: Guilford Press.

Garner, D. M., & Garfinkel, P. E. (1980). Socio-cultural factors in the development of anorexia nervosa. *Psychological Medicine, 10,* 647–656.

Garner, D. M., & Garfinkel, P. E. (Eds.). (1997). *Handbook of treatment for eating disorders.* New York: Guilford Press.

Garner, D. M., Garfinkel, P. E., & Bemis, K. M. (1982). A multidimensional psychotherapy for anorexia nervosa. *International Journal of Eating Disorders, 1,* 3–46.

Garner, D. M., Garner, M. V., & Rosen, L. W. (1993). Anorexia nervosa "restricters" who purge: Implications for subtyping anorexia nervosa. *International Journal of Eating Disorders, 13,* 171–185.

Garner, D. M., & Needleman, L. (1997). Sequencing and integration of treatments. In D. M. Garner & P. E. Garfinkel (Eds.), *Handbook of treatment for eating disorders* (pp. 50–66), New York: Guilford Press.

Garner, D. M., Olmsted, M. P., Davis, R., Rockert, W., Goldbloom, D., & Eagle, M. (1990). The association between bulimic symptoms and reported psychopathology. *International Journal of Eating Disorders, 9,* 1–15.

Garner, D. M., Rockert, W., Garner, M. V., Davis, R., & Olmsted, M. P. (1993). Comparison between cognitive-behavioral and short-term psychodynamic therapy for bulimia nervosa. *American Journal of Psychiatry, 150,* 37–46.

Garner, D. M., & Rosen, L. W. (1990). Anorexia nervosa and bulimia nervosa. In A. S. Bellack, M. Hersen, & A. E. Kazdin (Eds.), *International handbook of behavior modification and therapy* (pp. 805–817). New York: Plenum Press.

Garner, D. M., Rosen, L., & Barry, D. (1998). Eating disorders in athletes. In I. R. Tofler (Ed.), *Child and adolescent psychiatric clinics of North America* (Vol. 7, pp. 839–857). New York: Saunders.

Garner, D. M., Shafer, C. L., & Rosen, L. W. (1992). Critical appraisal of the *DSM-III-R* personality diagnostic criteria for eating disorders. In S. R. Hooper, G. W. Hynd, & R. E. Mattison (Eds.), *Child psychopathology: Diagnostic criteria and clinical assessment* (pp. 261–303). Hillsdale, NJ: Erlbaum.

Garner, D. M., Vitousek, K., & Pike, K. (1997). Cognitive-behavioral therapy for anorexia nervosa. In D. M. Garner & P. E. Garfinkel (Eds.), *Handbook of treatment for eating disorders* (pp. 94–144). New York: Guilford Press.

Garner, D. M., & Wooley, S. C. (1991). Confronting the failure of behavioral and dietary treatments for obesity. *Clinical Psychology Review, 11,* 729–780.

Gartner, A. F., Marcus, R. N., Halmi, K., & Loranger, A. W. (1989). *DSM-III-R* personality in patients with eating disorders. *American Journal of Psychiatry, 146,* 1585–1591.

Gillberg, G., Rastam, M., & Gillberg, C. (1995). Anorexia nervosa 6 years after onset: I. Personality disorders. *Comprehensive Psychiatry, 36,* 61–69.

Goodsitt, A. (1997). Eating disorders: A self psychological perspective. In D. M. Garner & P. E. Garfinkel (Eds.), *Handbook of treatment for eating disorders* (pp. 205–228). New York: Guilford Press.

Hatsukami, D., Mitchell, J. E., Eckert, E. D., & Pyle, R. (1986). Characteristics of patients with bulimia only, bulimia with affective disorder, and bulimia with substance abuse problems. *Addictive Behaviors, 11,* 399–406.

Herzog, D. B., Keller, M. B., Sacks, N. R., Yeh, C. J., & Lavori, P. W. (1992). Psychiatric morbidity in treatment-seeking anorexics and bulimics. *Journal of the American Academy of Child and Adolescent Psychiatry, 31,* 810–818.

Hoek, H. W. (1993). Review of the epidemiological studies of eating disorders. *International Review of Psychiatry, 5,* 61–74.

Hoek, H. W., Bartelds, A., Bosveld, J., Graff, Y., Limpens, V., Maiwald, M., & Spaij, C. (1995). Impact of urbanization on detection rates of eating disorders. *American Journal of Psychiatry, 152*(9), 1272–1278.

Holland, A. J., Sicotte, N., & Treasure, J. (1988). Anorexia nervosa: Evidence for a genetic basis. *Journal of Psychosomatic Research, 32,* 561–571.

Jaffe, A. C., & Singer, L. T. (1989). Atypical eating disorders in young children. *International Journal of Eating Disorders, 8,* 575–582.

Johnson, C., Tobin, D. L., & Dennis, A. (1990). Differences in treatment outcome between borderline and nonborderline bulimics at one-year follow-up. *International Journal of Eating Disorders, 9,* 617–627.

Klerman, G. L., Weissman, M. M., Rounsaville, B. J., & Chevron, E. (1984). *Interpersonal psychotherapy for depression.* New York: Basic Books.

Kreipe, R. E. (1995). Eating disorders among children and adolescents. *Pediatrics in Review, 16,* 370–379.

Lask, B., & Bryant-Waugh, R. (1997). Prepubertal eating disorders. In D. M. Garner & P. E. Garfinkel (Eds.), *Handbook of treatment for eating disorders* (pp. 476–483). New York: Guilford Press.

Leitenberg, H., Rosen, J. C., Wolf, J., Vara, L. S., Detzer, M. J., & Srebnik, D. (1994). Comparison of cognitive-behavior therapy and desipramine in the treatment of bulimia nervosa. *Behavior Research and Therapy, 32,* 37–45.

Levin, A. P., & Hyler, S. E. (1986). *DSM-III-R* personality diagnosis in bulimia. *Comprehensive Psychiatry, 27,* 47–53.

McKisack, C., & Waller, G. (1997). Factors influencing the outcome of group psychotherapy for bulimia nervosa. *International Journal of Eating Disorders, 22,* 1–13.

Minuchin, S., Rosman, B. L., & Baker, L. (1978). *Psychosomatic families: Anorexia nervosa in context.* Cambridge, MA: Harvard University Press.

Mitchell, J. E., Raymond, N., & Specker, S. (1993). A review of the controlled trials of pharmacotherapy and psychotherapy in the treatment of bulimia nervosa. *International Journal of Eating Disorders, 14,* 229–247.

Oppenheimer, R., Howells, K., Palmer, R. L., & Chaloner, D. A. (1985). Adverse sexual experience in childhood and clinical eating disorders: A preliminary description. *Journal of Psychiatric Research, 19,* 357–361.

Patton, G. C., Johnson-Sabine, E., Wood, K., Mann, A. H., & Wakeling, A. (1990). Abnormal eating attitudes in London schoolgirls: A prospective epidemiological study. Outcome at 12 month follow-up. *Psychological Medicine, 20,* 383–394.

Piran, N., Lerner, P., Garfinkel, P. E., Kennedy, S. H., & Brouilette, C. (1988). Personality disorders in anorexia patients. *International Journal of Eating Disorders, 5,* 589–599.

Pope, H. G., & Hudson, J. I. (1989). Are eating disorders associated with borderline personality disorder? A critical review. *International Journal of Eating Disorders, 8,* 1–9.

Rastam, M. (1992). Anorexia nervosa in 51 Swedish adolescents: Premorbid problems and comorbidity. *Journal of the American Academy of Child and Adolescent Psychiatry, 31,* 819–829.

Raymond, N. C., Mitchell, J. E., Fallon, P., & Katzman, M. A. (1994). A collaborative approach to the use of medication. In P. Fallon, M. Katzman, & S. C. Wooley (Eds.), *Feminist perspectives on eating disorders* (pp. 231–250). New York: Guilford Press.

Russell, G. F. M., Szmukler, G. I., Dare, C., & Eisler, I. (1987). An evaluation of family therapy in anorexia nervosa and bulimia nervosa. *Archives of General Psychiatry, 44,* 1047–1056.

Selvini-Palazzoli, M. P. (1974). *Self-starvation.* London: Chaucer.

Sloan, G., & Leichner, P. (1986). Is there a relationship between sexual abuse or incest and eating disorders? *Canadian Journal of Psychiatry, 31,* 656–660.

Sohlberg, S., Norring, C., Holmgren, S., & Rosmark, B. (1989). Impulsivity and long-term prognosis of psychiatric patients with anorexia nervosa/bulimia nervosa. *Journal of Nervous and Mental Disease, 177,* 249–258.

Strober, M. (1997). Consultation and therapeutic engagement in severe anorexia nervosa. In D. M. Garner & P. E. Garfinkel (Eds.), *Handbook of treatment for eating disorders* (pp. 229–247). New York: Guilford Press.

Vitousek, K. B., & Orimoto, L. (1993). Cognitive-behavioral models of anorexia nervosa, bulimia nervosa, and obesity. In P. Kendal & K. Dobson (Eds.), *Psychopathology and cognition* (pp. 191–243). New York: Academic Press.

Walsh, B. T., & Garner, D. M. (1997). Diagnostic issues. In D. M. Garner & P. E. Garfinkel (Eds.), *Handbook of treatment for eating disorders* (pp. 25–33). New York: Guilford Press.

Whittal, M. L., Agras, W. S., & Gould, R. A. (1999). Bulimia nervosa: A meta-analysis of psychosocial and pharmacological treatments. *Behavior Therapy, 30,* 117–135.

Wilfley, D. E., Agras, W. S., Telch, C. F., Rossiter, E. M., Schneider, J. A., Cole, A. G., Stifford, L., & Raeburn, S. D. (1993). Group cognitive-behavioral therapy and group interpersonal psychotherapy for the nonpurging bulimic individual: A controlled comparison. *Journal of Consulting and Clinical Psychology, 2,* 296–305.

Wonderlich, S. A., Swift, W. J., Slotnick, H. B., & Goodman, S. (1990). *DSM-III-R* personality disorders in eating disorder subtypes. *International Journal of Eating Disorders, 9,* 607–616.

20

MARIBETH GETTINGER
REBECCA KOSCIK

Psychological Services for Children with Learning Disabilities

Definition and Prevalence of Learning Disability

Learning disability (LD) is the term used to describe a handicapping condition that interferes with a person's ability to store, process, or produce information. Learning disability affects both children and adults and results in a gap between an individual's "true" potential and his or her actual performance, leading to significant academic and social difficulties. The most obvious indication of a learning disability is academic failure, or achievement that is significantly lower than expected based on all other information about the person. That is, the low performance of individuals with LD is *not* due to below-average intelligence; visual, hearing, or motor impairment; or environmental, cultural, or economic disadvantage.

Many definitions of "learning disability" have been written over the past 20 years. The statutory definition of learning disability included in the Individuals with Disabilities Education Act (IDEA; U.S. Department of Education, 1997) states that the disability is a "disorder in one or more basic psychological processes involved in understanding or in using language, spoken or written, that may manifest itself in an imperfect ability to listen, speak, read, write, spell, or to do mathematical calculations" (p. 149). Despite disagreement in the field about diagnostic criteria and evaluation procedures, there is some agreement about major definitional components of learning disability. The first is the existence of what is called an "ability-achievement discrepancy." For individuals with LD, academic and learning problems persist in spite of normal or average intelligence. Although a discrepancy between an intelligence quotient (IQ) and achievement has been the major criterion for diagnosing LD, there is considerable variation in how the discrepancy may be derived and quantified. The second definitional component is the presence of a central nervous system dysfunction or information-processing disorder. Although the precise nature of the processing disorder varies across theoretical models, experts do agree that individuals with LD handle information differently than typical learners do; and, although they cannot be cured, children and adults with LD can be taught compensatory strategies. Third, the majority of current conceptualizations view learning disability as a lifelong condition that may co-occur with other handicapping conditions, including giftedness. Fourth, across all definitions, the hallmark of learning disabilities is the presence of intraindividual differences. Individuals with LD exhibit an uneven profile of development and skill across various ability and achievement domains. Finally, all perspectives emphasize that learning disabilities vary in terms of severity and pervasiveness and that LD designates a heterogeneous and highly diverse group of learners (Lerner, 2000).

The number of individuals estimated to have learning disabilities is largely dependent on the definition and measurement procedures used to identify the disorder. Estimates of the prevalence of LD in the general population have ranged from 2% to 30% (Hallahan, Kauffman, & Lloyd, 1996). Using the federal definition to formulate identification criteria, approximately 5% of the total public school population is identified as having LD (Lyon, 1996).

The prevalence of LD has increased dramatically in the last 20 years. The U.S. Department of Education has documented a rapid and steady increase in the number of children identified as having LD relative to all other students with disabilities. For example, in 1978, the population of students with LD constituted approximately 29% of all children with identified handicapping conditions; this number rose sharply to 45% by 1982. According to the *Twentieth Annual Report to Congress on the Implementation of the Individuals with Disabilities Education Act* (U.S. Department of Education, 1998), students with learning disabilities now represent over half of all students identified as needing special education services. Lyon (1996) further estimates that 80% of children identified as having LD experience their primary difficulties and discrepant achievement in the acquisition of basic reading skills.

Functional Characteristics and Consequences of Learning Disability

Numerous investigations have been conducted over the past two decades to identify behavioral, cognitive, and affective characteristics of learning disability. Academic factors, specifically academic underachievement, are among the first variables that come to mind when describing the functional characteristics of individuals with learning disabilities. People with LD have difficulty in one or more of the following areas: reading, spelling, writing, mathematics, and spatial concepts. The eligibility criteria in most states indicate that a student must be significantly below his or her grade or age peers in one or more of these areas of academic functioning (Hardman, Drew, & Egan, 1999). Students with LD frequently show significant intraindividual variability in their achievement across content domains. For example, a child with a specific disability in reading may be far behind his or her peers in reading yet achieve commensurate with peers in mathematics. In addition, individuals with LD often exhibit language problems that contribute to their overall low academic performance. Common language problems include listening difficulties, delays in oral language development, poor vocabulary development, and inadequate linguistic competence (Zigmond, 1993).

The most rapid growth in knowledge in recent years concerns the cognitive characteristics associated with learning disability (Wong, 1992). Although their cognitive abilities are "normal," students with LD often exhibit cognitive characteristics that may interfere with their acquisition and application of academic and social skills. Several cognitive processes that differentiate students with LD from their typically developing peers have been described in the research, including memory, attentional, metacognitive, and attribution processes.

Individuals with LD frequently exhibit problems in various aspects of short-term and long-term memory (Swanson, Cooney, & O'Shaughnessy, 1998). Classroom teachers often cite memory difficulties as the most common characteristic among their students with LD. Empirical research confirms teachers' identification of memory problems in students. Studies that compare samples of children with and without LD have focused on two specific aspects of memory — retrieval and retention of information and strategy utilization. First, children with LD exhibit difficulties on retrieval tasks in comparison with their non-LD, same-age peers. Their ability to retain and retrieve both verbal and nonverbal information often approximates that of younger, normally achieving children (Swanson & Trahan, 1990). Research focusing on long-term memory indicates that individuals with LD are also less successful in committing information to long-term memory (referred to as a "storage failure"). Working memory, which is required to connect information in short- and long-term memory, has also been implicated as a source of difficulty for many individuals with LD (Swanson et al., 1998).

Second, memory problems among individuals with LD can be attributed, in part, to a failure to use effective strategies to facilitate memory, such as active rehearsal and categorization of information. Memory problems also derive from limited motivation for engaging in intentional mental efforts, or executive control (Swanson et al., 1998; Torgesen, 1994). Executive control refers to the purposeful use of rules and strategies for learning (e.g., mnemonic aids, rehearsal, etc.) that focus attention on salient information to be remembered, as well as the ability to manipulate and organize information. Torgesen (1994) found that problems with memory are often associated with deficits in executive control functions.

Similar to memory difficulties, problems in attention have long been considered a critical functional characteristic of learning disability (Conte, 1991). Dykman, Ackerman, Clements, and Peters (1971) originally postulated that an attentional deficit underlies most learning disabilities. They employed a battery of experimental tests to assess various aspects of attention, including alertness, vigilance, and ability to focus. On all attentional measures, children with LD performed more poorly than did normally achieving children. Additional support for an attentional deficit has been offered in recent years by observational studies of classroom behaviors of students with LD (e.g., McIntosh, Vaughn, Schumm, Haager, & Lee, 1993). Children with LD spend significantly less time engaged in task-oriented behaviors and more time in non-task-oriented behaviors. Gerber (1988) suggested that even when students with LD exhibit optimal attention or on-task behavior during learning situations, they may have difficulty allocating attention efficiently to information within tasks. This may account for a slower rate of learning among students with LD.

Of major significance in the study of attention is the consistent finding that individuals with LD exhibit a lag in their selective attention, or the ability to identify and extract important information and salient aspects of a stimulus. Similar to findings from memory research, these studies show that children with LD do not spontaneously use strategies, such as verbal rehearsal and organization, that would enable them to perform successfully on selective attention tasks (Lerner, 2000; Swanson & Trahan, 1990; Torgesen, 1990). Students with LD also have been shown to differ significantly from peers without LD in both the quantity and quality of their inner speech, which serves to focus attention on salient information. Specifically, children with LD do not give themselves instructions with the same frequency or degree of accuracy in order to focus on the most critical task parameters (Torgesen, 1990).

The view that individuals with LD fail to use appropriate memory or attention strategies has received considerable empirical support over the last 15 years. We now understand, however, that individuals with LD may possess the necessary strategies but do not recognize situations or tasks for appropriate strategy use (Pressley, Woloshyn, et al., 1995). This type of difficulty falls within the domain of metacognitive processing. Metacognitive research focuses on an individual's awareness of specific strategies that are available for cognitive and academic performance. Many researchers suggest that students with LD lack an awareness of how their own cognitive processes can enhance learning (Brownell, Mellard, & Deshler, 1993; Montague & Applegate, 1993; Wong, 1991). Students with LD have been characterized as inefficient learners who are neither aware of the demands of academic tasks nor able to access strategies to approach tasks. According to Montague (1992), what may be lacking is the ability to recognize that one task is like another and that a strategy which was useful for one problem may be used or modified to solve another. In addition, individuals with LD have difficulty assessing their own ability to solve problems, monitoring their problem-solving or comprehension processes, and evaluating their performance for accuracy (Deshler, Ellis, & Lenz, 1996).

The memory, attentional, and metacognitive characteristics of individuals with LD have led researchers to conclude that individuals with LD fail to engage in intentional self-regulated learning that promotes success in academic and social situations. Self-regulated learners use their knowledge of strategies for accomplishing tasks efficiently (Zimmerman, 1994). In addition, self-regulated learners demonstrate motivation to employ their knowledge effectively. Individuals with learning disabilities often lack the ability to regulate their own thinking; they may not know how to gain new knowledge or how to remember what they have learned. In general, individuals with LD do not display the knowledge and behaviors that characterize self-regulated learners (Ellis, Deshler, Lenz, Schumaker, & Clark, 1991; Wong, 1992).

Self-regulation is closely linked to the concept of personal control, or global awareness of one's personal impact or efficacy, in individuals with LD. There is evidence that many individuals with LD exhibit "learned helplessness," or the belief that their efforts will not result in a designated outcome (Levine & Swartz, 1995). Researchers have concluded that students with LD are generally pessimistic about their ability to influence academic and social outcomes and may not derive feelings of self-efficacy from their accomplishments. In addition, individuals with LD are more likely to have a low self-concept, which, in turn, leads to fewer attempts to plan and implement successful approaches to tasks. In sum, they are prone to view themselves as helpless when faced with difficult academic, social, or problem-solving situations.

Another way to characterize this "helpless" style of personal control is passivity in learning style. Students with LD have learned to approach learning tasks in a passive rather than active manner. They may lack interest in learning because of their history of academic failures and frustrations. Not believing they can succeed, students with LD do know how to go about the task of learning. As a consequence, they have become passive and dependent as learners, a style that is consistent with learned helplessness (Wong, 1998).

Collective descriptions of the functional characteristics of learning disability have led researchers and clinicians away from searching for one underlying cognitive or behavioral deficit that accounts for low performance. Instead, research suggests that each deficiency, whether memory, attentional, metacognitive, or attributional, should be viewed as a complex process. Bender (1992) used the concept of "cognitive strategies deficiency syndrome" to summarize the characteristics and consequences associated with learning disability. Bender's perspective of a "syndrome" is important in that it underscores the fact that learning disability results in a constellation of functional characteristics and that each individual with LD exhibits a unique and highly individual pattern of behavioral and cognitive characteristics.

Developmental Progression of Learning Disability

At any stage in the developmental progression of learning disability, certain factors may be present, yet the developmental profile of each person may be different. Describing the developmental progression of learning disabilities in preschool-aged children is difficult in that few children are actually diagnosed as having a learning disability during their early education years. Often, children with learning problems at this age are described as having significant "developmental delays" or being "at risk" for later learning problems. Young children who are at risk for learning disability typically have poor fine and gross motor development, language delays, speech disorders, limited ability to attend to relevant stimuli, hyperactivity, and poor concept development (Barnett & Carey, 1992). They also exhibit deficits in preacademic skills, such as phonological awareness, sound blending and segmentation, rapid naming (recall of object names), letter names and associated sounds, and visual-perceptual integration (Lyon, 1996).

Three categories of risk factors have been linked with LD in preschool children: established risk, biological risk, and environmental risk (Shonkoff & Meisels,

1991). Children who have an established risk are children who were given a medical diagnosis at an early age that is indicative of a disability or developmental delay. Children with biological risk are those who have a mental or physical condition that is likely to evolve into a developmental delay, such as very low-birth-weight infants. Finally, children who experience environmental risk include children from impoverished backgrounds with a high probability for delayed development. Family factors, such as chaos, poverty, substance abuse, parental education, and neglect, represent some of the many factors associated with environmental risk.

Lerner (1997) noted that the presence of a learning disability during the elementary school years is usually seen through underachievement or failure in one or more basic academic areas such as reading, writing, and math. Elementary schoolchildren with LD may also be unable to sustain attention for any length of time and may exhibit weak fine and gross motor skills. Children with LD at this age typically experience social-emotional problems (such as low self-esteem) as a result of their continued academic failure. In addition, elementary school children with LD often struggle to make and maintain friendships.

As children with LD develop into adolescents, they continue to experience both academic and social-emotional problems (Kass & Maddux, 1993). Social-emotional problems, such as low self-esteem and limited number of friends, are often exacerbated by persistent academic struggles, social skill deficits, and the development of normative adolescent issues (e.g., self-concept issues, physical changes, independence, peer pressure, etc.). Characteristics that surface during adolescence as a result of the challenges associated with having LD include learned helplessness, a significant drop in confidence in one's ability to learn and succeed, low motivation to achieve, attention problems, and maladaptive behavior (Deshler et al., 1996).

Finally, as individuals with LD progress to adulthood, they experience continued reading difficulties and social problems. In addition, adults with LD may experience challenges in locating and/or keeping a job (Gerber & Reiff, 1995). In a review of studies of adults with LD, Smith (1988) noted that adults identified needs in the areas of developing and maintaining relationships, career guidance (job training, job-finding skills), substance use and dependence, finance management, and personal organization skills.

Empirically Supported Interventions

Research describing the nature of the functional characteristics of individuals with learning disability has contributed to an understanding of interventions that are successful in enhancing the performance of individuals with LD. Current research has focused on two types of intervention approaches for addressing the needs of individuals with LD, specifically (1) direct instruction or explicit teaching approaches and (2) cognitive and metacognitive intervention approaches.

Direct-Instruction Approaches

There are a variety of interpretations of the term *direct instruction*. Direct instruction, also referred to as explicit teaching, describes a treatment approach that is derived from research on effective teaching. Direct instruction concentrates on the acquisition of specific skills (academic as well as social) and involves structuring the environment to ensure mastery of these skills (Tarver, 1992). In a direct-instruction approach, the interactions between therapists and their clients are highly structured and sometimes scripted. Direct-instruction approaches share several important characteristics, including a direct focus on skills, a high degree of teacher/therapist direction, the use of a carefully sequenced set of skills to teach, and an emphasis on mastery of skills (Shapiro, 1996).

Behavioral analysis provides the theoretical framework for direct instruction. Behavioral analysis requires that teachers or therapists analyze tasks in terms of the specific skills needed to accomplish them. Intervention involves helping individuals acquire the skills they have not yet mastered. In contrast to an emphasis on thinking and metacognition, explicit instruction emphasizes skill acquisitions. Interventions focus on the task (not the cognitive characteristics of the learner) and on the behaviors needed to learn the task (not the cognitive or metacognitive processes involved). An explicit-instruction approach is founded on numerous behavioral principles that have been shown to be effective in bringing about positive behavior change. These include specifying the target behavior, modeling the appropriate behavior, providing practice opportunities and frequent feedback, measuring the target behavior repeatedly, and requiring a high level of mastery.

The effective teaching literature, which provides a strong empirical foundation for the direct-instruction model, has identified key principles and guidelines for teaching individuals with learning disabilities. Generally, techniques derived from this research emphasize active effort by the teacher or therapist to elicit as much active responding and engagement from clients as possible. Direct instruction requires careful sequencing of skills to be taught and attention to the amount and type of environmental structuring necessary to assure success, for example, modeling of correct responding, use of teacher signals to control attention, choral as well as independent responding, immediate corrective practice, and ample monitored practice. An explicit-teaching model generally includes five steps or phases: (1) specification of a behavioral objective; (2) an initial direct-instruction phase in which the teacher or therapist models a problem and, through task analysis, identifies the critical steps in a solving the problem or completing a task; (3) a teacher-guided practice phase; (4) an independent practice phase with multiple opportunities to "try out" the skill or solution, paired with immediate and corrective feedback; and (5) routine and systematic assessment of performance, with a targeted high level of mastery (80%–90% accuracy; Rosenshine, 1986).

Research on direct-instruction programs has documented the effectiveness of this approach for individuals with LD, especially for basic skill acquisition in literary skills (reading and writing). Explicit- or direct-instruction procedures have proven successful across age levels, ability levels, and curriculum domains (Gersten, Carnine, & Woodward, 1987; Swanson, Carson, & Saches-Lee, 1996; Tarver, 1994). A meta-analytic review of research on direct instruction revealed an average effect size of 0.81 for academic measures (White, 1988). Thus the research support for explicit instruction is quite strong for students with LD across multiple domains.

Despite this research support, there are some concerns and cautions about a direct-instruction approach. The dominant research and intervention focus in learning disabilities has been on the use of a direct-instruction approach for teaching academic and literacy skills. Basic skill acquisition relies heavily on repetitive drill-and-practice formats and teacher-directed instruction. This exclusive emphasis on basic skills has been criticized because of the lack of cognitively complex and meaningful problem-solving activities. Research suggests that individuals with LD may experience difficulties related to memory, organization, and problem solving, even when they have mastered basic skills via a direct-instruction approach. For example, students with LD often fail to generate spontaneously effective memorization strategies to retain information, they typically require more time than their nondisabled peers to achieve mastery, and they often do not know why they are memorizing information or in what context the information is meaningful. Although teaching basic skills to students with LD is essential, it does not allow them to learn complex knowledge and problem-solving skills. A solution to this problem has been the training of strategies and problem-solving skills in conjunction with teaching of basic skills (Gersten, 1998).

In recent years, direct-instruction research has expanded beyond the so-called basic academic skills to more cognitively complex tasks, such as critical reading and comprehension. Researchers have converged on an explicit model for strategy instruction. The underlying notion is that teaching a strategy is analogous to teaching an academic skill. A strategy (similar to a skill) must be taught in isolation, practiced to mastery, and then returned to an authentic context or tried out on actual school tasks. Explicit instruction of strategies occurs when teachers and instructional materials are explicit about what needs to be done or said or written. Explicit instruction provides structure or frameworks for students to use as they read, write, complete math problems, study independently, or engage in group activities.

There are four core principles of direct or explicit instruction of strategies. First, because individuals with LD often bring limited background knowledge to academic activities, they must be provided with a wide range of examples of the skill, concept, or problem-solving strategy to learn. Second, individuals with LD have a difficult time organizing information on their own. Therefore, explicit instruction involves providing models of proficient and organized performance, including step-by-step procedures to complete tasks. The third principle of explicit instruction is to provide experiences in which individuals must explain how they completed a task and why they made their decisions. Fourth, individuals with LD require frequent feedback and practice to retain information, as well as consistent support to remain engaged in learning activities (Gersten, 1998). These principles have contributed to the development of a four-step sequence of explicit teaching for strategies which involves (1) direct teaching and modeling of step-by-step strategy; (2) guided practice and feedback, with repeated opportunities to perform the strategy and obtain feedback; (3) gradual increase in student responsibility for executing the strategy, which involves helping students perform the strategy on their own and shifting the responsibility for using the strategy gradually from teachers to the students; and (4) use of adequate, systematic practice and application of the strategy with a range of examples (Shapiro, 1996).

In addition to making initial instruction as explicit and direct as possible, explicit instruction also involves scaffolding, guiding, and prompting by the teacher, therapist, or peers. Scaffolding refers to the direct assistance given to an individual between the initial introduction of new knowledge, skills, or strategies and the eventual self-directed application of the knowledge. Because individuals with LD often fail as independent or self-directed learners, scaffolding is an important intervention technique as part of an explicit-instruction approach that facilitates the transition from teacher direction to self-direction (Pressley, Hogan, Wharton-Mc-Donald, Mistretta, & Ettenberger, 1996).

Cognitive and Metacognitive Approaches

Interest in the development, application, and evaluation of cognitive and metacognitive therapies for individuals with LD has increased in the last 10 years, paralleling the accumulation of evidence identifying the cognitive characteristics associated with learning disability. In general, these approaches concentrate on "cognitively activating" individuals with LD and giving them personal control or responsibility for planning and implementing solutions to academic or social problems. The focus of cognitive and metacognitive therapies is on the covert thinking or internal processes that presumably underlie overt behavior. The hypothesized relationship among private speech, thinking, and behavior has been influential in the development and application of these approaches with individuals with LD. Although a variety of different instructional and therapeutic strategies fall under the label of cognitive and metacognitive approaches, four key treatment components may be incorporated into treatment approaches used for learning disability. These are: (1) self-instructional training, (2) self-monitoring, (3) problem-solving or cognitive-strategy training, and (4) metacognitive training (Wong, 1992).

SELF-INSTRUCTIONAL TRAINING   Self-instructional training (SIT) is based on the notion that individuals with LD can be taught to verbalize their cognitive processes and use these verbalizations to guide their academic and social behavior. SIT is a procedure in which individuals learn to silently verbalize questions, directions, and judgments that enhance their performance. Meichenbaum (1980) pioneered the use of this approach for students with LD. Training in SIT involves teaching individuals to do the following: (1) ask questions of themselves about the nature of a problem, the most effective approach to a task, the relevant stimuli or information, and the accuracy or quality of their performance; (2) give themselves self-instructions to guide performance; and (3) provide themselves with reinforcement and feedback (Davey & McBride, 1986; Graham & Harris, 1994). The specific questions and statements that are taught vary depending on the nature of the task or problem targeted for intervention and on the individual characteristics of the person (e.g., developmental status, language abilities, etc.). Typically, training follows a sequence of activities beginning with the therapist's demonstration of overt self-instruction and concluding with the client's covert self-instruction.

SELF-MONITORING   Self-monitoring of behavior is a cognitive component which is directed at increasing appropriate behavior associated with academic and social success. Self-monitoring may be conceptualized as involving two stages —

self-assessment and self-recording. Self-assessment refers to the act of evaluating one's own behavior to determine whether a particular target behavior has or has not occurred. Self-recording is the act of keeping a tally of how many times the target behavior has occurred. The majority of developmental and evaluative research concerning self-monitoring with students with LD has been conducted by Hallahan (1980) and his associates. They have studied the effects of self-monitoring on both attentional behavior and academic productivity. Several findings have emerged from this work. Self-monitoring during academic tasks does lead to an increase in attentional behavior and academic productivity. Furthermore, training in self-monitoring appears to be most effective when students are engaged in tasks for which they have the necessary prerequisite skills (Rooney & Hallahan, 1985).

PROBLEM-SOLVING STRATEGIES   Problem-solving or cognitive strategies are the techniques, principles, or rules that enable individuals to learn, solve problems, and complete tasks. The most comprehensive efforts to develop training programs that focus on problem-solving strategies have been those of Deshler and his colleagues (Deshler et al., 1996). The distinguishing characteristic of strategy approaches is the use of explicit, step-by-step training in the acquisition and use of particular learning or problem-solving strategies. The purpose in articulating and demonstrating a step-by-step strategy is to show individuals with LD how a thinking process can lead to accurate solutions or to demonstrate reasonable attempts at deducing an acceptable answer to a question. In demonstrating a strategy, the therapist makes each step clear to the client. This overt demonstration and guidance appears to be most important for individuals with LD, who do not intuitively devise strategies on their own. A key intervention component of a problem-solving or cognitive-strategy approach is to emphasize generalization. Over time, the focus of intervention must shift from teaching individuals to use a task-specific strategy to helping them focus on how strategies can be used to address similar problems in other domains. Cognitive- and problem-solving strategy instruction has been shown to improve the performance and strategic knowledge of individuals with LD across academic and social-emotional domains (Montague, 1992; Montague & Applegate, 1993; Pressley, Woloshyn, et al., 1995; Scruggs & Mastropieri, 1993).

METACOGNITIVE TRAINING   Students who lack problem-solving skills generally need explicit instruction in specific cognitive strategies to enhance their performance. In contrast, individuals who have a repertoire of problem-solving strategies but use them inefficiently or ineffectively may need metacognitive training to help them activate, select, and monitor their strategy use (Graham & Harris, 1994). Whereas cognitive problem-solving training provides students with strategies for learning, metacognitive approaches emphasize self-regulation and self-initiative. The fact that many children with LD must be told explicitly to use particular strategies suggests that their difficulty in learning lies, in part, in their lack of awareness of when and how to use strategies. Research indicates that improving self-awareness and teaching students with LD *how* to think is at least as important as teaching them *what* to think (Rooney & Hallahan, 1985). This conclusion has led to an increase in the development and evaluation of interventions designed to incorporate a metacognitive training component. For example, there have been significant efforts in applying metacognitive principles to interventions for children with reading disabilities. The goal of these approaches is to have children with LD think about the content of what they are reading. Training children to generate and direct questions to themselves about why they are reading the material and what they are understanding has been shown to have positive effects on overall comprehension (Wong, 1998). Metacognitive training has been applied to mathematics instruction (Montague & Bos, 1990; Montague, Bos, & Doucette, 1991) and to social skills as well. Smith, Finn, and Dowdy (1993), for example, described programs for individuals with social problems that focus on training them to think about their own behavior and to develop alternative ways of responding in problematic social situations.

The four components of cognitive and metacognitive interventions described here (self-instructional training, self-monitoring, problem-solving and cognitive-strategy training, and metacognitive skill development) have been integrated by researchers into programmatic approaches to improve the performance of students with learning disabilities. Six instructional programs which have demonstrated empirical support are listed and described briefly in Table 20.1. The general goal of these interventions is to help individuals with LD become more effective learners (Scheid, 1993; Scruggs & Wong, 1990).

TABLE 20.1   Instructional Programs that Incorporate Cognitive and Metacognitive Training

Strategies Intervention Model (Deshler, Ellis, & Lenz, 1996)	Eight instructional stages for teaching any given strategy. Focuses on both overt actions and cognitive behaviors.
Reciprocal Teaching (Palincsar & Brown, 1988)	Model for strategic reading. Teachers first teach and model summarizing, questioning, clarifying, and predicting. Then students use strategies in small group instruction and discussion.
Attributional Retraining (Groteluschen, Borkowski, & Hale, 1990)	Students receive effort-related feedback plus direct training in executive control strategies.
Strategic Content Learning (Butler, 1995)	Assess students' extant metacognitive skills. Build from what students know and show them how to work strategically and reflect on their work.
Self-Regulatory Strategy Development (Graham & Harris, 1994)	Approach to strategic writing. Goals for student are to master cognitive processes, develop positive attitudes about writing and their writing skills, and increase their ability to reflect and self-regulate while engaged in writing.
Transactional Strategies Instruction (Pressley, Brown, El-Dinary, & Afflerback, 1995)	Focuses on reading comprehension. Promotes self-directed processing, positive beliefs, and metacognitive understanding.

Summary

Overall, individuals with LD are not agile in organizing and prioritizing the academic and social information to which they are exposed. Their academic performance and social behavior are limited by an information base which is not easily accessed and which is further constrained by dependence on poorly defined and/or inflexible strategies. Additionally, they experience difficulty identifying and describing the processes they actually use to learn and to interact with others. Because of research highlighting these important characteristics of learning disability, there have been extensive efforts to develop both direct-instruction and cognitive-strategy approaches for this population. Despite the documented success of both approaches, it is important for educators and clinicians to consider what the use of interventions may or may not accomplish for their students and clients who have learning disabilities. Even with explicit teaching and the use of cognitive strategies, idiosyncratic learning styles and performance differences are present among individuals with LD. In other words, the use of direct-instruction and strategy approaches may not transform an individual with a learning disability into an expert, nor advance him or her to being strategy proficient or to achieving automaticity and mastery of basic skills. Interventions for individuals with LD are best designed in an individualized manner and implemented only after a comprehensive assessment of their unique learning needs. The purpose of such an assessment is to gather information to identify the level of basic skills individuals have achieved and the nature of current strategies they use to solve problems and complete tasks.

The individual nature of difficulties and characteristics of persons with LD also leads to the important conclusion that a scripted approach to either explicit-instruction or cognitive-strategy training may not be the best approach to intervention. The design of individualized interventions should consider the unique strategies and procedures that students with LD already utilize. The hope of intervention approaches is that clients will retain and generalize information they have acquired and will internalize strategies to use in place of their previously ineffective, disorganized, or inefficient thinking. Such a focus and treatment goal maximizes the potential for improved maintenance and generalization of change among individuals with LD.

REFERENCES

Barnett, D., & Carey, K. T. (1992). *Designing interventions for preschool learning and behavior problems*. San Francisco: Jossey-Bass.

Bender, W. N. (1992). *Learning disabilities: Characteristics, identification, and teaching strategies*. Needham Heights, MA: Allyn & Bacon.

Brownell, M. T., Mellard, D. F., & Deshler, D. D. (1993). Differences in learning and transfer performances between students with learning disabilities and other low-achieving students on problem-solving tasks. *Learning Disability Quarterly, 16,* 138–156.

Butler, D. L. (1995). Promoting strategic

learning by post-secondary students with learning disabilities. *Journal of Learning Disabilities, 28,* 170–190.

Conte, R. (1991). Attention disorders. In B. Y. L. Wong (Ed.), *Learning about learning disabilities* (pp. 60–103). San Diego, CA: Academic Press.

Davey, B., & McBride, S. (1986). The effects of question generation training on reading comprehension. *Journal of Educational Psychology, 78,* 256–262.

Deshler, D. D., Ellis, E. S., & Lenz, B. K. (1996). *Teaching adolescents with learning disabilities: Strategies and methods* (2nd ed.). Denver, CO: Love.

Dykman, R. A., Ackerman, P. T., Clements, S. D., & Peters, J. E. (1971). Specific learning disabilities: An attentional deficit syndrome. In H. R. Myklebust (Ed.), *Progress in learning disabilities* (Vol. 2, pp. 145–189). Orlando, FL: Grune & Stratton.

Ellis, E. S., Deshler, D. D., Lenz, B. K., Schumaker, J. B., & Clark, F. L. (1991). An instructional model for teaching learning strategies. *Focus on Exceptional Children, 23,* 1–24.

Gerber, M. M. (1988). Cognitive-behavioral training in the curriculum: Time, slow learners, and basic skills. In E. L. Meyen, G. A. Vergason, & R. J. Whelan (Eds.), *Effective instructional strategies for exceptional children* (pp. 65–79). Denver, CO: Love.

Gerber, P. J., & Reiff, H. B. (1995). *Learning disabilities in adulthood: Persisting problems and evolving issues.* Austin, TX: Pro-Ed.

Gersten, R. (1998). Recent advances in instructional research for students with learning disabilities: An overview. *Learning Disabilities Research and Practice, 13,* 162–170.

Gersten, R., Carnine, D., & Woodward, J. (1987). Direct instruction research: The third decade. *Remedial and Special Education, 8,* 48–56.

Graham, S., & Harris, K. (1994). The role and development of self-regulation in the writing process. In D. H. Schunk &

B. J. Zimmerman (Eds.), *Self-regulation of learning and performance: Issues and educational applications* (pp. 203–228). Hillsdale, NJ: Erlbaum.

Groteluschen, A. K., Borkowski, J. G., & Hale, C. (1990). Strategy instruction is often insufficient: Addressing the interdependency of executive and attributional processes. In T. Scruggs & B. Y. L. Wong (Eds.), *Intervention research in learning disabilities* (pp. 81–101). New York: Springer-Verlag.

Hallahan, D. P. (1980). Teaching exceptional children to use cognitive strategies. *Exceptional Education Quarterly, 1,* 1–12.

Hallahan, D. P., Kauffman, J. M., & Lloyd, J. W. (1996). *Introduction to learning disabilities.* Boston: Allyn & Bacon.

Hardman, M. L., Drew, C. J., & Egan, M. W. (1999). *Human exceptionality: Society, school, and family* (6th ed.). Boston: Allyn & Bacon.

Kass, C. E., & Maddux, C. D. (1993). *A human development view of learning disabilities: From theory to practice.* Springfield, IL: Thomas.

Lerner, J. W. (2000). *Learning disabilities: Theories, diagnosis, and teaching strategies* (8th ed.). Boston: Houghton Mifflin.

Levine, M. D., & Swartz, C. W. (1995). The unsuccessful adolescent. In Learning Disabilities Association of America (Ed.), *Secondary education and beyond: Providing opportunities for students with learning disabilities* (pp. 3–12). Pittsburgh, PA: Author.

Lyon, G. R. (1996). Learning disabilities. *The Future of Children: Special Education for Students with Disabilities, 6*(1), 54–76.

McIntosh, R., Vaughn, S., Schumm, J. S., Haager, D., & Lee, O. (1993). Observations of students with learning disabilities in general education classrooms. *Exceptional Children, 60,* 249–261.

Meichenbaum, D. (1980). Cognitive behavior modification with exceptional children: A promise yet unfulfilled. *Exceptional Education Quarterly, 1,* 83–88.

Montague, M. (1992). The effects of cognitive and metacognitive strategy instruction on mathematical problem solving of middle school students with learning disabilities. *Journal of Learning Disabilities, 25,* 230–248.

Montague, M., & Applegate, B. (1993). Middle school students' mathematical problem solving: An analysis of think-aloud protocols. *Learning Disability Quarterly, 16,* 19–30.

Montague, M., & Bos, C. (1990). Cognitive and metacognitive characteristics of eighth-grade students' mathematical problem-solving. *Learning and Individual Differences, 2,* 109–127.

Montague, M., Bos, C., & Doucette, M. (1991). Affective, cognitive, and metacognitive attributes of eighth-grade mathematical problem solvers. *Learning Disabilities Research and Practice, 6,* 145–151.

Palincsar, A. S., & Brown, A. L. (1988). Teaching and practicing thinking skills to promote comprehension in the context of group problem solving. *Remedial and Special Education, 9*(1), 53–59.

Pressley, M., Brown, R., El-Dinary, P. B., & Afflerback, P. (1995). The comprehension instruction that students need: Instruction fostering constructively responsive reading. *Learning Disabilities Research and Practice, 10,* 215–224.

Pressley, M., Hogan, K., Wharton-McDonald, R., Mistretta, J., & Ettenberger, S. (1996). The challenges of instructional scaffolding: The challenges of instruction that supports student thinking. *Learning Disabilities Research and Practice, 11,* 138–146.

Pressley, M., Woloshyn, V., & Burkell, J., Cariglia-Bull, T., Lysynchuk, L., McGoldrick, J. A., Schneider, B., Snyder, B. L., & Symons, S. (1995). *Cognitive strategy instruction that really improves*

children's academic performance (2nd ed.). Cambridge, MA: Brookline.

Rooney, K. J., & Hallahan, D. P. (1985). Future directions for cognitive behavior modification research: The quest for cognitive change. *Remedial and Special Education, 6*(2), 46–51.

Rosenshine, B. (1986). Synthesis of research on explicit teaching. *Educational Leadership, 43,* 60–69.

Scheid, K. (1993). *Helping students become strategic learners: Guidelines for teaching.* Cambridge, MA: Brookline Books.

Scruggs, T., & Mastropieri, M. (1993). Special education for the twenty-first century: Integrating learning strategies and thinking skills. *Journal of Learning Disabilities, 26,* 392–398.

Scruggs, T., & Wong, B. (1990). *Intervention research in learning disabilities.* New York: Springer-Verlag.

Shapiro, E. S. (1996). *Academic skills problems: Direct assessment and intervention* (2nd ed.). New York: Guilford Press.

Shonkoff, J., & Meisels, S.J. (1991). Defining eligibility for services under PL 99-457. *Journal of Early Intervention, 15,* 21–25.

Smith, J. (1988). Social and vocational problems of adults with learning disabilities: A review of the literature. *Learning Disabilities Focus, 4,* 36–58.

Smith, T. E. C., Finn, D. M., & Dowdy, C. A. (1993). *Teaching students with mild disabilities.* Philadelphia: Harcourt Brace Jovanovich.

Swanson, H. L., Carson, C., & Saches-Lee, C. M. (1996). A selective synthesis of intervention research for students with learning disabilities. *School Psychology Review, 25*(3), 370–391.

Swanson, H. L., Cooney, J. B., & O'Shaughnessy, T. E. (1998). Learning disabilities and memory. In B. Y. L. Wong (Ed.), *Learning about learning disabilities* (2nd ed., pp. 107–162). New York: Academic Press.

Swanson, H. L., & Trahan, M. (1990). Naturalistic memory in learning disabled children. *Learning Disability Quarterly, 13*, 82–89.

Tarver, S. G. (1992). Direct instruction. In W. Stainback & S. Stainback (Eds.), *Controversial issues confronting special education* (pp. 141–152). Needham Heights, MA: Allyn & Bacon.

Tarver, S. G. (1994). In search of effective instruction. *Effective School Practices, 13*(4), 23–32.

Torgesen, J. K. (1990). Studies of children with learning disabilities who perform poorly on memory span tasks. In J. K. Torgesen (Ed.), *Cognitive and behavioral characteristics of children with learning disabilities* (pp. 41–58). Austin, TX: Pro-Ed.

Torgesen, J. K. (1994). Issues in the assessment of executive function: An information-processing perspective. In G. R. Lyon (Ed.), *Frames of reference for the assessment of learning disabilities* (pp. 143–162). Baltimore: Brookes.

U.S. Department of Education. (1997). *Individuals with Disabilities Education Act Amendments of 1997*. Washington, DC: U.S. Government Printing Office.

U.S. Department of Education (1998). *Implementation of the Individuals with Disabilities Education Act: Twentieth Annual Report to Congress*. Washington, DC: U.S. Government Printing Office.

White, W. A. T. (1988). A meta-analysis of the effects of direct instruction in special education. *Education and Treatment of Children, 11*, 364–374.

Wong, B. Y. L. (1991). The relevance of metacognition to learning disabilities. In B. Y. L. Wong (Ed.), *Learning about learning disabilities* (pp. 231–256). San Diego, CA: Academic Press.

Wong, B. Y. L. (1992). On cognitive process-based instruction: An introduction. *Journal of Learning Disabilities, 25*, 150–152.

Wong, B. Y. L. (Ed.). (1998). *Learning about learning disabilities* (2nd ed.). New York: Academic Press.

Zigmond, N. (1993). Learning disabilities from an educational perspective. In G. R. Lyon, D. B. Gray, J. F. Kavanagh, & N. A. Krasnegor (Eds.), *Better understanding learning disabilities: New views from research and their implications for education and public policies* (pp. 251–272). Baltimore: Brookes.

Zimmerman, B. J. (1994). Dimensions of academic self-regulation: A conceptual framework for education. In D. H. Schunk & B. J. Zimmerman (Eds.), *Self-regulation of learning and performance: Issues and educational applications* (pp. 3–21). Hillsdale, NJ: Erlbaum.

PART V

System-Level Consultation

21

JANE CLOSE CONOLEY
COLLEEN A. CONOLEY

Systemic Interventions for Safe Schools

Polls taken of adult Americans indicate that youth violence is a top concern (Elam & Rose, 1995). The public is accurate in identifying American society as one of the more violent among industrialized countries. The rate of homicide among young adult men, for example, is many times higher in the United States than anywhere else in the developed world (Fingerhut & Kleinman, 1990). Estimates from the Department of Justice suggest that almost two million people are victims of violence every year, including 400 children each month who die from gunshot wounds (United States Department of Justice, 1996).

Children are affected by violence in their homes. A million substantiated cases of child abuse were reported in 1993 (National Committee to Prevent Child Abuse, 1994). The streets are not safe for many of the nation's young people, with young-sters reporting staying indoors because of daily gunfire, wearing bullet proof vests to venture out, or taking strategic paths to school to avoid violent or harassing encounters (Eron, Gentry, & Schlegel, 1994).

In such a context, schools and areas close to schools are not immune from danger. Three million crimes on or near campuses were reported in 1995 (United States Department of Justice, 1996), and students believe that many of their classmates bring weapons to school (Sheley, McGee, & Wright, 1992). Despite these alarming facts, only a small percentage of American children are actually touched by violence at school, but the educational implications for those children and the need to respond to and prevent the spread of violence have generated significant research effort.

As the institutions that serve almost all children and families, public schools are strategically positioned to mount prevention programs, link with other agencies in their preventive and remedial interventions, and be places of safety, caring, and nurturance for children and young people. To ignore the problem is to invite further infiltration of violence into school buildings and to make learning impossible for a significant number of children.

Psychological science and practice have extensive information to bring to bear on the goal of creating safer schools. This chapter will include descriptions of empirically supported prevention and intervention programs that can be delivered or coordinated by schools. Although the focus is schools, work with families, communities, and all the other systems that influence children is included. Violence in schools is due to a constellation of factors and can be prevented or reduced only through an ecological intervention plan.

The special focus of this chapter is on approaches that change the systems or processes within communities, school districts, buildings, and classrooms. Individual and family therapy treatment models are not considered. Multisystemic therapy is mentioned, however, as a very promising model that depends on change in many of the life spaces inhabited by children (Henggeler, Schoenwald, Borduin, Rowland, & Cunningham, 1998).

Primary and Secondary Prevention of Violence in Schools

Only early and comprehensive intervention with children, their families, and their social contexts is likely to eliminate student violence (Gentry & Eron, 1993; Capaldi & Patterson, 1987; Coie & Jacobs, 1993; Coie et al., 1993; Lochman, Coie, Underwood, & Terry, 1993; Patterson, 1982; Patterson, Reid, & Dishion, 1992; Reid, 1993). The available research and the cost to children, teachers, parents, and community members from violence in and around schools call on school personnel to find ways to implement school- or community-supported programs that will make a difference with families and their social contexts (Furlong & Morrison, 1994; Smith, 1990). In becoming implementation platforms, schools adopt a broader definition of their role, often not by singly adding services but by fostering creative partnerships with community agencies. Highly successful partnerships among schools, mental health agencies, municipal programs, and private volunteer programs provide ample evidence that such role amplification is possible (Oestmann & Walker, 1997).

Although aggressiveness, or conduct disorder, in children and youth is highly resistant to treatment, it is an ideal target for prevention. Much is known about how the behavior pattern appears from toddlerhood through adolescence; the relevant risk factors, antecedents, and mediators of its early development are known (e.g., Lyons-Ruth, Alpern, & Repacholi, 1993; Reid, 1993).

The major antecedents for serious risk of developing conduct disorder are the following:

1. Behavioral characteristics of the child—for example, difficult temperament; oppositional, attention-deficit, or hyperactivity problems
2. Ineffective parenting—for example, low involvement and harsh, irritable, or noncontingent discipline

3. A host of more distal factors—for example, divorce, social disadvantage, maternal depression and stress, substance abuse (Pope, Bierman, & Mumma, 1989, 1991; Reid, 1993).

These antecedents suggest that systemic preventive efforts fall into two categories. First, comprehensive parent training and preschool programs should be available to families. Second, policy efforts that reduce stress on families are absolutely necessary. These policy efforts would include: high quality day care; prenatal, maternal, and infant health programs; economic assistance, especially job training for single mothers; and social support for young parents. Services coordinated or offered by schools are more likely to be in the first category, but the second category of actions must be part of any comprehensive plan to reduce violence in American schools.

Once children enter kindergarten, preventive efforts become more complex (Reid, 1993). After the transition to school, factors likely to precipitate aggressive behavior exist in at least three settings: home, school, and peer group. A child who enters school without the social and cognitive skills necessary to navigate the setting is likely to experience academic failure and peer rejection. These events predict an increased risk for depressed mood and involvement in a deviant peer group. Both these outcomes increase the probability of a child's involvement with violence (Patterson, DeBaryshe, & Ramsey, 1989).

Parent Training

Children at risk for conduct disorder tend to emit problematic behavior at twice the rate of those not at risk (Bank, Marlow, Reid, Patterson, & Weinrott, 1991). Their mothers (as compared with control mothers) demonstrate twice the rate of aversive behavior toward their children (Patterson, 1982). It may be that families with oppositional children engage in a kind of daily warfare that prepares a child to continue with acrimonious transactions once school is entered (Reid, 1993). Specific training to reduce coercive verbal transactions has been effective with a wide variety of parent groups.

Parents also require education in how to manage their child's peer interactions and how to communicate with other adults regarding their child's behavior and needs (Gorski & Pilotto, 1993). Given that some parents may have antisocial, drug abusing, or violent backgrounds themselves and be suffering from an array of stresses (e.g., marital acrimony, economic hardship, mental illness, racism), they may have counterproductive parenting styles and be difficult to reach (Edleson & Peled, 1994).

The first and hardest obstacle to overcome when planning training for this group of parents is gaining their participation. Participation in training programs can be increased by initiating home visits to explain the program, offering incentives for participation, giving frequent reminders, using procedures for tracking families who move frequently, providing child care, telephoning participants to bolster learning of material, offering lively and on-time presentations and refreshments, encouraging high audience participation, and giving practical advice specific to problems and ages of children (Capaldi & Patterson, 1987; Dangel & Polster, 1984; Werth, 1995).

Many of the neediest families will not attend training. They may be less organized and less skilled at solving problems and taking advantage of resources than other families. It is likely that home visits, characteristic of many early childhood programs, are a necessary component to boost attendance. Although this approach is expensive, there is compelling evidence, for example, that African American children who experienced high-quality early intervention had lower school dropout rates and fewer arrests as adults while being more likely to own a home and not to be on welfare (Schweinhart & Weikart, 1993). These are obvious markers that individualized early intervention may save and even enhance community resources. Some researchers suggest that every dollar spent on early childhood programming results in seven dollars saved in later services (Schweinhart, Barnes, Weikart, Barnett, & Epstein, 1993).

Social and Cognitive Skills Training

In addition to teaching parents productive ways to respond to their children's behavior, their children must be taught positive skills for problem solving and social interactions with others. A child's social and cognitive skills are targets for prevention so that in-home and out-of-home interaction may enhance adjustment. As Patterson et al. (1992) suggest, "Repeated and reciprocated aggressive and coercive interactions with other youngsters escalates the development of aggressive behavior through the same negative reinforcement process as . . . in the parent-child interaction" (p. 117).

Social skills training that targets positive peer skills, anger management, and conflict resolution and that provides opportunities to practice the skills with peers who are not at risk is critical (Bierman et al., 1992; Bierman & Smoot, 1991; Bierman, Smoot, & Aumiller, 1993; Zigler, Taussig, & Black, 1992). Coie and his colleagues have illustrated that with African American boys, aggression and poor peer relations are highly predictive of later delinquency (Coie, Dodge, Terry, & Wright, 1991; Coie & Jacobs, 1993; Coie, Lochman, Terry, & Hyman, 1992; Pettit, Dodge, Bakshi, & Coie, 1990; Underwood, Coie, & Herbsman, 1992). In addition, the social structure of the boys' groups emerged fairly rapidly, with bullies, victims, and rejected young people assuming long-lasting roles. These findings suggest that early intervention across day care, primary grades, and other community settings is critical to preventing violence and aggression in schoolchildren.

Social skills training has been combined with moral education (Goldstein, 1999) to increase its effectiveness with aggressive children. This combination aims to assist the child in building empathy, solving problems, perceiving situations correctly, managing stress, using cooperative strategies, and understanding group process. Supportive models are important components of the training (Goldstein & Glick, 1994). This approach facilitates the development of more helpful internal cognitive models for children to use in interpreting their situations and making decisions about action related to the array of risk-taking behaviors.

The Positive Adolescents Choices Training (PACT; Hammond, 1991) is a social and behavioral skills approach that has been tested in schools and is particularly designed to reduce violence among African American youth. Given this population's disproportionate risk of becoming victims or perpetrators of violence, it is a prime target for secondary intervention. This program uses a series of videotapes titled "Dealing with Anger: Givin' It. Takin' It. Workin' It Out," making it fairly easy to implement in school contexts. The goals of the program are to build skills in giving negative feedback, reacting to anger, and negotiation.

It may be important to coordinate and combine parent training, social skills training, and moral education (Baker, Swisher, Nadenichek, & Popowicz, 1984). In combination, these are considerably more powerful than when implemented individually (Kazdin, 1993). Such combinations create the systemic change needed to promote peaceful behavior among children. A school context that is obviously shared by parents and teachers is considerably more powerful than two settings that are disengaged from each other (Lightfoot, 1978). When parents and teachers reinforce the social skills taught to children, the generalization of skills throughout a school day and across the home and school settings is strengthened. This reinforcement and modeling has important effects on child and adult behavior, adding to the nurturing quality of young peoples' environments.

Multisystemic Therapy

When primary or secondary prevention has been unsuccessful or untried, one approach for treating juvenile offenders who disrupt schools is multisystemic therapy (MST; Henggeler, Mihalic, Rone, Thomas, & Timmons-Mitchell, 1998). This is a highly structured, intensive, family- and community-based treatment that addresses the known determinants of serious antisocial behavior. The typical MST client is between 14 and 16 years old, lives in a single-parent home that is characterized by a variety of needs and problems, has multiple arrests, is deeply involved with delinquent peers, has serious problems at school, and abuses substances.

The effectiveness of MST is promising, but implementation of such an intense, individualized program presents challenges for schools (Borduin et al., 1995; Henggeler, Melton, & Smith, 1992; Henggeler, Melton, Smith, Schoenwald, & Hanley, 1993; Henggeler, Mihalic, et al., 1998). Successful and cost-effective programs have been launched in South Carolina, Missouri, and Washington State (Washington State Institute for Public Policy, 1998). Each of the programs represents a collaboration among several agencies (schools, probation, police, social services, and state education agencies) led by a specially trained mental health provider.

The mental health provider offers approximately four months of intensive, 24-hour availability to clients and the clients' systems. The provider identifies each client's individual and system needs and strengths. Interventions that focus on strengths (e.g., intelligence, social skills, and athletic ability) are implemented. Strengths in a school might include concerned personnel, good classroom and schoolwide management practices, positive after-school activities, cultural and community activities held at the school, or home and school partnership organizations (Henggeler, Mihalic, et al., 1998).

The role of parents is highlighted with continuous support for the parents to supervise the child, coordinate with the school, reduce their own antisocial behaviors, improve their parenting skills, and enhance their personal relationships. Interventions are action oriented and present focused. For example, an MST therapist might focus on interactions parents are having with schools to improve educational performance or on their efforts to disengage their child from a delinquent peer group.

The developmental needs of clients and their families form the basis of intervention planning. Both the age and social competence of young people and their parents affect the intervention. Daily effort and frequent reporting of results allows the providers to adjust procedures and keep the many systems involved with the client.

Schools that have been successful partners in multisystemic treatment approaches have altered their systems for responding to disturbed youth. Providers are added to their school-based mental health teams. Teachers and administrators remove opportunities for the client to interact with negative peers (e.g., through schedule changes, mentors, and after-school activities). All personnel make efforts to involve the parents. Teachers change instructional tasks and/or processes to improve academic achievement, and so on.

Although MST is an initially expensive approach that challenges usual treatment strategies, the ultimate cost of treatment is less expensive than that of out-of-home placements. These savings would not be realized by schools, of course; therefore state funding would have to be reorganized to reward school districts that commit to such intensive approaches to keep youngsters in schools.

Learning Communities

Baker (1998) argued persuasively that a young person's positive identification with the social context or community of the school is a buffer against violence. She cites the importance of a "goodness of fit" between the youngster and the various structures, expectations, and policies of a school. It is a challenge for school personnel to maintain the energy necessary to contribute to safe schools, even with the support of their leadership teams. Safe schools require coordinated action and mutual support among teachers and school leadership teams.

Effective school leadership is a powerful buffer against violence. A review of administrator practices related to increased school safety illustrated the importance of leadership behaviors (Goldstein & Conoley, 1997). For example, administrators of low-violence schools lead building- or systemwide efforts to reduce the number of irrelevant or oppressive rules that create explosive climates in schools. They organize groups of stakeholders into various school safety committees. Stakeholders are parents, young people, business leaders, health professionals, police, social service professionals, and members of the judiciary. These committees play a powerful role in promoting safety. High-impact and low-cost activities include:

1. Writing handbooks of student rights and responsibilities
2. Planning and practicing crisis situation responses
3. Involving public and private community organizations in the education of all children
4. Developing effective intelligence networks so that potentially problematic situations can be anticipated and defused

5. Continuously scanning the school environment for forces that may disrupt the focus on learning, harm the relationships that exist between the students and adults, or threaten the perception of shared control and investment in school and community well-being.

This agenda requires school principals and superintendents to be skilled negotiators and facilitators of community decision making and action. They must be experts at gathering needed resources to deal with complex problems. They also must, as pointed out by Hyman and Perone (1998), avoid victimizing young people in the name of discipline. These are jobs that require exceptional commitment, skill, and energy directed toward the success of every child, family, and teacher in a school system. The following case study may illustrate one school district's use of efforts led by administrators, teachers, and psychologists to increase school safety (Borgelt & Conoley, 1999):

Metropolitan growth and the location of some industry in the suburbs resulted in many new children entering a school district in a very short period of time. A number of disquieting issues became apparent. District personnel learned that approaches that had been successful in the past were failing the new population of students. One of the important problems the district identified was the negative publicity caused by a number of gang-related incidents and the dramatic rise in discipline referrals. At first the district personnel opted to put their energies into establishing alternative learning units (ALUs, i.e., self-contained classrooms) for acting out youngsters. An evaluation after three years indicated that these alternative classrooms were expensive, extremely disruptive, and had no effect on increasing the overall safety of the district. The level of disruption in the regular classrooms remained the same. Following the negative evaluation of the ALUs, the school psychologist, who was the pupil personnel director, suggested a systems approach to increasing school safety. Over the period of five years the use of survey research, identification of priorities, and an increase in human resources resulted in some dramatic improvement in school safety.

A survey of the types and frequency of violent events and discipline referrals that characterized each school building and the array of interventions that were used in response was completed. Feedback of results created a plan in which highly disturbing/dangerous situations were identified and analyzed for antecedent and consequent conditions. Surveys also indicated what the high frequency problems really were in contrast to the high visibility violence concerns. For example, most district discipline referrals were based on verbal insolence or disrespect, not physically intimidating situations.

The highest priority situations were identified. For example, in one high school fights were breaking out among students during class changes. The school implemented an array of strategies. Many of these did not require additional funding, but did require a change in the regular routines of the building:

1. Assigned more teachers to supervise the corridors
2. Involved the community police to establish a presence in the building
3. Adopted a block scheduling format that resulted in fewer transitions per day
4. Reconfigured freshman classrooms so that teachers moved among a cohort of students instead of students moving from class to class (Felner & Adan, 1988)
5. Replaced outdoor recreation with quiet reading times
6. Selected the most frequent instigators of hallway violence and required they stay in class until most of young people had left the hallways

7. Involved fathers and community fraternal organizations in visits to the school building so there were more adult men in halls as the students changed class
8. Remodeled some of the classroom walls into windows so that hallways were easily observed from the inside of classrooms

Several school safety committees assisted the schools in making the problem of violence a concern for all the stakeholders. Some of the approaches were aimed at empowering students to become responsible for safety. For example, one student group was trained as peer mediators. Another group of students was trained to implement a student court to hear cases of rule infractions (Noguera, 1995).

A group of administrators, teachers, and students analyzed school rules to insure that all were necessary and none needlessly oppressive. This team also wrote a "Handbook of Student Rights and Responsibilities."

A community group composed of parents, police, social service, business, and medical representatives was charged with developing strategies to increase safety for young people. They suggested the following: improved lighting around the buildings; more chaperones at social events; more extracurricular activities; extended school hours; implementation of skill enhancing programs for young people concerning drugs and alcohol; increased police presence before and after school in the vicinity of the school; and establishment of a dress code for the students. District and state grants were accessed to pay for the lighting and the increased staff to manage early morning and late afternoon activities. The counselors and school psychologists shared responsibility for the skills programs in alcohol and other drugs. The police provided additional neighborhood coverage and a school officer at no charge to the school.

The six-year evaluation of the plan indicated that despite a rapidly rising district census, there was no concomitant rise in violent incidents. In fact, the costs of repairing vandalism decreased by 50%; school fist fights decreased by 80% in the school that targeted that as its main priority; and overall district discipline referrals were reduced by 45%. The savings in real dollars and staff time were considered impressive.

Each strategy outlined above required many of the school professionals to adopt new roles. For example, school psychologists became very heavily involved in skills training and parent contacts. Many teachers were required to change their team memberships to allow for grade level teams in the junior and senior high schools instead of the more traditional content area teams. Coaches, physical education, and health educators created many new programs to involve large numbers of youngsters in extracurricular activities that emphasized safety and positive decision making.

The district continues to grow in diversity. The professionals now see the advantage of arranging for adult-focused systems interventions that do not rely solely on changing individual children (p. 720).

Instructional Systems for Safe Schools

Effective instruction is a key component of assisting children to form a meaningful identification with the school. When children are learning they participate in a wide range of activities and gain important skills that allow them to contribute to and benefit from a safe school environment.

It has been shown that cognitive skills help prevent violence. Children develop cognitive skills while studying English, social studies, math, and science. These skills help them reason their way through stressful and dangerous situations. Those with superior language skills and analytic abilities are less likely to use force to persuade and more likely to use creative and intellectual exercises to imagine and respect different points of view. They are also able to more clearly envision the consequences of certain actions and possess a greater repertoire of options to violent behavior. (Prothrow-Stith & Quaday, 1995, p. 23)

Academically successful students are rarely violent or drug abusing. The inverse relationship between school achievement and violence highlights an important aspect of the ecology of a safe school environment (Epstein, Kinder, & Bursuck, 1989; Scruggs & Mastropieri, 1986). Schools that are effective in keeping an academic focus for the great majority of the children have far fewer discipline problems than do schools that lack academic focus.

Most of the young people who are diagnosed as conduct disordered display externalizing behaviors (e.g., high levels of activity, cruelty, bullying) that adversely affect their educational performance as measured by standardized tests. Epstein et al. (1989) reviewed the literature on the academic status of violent adolescents. Reading difficulties and other learning disabilities are common among such children (Scruggs & Mastropieri, 1986). Children with behavioral deficits face a double jeopardy—they experience little success during their school days because of their deviance from both behavioral and learning norms.

Available research and reports of practice concerning aggressive young people focus on the process by which curriculum is delivered rather than the specific content of the curriculum. The academic interventions that appear to hold the greatest promise for increasing the academic performance of aggressive youth include tutoring, time-delay procedures, mnemonic instruction, and self-monitoring. The use of these instructional processes may be the basis for a classroom-based systemic intervention to increase safety by increasing academic achievement.

Tutoring

Tutoring is the delivery of instruction from one student to another. Tutoring has a number of benefits as an alternative instructional strategy to teacher-delivered instruction. A special case of tutoring is classwide peer tutoring (Greenwood, 1991). This approach may hold promise in helping generalization of positive effects of tutoring beyond the specific tutor/tutee interaction. Because it has been quite successful in reducing acting-out behaviors of students, it is described in some detail in the following paragraphs.

The work of Greenwood and his associates at the Juniper Gardens Children's Project, as well as others, has demonstrated the consistent effectiveness of classwide peer tutoring (CWPT). This classroom treatment has improved the academic performance of diverse groups of students across a variety of settings and academic subjects (e.g., Bell, Young, Blair, & Nelson, 1990; Greenwood, 1991; Greenwood, Delquadri, & Hall, 1989; Maheady, Harper, & Sacca, 1988). Classwide peer tutoring was developed as an instructional approach to increase students' active engagement in learning. The amount of time students are actively engaged in learning and their opportunity to respond has shown to be positively correlated with academic achievement. Low-socioeconomic-status children tend to experience an increased risk of low levels of academic engaged time and opportunities to respond, contributing to the problem of impaired achievement among this population. The CWPT system has been used primarily with low-income, inner-city elementary students in an attempt to improve their achievement (Greenwood, Terry, Utley, Montagna, & Walker, 1993). The process relies heavily on the principles of behavior analysis:

1. Positive reinforcement is given for correct responding and for following appropriate program procedures
2. Group contingencies are employed as teams of students compete against one another for points
3. Individual and team points and feedback regarding individual and team performances are posted publicly

Time-Delay Procedures

Although, historically, time delay was used primarily with students identified as developmentally disabled, more recently this method has been extended to students identified as behaviorally disordered and learning disabled.

"Time delay is a method for transferring stimulus control by changing the temporal interval between the natural cue and the teacher's prompt" (Cybriwsky & Schuster, 1990, p. 54). For example, "What is 9 × 5?" (natural cue) is immediately followed by the teacher-provided correct answer, "45" (controlling prompt). Gradually, a time delay between the question and teacher presentation of the answer is inserted, giving the student an opportunity to respond.

Cybriwsky and Schuster (1990) have found that the use of time-delay procedures was not only effective but required minimal teacher preparation and was surprisingly efficient. For example, only approximately one hour total time was needed to teach multiplication facts to a response rate of 100% correct. The use of constant time-delay procedures with students who typically experience academic failure may be especially beneficial. Students are likely to make fewer errors because they are repeatedly presented with the correct answer before they attempt to answer the question themselves. This potentially low rate of errors may help to provide the student with a positive academic experience, as well as promote more positive teacher-student interactions.

There are related techniques, such as teacher-presented sequential prompts (Schloss, Harriman, & Pfeifer, 1985), that also may be useful in increasing written products from disturbed students. The key element of this strategy is the support of the teacher through verbal cues to keep young people working so that they experience the success of completing work.

Mnemonic Instruction

Mastropieri, Emerick, and Scruggs (1988) investigated the effectiveness of teacher-developed and teacher-presented mnemonic instruction materials for students with serious emotional disorders. Students were taught through both mnemonic and traditional methods of instruction.

Students evidenced greater learning under the mnemonic condition, scoring on average 94.5% correct with mnemonic methods as compared with 58.8% correct under traditional instruction. Student reports indicated they preferred the mnemonic methods of learning to the traditional.

Self-Monitoring

Self-monitoring is another classroom technique that can improve the academic performance of students labeled as behaviorally disordered. McLaughlin, Burgess, and Sackville-West (1981) investigated two conditions of self-monitoring: self-recording and self-recording that included a check on the students' record by a match to the teacher's record. All students evidenced a higher percentage of correct answers during both treatment conditions as opposed to baseline average. Students who matched their records with the teacher reports evidenced the best improvement in their academic scores.

Summary

The incidence of violence and drug use in our schools demands a response. It is vital, however, to keep the problem of school violence in some perspective (Steinberg, 1996; Stout, 1995). The overwhelming majority of schoolchildren are not involved in or even affected by violence. Although there is cause for concern, there is no cause for panic among educators, families, or other community members. Drastic overreactions on the part of involved individuals that put narrow focus on schools and a punitive focus on children are unlikely to be effective (Noguera, 1995).

Serious attempts to increase school safety are likely best informed by attempts to build children's sense of community and psychological membership in schools (Baker, 1998). The survey reported by Furlong, Casas, Corral, Chung, and Bates (1997) supports this premise. Their findings linked the marginal, peripheral school identification of drug-abusing youngsters to increased levels of school violence. Children need safe places if they are to learn to be peaceful and contributing members of a society. Actual school/family/community partnerships must be constructed. These partnerships may be as varied as the individuals who compose them, but a shift toward shared and coordinated responsibility for child welfare is long overdue.

REFERENCES

Baker, J. A. (1998). Are we missing the forest for the trees? Considering the social context of school violence. *Journal of School Psychology, 36*, 29–44.

Baker, S. B., Swisher, J. D., Nadenichek, P. E., & Popowicz, C. L. (1984). Measured effects of primary prevention strategies. *Personnel and Guidance Journal, 63*, 459–463.

Bank, L., Marlow, J. H., Reid, J. B., Patterson, G. R., & Weinrott, J. L. (1991). A comparative evaluation of parent-training interventions for families of chronic delinquents. *Journal of Abnormal Child Psychology, 19*, 15–34.

Bell, K., Young, K. R., Blair, M., & Nelson, R. (1990). Facilitating mainstreaming of students with behavioral disorders using classwide peer tutoring. *School Psychology Review, 19*, 564–573.

Bierman, K. L., & Smoot, D. L. (1991). Linking family characteristics with poor peer relations: The mediating role of conduct problems. *Journal of Abnormal Child Psychology, 19*(3), 341–356.

Bierman, K. L., Coie, J. D., Dodge, K. A., Greenberg, M. T., Lochman, J. E., & McMahon, R. J. (1992). A developmental and clinical model for the prevention of conduct disorder: The FAST Track Program. *Development and Psychopathology, 4,* 509–527.

Bierman, K. L., Smoot, D. L., & Aumiller, K. (1993). Characteristics of aggressive-rejected, aggressive (nonrejected), and rejected (nonaggressive) boys. *Child Development, 64*(1), 139–151.

Borduin, C. M., Mann, B. J., Cone, L. T., Henggeler, S. W., Fucci, B. R., Blaske, D. M., & Williams, R. A. (1995). Multisystemic treatment of serious juvenile offenders: Long-term prevention of criminality and violence. *Journal of Consulting and Clinical Psychology, 63,* 569–578.

Borgelt, C., & Conoley, J. C. (1999). Psychology in the schools: Systems intervention cases. In T. Gutkin & C. R. Reynolds (Eds.), *The handbook of school psychology* (3rd ed., pp. 1056–1076). New York: Wiley.

Capaldi, D. M., & Patterson, G. R. (1987). An approach to the problem of recruitment and retention rates for longitudinal research. *Behavioral Assessment, 9,* 489–504.

Coie, J. D., Dodge, K. A., Terry, R., & Wright, V. (1991). The role of aggression in peer relations: An analysis of aggression episodes in boys' play groups. *Child Development, 62,* 812–827.

Coie, J. D., & Jacobs, M. (1993). The role of social context in the prevention of conduct disorder. *Development and Psychopathology, 5,* 263–275.

Coie, J. D., Lochman, J. E., Terry, R., & Hyman, C. (1992). Predicting early adolescent disorder from childhood aggression and peer rejection. *Journal of Consulting and Clinical Psychology, 60,* 783–793.

Coie, J. D., Watt, N. F., West, S. G.,

Hawkins, J. D., Asarnow, J. R., Markman, H. J., Ramey, S. L., & Shure, M. B. (1993). The science of prevention: A conceptual framework and some directions for a national research program. *American Psychologist, 48,* 1013–1023.

Cybriwsky, C., & Schuster, J. W. (1990). Using constant time delay procedures to teach multiplication facts. *Remedial and Special Education, 11,* 54–59.

Dangel, R. F., & Polster, R. A. (1984). *Parent training: Foundations of research and practice.* New York: Guilford Press.

Edleson, J. L., & Peled, E. (1994). Community responses to children of battered women. *Child, Youth, and Family Services Quarterly, 17,* 4–6.

Elam, S., & Rose, L. (1995). The 27th annual Phi Delta Kappan poll of the public's attitudes toward the public schools. *Phi Delta Kappan, 77,* 41–59.

Epstein, M. H., Kinder, D., & Bursuck, B. (1989). The academic status of adolescents with behavioral disorders. *Behavioral Disorders, 14,* 157–165.

Eron, L. D., Gentry, J. H., & Schlegel, P. (1994). *Reason to hope: A psychosocial perspective on violence and youth.* Washington, DC: American Psychological Association.

Felner, R. D., & Adan, A. M. (1988). The school transitional environment project: An ecological intervention and evaluation. In R. H. Price, E. L. Cowen, R. P. Lorion, & J. Ramos-McKay (Eds.), *14 ounces of prevention: A casebook for practitioners* (pp. 111–122). Washington, DC: American Psychological Association.

Fingerhut, L. A., & Kleinman, J. C. (1990). International and interstate comparisons of homicide among young males. *Journal of the American Medical Association, 27,* 3292–3295.

Furlong, M. J., Casas, J. M., Corral, C., Chung, A., & Bates, M. (1997). Drugs and school violence. *Education and Treatment of Children, 20,* 263–280.

Furlong, M. J., & Morrison, G. M. (1994). School violence and safety in perspective. *School Psychology Review, 23,* 139–150.

Gentry, J., & Eron, L. D. (1993). American Psychological Association Commission on Violence and Youth. *American Psychologist, 48*(2), 89.

Goldstein, A. P. (1999). *The Prepare curriculum: Teaching prosocial competencies.* Champaign, IL: Research Press.

Goldstein, A. P., & Conoley, J. C. (Eds.) (1997). *Handbook of interventions for school violence.* New York: Guilford Press.

Goldstein, A. P., & Glick, B. (1994). Aggression replacement training: Curriculum and evaluation. *Simulation and Gaming, 25,* 9–27.

Gorski, J., & Pilotto, L. A. (1993). Interpersonal violence among youth: A challenge for school personnel. *Educational Psychology Review, 5,* 35–61.

Greenwood, C. R. (1991). Classwide peer tutoring: Longitudinal effects on the reading, language, and mathematics achievement of at-risk students. *Reading, Writing, and Learning Disabilities, 7,* 105–123.

Greenwood, C. R., Delquadri, J. C., & Hall, R. V. (1989). Longitudinal effects of classwide peer tutoring. *Journal of Educational Psychology, 81,* 371–383.

Greenwood, C. R., Terry, B., Utley, C. A., Montagna, D., & Walker, D. (1993). Achievement, placement, and services: Middle school benefits of classwide peer tutoring used at the elementary level. *School Psychology Review, 22,* 497–516.

Hammond, R. (1991). *Dealing with anger: Givin' it. Takin' it. Workin' it out.* Champaign, IL: Research Press.

Henggeler, S. W., Melton, G. B., & Smith, L. A. (1992). Family preservation using multisystemic therapy: An effective alternative to incarcerating serious juvenile offenders. *Journal of Consulting and Clinical Psychology, 10,* 953–961.

Henggeler, S. W., Melton, G. B., Smith, L. A., Schoenwald, S. K., & Hanley, J. H. (1993). Family preservation using multisystemic treatment: Long-term followup to a clinical trial with serious juvenile offenders. *Journal of Child and Family Studies, 2,* 283–293.

Henggeler, S. W., Mihalic, S. F., Rone, L., Thomas, C., & Timmons-Mitchell, J. (1998). *Blueprints for violence prevention: Multisystemic therapy.* Boulder: University of Colorado at Boulder, Center for the Study and Prevention of Violence, Blueprints Publications.

Henggeler, S. W., Schoenwald, S. K., Borduin, C. M., Rowland, M. D., & Cunningham, P. B. (1998). *Multisystemic treatment of antisocial behavior in children and adolescents.* New York: Guilford Press.

Hyman, I. A., & Perone, D. C. (1998). The other side of school violence: Educator policies and practices that may contribute to student misbehavior. *Journal of School Psychology, 36,* 7–27.

Kazdin, A. E. (1993). Treatment of conduct disorder: Progress and directions in psychotherapy research. *Development and Psychopathology, 5,* 277–310.

Lightfoot, S. L. (1978). *World apart.* New York: Basic Books.

Lochman, J. E., Coie, J. D., Underwood, M. K., & Terry, R. (1993). Effectiveness of a social relations intervention program for aggressive and nonaggressive, rejected children. *Journal of Consulting and Clinical Psychology, 61,* 1053–1059.

Lyons-Ruth, K., Alpern, L., & Repacholi, B. (1993). Disorganized infant attachment classification and maternal psychosocial problems as predictors of hostile-aggressive behavior in preschool children. *Child Development, 64,* 572–585.

Maheady, L., Harper, G. F., & Sacca, K. (1988). A classwide peer tutoring system in a secondary resource room program for the mildly handicapped. *Journal of Research and Development in Education, 21,* 76–83.

Mastropieri, M. A., Emerick, K., & Scruggs, T. E. (1988). Mnemonic instruction of science concepts. *Behavioral Disorders, 14,* 48–56.

McLaughlin, T. F., Burgess, N., & Sackville-West, L. (1981). Effects of self-recording and self-recording plus matching on academic performance. *Child Behavior Therapy, 3*(2/3), 17–27.

National Committee to Prevent Child Abuse (1994). *Current trends in child abuse reporting and fatalities.* Chicago, IL: Author.

Noguera, P. A. (1995). Preventing and producing violence: A critical analysis of responses to school violence. *Harvard Educational Review, 65,* 189–212.

Oestmann, J., & Walker, M. B. (1997). Interventions for aggressive students in a public-school-based day treatment program. In A. P. Goldstein & J. C. Conoley (Eds.), *School violence intervention: A practical handbook* (pp. 160–188). New York: Guilford Press.

Patterson, G. R. (1982). *Coercive family process.* Eugene, OR: Castalia.

Patterson, G. R., DeBaryshe, B., & Ramsey, E. (1989). A developmental perspective on antisocial behavior. *American Psychologist, 44,* 329–335.

Patterson, G. R., Reid, J. B., & Dishion, T. J. (1992). *Antisocial boys.* Eugene, OR: Castalia.

Pettit, G. S., Dodge, K. A., Bakshi, A., & Coie, J. D. (1990). The emergence of social dominance in young boys' play groups: Developmental differences and behavioral correlates. *Developmental Psychology, 26,* 1017–1026.

Pope, A. W., Bierman, K. L., & Mumma, G. H. (1989). Relations between hyperactive and aggressive behavior and peer relations at three elementary grade levels. *Journal of Abnormal Child Psychology, 17,* 253–268.

Pope, A. W., Bierman, K. L., & Mumma, G. H. (1991). Aggression, hyperactivity, and inattention-immaturity: Behavior dimensions associated with peer rejection in elementary school boys. *Developmental Psychology, 27,* 663–672.

Prothrow-Stith, D., & Quaday, S. (1995). *Hidden casualties: The relationship between violence and learning.* Washington, DC: National Consortium for African American Children, Inc., and the National Health and Education Consortium.

Reid, J. B. (1993). Prevention of conduct disorder before and after school entry: Relating interventions to developmental findings. *Development and Psychopathology, 5,* 243–262.

Schloss, P. J., Harriman, N. E., & Pfeifer, K. (1985). Application of a sequential prompt reduction technique to the independent composition performance of behaviorally disordered youth. *Behavioral Disorders, 11,* 17–23.

Schweinhart, L. J., Barnes, H. V., Weikart, D. P., Barnett, W. S., & Epstein, A. S. (1993). *Significant benefits: The High/Scope Perry Preschool study through age 27* (High/Scope Educational Research Foundation Monograph No. 10). Ypsilanti, MI: High/Scope Press.

Schweinhart, L. J., & Weikart, D. P. (1993). Success by empowerment: The High/Scope Perry Preschool Study through age 27. *Young Child, 48,* 54–58.

Scruggs, T. E., & Mastropieri, M. A. (1986). Academic characteristics of behaviorally disordered and learning disabled students. *Behavioral Disorders, 12,* 184–190.

Sheley, J., McGee, Z., & Wright, J. (1992). Gun-related violence in and around inner-city schools. *American Journal of Diseases of Childhood, 146,* 677–682.

Smith, D. (1990). *Caught in the crossfire: A report on gun violence in our nation's schools.* Washington, DC: Center to Prevent Handgun Violence.

Steinberg, J. (1996, September 19). Data show school crime is dropping. *The New York Times,* p. B7.

Stout, D. (1995, May 19). Violence in schools said to rise. *The New York Times,* p. B3.

Underwood, M. K., Coie, J. D., & Herbsman, C. R. (1992). Display rules for anger and aggression in school-age children. *Child Development, 63,* 366–381.

United States Department of Justice. (1996). *FBI uniform crime reports: Crime in the United States.* Washington, DC: Author.

Washington State Institute for Public Policy. (1998). *Watching the bottom line: Cost-effective intervention for reducing crime in Washington.* Olympia, WA: Evergreen State College.

Werth, E. B. (1995). Family assessment in behavioral parent training for antisocial behavior. In J. C. Conoley & E. B. Werth (Eds.), *Family assessment* (pp. 101–130). Lincoln, NE: Buros Institute of Mental Measurements.

Zigler, E., Taussig, C., & Black, K. (1992). Early childhood intervention: A promising preventative for juvenile delinquency. *American Psychologist, 47,* 997–1006.

22

SANDRA L. CHRISTENSON
YVONNE GODBER

Enhancing Constructive Family-School Connections

An essential prerequisite for delivering psychological services for children and youth is an understanding of the power of the family-school relationship for child and adolescent outcomes. Whether family-school relationships are described as parent involvement, family-school partnerships, family support, or family-centered practices, the goals are to enhance success for students and to improve learning opportunities and outcomes for children and youth, including those that are academic, social, emotional, and behavioral in nature. Family-school interventions address both child-specific and system-level concerns and are primarily viewed as a preventive activity. However, family and school are two systems, albeit essential for children's development, that are used to operating autonomously. Family-school relationships are not synonymous with parent-teacher relationships. According to the Family Resource Coalition (1993), comprehensive programs consist of school readiness, parent involvement that empowers parents to take a role in education across grades K–12, and school-linked services designed to improve achievement by ensuring that the health and social needs of children are met. Smrekar (1994) noted that policymakers and educators have mostly ignored the nature of interactions between families and schools, concluding that this relationship was "the missing link in school-linked social service programs" (p. 422).

Despite many investigations of the impact of family-school relationships on children's learning in the past two decades, it is still considered an unresolved relationship (Christenson, 2000). However, regardless of the model selected (e.g., Comer, Haynes, Joyner, & Ben-Avie, 1996; Epstein, 1995a; Swap, 1993), successful programs subscribe to new principles: (1) no-fault interactions in which blame is not attributed to family or school because there is not a single cause for the presenting concern, (2) a nondeficit approach in which strengths of individuals are emphasized, (3) the importance of empowerment, by which families are actively involved in decision making and choices for their personal lives, and (4) an ecological approach in which there is recognition of the reciprocal influence between family and school contexts (Liontos, 1992).

Effective family-school relationships are about connections — specifically, connecting the two socializing forces in children's lives to enhance their academic, social, behavioral, and emotional development and consequently their educational experiences, learning, and progress in school. The focus is on creating a collaborative ethic, which refers to a fundamental way for families and schools to work together in which (1) the relationship or interface between families and schools is emphasized over the specific role that either should or could assume, and (2) problem solving provides a systematic, structured way of creating mutual support for interventions and activities that improve the educational experience for students, engage students as learners, or orient them to a more positive trajectory for development.

Findings from the Metropolitan Life Survey (1998), which surveyed over 1300 teachers and compared teacher opinions about family-school relationships with those from a decade ago, suggest that there are more opportunities today for teachers and parents to work together to improve the quality of education provided in public schools. Specifically, teachers are more willing to want parents to actively participate in school management and more likely to value parental involvement and support. They believe parents are more responsive when their children call on them for help. Most teachers (83%) would like to see the level of parent involvement increase. Inner-city teachers remain the most critical of the level of parental support shown for their schools; 95% of teachers would like parents to become more involved. Ratings of parent-teacher relations are lowest for those working in inner-city schools; 55% of teachers described the relationship as fair or poor. Although 79% of urban teachers believe schools are doing a good job of encouraging parent involvement in education, 61% believe that parents take too little interest in their child's education. When educators feel that they are reaching out to parents but that parents, in turn, are failing to support children's learning, it is easy to envision how a cycle of blame begins to emerge. Such statistics reveal an urgency in improving on current parent-teacher relationships.

In this chapter, we provide a review of the most seminal characteristics of constructive family-school relationships. We have been selective, choosing those findings and constructs that relate to roles for psychologists, whether they are based in school, clinics, or community sites. We describe 6 Cs to enhance the relationship, or what Fantuzzo and Mohr (in press) refer to as the "connects" between family and school. Next, we discuss four guidelines for enhancing family-school connections. Finally, we provide concluding remarks about psychologists' contributions to enhancing these connections.

The "Cs" of Constructive Connections

Context-Specific Nature of Relationships

Context is important in forming constructive relationships between families and schools. What works in one school (e.g., New York City) will not work in another (e.g., Albuquerque). What works for one family-school relationship will not work for another. This site-specific aspect to the development of family-school relationships was recognized by Kagan (1984), who, based on a comprehensive review of the parent involvement literature, concluded there was no one prescription. Rather, parents and educators, as cofacilitators of children's development, must ask: What forms of parent participation are desirable and feasible? and What strategies can be employed to achieve them? Family-school teams for establishing policies and practices that address concerns and needs of both family and school systems with respect to educating students are a defining feature of many models (Comer et al., 1996; Davies, 1991; Epstein, 1995a). Based on a needs assessment that represents the "voices of all," a menu of practices is tailored for the school. Clearly, two-way communication — dialogue, not monologue — is evident in the functioning of the family-school team. This team, among other things, is a vehicle for establishing a common language, mapping existing school- and community-based resources, and identifying student, family, and staff needs (Fetro, 1998).

Complex Relationships

Family-school relationships are complex because they represent the interface of two systems relevant for children's development. Pianta and Walsh's (1996) perspective that the child/family system is in transaction with the school system is consistent with Coleman's (1987) theory about home and school influences on the socialization of children. According to Coleman, home inputs include messages about effort, attitudes about the value of learning, and a sense of self as a learner. School inputs present the child with new experiences, specifically demands, opportunities and rewards. According to Coleman, the extent to which children experience optimal socialization experiences depends on the interaction of resources in home and school contexts. Families provide the "building blocks" that make learning possible and the social capital (i.e., amount of time for adult-child interaction concerning personal and academic matters) needed by schools to enhance learner outcomes. Constructive family-school relationships establish a partnership and shared meaning about children (Pianta & Walsh, 1996). A partnership is a common effort toward a shared goal, not delegating services to families and children that the school recommends (Seeley, 1985), services that may be perceived by the family as unimportant or irrelevant.

Centrality to Children's Development

The centrality of family-school relationships for intervening to enhance children's development and learning can no longer be ignored. Epstein (1995a) asserted, "If educators view children simply as students, they are likely to see the family as separate from school. That is, the family is expected to do its job and leave the education of children to the schools. If educators view children as children, they are likely to see both the family and community as partners with the school in children's education and development" (p. 701). Furthermore, teachers and schools alone are not capable of making students reach their full potential. This is not an indictment of them; rather, it is a fact of child and adolescent development (Oka-gaki & Sternberg, 1991).

Epstein's (1995a) six types of activities in a comprehensive framework for family-school partnerships (parenting, communicating, volunteering, home learning, shared decision making and governance, and community support) illustrate how parents can be involved in education without coming to school. In fact, she demon-strated that different types of activities result in different benefits for students, parents, and teachers. Although not all activities are associated with better academic outcomes, consulting with parents about parenting and use of home learning activities has been impressive in this regard. Rich (1987) referred to these as the "meat and potatoes" of parent involvement.

There is emerging evidence that interventions are more successful when syner-gistic in nature. For example, it has been shown that family-school relationships are essential to the programming for children with ADHD (August, Anderson, & Bloomquist, 1992), conduct disorders (Reid & Patterson, 1996; Webster-Stratton, 1993), social skills deficits (Sheridan, Kratochwill, & Elliott, 1990) and homework completion difficulties (Jayanthi, Sawyer, Nelson, Bursuck, & Epstein, 1995), as well as significant improvement in academic achievement (Hansen, 1986; Heller & Fantuzzo, 1993). In their School Development Program, Comer and his col-leagues (1996) established the goal of positive family-school-community relation-ships as the fostering of balanced development for children and youth across six developmental pathways: psychological, physical, language, ethical, cognitive, and social. Given this orientation, it should be clear that the interface of systems provides many opportunities to influence positively the life paths of students.

Consistency across Socializing Systems

The influence of family on children's development and learning is well researched and recognized (Hess & Holloway, 1984; Rutter, 1985; Wahlberg, 1984). In fact, it is not uncommon to read statements that the effect of the family is undisputed and family cannot be eliminated from planning for school reforms (Lewis & Hender-son, 1997). A number of studies have shown that family involvement in children's education promotes a variety of desirable outcomes for children, including higher academic achievement rates (Hickman, Greenwood, & Miller, 1995; Howe, Cham-bers, & Abrami, 1998), better attendance and more positive attitudes toward school (Henderson & Berla, 1994), and lower dropout rates (Rumberger, 1995). A recent review of family, school, and community correlates of positive indicators of stu-dents' school performance revealed six factors in home and school contexts that facilitate student success in school (Christenson & Christenson, 1998). There is evidence that students achieve more when both families and schools (represented primarily by teachers) set realistic expectations, provide a structure and routine for learning, enhance students' learning opportunities, support students' learning, establish positive relationships, and model learning.

Students benefit when families and schools provide students with consistent messages about schooling. For example, Phelan, Yu, and Davidson (1994) found that high school students, even those who describe their home, peer, and school contexts as congruent with respect to academic expectations, report psychosocial pressure and stress. However, those who reported their peer, school, and family worlds to be different experienced greater adversity in navigating across these borders of diverse messages. Students in this group reported a low probability of graduating from high school and perceived their personal futures as bleak. Also, Mordkowitz and Ginsburg (1987) studied poor Asian immigrant families who did not provide the same types of support typical of middle-class American families but whose children were successful in school. Their findings suggest that the convergence of family and school values about learning and children's performance and behavior is more important than the extent of family resources available or the specific activities families engage in to support children's learning. In fact, Mitrsomwang and Hawley (1993) found that the presence of three factors in homes was strongly associated with student achievement: strong, consistent values about the importance of education; willingness to help children and to intervene at school; and ability to become involved. The consistency in correlations across several studies of families with varying income and ethnic backgrounds is noteworthy.

Both home and school play a role. According to Bronfenbrenner (1991), families provide the informal education that is a powerful prerequisite to the formal education provided by schools. With respect to discussions of "at-risk" students, we concur with Pianta and Walsh (1996), who contend that lack of continuity between home and school is a risk factor which is often unaccounted for. The more consistency and the clearer the connections between learning at home and learning at school, the more likely positive educational outcomes will be attained (Christenson & Christenson, 1998). Sadly, the social and physical distance between teachers and parents, particularly in urban settings, is often great, thereby weakening any potential benefits of collaborative contact.

Communication as the Foundational Element

Two-way communication is necessary to coconstruct the "bigger" picture of the child's life. Too often, families and school personnel see the child in their respective environments and jump to conclusions about the child's behavior in the other environment. Although the situation specificity of child behavior is well documented, communication practices and time constraints reduce opportunity for dialogue and problem solving between families and schools (Christenson & Hirsch, 1998).

Communication is considered a key process that helps districts and schools strengthen support and plans for coordinated school health programs (Fetro, 1998). Other process variables are cooperation, coordination, and collaboration. An examination of the four processes suggests levels of family-school interaction that increase in intensity. Communication refers to sharing ideas among interested parties; cooperation refers to informal relationships among individuals who have related goals; coordination refers to regular contact among individuals with related goals for sharing resources, plans and needs; and collaboration refers to formal relationships among individuals who are committed to a common vision, mission, and goals. Regardless of the process used, professionals are challenged to see parents as active peers — not passive clients of services.

Collaborative Relationships

Described by Allport more than 30 years ago, three criteria for successful collaboration are remarkably relevant as families and schools strive to connect for the benefit of students. According to Allport (1954), there need to be: (1) equal status between participants (e.g., parents, teachers, students, psychologists, principals), (2) a common goal, and (3) adequate leadership and support (e.g., school district, state, federal levels). The elements of collaboration are not unrecognized by educators. Key elements of collaboration identified by teachers and parents of children with emotional problems were: mutual respect for skills and knowledge, honest and clear communication, open and two-way sharing of information, mutually agreed-upon goals, and shared planning and decision making (Vosler-Hunter, 1989). Similarly, Dunst, Johanson, Rounds, Trivette, and Hamby (1992) identified trust, open communication, mutual respect, active listening, and honesty as essential characteristics of the parent-professional relationship. Although it is relatively easy to list the elements of collaboration, it is more difficult to translate them to practice. In part this is due to time constraints. To date, the social and physical distance between home and school is one aspect of time; another part is limited time for dialogue and interaction. Complicating this picture is that we say we are "child-centered" but respond with an "institutional" perspective.

Guidelines for Constructive Connections

Too many families remain disconnected from the schooling process. Epstein (1995b) characterized a common scenario when she stated, "Most teachers do not know most parents' goals for their children, nor do they understand the information parents would like to have to be more effective at home. Most parents do not know what most teachers are trying to do each year in school nor about school improvement activities" (p. 9). Furthermore, many teachers do not understand the communities in which their students live (Morris & Taylor, 1998). Family-school contact is often restricted to 20-minute parent-teacher conferences or is made only when problems need to be addressed. Ironically, schools often blame parents for student failure when in fact the fault actually lies with the interface between home and school (Weiss & Edwards, 1992). Partnerships between families and schools cannot thrive under these conditions.

Recent legislative policies directly encourage, and even mandate, home-school collaboration and partnerships (Epstein, 1995b; National Educational Goals Report, 1998; Trusty, 1998). Amid such mandates, many schools face the challenge of defining and implementing effective family involvement strategies. Fruchter, Gullotta, and White (1992) concluded that effective programs differ in specific activities, but share four tenets: (1) parents are children's first teachers and have a lifelong influence on their values, attitudes, and aspirations; (2) children's educational success requires congruence between what is taught at school and values practiced at home; (3) most parents care deeply about their children's education and can provide substantial support if given specific opportunities and knowledge; and (4) schools must take the lead in eliminating or at least reducing traditional barriers to parent involvement. According to Hoover-Dempsey and Sandler (1997), how and when parents become involved with their children's school depends on three factors: namely, the degrees to which parents believe they should play a certain role, parental self-efficacy is enhanced with personal efforts, and opportunities that invite parents to participate are actively created.

Empowering families to participate in their children's education is an intentional, ongoing process centered in the local community (Delgado-Gaitan, 1991). It involves mutual respect, critical reflection, caring, and group participation, through which people lacking an equal share of valued resources gain greater access to and control over resources. Critical elements include inclusion and a sense of power in decision making. Families must feel they are integral members of the school. The skills and expertise of families are currently untapped in the prescribed roles typically established for parents in schools (i.e., volunteer, fundraiser, homework helper). Policies and practices need to reflect a positive view of families and a clear desire for family involvement.

Recommended strategies to enhance relationships between families, school personnel, and representatives from various agencies exist. For example, Ooms and Hara (1991) reported these partnership principles:

- Every aspect of the school building and general climate is open, helpful, and friendly to parents
- Communications with parents—whether about school policies and programs or about their own children—are frequent, clear, and two-way
- Parents are treated by teachers as collaborators in the educational process
- Parents' own knowledge, expertise, and resources are valued as essential to their children's success in school
- The school recognizes its responsibility to forge a partnership with all families in the schools, not simply those most easily available
- The school principal and other administrators actively express in words and deeds the philosophy of partnership with all families
- The school encourages volunteer support and help from all parents by providing a wide variety of volunteer options, including those that can be done from home and during nonwork hours
- The school provides opportunities for parents to meet their needs for information, advice, and peer support
- Parents' views and expertise are sought in developing policies and solving schoolwide problems; in some schools parents are given important decision-making responsibilities at a policy level
- Schools recognize that they can best help parents provide a home environment conducive to children's learning if they facilitate their access to basic and supportive services.

There are, however, no "models" for building parent and community support for school reforms because each school's situation is unique. "There is a common, immediate need, however, to mobilize parents and communities, hold everyone accountable for higher student learning and build the capacity of people to carry out critical reforms" (Lewis & Henderson, 1997, p. xi). Guidelines for creating constructive connections between families and schools include making relationships a priority, enhancing two-way communication, interacting in a responsive and personalized way, and using thorough and persistent efforts to engage families.

Make Relationships a Priority

Roles and responsibilities between professionals and members of the community have become outdated and stagnant. Yet Epstein and Lee (1995) found that families were generally satisfied with the ability of schools to supervise and educate their children. At the same time, about 17% of a national sample of 217 parents of school-aged children reported feeling unwelcome at school and described their contacts with school personnel as stressful and uncomfortable (Christenson, Hurley, Sheridan, & Fenstermacher, 1997). Over one third of the parents reported infrequent contacts, and 11% described contacts as leading to mistrust. Also, a disconcerting finding from the National Longitudinal Study of 1988 (Ingels et al., 1990) revealed that two thirds of families are disconnected from schools, lack specific information on their child's academic progress, and are unaware of how to support education at home. Nonetheless, educators often cling to their professional roles, complaining that they are not able to effectively execute the positions for which they have been trained. As a result, staff feel overwhelmed and frustrated, communities and community agencies are forced to deal with problems that have escalated undetected to dangerous levels, and families remain increasingly isolated and unsupported. The vicious cycle of blame and shame among families, communities, schools, and service providers has a tendency to spin faster and faster (Adelman & Taylor, 1998).

WELCOMING ENVIRONMENT   The importance of a welcoming climate for family participation has been articulately described (Batey, 1996), and the degree to which parents feel unwelcome or uncomfortable at school has been reported as a barrier to family involvement (Liontos, 1992). Although it is not always possible for school personnel to interact with a particular family before a crisis that demands attention and intervention occurs, the degree to which the school is welcoming to all families is a variable under the control of educators. Creating constructive connections with families requires a commitment at the building level to reach out to all families. Several researchers elucidated the effects of noncollaborative school climates on family-school relationships. For example, Swap's (1987) research suggested that "if the culture of the school devalues parent involvement . . . , it may be difficult for a teacher to take the time to work closely with the parents" (p. 16). Also, Dauber and Epstein (1993) concluded that teachers of urban students in grades K–8 who believe they share similar beliefs with parents about involvement make more contacts with parents who are perceived as hard to reach, find more ways to involve families, and are less prone to think that disadvantaged characteristics of the student population are a deterrent to learning. They also found that most school programs and practices do not support teachers' beliefs in the importance of family-school partnerships for children's learning. Levels of parent involvement were reduced when there were discrepancies between teachers and principals or colleagues about the importance of family involvement in education.

Edwards (1992) recommended these actions for school personnel to adopt when reaching out to uninvolved families: (1) explore what families want schools to accomplish, (2) devise practical and meaningful opportunities for involvement, (3) reach out to parents with warmth and sensitivity, (4) develop an ongoing program in which parents and staff are both teachers and learners, and (5) acknowledge that sharing power with parents is not abdication of one's professional leadership role. Building relationships with families requires professionals and systems to move from the parent-professional hierarchy Seeley (1985) referred to as "social service imperialism." To do this, professionals are urged to follow Swick and McKnight's (1989) suggestion to be approachable, sensitive, flexible, and dependable when working with families.

Tomlinson's (1996) list of strategies to help parents feel welcome as partners in their children's education serves as an excellent benchmark for school personnel to evaluate school practices. The recommended strategies are: communicate frequently with parents, engage in two-way communication with parents, provide a variety of activities for parents, meet with parents on their own turf, overcome barriers to parent participation, set up a parent or family resource center, establish the position of family or parent involvement coordinator, support staff in efforts to involve parents, and develop a sense of community. The dominant theme is inclusion, and it is well illustrated by the following statement:

> Perhaps more important to the creation of a welcoming atmosphere is to foster a sense of teamwork and community at your school. Find ways to allow families, staff, and students to get to know one another. Always show respect for parents' thoughts and concerns and expect respect in return. Emphasize your shared goal of providing children with a superior education. Don't limit parent participation to superficial activities. Help them with the complex issues they face in raising their children, and invite them to take part in the difficult decisions involved in governing your school. (Tomlinson, 1996, p. 8)

Welcoming school climates rectify any misconceptions of families and students held by school personnel. For example, family status variables, such as ethnicity or income level, are not acceptable explanations for students' achievement levels (Wahlberg, 1984). Also, Dauber and Epstein (1993) found that school programs and teacher practices that encourage and guide parent involvement were the strongest and most consistent predictors of parent involvement. Educators' practices were more important in determining levels of involvement than were parents' educational level, family size, marital status, or student grade level. Furthermore, parents' attitudes about the quality of their child's school were strongly correlated with the success of school practices to involve parents.

TRUST-BUILDING   Comer and his colleagues (1996) cautioned:

> Basic to any attempt to reach and involve parents—especially the least affluent and educated—is a climate of trust and openness to ideas. Parents sometimes avoid schools because they feel inadequate, unwelcome, threatened, or insecure due to their own past educational experiences and their children's present difficulties. We seize every opportunity to break down the barriers of mistrust by reaching out to parents in their communities through home visits, regular and positive telephone calls and memos, and networking through institutions such as churches. Little, if any, learning occurs for students when there is a climate of mistrust between the key socializing agents. (p. 50)

Furthermore, they believe that strong relationships are a prerequisite for students' growth and learning; parents and professionals, according to Comer, need to like each other. To find out if they like and trust each other enough to value joint collaboration, they must engage in ongoing, positive, and individualized interactions, what Weiss and Edwards (1992) referred to as climate-building activities. In fostering such opportunities to enhance the effectiveness of relationships, Christenson (1995) reminds us that "home-school collaboration is an attitude, not simply an activity" (p. 253).

Typically, parents are used to being told by professionals what they need to do. Unfortunately, they are also used to being blamed for their child's failure when in fact the fault frequently lies with the service system. Case overload, working with families in isolation, and lack of a coordinated service effort contribute greatly to this tendency of professionals to blame parents. Although we believe most professionals strive to act in the best interest of children and families, it is apparent that the manner in which institutions are structured and services are delivered contributes to mistrust and misunderstanding between even the most well-intentioned individuals. This situation affords neither families nor professionals opportunities to nurture relationships, what Davies (1991) called the "potential lubrication" (p. 380).

Examination of trust in the family-school relationship raises many questions about whether it is reasonable to expect meaningful family-school collaboration without adequate trust-building opportunities (Adams & Christenson, 1998). They found that parents whose children were in middle school in an urban education setting trusted teachers more than teachers trusted parents and that parent trust for teachers did not differ as a function of social strata, educational level, or ethnicity. High-trust parents were more involved in education than moderate- or low-trust parents. Our data on trust suggest that the elements of collaboration may be difficult, if not impossible, to implement, particularly if the partners are unknown to each other or when a child is demonstrating any deviance from the norm for expected school behavior. A relationship between family and school helps deter tense, conflictual interactions and increases joint problem solving when serious intervention, such as significant placement decisions for students or handling crises, is needed.

In sum, obstacles to effective relationships identified by the U.S. Department of Education include restricted opportunities for interaction, limited skills and knowledge about how to collaborate, and psychological and cultural barriers (Moles, 1993). To effectively and efficiently address the hopes, needs, and concerns of families, it is recommended that service providers evaluate how their individual practices build or block their ability to establish productive relationships with families (Cochran & Dean, 1991). However, just as families do not exist in a vacuum, professionals are constrained by institutional practices. Supportive leadership entails allocating both the necessary time and resources toward the development of opportunities for interactions to occur in which professionals and families come together as equals. School personnel must be sensitive to needs facing families and communities and receive ongoing professional training on collaborating with families. The concept of coordinating councils proposed by Adelman and Taylor (1998) facilitates regular opportunities for professionals to share information and collaboratively strategize how services can be powerfully individualized and coordinated. Families must be welcomed to the table as equals and know that they help determine who and which services could best support their child or family at this point in time. Also, we need to remember that creating trust with families takes time (Margolis & Brannigan, 1986).

Enhance Two-Way Communication

At the beginning of the new millennium, a common scenario is arguably the current state of affairs for family-school interactions. Home-school communication is infrequent, inconsistent, sparked by a problem, and initiated mostly by school personnel. When learning at home and learning at school are seen as two separate endeavors, school staff tend to try to solve problems alone first, without enlisting or even notifying families that their child is struggling. Once the problem escalates to unmanageable levels, parents may be asked to explain their child's behavior. Recommendations and plans are frequently developed by educators beforehand, without parent or student input. Such communication practices do not reinforce the belief that parents play a critical role and that mutual support of parents and teachers is essential for the learning and development of children and adolescents. Nor does this interactional pattern conceptualize concerns for children and youth from a systemic perspective, one in which concerns represent a problematic situation (not problematic individuals) that demands the attention of parents, educators, and students. Despite this common scenario, communication is theorized to be the foundation of all family involvement (Moles, 1993).

Channels for parents to initiate contact with school personnel are more limited and less clearly defined. Families often wait to be contacted by schools, under the premise that "no news is good news." When schools send infrequent messages home, families are forced to rely solely on the written matter to ascertain both content and tone of the message. Watkins (1997) found that the manner in which parents perceived communication from their child's teacher enhanced or decreased their home-school behavior; perceptions of teacher involvement significantly influenced frequency of contact more than child achievement levels or parent educational level and ethnicity. Ames (1993) emphasized the need for positive attitudes to be reflected in messages sent home because families are more likely to participate when there is a sense of hopefulness. McAfee (1993) noted that collaboration across family and school is dependent on communicating of the "right" message, namely that "mutual respect and interdependence of home, school, and community are essential to children's development" (p. 21). Furthermore, mutual understanding of the desired outcome, as well as consideration of the ecology of the community, student age and level of development, the attitudes and skills of school personnel, and available resources, influences implementation of effective home-school communication.

Families and schools must be able to share information and resources to resolve shared concerns and prevent problems from escalating. To achieve this, Christenson and Hirsch (1998) recommended six tangible mechanisms for including families and keeping communication channels receptive to family signals. They are:

- Strive to maintain a positive orientation to all communication between family and school (e.g., make good-news phone calls; invite and incorporate parent reactions to policies and practices; contact parents at the first sign on a concern; reframe language from problems to goals for students)
- Develop and publicize regular, reliable, varied two-way communication systems (e.g., systemwide family-school communication/assignment notebooks; use of a telephone tree, Thursday folders, and newsletters; and shared parent-educator contacts)
- Keep focus of communication on child's performance (e.g., shared parent-educator monitoring system; electronic technology; home-school notes; family-school meetings; bidirectional communication regarding classroom activities and student progress)
- Ensure that parents have needed information to support children's educational progress (e.g., orientation nights with follow-up contact for nonattendees; parent support groups and home visits; home-school contracts; curriculum nights; monthly meetings on topics of mutual interest)
- Create formal and informal opportunities to communicate and build trust (e.g., multicultural potlucks; grade-level bagel breakfasts; family fun nights; committees designed to address home-school issues; principal's hour)
- Underscore all communication with a shared responsibility between families and schools (e.g., share information about the curriculum of the home; discuss roles (i.e., as cocommunicators); adopt a team approach for setting mutual goals for supporting children as learners; implement shared practices (i.e., common language about conditions for children's success).

Professionals must treat families as they would like to be treated (Lindle, 1989). Nowhere is this more applicable than when dealing with ethnically and linguistically diverse families (Tharp, 1997), who are often forced to rely on their child to share school-related information:

> Differences in language, experience, and expectations can set the stage for a tremendous gap in communication between culturally different parents and school personnel . . . parents expected and wanted to trust the school and were more comfortable when relationships with professionals had a personal tone. . . . For many years the district's extensive use of written communication in English compounded these problems. Even when most letters and reports were sent in Spanish, their meaning was still not clear because of the use of educational jargon, the inadequate information and experiential base from which the parents operated, and because of the need for a more personalized style of communication. (Harry, 1992, p. 183)

Bandura's (1997) theory of personal self-efficacy proves useful in explaining why certain parents and teachers are more effective communicators and collaborators. Individuals with high personal self-efficacy are more likely to believe and to act on the belief that they can successfully reach a goal despite obstacles encountered. Teachers who have a high sense of self-efficacy reported a more favorable view of the benefits of family involvement and engaged in more family outreach (Hoover-Dempsey, Bassler, & Brissie, 1987). Parents who are confident in their abilities as parents and as teachers of their children are more likely to be involved in their children's schooling. Having an external locus of control reduces the likelihood that parents will share information and resources with children and teachers. Research conducted by Hoover-Dempsey and colleagues (1992, 1997) showed that parental self-efficacy and locus of control determine frequency and type of engagement more than other family status variables (e.g., income, employment, parent education). Interpersonal support was important for the manifestation of higher self-efficacy.

Families' willingness to work with professionals hinges in part on the degree to which they feel empowered. An environment that elicits and follows through on parent suggestions increases the likelihood that parents will feel comfortable sharing their ideas in the future, will see their participation as critically linked to their children's success, and will work to implement interventions and strategies suggested by professionals (Fruchter et al., 1992). In addition, school personnel must be optimistic when addressing presenting academic, behavioral, and psychological concerns for students.

Interact in a Responsive and Personalized Way

The realization that working in isolation leads to fragmented and duplicated services (Adelman & Taylor, 1998) and that children's learning is far more complex than the "ABCs and 1,2,3s" is a driving, unifying force when intervening with families facing difficult predicaments. Liontos (1992) reinforced the power of personal contact, suggesting home visits, small parent-teacher conferences oriented toward information sharing and mutual planning, regular phone calls, and personalized notes as successful strategies for reaching families with multiple risk factors. There is a welcome shift toward strengthening families, moving away from strategies that are failing families to those that increase likelihood of family success. Referred to as the *deficit model*, strategies that fail families include viewing the family in isolation, defining the family solely by structure, and responding only to crises. In contrast, the *capacity model* sees family and community as interdependent, defines family primarily by functions, and involves the entire community in prevention, aspiring to achieve positive outcomes for children and youth (Benson, 1997).

The capacity model is not routinely implemented in schools. According to Power and Bartholomew (1987), however, defining features of a collaborative family-school relationship include understanding the constraints of, establishing clear boundaries and authority in, and sharing information and voicing concerns about each system. A balanced relationship, in which parents are not in the role of professional educator and school personnel are not a parent substitute, is desired. Furthermore, if parents "squeak" or ask questions, they are not viewed as problem parents. There is a recognition that coconstructing the full picture of the child is necessary to understand child behavior and to intervene comprehensively and effectively. Borrowed from Piaget (1965), cooperating means striving to attain a

common goal while coordinating one's own feelings and perspective with a consciousness of another's feelings and perspective. Implementing a capacity model
requires perspective taking, which can be actively practiced by employing these
questions during information-sharing and problem-solving interactions: What is
the issue? What do I need to say about the issue? What do I need to understand
from others about the issue? and How can we develop a better policy or practice?
A positive plan of action satisfies the desires of students, teachers, and parents
(Christenson & Hirsch, 1998).

Bronfenbrenner (1991) postulated that parents and educators must be treated
as equals because both contribute in major ways to the education of children and
youth. However, to succeed, the partnership must be based on mutual trust and
respect, with educators taking the lead to nurture these key ingredients of collaboration. The work of McWilliam, Tocci, and Harbin (1998) in early intervention
offers a promising direction for service delivery in grades K–12. They define family-
centered practice as a friendly, respectful partnership with families that provides
emotional and educational supports, opportunities to participate in service delivery
and to make decisions, and activities to enhance family members' capacities to carry
out their self-determined roles. Dimensions of family-centered practice include: a
family orientation, positiveness ("Thinking the best of families"), sensitivity ("In the
parents' shoes"), responsiveness ("Doing whatever needs to be done"), friendliness
("Treating parents as friends"), and being a resource for children and community
services.

It is often recommended that school personnel listen to families and strive to
understand their concerns. When are families really asked what they want and
need to help their children succeed? All too often, this question, if asked, is asked
in a pro forma fashion; under the best scenario it sounds superficial, under the
worst it sounds condescending. Christenson and colleagues (1997) investigated
the relationship between 33 parent-involvement activities desired by parents and
the degree to which these activities were rated as feasible by school psychologists.
Items endorsed most strongly by parents reflected a common theme found in the
literature: Parents want schools to share more information on children's development and school policies and procedures and want teachers to provide suggestions
on how to support children's school performance at home. The activities parents
most desired were characterized by more time to interact with teachers and school
psychologists about children's social skills, academic performance, behavior, and
mental health. Overall, ratings of parents' desires were consistently higher than
school psychologists' ratings of feasibility for implementation, suggesting that
parents want more and varied involvement than viewed readily possible in schools.
Clearly, new roles for parents in education and schooling must be formed for and
with families.

The labeling of parents as resistant is a highly questionable, although common,
practice. The challenge of empowerment, which refers to removing obstacles to
ensure equal opportunity, is not to demonstrate that families differ but to show
"how supports tailored to reflect these differences are helpful to different kinds of
families in different ways" (Cochran, 1987, p. 22). The process of empowerment
consists of three levels: building parents' sense of self-efficacy, creating opportun-

ities for parents to form relationships with teachers, and asking parents to take social action (e.g., governance). According to the model developed by Dunst and Trivette (1987), it is assumed that help seekers (parents) are competent or have the capacity to be competent in solving their problems when given resources, skills, and opportunities with support from the help giver (psychologists, educators). More recently, Fantuzzo and Mohr (in press) described the resiliency, partnership-directed approach for building positive connections with parents in Head Start. Partnership, defined as *shared commitments + shared ideas + shared actions*, reinforces the critical nature of coconstruction of a plan of shared action and eliminates the tendency to categorize parents as resistant that is evident in some parent training efforts (Patterson & Chamberlain, 1994).

From preventive to conflict-resolution strategies, our goal is to find what works for problematic situations (home and schools), not problematic individuals (educators, students, or parents). Through encouraging personal contact and consistently sending positive, solution-oriented, optimistic messages, families will be more empowered to join the problem-solving table (Christenson & Hirsch, 1998). The success of this approach is contingent on professionals' ability to share power and their traditional authority status with parents. Harry (1992) recommended restructuring the parent-professional discourse by developing meaningful roles for parents that tend to achieve a balance of power across family and school. Specifically, she described roles for parents as assessors, presenters of reports, policymakers, and advocates and peer supports. Her work with culturally diverse families whose children were in special education illustrates the importance of giving official channels for reciprocal rather than one-way discourse about students' education.

Engage Parents with Thorough and Persistent Efforts

Consider the children and families with whom psychologists work in varied settings. Economic, social, emotional, and/or behavioral issues often fill their lives. Sometimes families are unwilling or mandated to meet, are defensive or in denial after a long history of negative interactions with schools and social service institutions, and may not see the service provider as able to address problems facing their family or community. Pervasive, encompassing, and consuming difficulties affect all aspects of their children's lives — at home, in the neighborhood, and at school. Repeated negative experiences cause feelings of guilt, shame, inadequacy, failure, and hopelessness. Complicated by institutional and cultural barriers, the possibility of establishing a positive relationship often seems nearly impossible. Unfortunately, the status quo with some families tends to be crisis oriented. These situations are not conducive to the development of trusting relationships. Arguably, the focus on these families has taken a deficit approach for far too long.

Developing relationships with families is vital. This does not necessarily mean increasing the number of times one meets with each family. In fact, Patrikakou and Weissberg (1999) found that the quality of parent-teacher relationships rather than the quantity of contacts was associated with improved student achievement and behavior. Similarly, Adams and Christenson (1998) found that satisfaction, not frequency, of parent-teacher interaction was a predictor of trust between family and school. Too often educators want to solve the problem quickly and in their own way. Too often they are focused on solutions rather than on the interaction process that can yield a sound product (i.e., an action plan). The ability to enhance the quality of the relationship with families depends on professionals' subtle and active attempts to build a trusting relationship—a connection for children and youth—through thorough and persistent efforts.

Recommended practices are prevention-oriented and generally characterized by planning the relationship in advance, charting a common course together, enhancing trust over time, and engaging in ongoing dialogue about the student's performance. Additionally, they are solution-oriented and focus on mesosystemic intervention. For example, Comer's School Development Program illustrates the power of relationships at a systems level (Comer et al., 1996). This school-based model consists of three teams (parent, school planning and management, and student and staff support), three operations (comprehensive school plan, staff development, and periodic assessment and modification), and three guiding principles to create a positive school climate for learning. The principles are: (1) consensus—decisions made in this way; (2) collaboration—viewpoints of team members are heard and respected; and (3) no fault—time is not wasted on unproductive blaming. Shared accountability across family and school to promote academic and social growth for students is emphasized by answering the question, How can we work together to improve student performance? Recently, coordinated school health programs add the important dimension of coordination of services described by Adelman and Taylor (1998) as the coordinating council and by Fetro (1998) as the healthy school team.

The benefits of using structured problem-solving approaches to join with families for the purpose of mutually designing interventions across multiple contexts receives much attention in the literature and includes family school meetings (Weiss & Edwards, 1992), family-school consultation (Carlson, Hickman, & Horton, 1992), and parent-educator problem solving (Christenson, 1995). The most highly researched approach is conjoint behavioral consultation (CBC). The process of CBC (Sheridan, Kratochwill, & Bergan, 1996) entails four separate stages in which professionals and families work together to identify and solve academic, social-emotional, or behavioral concerns for students: problem identification, problem analysis, implementation, and evaluation.

These approaches share four principles: joint ownership of the responsibility for change and solution; clear but flexible roles and responsibilities in supporting children and youth; willingness to investigate and understand different perspectives between family and school; and professional helping that focuses on principles of empowerment and cooperating (as described previously) with families. Structured problem solving is also necessary when psychologists must employ nonadversarial approaches to resolve conflict (Christenson & Hirsch, 1998; Swap, 1993).

Another example is found in Check and Connect, a model designed to promote student engagement with school for youth at high risk for dropping out (Sinclair, Christenson, Evelo, & Hurley, 1998). A monitor systematically checks students' risk for dropping out and connects students to individualized interventions in a timely fashion. The approach is based on enhancing the strengths and connections between home, school, and community through relationship building, problem solving, and persistence. Project personnel continue to postulate that the unique feature of the Check and Connect procedure is not the intervention per se but the fact that the interventions are facilitated by monitors who are trusted and known by students and families. Monitors demonstrate concern for students and families persistently and consistently over time.

Families differ in terms of knowledge, skills, time, and resources available to them; they are unique and have their own assets and difficulties. Families whose children are labeled in the same ways (e.g., ADHD, conduct disorder, depressed) are very different from one another. Although similar issues may be at hand across families, an unwavering prescriptive approach fails to acknowledge and build on individual strengths and the potential that exists within a specific family.

Summary

Implementation of these four guidelines for creating constructive connections between families and schools are based in several theoretical and empirical contributions evident in psychology, including the importance of the person-environment fit, resiliency, cognitive-behavioral interventions, and evaluation of whether the program is having the intended effect on the intended population. In this chapter, we summarized the literature on family-school relationships by focusing on connections, specifically the Cs of constructive connections: context, centrality, complexity, consistency, communication, and collaboration.

Constructing sustaining relationships across family and school for the engagement with learning and healthy development of children and youth is a philosophy rather than a set of activities. The Search Institute (1994) also suggested that family-school relationships to promote the success of youth can be represented by the term CONNECT, where C = Customize, O = Overcome logistical barriers, N = New practices, N = New understanding, E = Expand options, C = Create relationships, and T = Team. Although there are no exact formulas, we suggest that psychologists can make a significant contribution to enhancing constructive relationships by heeding this advice. Furthermore, the significant contributions from the early intervention literature, especially family-centered practices, are highly relevant and sorely needed for application in elementary and secondary schools. Including parents by inviting their assistance and ensuring meaningful roles for their participation, fostering parental self-efficacy, reaching uninvolved families, maintaining a solution-oriented approach, and implementing mesosystemic interventions offer much promise for addressing the psychological and educational needs of children and youth.

REFERENCES

Adams, K. S., & Christenson, S. L. (1998). Differences in parent and teacher trust levels: Implications for creating collaborative family-school relationships. *Spe-*

cial Services in the Schools, 14(1/2), 1–22.

Adelman, H. S., & Taylor, L. (1998). Mental health in schools: Moving forward. School Psychology Review, 27(2), 175–190.

Allport, G. W. (1954). The nature of prejudice. Reading, MA: Addison-Wesley.

Ames, C. (1993). How school-to-home communications influence parent beliefs and perceptions. Equity and Choice, 9(3), 44–49.

August, G. J., Anderson, D., & Bloomquist, M. L. (1992). Competence enhancement training for children: An integrated child, parent, and school approach. In S. L. Christenson & J. C. Conoley (Eds.), Home-school collaboration: Enhancing children's academic and social competence (pp. 175–192). Silver Spring, MD: National Association of School Psychologists.

Bandura, A. (1997). Self-efficacy: The exercise of control. New York: Freeman.

Batey, C. S. (1996). Parents are lifesavers: A handbook for parent involvement in the schools. Thousand Oaks, CA: Corwin Press.

Benson, P. (1997). All kids are our kids: What communities must do to raise caring and responsible children and adolescents. San Francisco: Jossey-Bass.

Bronfenbrenner, U. (1991). What do families do?: 1, Teaching Thinking and Problem Solving, 13(4), 1, 3–5.

Carlson, C. I., Hickman, J., & Horton, C. B. (1992). From blame to solutions: Solution-oriented family-school consultation. In S. L. Christenson & J. C. Conoley (Eds.), Home-school collaboration: Enhancing children's academic and social competence (pp. 193–213). Silver Spring, MD: National Association of School Psychologists.

Christenson, S. L. (1995). Supporting home-school collaboration. In A. Thomas & J. Grimes (Eds.), Best practices in school psychology III (pp. 253–267). Washington, DC: National Association of School Psychologists.

Christenson, S. L. (2000). Families and schools: Rights, responsibilities, resources, and relationship. In R. C. Pianta & M. J. Cox (Eds.), The transition to kindergarten (pp. 143–177). Baltimore: Brookes Publishing.

Christenson, S. L., & Christenson, C. J. (1998). Family, school, and community influences on children's learning: Creating conditions for success (Report No. 1). Minneapolis, MN: University of Minnesota Extension Service, Live and Learn Project.

Christenson, S. L., & Hirsch, J. (1998). Facilitating partnerships and conflict resolution between families and schools. In K. C. Stoiber & T. R. Kratochwill (Eds), Handbook of group interventions for children and families (pp. 307–344). Boston: Allyn & Bacon.

Christenson, S. L., Hurley, C. M., Sheridan, S. M., & Fenstermacher, K. (1997). Parents' and school psychologists' perspectives on parent involvement activities. School Psychology Review, 26(1), 111–130.

Cochran, M. (1987). The parental empowerment process: Building on family strengths. Equity and Choice, 4(1), 9–23.

Cochran, M., & Dean, C. (1991). Home-school relations and the empowerment process. Elementary School Journal, 91, 261–270.

Coleman, J. S. (1987). Families and schools. Educational Researcher, 16(6), 32–38.

Comer, J. P., Haynes, N. M., Joyner, E. T., & Ben-Avie, M. (1996). Rallying the whole village: The Comer process for reforming education. New York: Teachers College Press.

Dauber, S. L., & Epstein, J. L. (1993). Parents' attitudes and practices of involvement in inner-city elementary and middle schools. In N. F. Chavkin (Ed.), Families and schools in a pluralistic society (pp. 53–71). Albany, NY: State University of New York Press.

Davies, D. (1991). Schools reaching out:

Family, school, and community partnerships for student success. *Phi Delta Kappan, 72*(5), 376–382.

Delgado-Gaitan, C. (1991). Involving parents in the schools: A process of empowerment. *American Journal of Education, 100*(1), 20–46.

Dunst, C. J., Johanson, C., Rounds, T., Trivette, C. M., & Hamby, D. (1992). Characteristics of parent-professional partnerships. In S. L. Christenson & J. C. Conoley (Eds.), *Home-school collaboration: Enhancing children's academic and social competence* (pp. 157–174). Silver Spring, MD: National Association of School Psychologists.

Dunst, C. J., & Trivette, C. M. (1987). Enabling and empowering families: Conceptual and intervention issues. *School Psychology Review, 7*, 77–94.

Edwards, P. A. (1992). Strategies and techniques for establishing home-school partnerships with minority parents. In A. Barona & E. Garcia (Eds.), *Children at-risk: Poverty, minority status, and other issues in educational equity* (pp. 217–236). Silver Spring, MD: National Association of School Psychologists.

Epstein, J. L. (1995a). School/family/community partnerships: Caring for the children we share. *Phi Delta Kappan, 76*(9), 701–712.

Epstein, J. L. (1995b). Perspectives and previews on research and policy for school, family, and community partnerships. In A. Booth & J. Dunn (Eds.), *Family-school links: How do they affect educational outcomes?* (pp. 209–246). Hillside, NJ: Erlbaum.

Epstein, J. L., & Lee, S. (1995). National patterns of school and family connections in the middle grades. In B. Ryan, G. R. Adams, T. P. Gullotta, R. P. Weissberg, & R. L. Hampton (Eds.), *The family-school connection: Theory, research, and practice* (pp. 108–154). Thousand Oaks, CA: Sage.

Family Resource Coalition (1993). Family support and school-linked services. *Report, 12*(3&4), 4–50.

Fantuzzo, J. W., & Mohr, W. (in press). Pursuit of wellness in Head Start: Making beneficial connections for children and families. In D. Cicchetti, J. Rapaport, I. Sandler, & R. Weissberg (Eds.), *The promotion of wellness in children and adolescents.* (pp.) New York: Sage.

Fetro, J. V. (1998). Implementing coordinated school health programs in local schools. In E. Marx & S. F. Wooley (Eds.), *Health is academic* (pp. 15–42). New York: Teachers College Press.

Fruchter, N., Gullotta, A., & White, J. L. (1992). *New directions in parent involvement.* Washington, DC: Academy for Educational Development.

Hansen, D. A. (1986). Family-school articulations: The effect of interaction rule mismatch. *American Educational Research Journal, 23*(4), 643–659.

Harry, B. (1992). *Cultural diversity, families, and the special education system: Communication and empowerment.* New York: Teachers College Press.

Heller, L. R., & Fantuzzo, J. W. (1993). Reciprocal peer tutoring and parent partnership: Does parent involvement make a difference? *School Psychology Review, 22*(3), 517–534.

Henderson, A. T., & Berla, N. (1994). *A new generation of evidence: The family is critical to student achievement.* Washington, DC: National Committee for Citizens in Education.

Hess, R. D., & Holloway, S. D. (1984). Family and school as educational institutions. In R. D. Parke, R. N. Emde, H. P. McAdoo, & G. P. Sackett (Eds.), *Review of child development research: Vol. 7. The family* (pp. 179–222). Chicago: University of Chicago Press.

Hickman, C. W., Greenwood, G., & Miller, M. D. (1995). High school parent involvement: Relationships with achievement, grade level, SES, and gender. *Journal of Research and Development in Education, 28*(3), 128–134.

Hoover-Dempsey, K. V., Bassler, O. C., & Brissie, J. S. (1987). Parent involvement: Contributions of teacher efficacy, school socioeconomic status, and other school characteristics. *American Educational Research Journal, 24*(3), 417–435.

Hoover-Dempsey, K. V., Bassler, O. C., & Brissie, J. S. (1992). Explorations in parent-school relations. *Journal of Educational Research, 85*(5), 287–294.

Hoover-Dempsey, K., & Sandler, H. M. (1997). Why do parents become involved in their children's education? *Review of Educational Research, 67*(1), 3–42.

Howe, N., Chambers, B., & Abrami, P.C. (1998). The effects of an academic restructuring program on parental attitudes and behaviors. *Alberta Journal of Educational Research, 44*(1), 106–110.

Ingels, S. J., Abraham, S., Rasinski, K. A., Karr, R., Spencer, B. D., & Frankel, M. R. (1990). *NELS:88 base-year data file user's manuals.* Washington, DC: U.S. Department of Education, Office for Educational Research and Improvement/National Center for Educational Statistics.

Jayanthi, M., Sawyer, V., Nelson, J. S., Bursuck, W. D., & Epstein, M. H. (1995). Recommendations for homework-communication problems: From parents, classroom teachers, and special education teachers. *Remedial and Special Education, 16*(4), 212–225.

Kagan, S. L. (1984). *Parental involvement research: A field in search of itself* (Report No. 8). Boston, MA: Institute for Responsive Education.

Lewis, A. C., & Henderson, A. T. (1997). *Urgent message: Families crucial to school reform.* Washington, DC: Center for Law and Education.

Lindle, J. C. (1989). What do parents want from principals and teachers? *Educational Leadership, 47*(2), 8–10.

Liontos, L. B. (1992). *At-risk families and schools: Becoming partners.* Eugene, OR: University of Oregon, College of Education (ERIC Document Reproduction Service No. 342 055).

Margolis, H., & Brannigan, G. (1986).

Building trust with parents. *Academic Therapy, 22*(1), 71–74.

McAfee, O. (1993). Communication: The key to effective partnerships. In R. C. Burns (Ed.), *Parents and schools: From visitors to partners* (pp. 21–34). Washington, DC: National Education Association.

McWilliam, R. A., Tocci, L., & Harbin, G. L. (1998). Family-centered services: Service provider's discourse and behavior. *Topics in Early Childhood Special Education, 18*(4), 206–221.

Metropolitan Life Survey (1998). *The American teacher 1998: Building family-school partnerships: Views of teachers and students.* New York: Harris.

Mitrsomwang, S., & Hawley, W. (1993). *Cultural adaptation and the effects of family values and behavior on the academic achievement and persistence of Indo-Chinese students* (Report #R 117E00045). Washington, DC: Office of Educational Research and Improvement, U.S. Department of Education.

Moles, O. (1993). Collaboration between schools and disadvantaged parents: Obstacles and openings. In N. Chavkin (Ed.), *Families and schools in a pluralistic society* (pp. 21–49). Albany, NY: State University of New York Press.

Mordkowitz, E., & Ginsburg, H. P. (1987). Early academic socialization of successful Asian-American college students. *Quarterly Newsletter of the Laboratory of Comparative Human Cognition, 9,* 85–90.

Morris, V. G., & Taylor, S. I. (1998). Alleviating barriers to family involvement in education: The role of teacher education. *Teaching and Teacher Education, 14*(2), 219–231.

National Education Goals Report (1998). *Building a nation of learners.* ERIC Document Reproduction Service No. 421 553) Washington, DC: U.S. Government Printing Office.

Okagaki, L., & Sternberg, R. J. (1991). *Directors of development: Influences on the development of children's thinking.* Hillsdale, NJ: Erlbaum.

Ooms, T., & Hara, S. (1991). *The family-school partnership: A critical component of school reform.* Washington, DC: The Family Impact Seminar.

Patrikakou, E. N., & Weissberg, R. P. (February, 1999). The seven P's of school-family partnerships. *Education Week, 18*(21), 34, 36.

Patterson, G. R., & Chamberlain, P. (1994). A functional analysis of resistance during parent training therapy. *Clinical Psychology: Science and Practice, 1*(1), 53–70.

Phelan, P., Yu, H. C., & Davidson, A. L. (1994). Navigating the psychosocial pressures of adolescence: The voices and experiences of high school youth. *American Educational Research Journal, 31*(2), 415–447.

Piaget, J. (1965). *The moral judgment of the child.* London: Free Press.

Pianta, R., & Walsh, D. B. (1996). *High-risk children in schools: Constructing sustaining relationships.* New York: Routledge.

Power, T. J., & Bartholomew, K. L. (1987). Family-school relationship patterns: An ecological assessment. *School Psychology Review, 16,* 498–512.

Reid, J. B., & Patterson, G. R. (1996). Early prevention and intervention with conduct problems: A social interactional model for the integration of research and practice. In G. Stoner, M. R. Shinn, & H. M. Walker (Eds.), *Interventions for achievement and behavior problems* (pp. 715–739). Bethesda, MD: National Association of School Psychologists.

Rich, D. (1987). *Schools and families: Issues and actions.* Washington, DC: National Education Association.

Rumberger, R. W. (1995). Dropping out of middle school: A multilevel analysis of students and schools. *American Educational Research Journal, 32*(3), 583–625.

Rutter, M. (1985). Family and school influences on behavioral development. *Journal of Child Psychology and Psychiatry, 26*(3), 349–368.

Search Institute (1994). Connecting schools and families. *Source, 10*(3), 1–3.

Seeley, D. S. (1985). *Education through partnership.* Washington, DC: American Enterprise Institute for Public Policy Research.

Sheridan, S. M., Kratochwill, T. R., & Bergan, J. R. (1996). *Conjoint behavioral consultation: A procedural manual.* New York: Plenum Press.

Sheridan, S. M., Kratochwill, T. R., & Elliott, S. (1990). Behavioral consultation with parents and teachers: Applications with socially withdrawn children. *School Psychology Review, 19,* 33–53.

Sinclair, M. F., Christenson, S. L., Evelo, D., & Hurley, C. (1998). Dropout prevention for high-risk youth with disabilities: Efficacy of a sustained school engagement procedure. *Exceptional Children, 65*(1), 7–21.

Smrekar, C. (1994). The missing link in school-linked social service programs. *Educational Evaluation and Policy Analysis, 16*(4), 422–433.

Swap, S. M. (1987). *Enhancing parent involvement in schools.* New York: Teacher's College Press.

Swap, S. M. (1993). *Developing home-school partnerships: From concepts to practice.* New York: Teachers College Press.

Swick, K. J., & McKnight, S. (1989). Characteristics of kindergarten teachers who promote parent involvement. *Early Childhood Research Quarterly, 4,* 19–29.

Tharp, E. K. (1997). Increasing opportunities for partnerships with culturally and linguistically diverse families. *Intervention in School and Clinic, 32*(5), 261–269.

Tomlinson, S. G. (1996). *Welcoming parents at your school: Strategies that work.* Washington, DC: Office of Educational Research and Improvement.

Trusty, J. (1998). Family influences on educational expectations of late adolescents. *Journal of Educational Research,*
91(5), 260–270.

Vosler-Hunter, R. W. (1989). Families and
professionals working together: Issues
and opportunities. *Focal Point,* 4(1),
1–4.

Wahlberg, H. J. (1984). Families as partners in educational productivity. *Phi
Delta Kappan,* 65, 397–400.

Watkins, T. J. (1997). Teacher communications, child achievement, and parent
traits in parent involvement models.
Journal of Educational Research, 91(1),
3–14.

Webster-Stratton, C. (1993). Strategies for
helping early school-aged children with
oppositional defiant and conduct disorders: The importance of home-school
partnerships. *School Psychology Review,*
22(3), 437–457.

Weiss, H. M., & Edwards, M. E. (1992).
The family-school collaboration project:
Systematic interventions for school improvement. In S. L. Christenson &
J. C. Conoley (Eds.), *Home-school collaboration: Enhancing children's academic and social competence* (pp.
215–243). Silver Spring, MD:
National Association of School Psychologists.

INDEX